# CARDIAC SPECT IMAGING

## SECOND EDITION

# CARDIAC SPECT IMAGING

## SECOND EDITION

*Editors*

## E. GORDON DePUEY, M.D.

*Professor*
*Department of Radiology*
*Columbia University College of Physicians and Surgeons*
*Director*
*Division of Nuclear Medicine*
*Department of Radiology*
*St. Luke's-Roosevelt Hospital*
*New York, New York*

## ERNEST V. GARCIA, Ph.D.

*Professor and Vice Chairman for Research*
*Department of Radiology*
*Emory University School of Medicine*
*Atlanta, Georgia*

## DANIEL S. BERMAN, M.D.

*Professor of Medicine*
*University of California at Los Angeles School of Medicine*
*Director, Nuclear Cardiology*
*Cedars-Sinai Medical Center*
*Los Angeles, California*

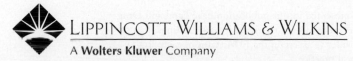

LIPPINCOTT WILLIAMS & WILKINS
A **Wolters Kluwer** Company
Philadelphia • Baltimore • New York • London
Buenos Aires • Hong Kong • Sydney • Tokyo

*Acquisitions Editor:* Joyce-Rachel John
*Developmental Editor:* Pamela Sutton
*Production Editor:* Janice G. Stangel
*Manufacturing Manager:* Benjamin Rivera
*Cover Designer:* Patty Gast
*Compositor:* Lippincott Williams & Wilkins Desktop Divison

Printed in China

Library of Congress Cataloging-in-Publication Data

Cardiac SPECT imaging / editors, E. Gordon DePuey, Ernest V. Garcia, Daniel S. Berman.—2nd ed.
      p. ; cm.
   Includes bibliographical references and index.
   ISBN 0-7817-2007-9
      1. Heart—Tomography. 2. Heart—Radionuclide imaging. I. DePuey, E. Gordon. II. Berman, Daniel S. (Daniel Sholom), 1944- III. Garcia, Ernest V.
      [DNLM: 1. Heart—radionuclide imaging. 2. Tomography, Emission-Computed, Single-Photon. 3. Heart Diseases—radionuclide imaging. WG 141.5.R3 C2672 2000]
   RC683.5.T66 C37 2000
   616.1'207575—dc21

                                                                      00-060557

   Care has been taken to confirm the accuracy of the information presented and to describe generally accepted practices. However, the authors, editors, and publisher are not responsible for errors or omissions or for any consequences from application of the information in this book and make no warranty, expressed or implied, with respect to the currency, completeness, or accuracy of the contents of the publication. Application of this information in a particular situation remains the professional responsibility of the practitioner.

   The authors, editors, and publisher have exerted every effort to ensure that drug selection and dosage set forth in this text are in accordance with current recommendations and practice at the time of publication. However, in view of ongoing research, changes in government regulations, and the constant flow of information relating to drug therapy and drug reactions, the reader is urged to check the package insert for each drug for any change in indications and dosage and for added warnings and precautions. This is particularly important when the recommended agent is a new or infrequently employed drug.

   Some drugs and medical devices presented in this publication have Food and Drug Administration (FDA) clearance for limited use in restricted research settings. It is the responsibility of the health care provider to ascertain the FDA status of each drug or device planned for use in their clinical practice.

                                 9  8  7  6  5  4  3  2  1

*To Dr. John A Burdine, for his leadership in Nuclear Medicine,*
*and personally for his guidance, love, and an occasional kick in the pants.*
*EGD*

*To Evan, Meredith and Terri—the loves of my life.*
*EVG*

*To Dr. Dean T. Mason, whose mentoring*
*provided the sine qua non for my academic career.*
*DSB*

# CONTENTS

# CONTRIBUTING AUTHORS

**Joseph S. Areeda, B.A.** Department of Nuclear Medicine, Cedars-Sinai Medical Center, 8700 Beverly Boulevard, Los Angeles, California 90048

**Timothy M. Bateman** Cardiovascular Consultants, Mid-America Heart Institute, 4401 Wornall Road, Kansas City, Missouri 64111

**Jeroen J. Bax** Cardiologist, Department of Cardiology, Leiden University Medical Center, 2 Albinusdreef, Leiden, 2333ZA, The Netherlands

**Daniel S. Berman, M.D.** Professor of Medicine, UCLA School of Medicine; Director, Nuclear Cardiology, Cedars-Sinai Medical Center, 8700 Beverly Boulevard, Los Angeles, California 90048

**James A. Case** Cardiovascular Consultants, Mid-America Heart Institute, 4401 Wornall Road, Kansas City, Missouri 64111

**C. David Cooke, M.S.E.E.** Assistant Professor, Department of Radiology, Emory University School of Medicine, 1364 Clifton Road NE, Atlanta, Georgia 30322

**James R. Corbett, M.D.** Director, Cardiovascular Nuclear Medicine; Professor, Department of Radiology and Internal Medicine, University of Michigan Medical Center, 1500 E. Medical Center Drive, Ann Arbor, Michigan 48109-0028

**S. James Cullom, Ph.D.** Clinical Physicist, Cardiovascular Consultants, PC, 4330 Wornall Road, Suite 2000, Mid-America Heart Institute, 4401 Wornall Road, Kansas City, Missouri 64111

**E. Gordon DePuey, M.D.** Professor, Department of Radiology, Columbia University College of Physicians and Surgeons, Director, Division of Nuclear Medicine, Department of Radiology, St. Luke's-Roosevelt Hospital, 1111 Amsterdam Avenue, New York, New York 10025

**Tracy L. Faber, Ph.D.** Assistant Professor of Radiology, Division of Nuclear Medicine, Emory University School of Medicine, 1364 Clifton Road NE, Atlanta, Georgia 30322

**Edward P. Ficaro, Ph.D.** Assistant Research Scientist, Department of Radiology, University of Michigan Medical Center, 1500 East Medical Center Drive, Ann Arbor, Michigan 48109

**James R. Galt, Ph.D.** Assistant Professor, Department of Radiology, Emory University School of Medicine; Director of Nuclear Medicine Physics, Division of Nuclear Medicine, Emory University Hospital, 1364 Clifton Road NE, Atlanta, Georgia 30322

**Ernest V. Garcia, Ph.D.** Professor and Vice Chairman for Research, Department of Radiology, Emory University School of Medicine, 1364 Clifton Road NE, Atlanta, Georgia 30322

**Guido Germano, Ph.D.** Director, Nuclear Medicine Physics, Cedars-Sinai Medical Center; Associate Professor of Radiological Science, University of California at Los Angeles School of Medicine, 10833 LeConte Avenue, Los Angeles, California 90024

**Rory Hachamovitch, M.D.**   Co-Director, Technology Evaluation Center; and Associate Professor, Department of Health Policy and Management, Emory University, 1518 Clifton Road NE, Atlanta, Georgia 30322

**Sean W. Hayes, M.D.**   Department of Cardiology/Nuclear Medicine, Cedars-Sinai Medical Center, 8700 Beverly Boulevard, Los Angeles, California 90048

**Gary Heller**   Division of Nuclear Medicine, Department of Radiology, St. Luke's-Roosevelt Hospital, 114th Street and Amsterdam Avenue, New York, New York 10025

**Jamshid Maddahi, M.D.**   Professor of Molecular and Medical Pharmacology (Nuclear Medicine), University of California at Los Angeles School of Medicine, 10833 LeConte Avenue, Los Angeles, California 90024

**Kenneth J. Nichols, Ph.D.**   Associate Research Scientist, Division of Cardiology, Columbia University, 622 West 168th Street, New York, New York 10032

**Alan Rozanski, M.D.**   Professor of Medicine, Columbia University College of Physicians and Surgeons; and Director, Nuclear Cardiology, St. Luke's-Roosevelt Medical Center, 1111 Amsterdam Avenue, New York, New York 10025

**Martin P. Sandler**   Professor and Vice-Chairman, Department of Radiology and Radiological Sciences, Vanderbilt University School of Medicine, Nashville, Tennessee 37232

**Leslee J. Shaw, Ph.D.**   Associate Professor, Department of Health Policy and Management, Emory University; Co-Director of Outcomes Research, Department of Medicine, Emory University Hospital, 318 Woodruff Research Building, Atlanta, Georgia 30322

**Raymond Taillefer, M.D., F.R.C.P., A.B.N.M.**   Professor, Departments of Radiology and Nuclear Medicine, Université dé Montréal; and Chief, Department of Nuclear Medicine, Centre Hospitalier De l'Universite de Montreal, Hôtel-Dieu, 3840 St. Urbain, Montreal, Quebec H2W 1T8, Canada

**Kenneth F. Van Train, M.S.**   Director of Computer Research and Development, Department of Medical Physics and Imaging, Cedars-Sinai Medical Center, 8700 Beverly Boulevard, Los Angeles, California 90048-1805

**Frans C. Visser, M.D.**   Professor, Department of Cardiology, Academic Hospital Vrÿe Universiteit, 1117 de Boelelaan; Vice-Director, Institute for Cardiovascular Research-Vrÿe Universiteit, 7 Vander Boechorststraat, Amsterdam 1081BT, The Netherlands

**Siu-Sun Yao**   Assistant Professor of Clinical Medicine, Columbia University College of Physicians and Surgeons; and Co-Director, Nuclear Cardiology and Cardiac Stress Testing, St. Luke's-Roosevelt Medical Center, 1111 Amsterdam Avenue, New York, New York 10025

# PREFACE

Since the publication of the first edition of this book, there has been a steady increase in the number of myocardial perfusion SPECT studies performed worldwide. Planar imaging has almost been completely replaced by tomography. Clinically, perfusion SPECT maintains its role as the most accurate noninvasive imaging modality to detect and characterize the physiologic significance of coronary artery disease.

Numerous technical advances have further improved the reliability and diagnostic accuracy of myocardial perfusion SPECT. These advances are highlighted in the first part of this book entitled "General Considerations." These technical advances include more sophisticated quantitative techniques to characterize perfusion abnormalities, quantitation of ventricular function from gated SPECT, attenuation correction, and the introduction of new radiopharmaceuticals. Empowered by all of these improvements, our efforts to assure accurate and reliable imaging must be redoubled through rigorous quality control. In Section I, as well as through the remainder of the book, these important quality control mechanisms are emphasized.

The clinical role of cardiac SPECT, which now accurately assesses both myocardial perfusion and function, has also greatly expanded since the publication of the first edi-tion. These applications are highlighted in the second part of the book entitled "Clinical Considerations." The additional ability of perfusion SPECT to risk stratify patients with known or suspected coronary artery disease has afforded it an important role as a cost-effective "gatekeeper" to determine which patients benefit from cardiac catheterization and revascularization. Modification of scintillation cameras to image 511 KeV photons has expanded the role of SPECT in the determination of myocardial viability. The widespread availability of multiheaded detector systems and the introduction of sophisticated software have also expanded the role of SPECT to gated blood pool imaging to evaluate left and right ventricular function.

This book will serve as a reference for physicians interpreting cardiac SPECT as well as for physicians referring patients for diagnostic imaging. Moreover, the expanded technical sections should benefit technologists and basic scientists.

The editors gratefully acknowledge the efforts of the contributing authors and our research teams and clerical support staffs, all of whom have dedicated their time and effort to make this book possible.

*E. Gordon DePuey, M.D.*

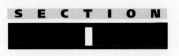

# GENERAL CONSIDERATIONS

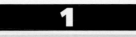

# PRINCIPLES OF CARDIAC SPECT

## S. JAMES CULLOM

Myocardial perfusion single photon emission computed tomography (SPECT) is a widely utilized noninvasive imaging modality for the diagnosis and management of coronary artery disease. This modality permits three-dimensional assessment and quantitation of the perfused myocardium and functional assessment through electrocardiogram (ECG)-gating of the perfusion images. The clinical success of this modality relies largely on a well-established infrastructure supporting the understanding of physical principles, technical limitations, and quality assurance requirements. This chapter describes the physics and technical aspects of SPECT imaging, including practical considerations for optimal clinical utilization.

## PLANAR AND TOMOGRAPHIC IMAGING

The strength of SPECT is largely derived from the three-dimensional (volumeric) nature of its images compared with the two-dimensional projections of planar perfusion imaging. Whereas planar image values are composed of the superposition of the attenuated activity from sources along a line through the patient, SPECT permits three-dimensional interactive assessment of the perfused volume. Regional and global perfusion patterns as well as cardiac shape information and more recently functional information from ECG-gated SPECT can be derived and quantified by selective interrogation of appropriate planes through the myocardium (1,2). Tomography permits separation of target regions from overlying structures. It is the primary attribute associated with improved diagnostic results over planar imaging and quantitation in early clinical studies (3) and the broad acceptance of this imaging modality clinically.

An important quantity related to the diagnostic value is the target-to-background ratio. Figure 1.1A illustrates how tomography permits improved target-to-background by allowing extraction of the plane of interest from surrounding structures. Note that the target counts are the same but background counts are reduced. Figure 1.1B illustrates this principle in a technetium 99m ($^{99m}$Tc)-sestamibi stress SPECT short-axis compared with a corresponding left anterior oblique (LAO) planar view where improved features such as left ventricular cavity visualization and minimized background structure can be appreciated. Quantitation of myocardial perfusion and function is greatly improved as algorithms can be directed to analyze image data more directly associated with the heart.

## IMAGING SYSTEMS AND IMAGE QUALITY

The clinical value of an imaging technique is dependent on the quality of the images. Image quality reflects all factors in the imaging chain including patient- and tracer-related factors, intrinsic detector properties, quality control, processing, and display. SPECT systems are modeled as linear systems and can be characterized by the response to a point or line source of activity (4). The point spread function (PSF) is used to relate the point distribution to its image (4). It can be visualized by the shape of high-count profiles of the point source image. Image noise resulting from the statistical nature of the emission process is considered separately from the PSF. Figure 1.2 illustrates the PSF and characterizes the blur of the system.

Two practical measures of image quality that can be related to the PSF are spatial resolution and contrast resolution. Spatial resolution describes how well an imaging system can separate two distinct point objects. Separability is dependent also on the observer. The minimal distance required defines the spatial resolution often expressed in millimeters. The full width at half-maximum (FWHM) of the profile is commonly reported as a measure of spatial resolution. Spatial resolution is related to the edges or boundaries in an image important for assessing dimensions in the image such as cavity size, defect extent, cardiac shape, and wall thickness. Intrinsic spatial resolution is the contribution to the total resolution by the detector alone (no colli-

S. J. Cullom: Cardiovascular Consultants, Mid-America Heart Institute, Kansas City, Missouri 64111.

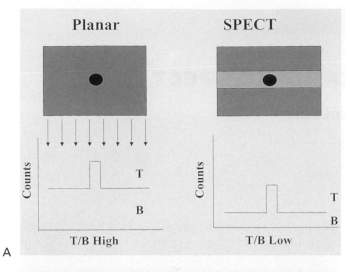

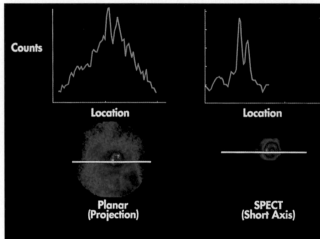

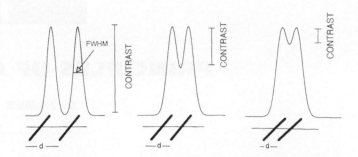

**FIGURE 1.2.** Illustration of spatial resolution (FWHM) and the relationship to contrast resolution. The point spread function (PSF) is described by the profile of the image of a point source and represents the blur of the system. Spatial resolution (d) is defined as the minimal distance at which two objects can be distinguished as discrete objects. For lesions with characteristic dimensions close to the spatial resolution of a SPECT system, detection can be impaired. Likewise, as spatial resolution improves, the ability to resolve smaller objects improves.

**FIGURE 1.1. A:** Illustration of improved contrast resolution obtained with single photon emission computed tomography (SPECT) compared with planar projection imaging. **B:** Planar left anterior oblique (LAO) and short-axis image of technetium 99m (99mTc)-sestamibi stress study illustrating improved target-to-background with SPECT. (From DuPont Pharmaceutical, Medical Imaging Division. *Principles of Myocardial Perfusion SPECT Imaging* 1994, 2000, with permission.)

mation). The specification for most modern detectors is 3 to 5 mm FWHM, whereas collimated values are in the range of 7 to 10 mm for planar imaging and 12 to 16 mm for SPECT.

Contrast refers to a measure of relative values in the image usually associated with distinct objects. Contrast resolution describes how well the imaging system responds to the true or inherent contrast in the object. For example, if uptake in a perfusion defect is one-half that of the surrounding normally perfused myocardium, contrast resolution will determine how accurate that value is represented in the image. Contrast resolution is related to the full width at tenth-maximum (FWTM) of the PSF and dictates how counts in the source are spread into surrounding planes during imaging. Spatial resolution

and contrast resolution are largely independent but both contribute to the assessment of image quality and convey important information to the clinician. Many important and unique properties of SPECT result from the effects of the PSF on the true tracer distributions.

## RADIONUCLIDE PROPERTIES AND IMPORTANCE TO IMAGE QUALITY

Image quality is dependent on the physical properties of the radionuclides used for imaging. Essentially all cardiac perfusion SPECT studies are acquired with either 99mTc-based agents (99mTc-sestamibi, 99mTc-tetrofosmin, 99mTc-teboroxime) or thallium-201 (201Tl) (5,6). Other radionuclide applications to cardiac SPECT include iodide 123 in the form 123I-methoxyiodobenzylguanidine (MIBG) to assess cardiac denervation (7) and indium-111 antimyosin to image necrotic myocardium from infarct or ischemic injury (8). More recently, SPECT with high-energy collimation has been applied to image fluorodeoxyglucose (18FDG) at 511 keV for glucose utilization and viability (9).

Image quality is dependent on the energy of the emissions from these radionuclides and their interaction in the detector. Gamma cameras rely on the scintillation that results when a photon is absorbed in the crystal (10). The light produced from the scintillation is processed electronically to record the energy and spatial location of the detected photon. Crystals used in essentially all gamma cameras are NaI-based with doping by various compounds, most notably thallium, to enhance the light-producing properties at scintillation (10). The dominance of 99mTc as a radiolabel in nuclear medicine has influenced the migration to thinner crystal design (¼- to ⅜-inch) to be optimal for responding to the 140 keV photons. Thinner crystals systems are less sensitive, as photons are less likely to penetrate the crystal and not be detected. However, they localize the scintillation event better and are associated with improved spatial resolution. Recently, thicker crystals (½- to ¾-inch) to image the 511-keV annihilation photons of positron emitting tracers have become available. These permit increased sensitivity for 511 keV but reduce the spatial resolution of lower energy emissions, although this can be offset by improved energy resolution of modern detectors (described below) (11).

## SPECT DATA ACQUISITION

Acquisition protocols in SPECT seek to obtain a set of projections sufficient for tomographic reconstruction. Three primary modes are currently used for conventional SPECT data acquisition: step and shoot, continuous, and continuous step and shoot. The most common mode of acquisition used today is the step-and-shoot mode (12). In this mode, the detectors move to predefined positions at discrete angles along the orbital path, acquire planar images for a fixed time, and then move to the next position. While translating to the next position, the detector does not record counts into the images with this mode. The time required to move between angles is important to imaging efficiency. Older systems can have values as much as 7 sec, while newer systems are as small as 1-2 sec (for a 20-second/view study). If counts are recorded into the images as the detector repositions itself to the next angle, the mode is referred to as continuous step and shoot. This mode provides a modest improvement in the rate at which a study can be acquired. The counts acquired during motion are associated with one of the discrete projection images. Spatial resolution is decreased slightly by the motion of the detector, although the amount is usually minimal as it only impacts a small percentage of the counts. A third mode referred to as continuous acquisition is characterized by the continuous movement of the detector about the patient. Counts are acquired continuously to form the projections and are periodically binned in to the discrete angles specified in the acquisition protocol. Note that all modes result in a discrete set of projection images associated with angular positions. This mode has modest spatial resolution decrease, although the blur from motion relative to the spatial resolution is small, and therefore, sensitivity is gained at the expense of a modest loss of spatial resolution.

## COLLIMATION AND DETECTOR ORBIT

Mechanical collimation of gamma camera detectors is required to localize the line of emission of photons for tomographic reconstruction (Fig. 1.3). This is achieved at great cost to system sensitivity (counts/μCi/min in a standard geometry) as only a few percent of the photons are emitted in a direction that will permit detection. Collimators are typically constructed of lead or similar materials with high atomic number, which act as good absorbers of photons. Several geometries have been proposed for cardiac SPECT collimation including parallel, convergent, and asymmetric arrays (13). Most systems today utilize parallel hole or convergent geometry in the form of a fan beam or an asymmetric fan beam. Figure 1.3 illustrates the principle of collimation for parallel hole geometry most commonly used in nuclear medicine imaging. The geometry and specifications of the array determines the effect on system sensitivity and is the largest factor influencing spatial resolution. The geometric influence of the collimator on system spatial resolution is two to four times that of the intrinsic (3- to 5-mm) component.

A fundamental principle of collimation is the trade-off between system sensitivity and spatial resolution. This has important implications for SPECT image quality as the orbit about the patient causes the detector to be, at times, at different distances from the heart. Collimators are characterized by the hole length, hole diameter (or bore for more general hole shapes), number of holes per unit area, and septal thickness (amount of material between the holes). Higher resolution collimators tend to have longer hole length and smaller bore. High-energy collimation as for 511 keV has large, thick septa to minimize penetration of high-energy photons. Increasing the hole length or reducing the bore decreases the solid angle through which photons emitted from a point in the patient can reach the detector, thereby reducing sensitivity (Fig. 1.3). Photons that are incident on the septa are largely absorbed for the low energies used in cardiac SPECT, although a small percentage may penetrate the septa leading to an increase of the FWTM value. The

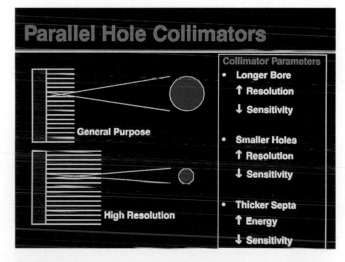

**FIGURE 1.3.** The principle of parallel hole collimation. The geometric effect of reduced spatial resolution with increasing distance to the detector is illustrated. Low-resolution collimators are characterized by shorter hole length compared with high-resolution collimation.

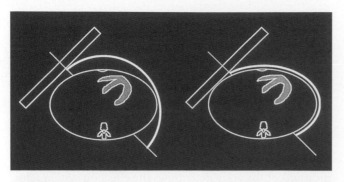

**FIGURE 1.4.** Illustration of circular and noncircular (elliptical) orbits for cardiac SPECT and the relation between the detector surface and distance to the heart.

amount of septal penetration increases with increasing photon energy, and therefore, reduced contrast resolution can be expected with higher energy tracers.

As the distance of the source to the detector increases, spatial resolution decreases (FWHM increases). Distance-dependent spatial resolution is a result of the collimator geometry and contributes to an inconsistency in the projection as the heart is at different distances from the detector as it orbits the patient. Therefore, the reconstructed image is a weighted composite of these different spatial resolution values. SPECT orbits may be broadly classified as circular and noncircular, including elliptical and other eccentric orbits. With the circular orbits, the detector is at a fixed distance from the center of rotation for all angles. The heart is on average farther from the detector over all the projection angles, leading to reduced spatial resolution but less variability with angular projection. Noncircular orbits can at times be closer to the heart for some views and therefore have improved spatial resolution for these views (Fig. 1.4). However, this is obtained at the expense of increased variability in spatial resolution, which is a potential source of artifacts (14,15). Circular orbits have been recommended by the ASNC guidelines (16) but noncircular orbits may be required for attenuation correction methods to prevent body truncation (Chapter 6). Perhaps most important is that a consistent approach to orbit selection be used. Both rest and stress components of SPECT studies should utilize the same orbital type and repeat studies on the same patient should attempt to be acquired with the same orbits. If not, orbital variations should be taken into consideration during interpretation.

### 180- and 360-Degree Orbital Acquisition

The predominant acquisition orbit for cardiac perfusion SPECT has become the 180-degree right anterior oblique (RAO)–left posterior oblique (LPO) orbit, although 360-degree orbits were promoted in early investigations (17). The relative merit of these two approaches was debated early

in the development of SPECT (18,19), and the use of 180-degree acquisition has been largely influenced by the predominant development of dual 90-degree detector systems (13). Improved defect contrast and improve signal-to-noise values are obtained with 180-degree orbits, particularly for $^{201}$Tl (19). This is attributed to the poor spatial resolution of the posterior views where the heart is further from the detector, and the additional scatter and attenuation from these views, both of which degrade image quality. Reconstructed images from 180-degree orbits are reported to have a slight distortion in the transverse plane attributable to variable spatial resolution and nonuniform attenuation by the thorax (20,21). With 360-degree orbits, spatial resolution is reduced compared with 180-degree acquisition, as the opposing view is combined in the reconstruction, forming an effective resolution equal to the geometric mean of the two values (21). This operation yields spatial resolution that is less variable across the transverse plane. Despite these considerations, 180-degree acquisition has become the standard for cardiac SPECT imaging, particularly for dual-detector 90-degree systems (16).

### TOMOGRAPHIC IMAGE RECONSTRUCTION

The clinical imaging problem to be solved is the determination of the three-dimensional distribution of tracer uptake from the projection image data. Many algorithms have been proposed for tomographic reconstruction in SPECT; however, the filtered backprojection (FBP) algorithm remains the most widely implemented (essentially all systems) except in the area of new attenuation correction methods. Although this algorithm has well described technical limitations, it remains the most understood and standardized.

Filtered backprojection can be viewed as a two-step process: filtering of the data and backprojection. The information used to generate the image on a given transverse plane corresponds to a unique row of pixel values in the projections. Data from adjacent planes may contribute to a given plane from photon scatter and spatial resolution, but FBP assumes that all counts originated on the plane being reconstructed. The three-dimensional volume is obtained from stacking of the individual transverse planes after reconstruction. The FBP process can be illustrated by considering reconstruction of a point source on a single transverse plane (Fig. 1.5). In SPECT, the measured projection values are proportional to the linear superposition of attenuated activity along lines through the patient defined by the collimator geometry. The backprojection step assigns these projection values to all points along the line of acquisition defined by the collimator through the image plane that intersects the pixels of the tomographic matrix. This operation is repeated for all pixels and for all angles. Additional shape information is contributed to the image as the back-

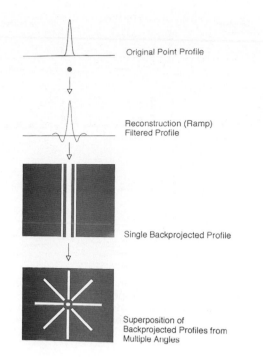

**FIGURE 1.5.** Filtered backprojection reconstruction. Filtering of the projection data with the ramp filter creates negative values in the profile necessary for accurate cancellation of other angular contributions in the image required for image accuracy. The angular components are combined by linear superposition of the data from all projections.

projected values from successive angles intersect in the image and are combined by linear superposition. With successive angular contributions, the object (point) definition improves, and an estimate of the true distribution emerges. Distributed objects (more than a single point) are obtained by a linear superposition of the contributions from the individual points.

Although conceptually illustrative, backprojection is not sufficient for accurate reconstruction. Without modification, a star artifact is produced that results from improper cancellation of angular contributions (22). The object is distorted and important edge information is not recovered. Therefore, filtered backprojection is used in practice and includes a preprocessing step with a ramp filter (23,24). The ramp filter provides the proper transformation of data from the projection coordinate system into the patient coordinate system. The ramp-filtered projections are characterized by enhancement of edge information and the introduction of negative values (or lobes) in to the filtered projections. Superposition in the backprojection process with these negative values cancels portions of other angular contributions. This process dictates a minimal angular sampling requirement to ensure that proper cancellation can be obtained and becomes part of the acquisition protocol. Insufficient cancellation from angular contributions can often be observed in clinical studies outside of the central

image region where radial blurring or streaking appears and increases toward the periphery of the image. In correctly sampled and reconstructed studies, this streaking is not present. The appearance is an important quality control indicator for proper protocol implementation.

## Noise Filtering: Spatial and Frequency Domain Approaches

Image noise resulting from statistical variations in the photon emission and detection process limits image quality by introducing random variations on image values. The random variations are Poisson distributed with the mean value equal to the true pixel value (10). Filtering operations are mathematical operations applied to the image data to minimize the effects of noise. Filtering can be performed in the spatial domain (calculations directly on the pixels) or in the frequency domain after mathematical transformation with the Fourier transform (23,24). This transformation produces fundamental components of the image in terms of periodic sine and cosine curves with associated frequencies, amplitudes, and phases. This set of values composes the Fourier spectrum of the image, and therefore, the frequency domain representation is sometimes referred to as the spectral domain. Figure 1.6 illustrates the Fourier decomposition for a simple one-dimensional square-wave profile with the more significant components shown below the profile. The amplitude component describes the relative strength or energy associated with a particular frequency value and is

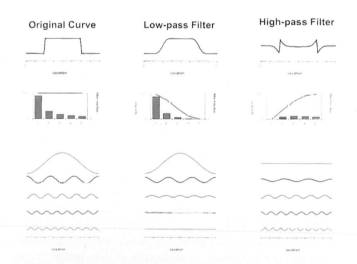

**FIGURE 1.6.** Fourier decomposition of a simple square-wave profile to the spectral components. Shown are only the lower frequency components. The concept can be extended to two-dimensional images. A characteristic of most Fourier decompositions is that the energy or amplitude of the components decrease with increasing frequency. The original profile can be obtained by summation of the components as specified by the spectrum. (From DuPont Pharmaceutical, Medical Imaging Division. *Principles of Myocardial Perfusion SPECT Imaging* 1994, 2000, with permission.)

graphically represented by the height of the component curve to the horizontal axis. The phase parameter describes the relative position or shift of the component curve with respect to a point of reference. If certain mathematical conditions are met, the original image can be obtained from the components by linear superposition of the sine and cosine curves with the proportions of each described by the amplitude and phase for each value. The advantage of this approach is the ability to alter components of the image that correspond to specific image features independent of the other components. The objective of filter design is to optimize image quality by minimizing noise while minimizing the loss of spatial resolution.

The frequency values for the sine and cosine components describe the number of cycles per unit distance in the image. For an image matrix of $N \times N$ pixels (64 or 128 for most nuclear images), there are $(N/2) + 1$ discrete frequency values (33 or 65, respectively). Frequency values are expressed in units of cycles per pixel, cycles per unit distance, or as a fraction of the highest frequency value obtainable, the Nyquist frequency. The Nyquist frequency is determined by the pixel dimensions and is calculated as $1/2x$ where $x$ is the pixel size. Nonsquare pixels have corresponding Nyquist values for each dimension. The frequency-domain representation can be used to separate the desired structure or important detail in an image from the noise. The random nature of noise from pixel to pixel is represented equally in amplitude at all frequencies but dominates in the higher frequency components of the spectrum where object components are diminished. These same higher frequency components contain the details or edges in the image that may contain important diagnostic information. Therefore, it is increasingly difficult to exactly discriminate the object and noise components beyond a certain frequency value that is dictated by the amount of noise in the image. Some image details are unavoidably removed or reduced in the filtering process, and balancing of these two objectives is an important goal of optimal filter design.

The common method for reducing noise in nuclear medicine images is the application of low-pass or smoothing filters. As their name implies, these filters preserve or pass, in a weighted fashion, the lower and mid-range frequency components of an image, which contains the important diagnostic information. The filtering operation can be accomplished by simply multiplying the respective components of the filter in the frequency representation by the respective frequency components of the image. This idea is illustrated in Fig. 1.7.

The frequency domain representation of the low-pass filters has values that range from 1.0 at the zero frequency value to a lower value at the Nyquist frequency. The original image components are preserved (1.0), reduced (<1.0), or removed (0.0) depending on the values of the filter component for each frequency. The frequency representation of the filtered image is then used in an inverse Fourier transforma-

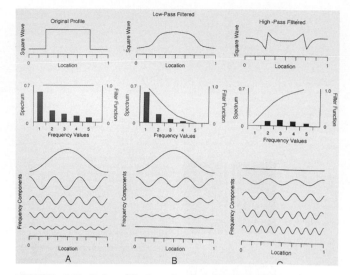

**FIGURE 1.7.** Noise filtering in the frequency domain. The respective components of the spectral representation of the filter and the spectral components of the image are multiplied together. The filtered image is obtained by inverse Fourier filtering.

tion to obtain the new image. The low-pass filtered image is generally characterized by a smoother appearance compared with the original, and its edges are slightly blurred, reflecting a decrease in spatial resolution. These filtered images can be used in the reconstruction, in place of the original projection images. An important objective is to apply filtering in a symmetric (isotropic) fashion such that image information is not preferentially changed in a specific direction.

Two low-pass filters commonly used are the Hanning and Butterworth filters and have parameters that can be adjusted to define the trade-off between preservation of spatial resolution and noise reduction. The Hanning filter is simpler than the Butterworth filter, having only a single parameter to describe its shape, referred to as the cutoff frequency. The filter is forced to be 0 at this frequency. The Hanning is a raised cosine function that has normalized value of 1.0 at the zero frequency value and 0.0 at the cutoff frequency. The effect of various cutoff values on filter shape and image quality is shown in Fig. 1.8.

The Butterworth filter has two parameters to specify its properties. The order influences the extent to which the low to mid-range frequency components are preserved, as the filter is maximally 1.0 in this range. Frequently, power is used in place of order, and it is equal to twice the order. A second parameter, the critical frequency, is defined so that the filter has a value of 0.707 (square root of 2) at this frequency. Together these two values determine the shape of the filter in the frequency domain (Fig. 1.9). As with the Hanning, the Butterworth rolls off to suppress noise at the higher frequencies. Filtering parameters are not well standardized across manufacturers with respect to filter values and units. Therefore, care should be exercised in their implementation.

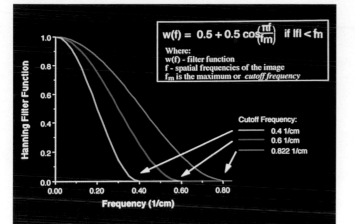

**FIGURE 1.8.** Illustration of the Hanning filter and the impact of changing the cutoff frequency on image quality. (From DuPont Pharmaceutical, Medical Imaging Division. *Principles of Myocardial Perfusion SPECT Imaging* 1994, 2000, with permission.)

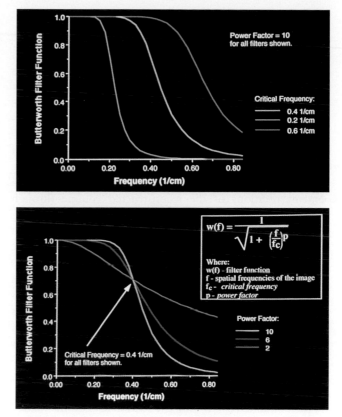

**FIGURE 1.9.** Illustration of the Butterworth filter and the impact of changing the critical frequency and order independently on image quality. (From DuPont Pharmaceutical, Medical Imaging Division. *Principles of Myocardial Perfusion SPECT Imaging* 1994, 2000, with permission.)

Filtering can be performed as a prereconstruction step (filtering of projections), during reconstruction, or after reconstruction (filtering of the transverse images). The prereconstruction option is the most commonly implemented in commercial systems and standardized protocols. An advantage of the Fourier approach to filter implementation is that multiple filtering operations can be performed very efficiently by concatenating the individual filters. As outlined in the previous section on image reconstruction, filtered backprojection requires ramp filtering and is performed along the one-dimensional projection profiles in the transverse plane. Ramp and noise filtering can be accomplished efficiently by multiplying the frequency domain values of the ramp filter by the corresponding values for the noise filter, forming a composite set of filter coefficients that may then be applied to the image spectral data.

High-pass and band-pass filters are other filter types used in nuclear medicine. A high-pass filter is characterized by values less than 1.0 at the lower frequencies, with larger values for the higher frequencies. The higher frequency components of the image are therefore amplified relative to the others. The filtered image will appear to have enhanced edges to a degree that depends on the shape of the filter. The ramp filter is an example of a high-pass filter used in nuclear medicine. High-pass filters are sometimes used in postreconstruction processing to define boundaries of specific regions for quantitation or volume determination. The frequency representation of band-pass filters are greater in magnitude for a region or band of the spectrum, which amplifies these frequencies relative to those outside of this band.

Another class of filters, referred to as restoration or resolution recovery filters, has frequency values that may be greater than 1.0 for some range of frequency values, usually in the low to mid-range values (25,26). The higher frequency values of the filter roll-off to act as low-pass filters in the high-frequency region. Images filtered in this way have correspondingly low- and mid-range values amplified or restored, since they are multiplied by values greater than 1.0. The frequency domain representation of the PSF, known as the modulation transfer function (MTF), is used in the design of these filters, which therefore attempt to compensate for these effects of system blur. With restoration filters, image contrast, which is determined largely by the mid-range frequency component, is improved while noise is simultaneously suppressed.

The amount of noise in an image, and therefore the degree of filtering, will vary with image counts. Optimal filtering protocols are determined from measurements of the imaging system response to controlled phantom studies, followed by validation of filtering in clinical trials. Deviating from recommended filtering protocols requires a careful understanding of the relationship between noise and resolution, and may significantly affect the quantitative outcome. Therefore, strict adherence to filtering protocols is important for image quality, standardization, and optimal quantitation as algorithms are validated for specific filtering protocols and parameters.

## Oblique Axis Reorientation

Once the transverse planes are reconstructed, the tracer distribution on other planes can be obtained by reorientation of the images (27). This provides enhanced opportunity to evaluate the spatial extent and characteristics of the perfused myocardium. The natural planes for the heart are the vertical long and horizontal long and short axes. The American College of Cardiology (ACC) has established guidelines for standardized display of the reconstructed images of the myocardium (28).

Reorientation is obtained by two sequential and independent rotations of the reconstructed volume through manually or automatically (29) selected angles. First, a single axis is chosen by the operator or automated algorithm from the apex to the center of the base, in an approximate midventricular transverse plane in which the ventricle is well visualized (Fig. 1.10). The reconstructed volume is then rotated through the angle defined by the selected axis and an axis of the reconstructed matrix. A second axis is then chosen on a representative midventricular image from this rotated set. A second rotation angle of the volume is therefore defined and executed. After rotation through this angle, the reconstructed matrix is aligned along the long axis of the heart. Vertical, horizontal, and short axis images are then obtained by viewing the natural axes of this rotated volume matrix.

Reorientation of the images facilitates qualitative and quantitative evaluation of perfusion and function by exploiting the symmetry of the normal left ventricle in the standardized display. The same reorientation standard is applied to ECG-gated images as well. Improper selection of the angles, placement of axes for reorientation, or improper slice selection limits at the base and apex can result in artifacts in the reoriented images (30,31). When quantified with normal database techniques, these problems can cause misalignment of segments between the database and patient study and therefore should be avoided when possible (32,33).

## Physical Factors Influencing SPECT Quality

Physical interactions of photons in the patient by Compton scattering or photoelectric absorption and the effect of spatial resolution by the collimated detector are significant factors affecting the quality of SPECT images. This section describes their relevant technical importance to cardiac SPECT.

## Photon Scatter

Photons can interact via Compton scattering in the patient and detector prior to detection (Fig. 1.11). These photons change direction and can lose a portion of their energy as they interact with orbital electrons in the tissue and can be detected in planes adjacent or remote to their plane of origin. The effect of including these photons in the image is reduced contrast resolution and quantification. The loss of

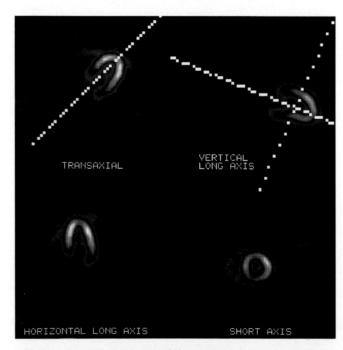

**FIGURE 1.10.** Reorientation of the transverse images to generate the vertical, horizontal, and short-axis images.

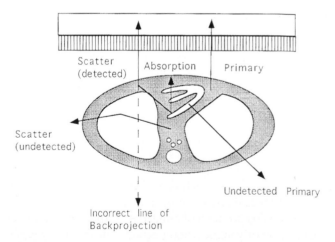

**FIGURE 1.11.** Photon interactions in the patient including Compton scattering and photoelectric absorption. Compton scattered photons (if detected) cause a loss of contrast resolution due to mispositioning of the events in the tomographic plane with conventional reconstruction algorithms. Photoelectric absorption causes quantitative errors in the profiles that depend on the amount and properties of the tissue between the source and detector. These two factors together are the source of attenuation artifacts in cardiac perfusion SPECT.

directional information leads to the misregistration of counts in the projection images, as reconstruction assumes these counts originate along the line defined by the collimator.

The gamma camera's ability to discriminate photopeak photons from scattered photons with reduced energy relies on the intrinsic energy resolution of the detector. It is quantified as the FWHM of the photopeak energy spectrum and expressed as a percentage of the photopeak energy. Typical values are 7% to 12% for the 140-keV energy of $^{99m}$Tc.

The physics of Compton interactions states that the energy loss changes slowly with increasing scattering angle (10). So-called "small-angle scatter" is the most abundant in the photopeak window and is therefore the most difficult to discriminate by the detector as the energy difference between it and the photopeak is small compared to the uncertainty defined by the intrinsic energy resolution. For example, in the 140-keV, 20% energy window commonly used for $^{99m}$Tc imaging, photons may scatter by as much as 54% in a single interaction and still be detected in the energy window (34). It may be somewhat less in newer systems with improved energy resolution, but is still a significant limitation. Some commercial systems with superior energy resolution recommend a 15% energy window width with $^{99m}$Tc to take advantage of this ability. Photons may also be scattered by such a large angle that they are never detected. In this case, projection values are underestimated, leading to errors in image reconstruction.

The proportion of scatter in the photopeak image increases for lower photopeak energies. The 72-keV, 20% energy window commonly used with $^{201}$Tl contains a mixture of photopeak (Hg x-rays) and scatter energies that cannot be sufficiently discriminated by the detector. This has been a fundamental limiting factor in image quality and scatter correction methods for $^{201}$Tl.

## Photon Attenuation

Attenuation of photons in the patient is regarded as the most significant factor affecting image quality and quantitative tracer distribution in SPECT (31,35). Attenuation refers to the combined effects of photoelectric absorption and Compton scattering. The former occurs when a photon interacts with an orbital electron in the tissue and the total energy of the photon is lost (Fig. 1.11). Absorption of photons via the photoelectric effect is dependent largely on the atomic number of the medium as $1/Z^3$. Therefore, material such as lead provides a very high level of attenuation, which is the reason it is used for shielding of photons. Attenuation artifacts in the image can result from the nonuniform attenuation properties of the thorax that are well described as a significant factor in reduced specificity and sensitivity of cardiac perfusion SPECT (31,36).

It is important to distinguish between the terms *absorption* and *attenuation*. The latter includes the effect of Compton scattering. Attenuation of photons is described quantitatively by the linear attenuation coefficient (37). Attenuation coefficients are commonly expressed in units of cm$^{-1}$ and define the number of photons removed from a beam of photons of a specific energy per unit length.

The values for the attenuation coefficient depend on the proportion of scattered photons counted in the photopeak window. Narrow-beam attenuation coefficient values do not include the effects of scatter (photoelectric absorption only) (37). Broad-beam attenuation values include scatter and therefore depend on the geometry of the measurement (37). For clinical imaging, broad-beam values are more appropriate, since the regions imaged are distributed. Detectors do not adequately reject scattered photons. For $^{201}$Tl, narrow- and broad-beam attenuation coefficients in soft tissue are approximately 0.21 and 0.18 cm$^{-1}$, respectively. For $^{99m}$Tc, these values are 0.15 and 0.12 cm$^{-1}$ (37). Both quantities are less for higher energy emissions. A common practice in nuclear medicine has been to use a broad-beam value to correct for attenuation, which partially compensates for scatter. This approximation does not work in cardiac applications, owing to the variable tissue composition of the thorax.

Attenuation causes the number of photons incident on the medium to decrease exponentially with the source depth in the medium. A half-value layer (HVL), analogous to the half-life of radionuclides, defines the thickness of material required to attenuate the number of photons by 50%. For $^{201}$Tl (72 keV), the HVL is approximately 3.6 cm$^{-1}$ and for $^{99m}$Tc (140 keV) approximately 4.6 cm$^{-1}$. In general, the HVL decreases with increasing photon energy. For cardiac SPECT, this implies that as regions are eclipsed by larger amounts or more dense amounts of tissue, they will be attenuated more. This causes features such as the nonuniform myocardial wall ratios expected in normal scans.

## Imaging System Resolution

Spatial resolution was defined in an earlier section. The limitations of collimation and other factors yield system resolution that is finite (FWHM is nonzero). Moreover, spatial resolution is relatively poor compared to other diagnostic imaging modalities. Additionally, spatial resolution is nonstationary or variable with the distance of the source from the detector due to the effects of collimation. These factors have important implications for the quality of myocardial SPECT perfusion images.

The FWHM values are on the order of the characteristic size of the myocardial walls (1 to 2 cm). Finite resolution effects are important to cardiac SPECT and refer to the strong dependence of measured maximal count values on the ratio of object size and spatial resolution values (38,39). Figure 1.12 illustrates this relationship. The origins lie in the shape of the PSF. Qualitatively speaking, objects with characteristic dimensions on the order of the size of the FWHM have maximal count values that are influenced largely by the source only. As the object increases in size beyond this value, the counts measured at a point are influenced more by sources distant from the point of measurement. As the object size increases even more, the point of measurement is no longer affected significantly, as the tails of the PSF do not extend that far. This creates the functional relationship shown in Fig. 1.x. Accordingly, as spatial resolution improves, counts from adjacent regions are less likely to influence each other (better separability). Finite spatial resolution is significant when the object is less than twice the spatial resolution value (38,39). The importance of limited resolution for visual interpretation of cardiac SPECT images has been described in detail (15,39). Determination of whether a region of decreased activity in the myocardial wall is due to hypoperfusion or from reduced thickness is a consequence of finite resolution effects. Maximal count circumferential profile sampling, used widely for quantitation of myocardial perfusion, is dependent on the finite resolution effect (33,34).

The object size and resolution relationship has been used to great advantage in ECG-gated cardiac perfusion studies (2). As the wall of the myocardium thickens over the cardiac cycle, the relative maximal count changes from end-diastole to end-systole and is proportional to the change in thickness of the myocardial wall; it is a count-based measure of myocardial thickening (40). Thickening evaluation by ECG-gated SPECT can also be used to differentiate atten-

uation artifacts from true defects in patients without previous myocardial infarction (41).

Another important factor affecting count values in myocardial perfusion SPECT is the partial volume effect (42). This is sometimes confused with the effect of finite spatial resolution, but it is related to the limitations resulting from digital sampling of the image with pixels that are of finite size. By definition, pixel values in an image represent the integrated value of activity under the area described by the pixel. When the activity concentration changes across the image, the pixel size must be sufficiently small to capture this information as sampling integrates counts. Otherwise, this information is lost through integration into the pixel. This process is independent of spatial resolution, although spatial resolution limits the rate of change of image values. Minimal pixel size is limited as count density decreases with decreasing pixel size and statistical noise variations increase. Maximal pixel size is limited by sampling requirements to accurately represent the details of the object in the image. Current investigations are focusing on methods to correct for the effects of partial volume and spatial resolution (42).

## QUALITY CONTROL

Quality control is paramount for the optimal utility of SPECT imaging. This section describes some important quality control considerations for SPECT, including instrumentation, and laboratory operation factors.

### Instrumentation Performance

Standardized guidelines exist for the performance of gamma cameras for SPECT imaging and are an essential part of laboratory quality control and for meeting the requirements of laboratory accreditation (43,44). The National Electrical Manufacturers' Association (NEMA) publishes protocols that describe a basis for assuring standardized measurement criteria for comparison of individual manufacturer specifications (43). These protocols are comprehensive and may be difficult to apply for some systems or laboratories. The following sections represent important (but not complete) considerations for quality control of cardiac SPECT. The references cited should be consulted as part of a comprehensive quality assurance program for the laboratory.

### Flood Field Uniformity

It is assumed that the detection of photons occurs uniformly across the surface of the detector. Variations in electronic response or collimator damage may cause nonuniform recording of events (Fig. 1.13). Significant nonuniformity can cause characteristic ring artifacts in the transverse planes of the SPECT study (45). These artifacts may not be

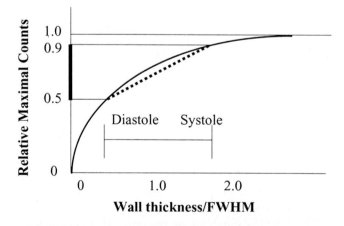

**FIGURE 1.12.** Illustration of the relationship between maximal measured image counts and the dependence on the relative values of the characteristic object dimensions and the spatial resolution [full width at half maximum (FWHM)] of the imaging system. For electrocardiogram (ECG)-gated SPECT, the dependence of regional image intensity that is related to thickening is shown. As the object becomes large or small relative to the FWHM, maximal counts increase or decrease, respectively, and therefore are proportional to regional thickening.

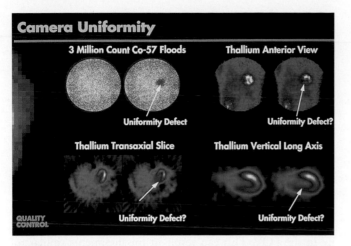

**FIGURE 1.13.** Illustration of the origin of ring artifacts in SPECT. The nonuniformity is at a fixed distance from the center of rotation in circular orbits, thereby tracing out this structure in the image plane. Artifacts with noncircular orbits may be less subtle. (From DuPont Pharmaceutical, Medical Imaging Division. *Principles of Myocardial Perfusion SPECT Imaging* 1994, 2000, with permission.)

detectable in the oblique planes but potentially may influence image quality and interpretation (Fig. 1.13). Uniformity artifacts in general are less detectable in low-count images where statistical noise variations may conceal subtle artifacts as in [201]Tl or low-count [99m]Tc images.

Flood field uniformity is a standard measure of detector response to a uniform flux of photons. Flood field uniformity can be evaluated intrinsically (no collimator) and extrinsically (with the collimator): The former represents a baseline response of the detector operations and is often performed by the field service engineer or physicist; the latter is collimator-specific and should be performed on each day that SPECT is performed. The preferred method for extrinsic evaluation is to place a cobalt 57 (122-keV) sheet source on the collimated detector and acquire a minimum of 3 to 5 million counts daily. Fillable flood sources are commercially available and can also be used, but they may have limitations due to poor rigidity or other factors that cause nonuniform concentration or filling. Periodic high-count (15 to 30 million) acquisitions should also be performed to detect more subtle nonuniformity including collimator damage.

Uniformity is measured over the useful field of view (UFOV) and central field of view (CFOV). Values are reported for differential (local measurement) and integral values (global measurement). A rule of thumb is that values for any of these parameters beyond 5% should be noted, and the detector observed for possible continued problems. Values over 6% are reason for concern, and the field service engineer should be contacted. These values should be recorded daily and monitored to detect trends and to evaluate the stability of the system.

## Center of Rotation

The earlier discussion on image reconstruction stressed the importance of alignment between the acquired projections throughout the study acquisition. This requires that the detector is properly calibrated electronically and mechanically to the center of rotation (COR) of the system (45). Errors in COR can cause a reduction in image quality and potentially severe artifacts (Fig. 1.14). COR errors of 0.5 pixels or less are generally considered acceptable. Greater errors in any direction are cause for concern, and field service should be performed. COR assessment is also collimator and photon energy dependent. The standard measurement is performed with a small (point) source of [99m]Tc that is imaged tomographically, from which automated algorithms compute the difference between true and measured COR and subsequently reported to the user. These values should also be recorded and monitored for baseline assessment of performance.

## System Sensitivity

An important consideration for SPECT is the system sensitivity (counts/minute/μCi) (43), which is a measure of how efficiently the gamma camera measures the image data. For single- and multidetector systems, it has different implications. Poor system sensitivity for a single-detector system may reduce the rate at which counts can be acquired, but the error is relatively the same in all views, and although image noise will increase, structural artifacts will not result. Differences in this value between detectors on a multidetector system can be a source of inconsistency and potential artifacts (46,47). System sensitivity of the detectors in a

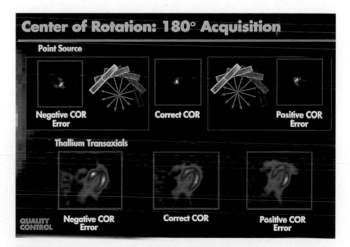

**FIGURE 1.14.** Center of rotation (COR) and its relationship to alignment of projection data for tomographic reconstruction. Significant misalignment can cause image artifacts resembling perfusion defects. (From DuPont Pharmaceutical, Medical Imaging Division. *Principles of Myocardial Perfusion SPECT Imaging* 1994, 2000, with permission.)

multidetector system should be within 2% of one another. System sensitivity is a NEMA standard and should be verified as part of the quality assurance protocol.

## Energy Peaking

Prior to study acquisition, the appropriateness and accuracy of the energy window used for imaging should be checked visually to ensure proper placement. Deviations from recommended values are potential sources of artifact (11). Mispositioning of the energy window can cause nonuniformity in the detector response, as energy calibrations factors are energy specific. Significant errors in energy window placement can cause photons from irrelevant regions of the spectrum to be imaged and degrade image quality, potentially requiring the study to be repeated or rescheduled.

## Patient Motion

Many patient-related factors can affect SPECT image quality. Patient motion is a frequent and significant limitation in all patient populations. A requirement of SPECT reconstruction algorithms is that the spatial distribution of the radiopharmaceutical is constant in time and space. This assumption is invalid when the patient moves during the study or the heart moves within the patient, which can lead to image quality degradation and detectable artifacts if the motion is significant (48,49).

The impact of patient motion on image quality during SPECT data acquisition can be understood in terms of filtered backprojection reconstruction. When motion occurs, the backprojected rays will not intersect correctly, and the necessary superposition will not occur. If the motion is minor (generally less than half a pixel in a $64 \times 64$ matrix), the result is a slight loss of spatial and contrast resolution that can usually be tolerated clinically. With more extensive motion (more than half a pixel and/or in multiple frames), artifacts can appear in which the distribution appears discontinuous or "broken," and can resemble patterns characteristic of disease. Patient motion is commonly detected by visual evaluation of the rotating planar projection images (31). Motion can occur in any direction or combination of directions including parallel to the camera axis (patient shifts upward or downward), rotation of the patient about or parallel to the system axis, translation away from the system axis, and relative upward movement of the heart within the thorax, or "cardiac creep," after exercise stress $^{201}$Tl (50). Rotational motion and motion perpendicular to the detector surface are difficult to detect. Movement parallel to the axis of rotation can usually be detected as an upward or downward deviation of the center of mass of the myocardium from a horizontal reference line in rotating projection images.

There are methods for correcting motion effects along the axis of rotation (51,52). They generally involve tracking the center of the myocardium and other features through the projection images and comparing the measured data to what would be expected in the absence of the motion. They can be manual or automated. An adjustment or translation of the projection data to the correct position is made prior to reconstruction. Automated tracking algorithms generally consider activity within the entire field of view, and anomalous activity, such as from tracer uptake by the bowel or gallbladder, can therefore introduce error into the correction. These algorithms are specific to the radionuclide and to the type of study, and should be applied appropriately. Corrected projection sets must be carefully examined after correction to ensure consistent results before proceeding with the reconstruction. Cardiac creep is detected as an upward deviation of the myocardium from a horizontal reference line in rotating projection images where there is no other apparent shift in activity in the FOV. This can result in misalignments similar to those from other types of patient motion. Delaying imaging for a few minutes after exercise stress can significantly reduce the amount of cardiac creep and improve image quality (50).

## REFERENCES

1. DePasquale EE, Nody AC, DePuey EG, et al. Quantitative rotational thallium-201 tomography for identifying and localizing coronary artery disease. *Circulation* 1988;77:316–327.
2. Chua T, Kiat H, Germano G, et al. Gated technetium-99m sestamibi for simultaneous assessment of stress myocardial perfusion, post-exercise regional ventricular function and myocardial viability. Correlation with echocardiography and rest thallium-201 scintigraphy. *J Am Coll Cardiol* 1995;23(5): 1107–1114.
3. Kiat H, Berman DS, Maddahi J. Comparison of planar and tomographic exercise thallium-201 imaging methods for the evaluation of coronary artery disease. *J Am Coll Cardiol* 1989;13 (3):613–616.
4. King MA, Schwinger RB, Penney BC. Variation of the count-dependent Metz filter with imaging system modulation transfer function. *Med Phys* 1986;13(2):139–149.
5. Berman DS, Kiat H, Maddahi J. The new 99mTc myocardial perfusion imaging agents: 99mTc-sestamibi and 99mTc-teboroxime. *Circulation* 1991;84(3):17–21.
6. Strauss HW, Harrison K, Langan JK, et al. Thallium-201 for myocardial imaging. Relation of thallium-201 to regional myocardial perfusion. *Circulation* 1975;51(4):641–645.
7. Strantun MS and Zipes DP. Nuclear imaging of cardiac autonomic innervation and receptors: focus on metaiodogenzylguanidine. In: Gerson MC. *Cardiac nuclear medicine.* New York: McGraw-Hill, 1991:603–613.
8. Khaw BA, Yasuda T, Gold HK, et al. Acute myocardial infarct imaging with In-111-labeled monoclonal antimyosin fab. *J Nucl Med* 1987;28(11):1671–1678.
9. Sandler MP, Bax JJ, Patton JA, et al. Fluorine-18-fluorodeoxyglucose cardiac imaging using a modified scintillation camera (review). *J Nucl Med* 1998;39(12):2035–2043.
10. Sorenson JA, Phelps ME. *Physics in nuclear medicine.* Philadelphia: WB Saunders, 1987.
11. Baron JM, Chouraqui P. Myocardial single-photon emission computed tomographic quality assurance. *J Nucl Cardiol* 1996;3:157–166.
12. Bieszk JA, Hawman EG. Evaluation of SPECT angular sampling effects: continuous versus step-and-shoot acquisition. *J Nucl Med* 1987;28:1308–1314.
13. Galt JR, Germano G. Advances in instrumentation for cardiac

SPECT. In: DePuey EG, Berman DS, Garcia EV, eds. *Cardiac SPECT imaging*. New York: Raven Press, 1995:91–102.

14. Maniawski PJ, Morgan HT, Whackers FJTh. Orbit-related variation in spatial resolution as a source of artifactual defects in thallium-201 SPECT. *J Nucl Med* 1991;32(5):871–875.

15. Garcia EV, Cooke CD, Van Train KF, et al. Technical aspects of myocardial SPECT imaging with technetium-99m sestamibi. *Am J Cardiol* 1990;66(13):23E.

16. Garcia EV, ed. Imaging guidelines for nuclear cardiology procedures, part 1. *J Nucl Cardiol* 1996;3:GG3–45.

17. Go RT, MacIntyre WJ, Houser TS, et al. Clinical evaluation of 360° and 180° data sampling techniques for transaxial SPECT thallium-201 myocardial perfusion imaging. *J Nucl Med* 1985;26:695–706.

18. Hoffman EJ. 180° compared with 360° sampling in SPECT. *J Nucl Med* 1982;23:745–746.

19. Maublant JC, Peycelon P, Kwiatkowski F, et al. Comparison between 180° and 360° data collection in technetium-99m MIBI SPECT of the myocardium. *J Nucl Med* 1989;30:295–300.

20. Eisner RL, Nowak DJ, Pettigrew R, et al. Fundamentals of 180° reconstruction in SPECT imaging. *J Nucl Med* 1986;27:1717–1728.

21. Knesaurek K, King MA, Glick SJ, et al. Investigation of causes of geometric distortion in 180° and 360° angular sampling in SPECT. *J Nucl Med* 1989;30:1666–1675.

22. Brooks RA, DiChiro G. Principles of computer assisted tomography (CAT) in radiographic and radioisotopic imaging. *Phys Med Biol* 1976;21(5):689–732.

23. Galt JR, Hise LH, Garcia EV, et al. Filtering in frequency space. *J Nucl Med Tech* 1986;14:152–162.

24. Zubal IG, Wisniewski G. Understanding Fourier space and filter selection. *J Nucl Cardiol* 1997;4(3):234–243.

25. King MA, Schwinger RB, Doherty PW, et al. Two dimensional filtering of SPECT images using the Metz and Wiener filters. *J Nucl Med* 1984;25:1234–1240.

26. Boulfelfel D, Rangayyan RM, Hahn LJ, et al. Prereconstruction restoration of myocardial single photon emission computed tomography images. *IEEE Trans Med Imaging* 1992;11(3):336–341.

27. Borello JA, Clinthorne NH, Rogers WL, et al. Oblique-angle tomography. A restructuring algorithm for transaxial tomographic data. *J Nucl Med* 1981;22:471–473.

28. The Cardiovascular Imaging Committee, American College of Cardiology. Standardization of cardiac tomographic imaging. *J Am Coll Cardiol* 1992;20:255–256.

29. Germano G, Kiat H, Kavanagh PB, et al. Automatic quantification of ejection fraction from gated myocardial perfusion SPECT. *J Nucl Med* 1995;36:2138–2147.

30. O'Brien A, Gemmell H. Effectiveness of oblique section display in thallium-201 myocardial tomography. *Nucl Med Commun* 1986;7:609–616.

31. DePuey EG, Garcia EV. Optimal specificity of thallium-201 SPECT through recognition of imaging artifacts. *J Nucl Med* 1989;30:441.

32. Eisner RL, Tamas MJ, Cloninger K, et al. Normal SPECT thallium-201 bull's-eye display: gender differences. *J Nucl Med* 1988;29(12):1901–1909.

33. Garcia EV, Van Train K, Maddahi J, et al. Quantification of rotational thallium-201 myocardial tomography. *J Nucl Med* 1985;26:17–26.

34. Jaszczak RJ, Greer KL, Floyd CE, et al. Improved SPECT quantitation using compensation for scattered photons. *J Nucl Med* 1984;25:893–900.

35. Tsui BMW, Zhao XD, Gregoriou GK, et al. Quantitative cardiac SPECT reconstruction with reduced image degradation due to patient anatomy. *IEEE Trans Nucl Sci* 1994;41(6):2838–2844.

36. Corbett JR, Ficaro EP. Clinical review of attenuation-corrected cardiac SPECT. *J Nucl Cardiol* 199;6:54–68.

37. Harris CC, Greer KL, Jaszczak RJ, et al. Tc-99m attenuation coefficients in water-tilled phantom determined with gamma cameras. *Med Phys* 1984;11(5):681–685.

38. Hoffman EJ, Huang SC, Phelps ME. Quantitation in positron emission computed tomography: I. Effect of object size. *J Comput Assist Tomogr* 1979;3:299–308.

39. Galt JR, Garcia EV, Robbins WL. Effects of myocardial wall thickness on SPECT quantification. *IEEE Trans Med Imaging* 1990;9(2):144–150.

40. Cooke CD, Garcia EV, Cullom SJ, et al. Determining the accuracy of calculating systolic wall thickening using a fast fourier transform approximation: A simulation study based on canine and patient data. *J Nucl Med* 1994;35;1185–1192.

41. DePuey EG, Rozanski AR. Using gated technetium-99m-sestamibi SPECT to characterize fixed defects as infarct or artifact. *J Nucl Med* 1995;36:952–955.

42. Hutton BF, Osiecki A. Correction of partial volume effects in myocardial SPECT. *J Nucl Cardiol* 1998;5(4):2–13.

43. National Electrical Manufacturers' Association. *Performance measurements of scintillation cameras.* NEMA standards publication NU 1-1994. National Electrical Manufacturers' Association, 1994.

44. Hines H, Kayayan R, Colsher J, et al. National Electrical Manufacturers' Association recommendations for implementing SPECT instrumentation quality control. *J Nucl Med* 2000;41(2):383–389.

45. Nichols KJ, Galt JR. Quality control for SPECT imaging. In: DePuey EG, Berman DS, Garcia EV, eds. *Cardiac SPECT imaging*. New York: Raven Press, 1995:21–48.

46. Fahey FH, Harkness BA, Keyes JW Jr, et al. Sensitivity, resolution and image quality with a multi-head SPECT camera. *J Nucl Med* 1992;33(10):1859–1863.

47. Faber TL. Multiheaded rotating gamma cameras in cardiac single-photon emission computed tomographic imaging. *J Nucl Cardiol* 1994;1(3):292–303.

48. Friedman J, Berman DS, Van Train KF, et al. Patient motion in Tl-201 myocardial SPECT imaging. An easily identified frequent source of artifactual defect. *Clin Nucl Med* 1988;13(5):321–324.

49. Botvinick EH, Zhu YY, O'Connell WJ, et al. A quantitative assessment of patient motion and its effect on myocardial perfusion SPECT images. *J Nucl Med* 1993;34:303–310.

50. Friedman J, Van Train K, Maddahi J, et al. "Upward creep" of the heart: a frequent source of false-positive reversible defects on Tl-201 stress-redistribution SPECT. *J Nucl Med* 1989;30:1718–1722.

51. Eisner RL, Noever T, Nowak D, et al. Use of cross-correlation function to detect patient motion during SPECT imaging. *J Nucl Med* 1987;28(1):97–101.

52. Germano G, Chua T, Kavanagh PB, et al. Detection and correction of patient motion in dynamic and static myocardial SPECT using a multi-detector camera. *J Nucl Med* 1993;34(8):1349–1355.

53. Graham LS. Quality control for SPECT systems. *Radiographics* 1995;15(6):1471–1481.

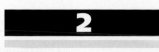
# QUALITY CONTROL FOR SPECT IMAGING

KENNETH J. NICHOLS
JAMES R. GALT

## CAMERA QUALITY CONTROL IN SINGLE PHOTON EMISSION COMPUTED TOMOGRAPHY

### Rationale for Quality Control

The foremost reason to perform quality control (QC) testing of medical imaging equipment is to assure the provision of the best possible diagnostic service to the patient population. But there are additional reasons, not the least of which is the satisfaction of legal requirements. Laws governing the medical use of isotopes are derived from the Nuclear Regulatory Commission (NRC) regulations as specified in Title 10 of the Code of Federal Regulations, especially Parts 20 and 35, and are based on the recommendations of the National Committee on Radiation Protection (1). In "agreement states," the state government licenses and regulates the use of isotopes, and those states' laws may be even more restrictive than those of the NRC. In a few localities, the city government's statutes must be satisfied as well as the state's. Some city governments contain additional departments, such as an office of electrical safety, the requirements of which also must be met. Furthermore, the Joint Committee on the Accreditation of Hospital Organizations has guidelines dealing with the use of medical isotopes and associated radiation measuring and imaging equipment. The requirements of all of these regulatory agencies must be satisfied.

Users must familiarize themselves with the details specified by the radiation license as to how to conduct quality assurance tests on equipment. While some radiation licenses may direct that QC recommendations of the equipment manufacturers be followed, other licenses detail the frequency and methods by which each procedure must be

accomplished. It is important to comply with all of the regulations relevant to a particular facility, but the ultimate goal of any QC program is the production of high-quality images as one aspect of good medical practice.

### Planar Gamma Camera Quality Control

Quality control for single photon emission computed tomography (SPECT) gamma cameras begins with diligent quality assurance procedures appropriate to ordinary planar scintillation cameras. On each day a machine is to be used, this consists of "peaking" the camera for the relevant energies and obtaining floods. If the principal application is cardiac imaging then primarily technetium 99m ($^{99m}$Tc) and thallium 201 ($^{201}$Tl) should be used, but if the same gamma camera will be used for procedures involving other isotopes, then the machine must be peaked for those as well. These tests indicate whether automatic peaking circuitry is working properly, if the peak appears at the correct energy, and if the shape of the spectrum is correct. A further benefit can be the detection of accidental contamination of the camera by an isotope used during some previous medical imaging procedure. Photographs of spectra should be taken and stored.

#### Daily Flood Uniformity Tests

Accompanying each spectrum will be photographs of the camera's flood fields. The preferred method is that these be acquired intrinsically, i.e., without any collimators. However, for some multidetector systems, the geometric arrangement of detectors is such that performing intrinsic floods can be difficult or even impossible, in which case the manufacturer will have made other provisions, such as evaluating uniformity with extrinsic flood fields (i.e., acquired with a collimator) and a radioactive sheet source. But for single-detector cameras, these floods will be performed typically with a small source approximating a point, placed in an easily reproducible geometry with respect to the detector, such as by means of a tripod to hold the source (Fig. 2.1).

K. J. Nichols: Nuclear Cardiology, Department of Medicine, College of Physicians and Surgeons, Columbia University, New York, New York 10032.

J. R. Galt: Department of Nuclear Medicine, Emory University School of Medicine, Atlanta, Georgia 30322.

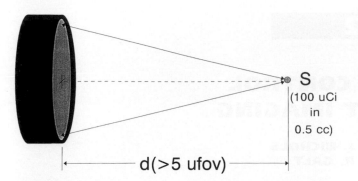

**FIGURE 2.1.** Intrinsic flood field data acquisition can be performed using a source, *S*, of 100 μCi in a 0.5-cc volume as an approximation to a point source. The distance, *d*, of the source to the detector should exceed five uniform field of view (ufov) diameters. The source should be placed directly over the center of the detector.

To implement this procedure, a small amount of isotope (100 μCi) is placed in a small volume (0.5 cc) in the bottom of a narrow tube, such as a test tube. Irregularly shaped sources should be avoided, as these can produce floods that mistakenly appear to be nonuniform even when machinery is functioning properly. It is important to not present the camera's electronics with too high a count rate, or else the circuitry that performs the energy correction will not be able to respond rapidly enough, and photomultiplier (PM) tube patterns will appear inappropriately on the floods. Therefore, as a rule of thumb, count rates should be kept below 20 thousand counts per second (kcps). The source-to-detector distance should exceed five times the crystal's useful field of view (UFOV) diameter, usually considered to be the central 50% to 60%, unless the manufacturer has explicitly provided software to compensate for the geometric variation from the center to the edge of the crystal. If available, a lead ring to shield the outermost tubes from the radiation should be used. Flood fields should be acquired as $64^2$ matrices using a 20% energy window for 2- to 5-million (M) counts. Typically, a minimum of 2.5-M counts should be acquired for a circular detector and 4 M for a rectangular detector (2). If possible, flood images both with and without correction circuitry turned on should be acquired, preferably daily but at least monthly.

Rather than rely on visual assessment of flood images in evaluating uniformity, two kinds of flood uniformity parameters should be computed, with a minimum of collected counts of 4,500/cm² (2). The National Electrical Manufacturers' Association (NEMA) standards (3) specify that the flood field first be smoothed with a nine-point smoothing filter of kernel 4:2:1. Then "integral uniformity" measures contrast over a large area of the detector and is computed from the smoothed flood image as:

$$\text{Integral Uniformity} = \pm100\% \times \frac{\text{Max} - \text{Min}}{\text{Max} + \text{Min}}$$

where "Max" is the maximum count, and "Min" is the minimum count found in any pixel within the specified area. "Differential Uniformity" is defined for small neighborhoods of contiguous pixels in a row or column as:

$$\text{Differential Uniformity} = \pm100\% \times \frac{\text{Max} - \text{Min}}{\text{Max} + \text{Min}}$$

where now the maximum and minimum pixel counts are confined to any five-pixel row (*x* direction) or column (*y* direction) of the digital image (3). Thus, integral uniformity is a global parameter while differential uniformity is a local measurement and is more reflective of the rate of change of local nonuniformities. These parameters are computed for both the UFOV and for the central field of view (CFOV), generally taken to be the central 25% to 30% of detector area. Because it is not possible to balance electrical current generated by PM tubes at the crystal's periphery with current from the interior tubes, the edge of the field of view always appears brighter than the interior in a phenomenon known as *edge packing,* and consequently, uniformity values are not computed for the outer 10% to 20% of detector area. For a gamma camera that will be used for tomography, these numbers should not exceed 4% for corrected flood fields (Fig. 2.2). If any of the numbers exceed 10% for an uncorrected flood field, the machinery may need to be serviced, if it is unlikely the correction circuits will handle adequately deviations larger than this. It is useful to graph the uniformity measurements versus time on a monthly basis (Fig. 2.3), as these will readily demonstrate

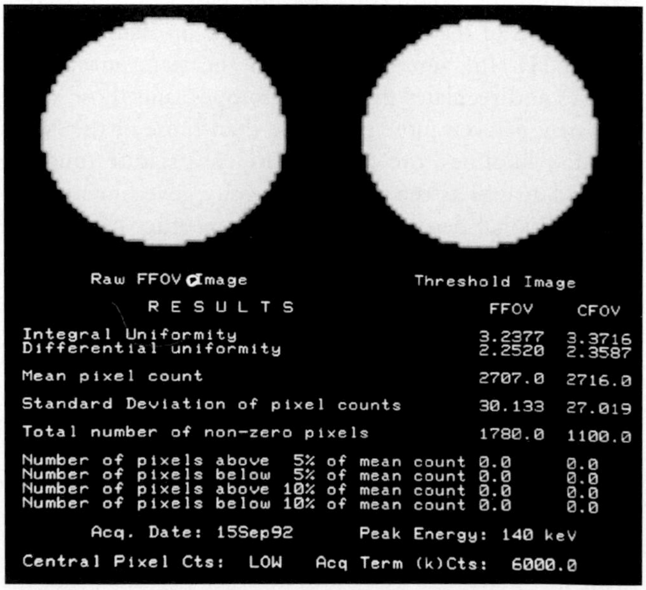

|                                    | FFOV   | CFOV   |
| ---------------------------------- | ------ | ------ |
| Raw FFOV image / Threshold Image   |        |        |
| **RESULTS**                        |        |        |
| Integral Uniformity                | 3.2377 | 3.3716 |
| Differential uniformity            | 2.2520 | 2.3587 |
| Mean pixel count                   | 2707.0 | 2716.0 |
| Standard Deviation of pixel counts | 30.133 | 27.019 |
| Total number of non-zero pixels    | 1780.0 | 1100.0 |
| Number of pixels above  5% of mean count | 0.0 | 0.0 |
| Number of pixels below  5% of mean count | 0.0 | 0.0 |
| Number of pixels above 10% of mean count | 0.0 | 0.0 |
| Number of pixels below 10% of mean count | 0.0 | 0.0 |

Acq. Date: 15Sep92      Peak Energy: 140 keV

Central Pixel Cts: LOW      Acq Term (k)Cts: 6000.0

**FIGURE 2.2.** Tabulations of integral and differential uniformity values for the central field of view and useful field of view are shown beneath a typical intrinsic flood field *(upper left)* along with an enhanced representation of the same flood field *(upper right).* All of the uniformity values are beneath 4%, and no pixels are above 5% of the mean count rate, nor are any beneath 5% of the mean, which represents typical results for an acceptable intrinsic flood.

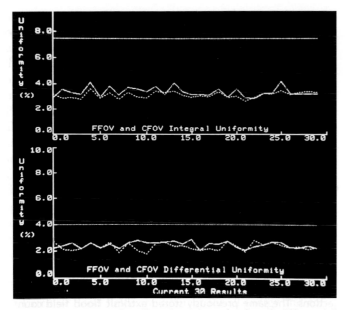

**FIGURE 2.3.** Integral uniformity values *(top)* and differential uniformity values *(bottom)* are plotted versus time for a 30-day period. Both full field of view (FFOV) and central field of view (CFOV) uniformity values are graphed.

sudden variations from normal, as well as show the development of time trends, indicative of a progressively worsening condition of the machinery.

### Daily Gamma Camera Sensitivity Measurement

By measuring the activity of the source used for the intrinsic flood field with a dose calibrator, it is possible to compute detector sensitivity, expressed in terms of counts per minute per μCi per meter from the center of the camera detector:

$$\text{Sensitivity} = C/(t{\cdot}A{\cdot}d^2)$$

for count rate $C$, time of acquisition $t$, activity $A$, and source-to-detector distance $d$. It is suggested that this be computed as a normal part of the daily QC. A convenient means of measuring sensitivity is by recording the time needed to acquire the 2-M count intrinsic flood using a source of known activity.

A frequent cause of daily flood field instabilities is PM tube drift, meaning that either the voltage supplied to the tube or the current produced by the tube is varying with time. This can have the effect of causing the energy correction circuitry to perform more computations than usual for the "balancing" of tubes, thereby resulting in an abnormal decrease in detector sensitivity. Generally, detector sensitivity should not vary from day to day by more than a few per cent. Flood fields should be examined to see if any tubes are visible, and if so, whether they appear to be more prominent than on previous days. Particular attention should be

paid to a single tube becoming more visible over a period of a few days, as this indicates the tube is drifting progressively further out of alignment from the others. The flood images should also be examined to determine if the blanking circuits (if any) are functioning to suppress the display of counts from the outermost tubes.

### Weekly Linearity and Resolution Assessment

Weekly QC of all single-detector gamma cameras should include linearity assessment with a bar phantom. It is inadvisable to image bar phantoms extrinsically because the pattern of lead holes and septa of the collimators often interfere with the bars to produce artifactual moire patterns. Therefore, bar phantoms usually are acquired intrinsically, using the same point source as for intrinsic flood fields. The point source should be greater than five UFOV diameters from the center of the unshielded detector, and the bar phantom should be placed as near to the crystal as is practical, consistent with protecting the crystal.

Commercially available bar phantoms include PLES ("parallel line equally spaced") bar phantoms, quadrant phantoms, and orthogonal hole phantoms. Quadrant phantoms contain four different sizes of bars, and if one of these is used, it should be rotated four times, so that the quadrant with the most closely spaced bars is imaged over the entire usable surface of the crystal. To have all four bar sizes sampled in both $x$ and $y$ directions, the bar phantom may be turned over and imaged four times again. It is generally sufficient to do this over an 8-week cycle with the eight different possible bar phantom orientations.

While barrel effects and pin-cushion effects are always present, particularly in older cameras (4), bar phantom images should be examined for the appearance of unusual wavy lines and local loses in spatial resolution (i.e., localized inability to resolve the bars). Most probably, any striking abnormalities will be due to PM tube drift. Additionally, bar phantom images provide some indication of the camera's intrinsic spatial resolution. For example, if a set of 4-mm bars for a particular phantom cannot be resolved but a set of 7-mm bars can be, then the intrinsically resolvable bar size lies somewhere between these two values (Fig. 2.4). The relationship between resolution as expressed by the full width at half maximum (FWHM) of the profile of a line spread function and the bar size that is just barely resolvable is (2,4):

$$\text{Resolution (in mm)} = 1.7 \times \text{bar size (in mm)}$$

In addition, the use of digitized bar phantom images provide pixel size information, which may be needed for applications such as tomographic attenuation compensation. While orthogonal hole phantoms have the advantage of not needing to be rotated and repeated, they have the disadvantage of having only one spatial dimension, and therefore are less useful in providing intrinsic resolution infor-

If there are several options of using either line sources, capillary tubes, or point sources, then extended line sources should be employed because these images can also be used for assessment of system tomographic spatial resolution, as described below. Line sources will be loaded with a typical amount of activity of 100 μCi in a volume of 0.5 cc and alignment of the line source with the computer's *y*-axis is most easily accomplished by sequential imaging of the source until it clearly falls at the same *y* location from the top to the bottom of the image matrix when the detector is positioned looking straight down at the imaging table.

### Quarterly Multipurpose SPECT Phantom Evaluation

The use of multipurpose Plexiglass phantoms, the cavities of which can be filled with radioactive liquid, constitutes the major component of quarterly QC of SPECT systems (Fig. 2.7). Both Plexiglas and water have attenuation and scattering properties similar to tissue, and therefore, phantoms composed of them approximate realistic clinical scattering and attenuation imaging conditions. In general, it makes sense to test three dimensionally machinery that is used for three-dimensional imaging, and the multipurpose Plexiglas phantoms that are available from several companies provide one means for doing this (14). In the process of imaging these phantoms, the limits of machine capability become apparent, and a standard is established against which future performance can be judged. As an example, if at some point ^99mTc-sestamibi perfusion tomograms from a particular camera seem to be of a less high technical quality than those acquired in previous days, comparing a new acquisition of a multipurpose phantom to that acquired as part of the quarterly QC tests will facilitate the separation of machin-

ery problems from other aspects of the total imaging process, such as poor injection technique. In addition to evaluating performance of an imaging system to reconstruct emission data, these are now also used to assess the effectiveness of transmission scans using external radioactive line sources (15).

Generally speaking, multipurpose Plexiglas phantoms include several removable cold rod sections. In one version of these phantoms solid rods are arranged in hexagonal divisions, ranging in size from a maximum diameter of 12.7 mm down to a minimum diameter of 4.8 mm, and removable spheres representing cold lesions can be used as well, ranging in size from 31.8 mm down to 9.5 mm (Fig. 2.7). Elliptical containers and arrangements of solid rods of different sizes are also commercially available from several companies.

Because the aim of using multipurpose Plexiglas phantoms is to determine the limits of resolution of the machinery, high activities (20–30 mCi) and fine sampling ($128^2$ matrices and 128 projections over 360 degrees) are employed, and customarily acquisitions are performed at typical ^99mTc energy settings of 140 keV with a 20% energy window. It is important that the detector come as close to the cylinder as possible throughout the entire 360-degree rotation, and that the phantom and detectors be centered and leveled as well as possible. Because some protocols require all slices containing rods to be summed for higher counting statistics, it is imperative that the phantom's axis align with the camera's AOR.

These phantoms often are assembled with the spheres in the top half of the cylindrical container and solid rods in the bottom half of the container, in which case transverse reconstructions are performed for three distinct volumes: the entire bottom half of the container for the cold rods, a

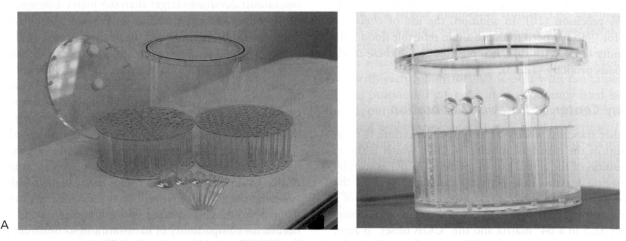

A                                                                                              B

**FIGURE 2.7.** A disassembled multipurpose Plexiglas single photon emission computed tomography (SPECT) phantom is shown *(left)*. It consists of a cylindrical tub, two inserts each having six different sizes of solid rods, and six solid spheres of different sizes. A typical configuration of the assembled phantom is shown on its side *(right)*, with spheres occupying the top half of the tub phantom and a solid rod insert placed in the bottom of the tub.

single 6-mm slice through the center of the cold spheres, and as large a volume as possible of the vacant uniform section above the spheres. Each of these volumes are reconstructed into a single transverse tomographic section. Another way to use the phantom is to just image the radioactive cylinder with no rods or sphere inserts, and reconstruct each transverse section as one-pixel-thick sections. The optimal attenuation correction and filtering algorithms of the computer are used, defined by those that provide the highest contrast cold rod images while simultaneously generating uniform images of the lowest noise-to-signal ratio. The rod inserts of the multipurpose phantoms provide an appreciation of effective tomographic system resolution varying from the surface to deep within the phantom.

If used to evaluate the performance of a SPECT system's scanning source transmission correcting ability, transmission uniformity and spatial resolution should be recorded. These should vary little from one time to the next, and deviations from baseline values can be used to recognize errors due to incorrect blank scale factors or crosstalk measurements, collimator misalignments, and inadequate transmission counts, such as result from using a transmission source beyond its useful half-life (15).

## Quarterly Line Source SPECT Resolution Tests

Line source data produces an even better determination of tomographic spatial resolution than that provided by multipurpose SPECT phantom measurements. With the source parallel to the AOR, a high-resolution tomogram should be acquired and reconstructed into transverse slices. As with the multipurpose Plexiglas phantom acquisition, this will consist of a line source or capillary tube filled with a high specific activity (e.g., 10 mCi of $^{99m}$Tc in 0.5 cc of water). Data should be acquired into $128^2$ matrices at 128 projections over 360 degrees, with high-resolution collimation and with the detector 10 to 20 cm from the source. For a planar image, not less than 100,000 counts should be acquired, and total tomographic counts should exceed 0.5 M counts in order to have adequate counting statistics to compare FHWM values of curves of planar images to those of tomographic transaxial slices (16).

The characteristics of the curve passing through the middle of the point-like transverse section of the reconstructed line source should be similar to the profile through a planar image of the same line source imaged at the same distance from the collimator (Fig. 2.8). One should determine and record the FWHM curve parameter. To characterize system spatial resolution more completely, it is necessary to compute the modulation transfer function from the reconstructed line spread function (17), the characteristics of which depend on the collimator, isotope, and reconstruction filters used.

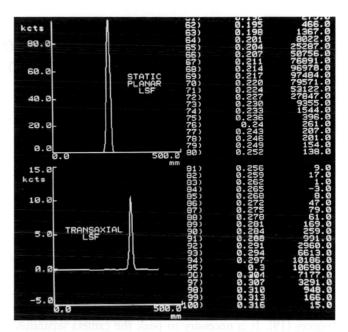

**FIGURE 2.8.** Profiles and numerical expressions of the line spread function of a planar image of a line source are shown *(top)*, as are the corresponding plots and numerical listings for the profile through the center of the transverse tomographic reconstruction of the same line source *(bottom)*. Plots display total counts versus pixel locations within the image matrices. Columns of numerical listings are in order of pixel number, distance location in millimeters, and counts at each pixel location.

## Organ Phantoms

It is advisable to have additionally elliptical multipurpose phantoms and phantoms relevant to the clinical setting of the laboratory in which the SPECT camera is used, such as cardiac phantoms (Fig. 2.9), liver phantoms, brain phan-

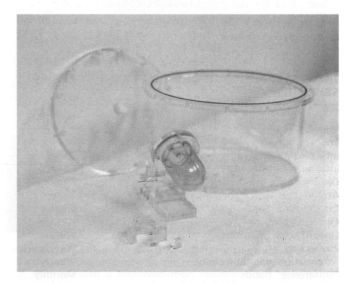

**FIGURE 2.9.** A cardiac phantom is shown, consisting of an elliptical tub, simulated lesion chambers that can be filled with any desired concentration of radioactivity, and a cardiac insert having both a left ventricle chamber and a myocardial chamber.

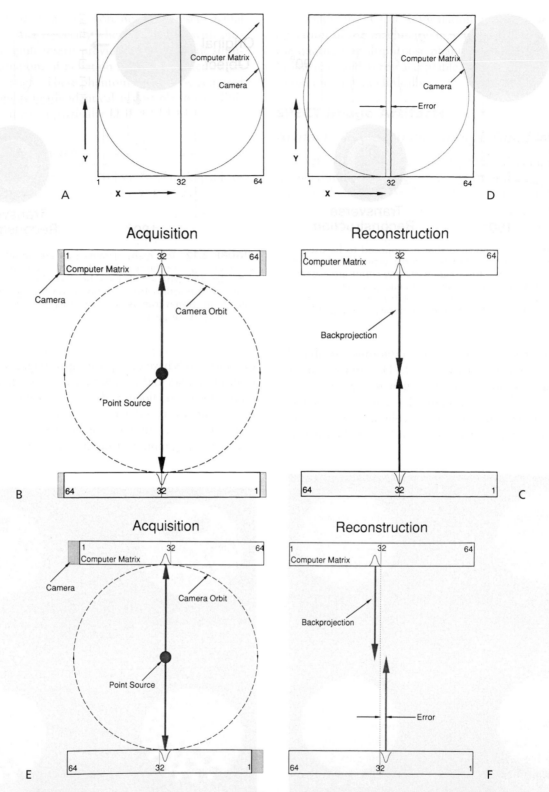

**FIGURE 2.14.** When machinery is properly calibrated, the digitized image matrix *(square)* exactly corresponds to the actual field of view *(circle)* **(A)**, in which case, gamma rays emitted by a point source positioned at the axis of rotation will be registered at the central pixel of every projection **(B)**, and consequently, rays centered at the middle pixel will be properly projected back into the center of the transverse slice during the reconstruction process **(C)**. However, if the computer matrix does not correspond to the field of view **(D)**, and this difference is not taken into account, then a point source placed at the axis of rotation will incorrectly be registered at the wrong pixel location **(E)**, and when this information is reconstructed, the rays will not meet at the center of the transverse reconstruction **(F)**.

part in whether or not the artifacts are actually visible. Ring artifacts are most obvious on high-count multipurpose phantom acquisitions, where several million total counts can be acquired. They are less likely to be apparent in $^{99m}$Tc–methoxy isobutyl isonitrile (MIBI) tomograms consisting of a total of a few million counts and highly unlikely to be seen in $^{201}$Tl tomograms consisting of fewer than 0.5-M counts.

## Artifacts Due to Incorrect COR Information

The other most common source of backprojection artifacts arises from incorrect COR information. COR measurements and corrections are important due to the methods by which the computer's backprojection algorithm is implemented (27). A properly calibrated machine maps point source *x* positions as a sinusoid as the detector rotates about the AOR. But correct knowledge of source distance from the AOR can be determined only if the COR itself is known (Fig. 2.14). Ideally, this will be at *x* location = 32.5 pixels in an image spanned by 1 to 64 pixels. If the COR is actually offset from the ideal value, and no correction is made for this fact, then every view that the camera receives is incorrectly offset by this amount. Thus, when the backprojector is instructed to produce a transaxial reconstruction of the point source, it will not backproject rays through the correct positions.

This is most easily demonstrated for a point source. It is obvious that backprojections of its image should all converge at the position in space where the source is located relative to the camera. But if the COR information is erroneous, each projection will be offset by the same amount, and the transaxial reconstruction of the point source will

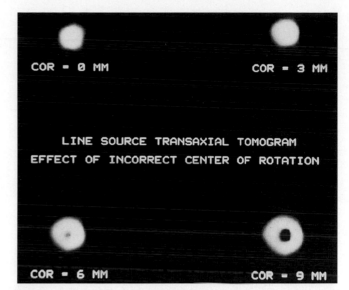

**FIGURE 2.16.** The transverse reconstructions of the same line source data are shown using the correct center of rotation offset information (COR = 0 mm), and with varying degrees of incorrect COR information. In these 128² images, 3.1 mm represents one pixel.

result in a ring (Fig. 2.15). Since every location of the original radiating object may be regarded as a point source, all points become blurred as they are mapped into rings during transverse reconstruction (Fig. 2.16). Thus, tomographic spatial resolution is degraded, as can be appreciated from examination of the reconstructed rods of a multipurpose Plexiglas phantom (Fig. 2.17). When the true distrib-

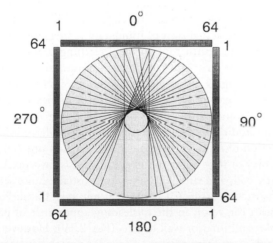

**FIGURE 2.15.** When the computer is provided with an incorrect constant center of rotation offset of the matrix registration information, the rays seen by the camera at each projection are offset from the center and projected back to form a ring in the transverse slice, even if the input data was emitted by a point source.

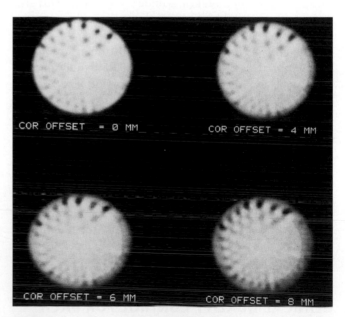

**FIGURE 2.17.** The summed transverse section containing the solid rods of a multipurpose SPECT phantom are shown, with both correct center of rotation offset information (COR = 0 mm), and with varying degrees of incorrect COR information. In these 128² images, 3.1 mm represents one pixel.

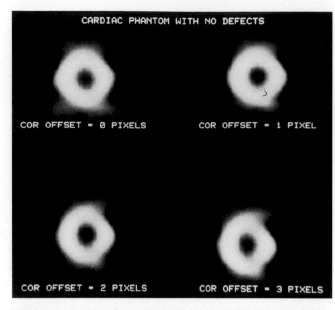

**FIGURE 2.18.** Data from the same cardiac phantom simulating a thallium 201 ($^{201}$Tl) myocardial perfusion study with no myocardial defects were reconstructed into short-axis slices with the correct center of rotation offset information (COR = 0 pixels) and with varying degrees of incorrect center of rotation information. Notice that in the most extreme case, anterior and inferior wall defects incorrectly appear, with activity incongruously appearing to stream away from the ventricular center, a striking nonphysiologic image artifact pattern.

ution of activity is cylindrical, such as for the myocardium, then incorrect COR information can result in transverse reconstructions in which the activity is mistakenly mapped into two halves of a broken cylinder (Fig. 2.18). This artifactual pattern could be misinterpreted as paired anterior and inferior wall myocardial perfusion defects.

The artifacts just described represent things to look for on the quarterly QC images of line sources, multipurpose phantoms, and organ phantoms. The appearance of circular artifacts indicates problems with collimators or with the way the correcting floods are stored or used, or is a clue that the wrong flood field is being applied by the software. The use of a multidetector system can provide a considerable improvement in count rate and resolution, but only if QC is performed satisfactorily so that one can be confident that the multiple heads truly are better than one. These additional necessary checks include comparisons of imaging characteristics of the individual detectors to those of the combined information from all detectors, and are discussed below (see Multidetector SPECT Systems).

## CLINICAL QUALITY CONTROL FOR EACH PATIENT PROCEDURE

All of the QC procedures described above will help reduce the frequency of misdiagnosis due to technical problems

but will not eliminate them. Ongoing clinical QC is needed as well. This includes preventing, identifying, and compensating for imaging artifacts, including motion of the patient, movement of the heart within the patient, and breast and prosthesis artifacts. To obtain optimal images, attention must be paid to technical factors such as minimizing the distance of the detector to the patient, correctly leveling the detector, repositioning repeated scans on the same patient in the same way, positioning consistently among different patients, and avoiding outright errors such as failing to repeak the camera between procedures that use different isotopes.

## Patient Motion

The most common source of misalignment in myocardial tomographic imaging is patient motion (28–30). The imaging procedure always should be explained to patients prior to data collection, and they should be advised as to the necessity of remaining immobile. Diligent monitoring of the patient throughout the acquisition is essential (2). The most common cause of motion is patient fatigue, and the use of arm supports, whole body restraints, and biplane cameras for cardiac imaging are recommended to reduce the frequency of patient motion, but these measures are not always sufficient. Therefore, to help recognize and quantify the extent of motion, some laboratories apply marker sources holding a few microcuries of activity taped to the patient's skin. These can be attached near the patient's throat or below the sternum, or both. However, these do not always correspond to the independent motion of the heart itself, such as can arise from diaphragmatic alterations.

One type of motion artifact is "upward creep," in which the heart is slowly displaced over a period of minutes upward by diaphragmatic relaxation following strenuous exercise (31). For this reason, 10 to 15 minutes should be allowed to elapse between the injection of $^{201}$Tl at peak stress and the actual start of tomographic imaging, to allow the patient to return to a normal breathing pattern. Compensating for this form of cardiac motion represents the most challenging situation, and often may prove impossible, since there is no abrupt alteration of heart location from one tomographic projection angle to the next. Of the various studies performed dealing with the detection and correction of motion patterns, it appears that one 6.4-mm pixel may or may not result in misdiagnosis; two pixels frequently will, and three or more pixels usually cause serious reconstruction artifacts (32–34). Simple axial translation of the heart can result in the misleading appearance of paired anterior and inferior wall defects (Fig. 2.19). However, the particular artifact pattern depends on the projection angle(s) at which motion occurred as well as the magnitude and direction of the displacements (33).

In addition, for those cameras equipped with attenuation correcting machinery, it is crucial that patient motion be

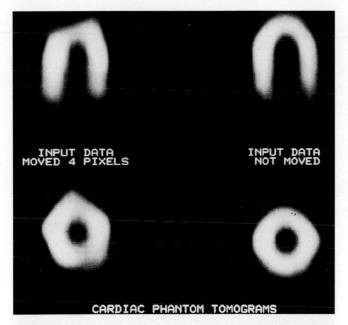

**FIGURE 2.19.** A cardiac phantom filled with [201]Tl was moved axially and sinusoidally by a total amount of four pixels, with no lateral translation, such as can occur when a patient's diaphragm moves erratically and uncontrollably. This resulted in anterior and inferior wall defects *(left)*, even though the phantom contained no defects and when reconstructed without simulated motion showed a uniform distribution of activity *(right)*.

minimized between emission and transmission images if these are not acquired simultaneously. Transverse and axial shifts of three pixels between the two studies have been found to produce artifactual myocardial defects by up to 35% (20), and relative displacements of only one pixel have been reported to decrease myocardial counts regionally of up to 15% (35). Similar effects have been observed in relation to SPECT tumor imaging (36). While systems that acquire both attenuation and emission studies simultaneously should be free of these problems, it is necessary to verify that gamma rays of the two energies are registered similarly or else the same types of artifacts would be expected. This is a further reason to use the same multipurpose Plexiglas phantom to assess the ability of the gamma camera to properly reconstruct both emission and attenuation data (15).

## Motion Correction Algorithms

Some methods for semiautomatically detecting and compensating for motion that have been reported in the literature include "cross-correlation" and "diverging squares" techniques. Cross-correlation approximates the distance shifted between successive planar images by performing parabolic fits between peaks and neighboring points of the correlation functions:

$$CN_N(S) = \Sigma(P_N(j) \cdot P_{N-1}(j + S))$$

where CN is the measure of cross-correlation, $P_N$ is the summed transaxial or axial profile, $P_{N-1}$ is the summed profile of an adjacent frame, $j$ is the profile index, and $s$ is relative pixel offset (29). "Diverging squares" tracks the coordinates of the heart center by beginning with an operator-positioned $10 \times 10$ square over the initial tomogram and then finding the $20 \times 20$ square encompassing the heart with the highest count rate, upon considering successively larger squares (37).

### Visual Review of Motion

Generally speaking, detecting and compensating for axial motion in the AOR direction is easier than discerning lateral motion in the plane normal to the rotation axis. Some studies found that detecting motion visually is accurate for more than one 3.2-mm pixel of axial displacement and for more than two 3.2-mm pixels of lateral displacement, but not sufficiently accurate for displacements smaller than these amounts (38).

The cinematic playback of tomographic data should always be examined before the patient leaves the department, and if severe motion is observed, then data acquisition should be repeated. If it is impractical to repeat the study, then automated correction algorithms should be attempted, but it is important to again review the results of such corrections and to reject them if for any reason the automated programs are deemed to have failed. In the event that data cannot be reacquired and automated motion corrections have clearly failed, the only recourse is to correct the motion manually, frame by frame if necessary, and again review the cinematic playback of the manually translated images. In examining the short-axis reconstructions and polar perfusion maps of data that must be moved, if the results appear normal, then it is unlikely that the original data contain perfusion abnormalities. But if the results are abnormal, and particularly if the observer is unsure as to the success of the motion correction, then the study should be discarded.

### Patient Positioning

It is important for the technologist to maintain consistency of setup from one patient to another, so that the physician may depend on having uniformity among acquisitions. It is even more important to image the same patient as nearly identically as possible between one scan and another, such as for [201]Tl rest-redistribution studies, [201]Tl reinjection protocols, and 2-day [99m]Tc-sestamibi protocols. Especially important in assisting the technologist to achieve reproducible patient setups is the recording of relevant information such as table height and table offset. In some laboratories, the first view of projection data of a previous scan is displayed on the computer during setup for a subsequent study, and the patient is sequentially repositioned while the computer screen is switched between stored images and current incoming signals until incoming data roughly match the stored data.

### Breast Artifacts

Consistent repositioning is most important for female patients with large breasts. Since there is some leeway in how breasts can be positioned, it is important that they be positioned the same for all tomographic data sets acquired for the same patient. Particularly in patients with large breasts, it is advantageous to image the patient with the bra removed, as this helps to distribute the breast tissue more nearly uniformly between the heart and the detector. Obviously, if a patient is imaged without a bra for one tomographic study, she should be setup similarly without a bra for subsequent perfusion tomograms. Attenuation artifacts will inevitably arise for such patients, but at least the physician who reads the studies will not be additionally confused by the shifting of the breast shadow between rest and stress studies.

The most pernicious situation is for a breast shadow to obscure the anterior wall of a stress study, but then to appear more laterally in the delay study of a [201]Tl tomogram, and so cause less attenuation on the delayed study. Such a pattern could easily be misinterpreted as a reversible anterior defect. An invaluable aid to recognizing these false patterns is to review the cinematic playback of the original tomographic data of both stress and delay studies, viewed simultaneously.

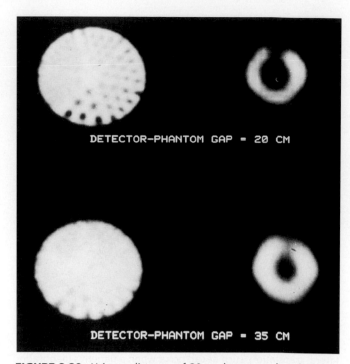

**FIGURE 2.20.** Using a distance of 20 cm between the phantom edge and the detector, the solid rod insert of a multipurpose SPECT phantom was acquired *(top left)*, as was the cardiac phantom containing a 2-cm-long 100% defect *(top right)*. Both phantoms contained [99m]Tc in water. These phantoms were also acquired with a larger detector-to-phantom gap of 35 cm and the resulting short-axis slices are displayed *(bottom)*. At the larger distance, the simulated myocardium is considerably blurred and the simulated myocardial defect much less distinct compared to the acquisition performed for the smaller distance from detector to phantom.

### Optimal Camera Setup

Of the different aspects of patient setup, one of the most important to the acquisition of optimal images for a given patient is minimizing the distance between the detector and the organ to be imaged, because spatial resolution falls off as the distance from the surface of any parallel hole collimator increases (39). In the case of cardiac scans with single-detector gamma cameras, this generally means doing one's best to minimize the distance in the left anterior oblique projection. The most propitious circumstance is the imaging of patients who are so thin that the limiting factor is the width of the imaging table, so that the closest the camera can approach is the table edge in the left posterior oblique (LPO) position. But this is rarely the case, and usually it is necessary to lower the imaging table from its central position until the heart is in the center of the field of view in the lateral position, and then back the camera away from the edge of the table in the LPO position. However, one should obtain the manufacturer's recommendations as to how to optimize acquisitions for a particular machine. An examination of phantoms acquired at two different radii reveals considerable degradation of image resolution at the larger radius (Fig. 2.20).

It also is important that the detector head be leveled in the anterior position before commencing the scan, and this is done most reliably with a carpenter's level (27). Failure to do so will provide the backprojection circuitry with mixtures of image projections from different planes normal to the AOR, whereas these circuits and software are usually designed to handle data only from within these planes. This also will result in diminished image contrast and degraded resolution (Fig. 2.21).

It is crucial that the SPECT system have the correct pulse height analyzer settings corresponding to the injected isotope. There are several clinical circumstances in which energy peaking errors can occur, such as in switching back and forth between [201]Tl and [99m]Tc-sestamibi patients, or scanning a [99m]Tc-sestamibi patient following acquisition of the weekly [57]Co extrinsic flood. Incorrect energy peaks result in the acquisition of Compton scatter photons rather than those of the photopeak, and the consequence will be tomograms of greatly reduced count rate, contrast, and spatial resolution compared to what it would have been had the camera been peaked properly (Fig. 2.22). Typical acquired myocardial counts should be 10,000 to 30,000 for

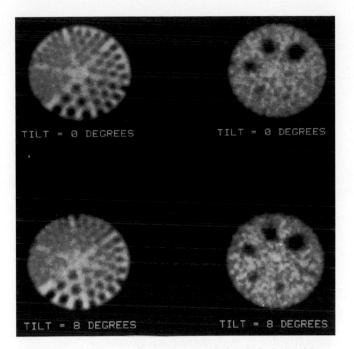

**FIGURE 2.21.** With the detector properly leveled, the multipurpose phantom was acquired on the technetium 99m ($^{99m}$Tc) window using both the solid rod inserts *(upper left)* and the solid spheres *(upper right)*. The effect of improperly tilting the detector by 8 degrees is demonstrated *(lower left and right)*, in which it can be seen that the solid rods are less easily resolved, especially near the phantom's center, and that the edges of the solid spheres appear to be less distinct.

$^{201}$Tl and 20,000 to 80,000 for $^{99m}$Tc-sestamibi in order to obtain clinically useful information (2).

Problems also arise when one unknowingly acquires a tomogram at an abnormally high count rate. In that case, the stored intrinsic and extrinsic flood fields will differ from the pattern of tubes that appears during the onset of paralysis of the camera electronics. This problem can be particularly difficult to detect if count rates are higher for some projections than for others, although drastic alterations of the upper and lower display window thresholds might be attempted to reveal the tube patterns. The resulting circular ring artifacts and resolution deterioration are similar to those that occur when the incorrect energy window is used to acquire a tomogram (Fig. 2.22).

Other obvious abnormalities can occur from incorrect blocking of essential image information. Examples of these are the stark attenuation shadows of metal electrocardiogram (ECG) electrodes as they appear on tomograms. These can produce vivid, high-contrast streak artifacts on transverse tomograms and create the false impression of localized perfusion defects, and would be especially troublesome if the artifact were to appear on a stress tomogram but not on the resting study (due to differences of patient setup), creating the mistaken impression of reversible defects. Occasional equipment failure of various forms in which the counts of several projections are accidentally dropped also can ruin a study (Fig. 2.23). These problems are readily detected by viewing the cinematic playback of original rotating data.

## Gating Quality Assurance

Increasingly, R-wave gating is performed in conjunction with myocardial SPECT, so that gated SPECT now accounts for the majority of nuclear cardiology procedures. A three-lead ECG monitor is used most commonly with a left-to-right lead, or "lead I." Technologists always should review the tracing prior to data acquisition, and verify that the heart rate is stable and that the heart rate reported by

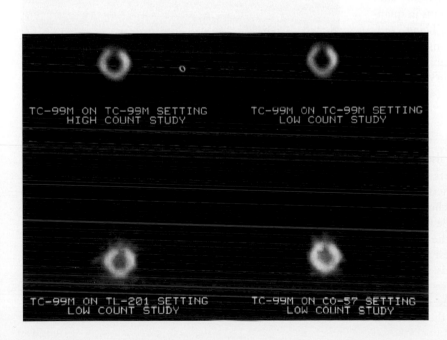

**FIGURE 2.22.** The cardiac phantom was loaded with $^{99m}$Tc and a 2-cm-long 100% anterior defect. The anterior defect appears well visualized *(upper left)* when the camera was correctly set to the $^{99m}$Tc energy settings. When acquired on either $^{201}$Tl *(lower left)* or $^{57}$Co *(lower right)* settings, the defect is less distinct and the uniform portion of the myocardial phantom considerably blurred. To show that the diminution of contrast was due to scattered photons rather than to the decreased signal-to-noise ratio of the lower counts acquired in the wrong energy window, the phantom was also imaged for the $^{99m}$Tc window for the same number of counts as were obtained for the $^{201}$Tl acquisition *(upper right)*.

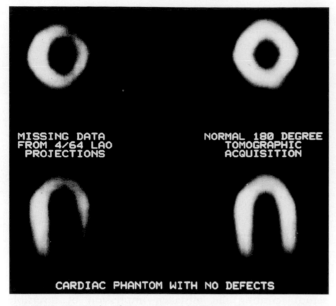

**FIGURE 2.23.** *Right:* Short-axis and horizontal long-axis sections through the mid-ventricular portion of a 180-degree [201]Tl tomogram of a cardiac phantom having no defects. *Left:* The same slices through the tomographic data sets of the same phantom data reconstructed in the same fashion but with four left anterior oblique projections missing from the 64-projection study. The reconstruction of the data with incorrectly lost data thus has the false appearance of a large lateral wall myocardial defect.

the monitor agrees with that of the acquisition computer (40). Mechanisms for handling variable hearts rates do exist and vary among manufacturers, including multiplying cinematic tomographic frames that are late in the R-R cycle by a scaling factor if these are count deficient, even though this can lead to severe distortion of the data if counts are quite low (41). Sometimes patients begin the data acquisition session in sinus rhythm but then develop an arrhythmia later in the study. This can cause a number of problems in quantifying cardiac parameters, the most sensitive being computed wall thickening. For this reason, it is important to examine graphically the counts versus projection curves of all eight (or 16) individual gated tomograms in order to be alerted to possible gating error contamination (42).

## Data-Processing Quality Control

Quality assurance of data processing is also of paramount importance. While some manufacturers offer completely automated processing packages, others' software requires the technologist to make several choices as to approximate symmetry axes of the left ventricle (LV). Typically, a first choice is of the angle that bisects the LV as seen in the transaxial view demonstrating the widest ventricular cavity; from this choice the vertical long-axis images are reoriented. Next, the slice is chosen that shows the largest LV cavity, and the line is drawn dividing the cavity into anterior and posterior territories, from which the short-axis

and horizontal long-axis images are formed. Finally, on the central vertical long-axis image, the user chooses the apical and basal short-axis images to be used in generating the polar perfusion maps.

As shown in Figs. 2.24 to 2.26, inappropriate axis choices produce misleading reoriented images. Part of QC consists of viewing these axes superimposed on the chosen slices, with particular attention paid as to whether both the slice numbers and angles chosen were optimal. For instance, the incorrect choice of the LV axis in the transverse slice of the simulated [99m]Tc-sestamibi delay image of Fig. 2.24 leads to peculiar orientations of the slices as seen on the vertical long-axis images of Fig. 2.25. Also, an examination of reoriented images should be revealing. In Fig. 2.25, the delayed vertical long-axis image does not demonstrate clearly a flaring out toward the base as it should. Nor, in Fig. 2.26 do the resulting short-axis slices appear to be round uniform concentric circles, but rather elongated ellipses. None of these peculiarities are due to the cardiac phantom used to create the images of Figs. 2.24 to 2.26 but are solely due to the incorrect axis choices.

It also is important to make correct choices as to the apical and basal myocardial slices to be used in generating polar perfusion maps. The apical slice should be the first one showing a ventricular cavity, and the basal choice should be that slice at which the myocardium is visible in

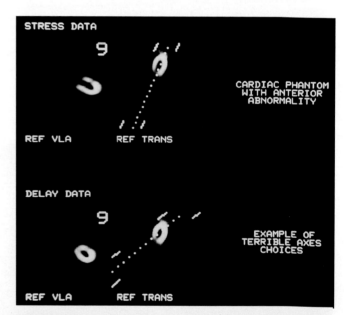

**FIGURE 2.24.** *Top:* The operator-chosen line bisecting the simulated left ventricle of the cardiac phantom and resulting vertical long-axis mid-ventricular slice are shown. The cardiac phantom with a 2-cm-large anterior defect was loaded with [99m]Tc and count rates of "stress" and "rest" data were acquired to emulate a [99m]Tc-sestamibi 1-day protocol. *Bottom:* The same input data were used, but on the "delay" data an inappropriate choice was made for the transverse axis. Note that the vertical long-axis tomogram generated by this choice does not well represent the base of the heart.

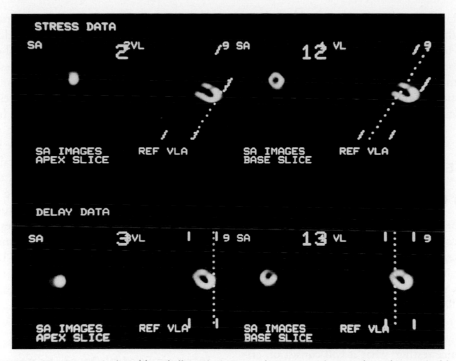

**FIGURE 2.25.** *Top:* Apical and basal slices choices are shown superimposed on the vertical long axis simulated stress data generated from the axis choice from Fig. 2.24. *Bottom:* Apical and basal slice choices are displayed on the simulated delay images, at orientations inconsistent with the ventricular axis.

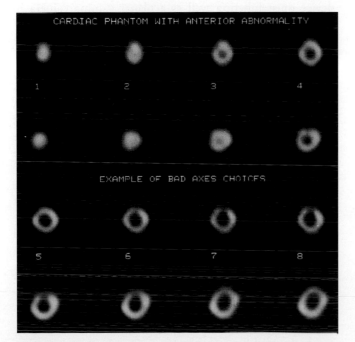

**FIGURE 2.26.** Paired short-axis slices of the simulated $^{99m}$Tc-sestamibi stress-rest study of Fig. 2.24 are shown. The uppermost row shows the first four short-axis slices of the "stress" study, beneath which are the corresponding first four slices of the "delay" study, followed in the third row by the next four slices of the "stress" study, etc. Note the appearance of the 2-cm defect in the stress simulations in slices 6 to 8, and the appearance of the defect to a lesser degree in slices 4 to 6 of the "delay" simulation. Note also that the "delay" short-axis slices are eccentrically shaped.

the lateral wall but absent in the septal location, as illustrated in the simulated stress images of Fig. 2.25. Choosing limits too far beyond the apex or too far beyond the base will result in these regions incorrectly seeming to be abnormally underperfused when compared against databases of normal patients. However, selection within the cavity of too few slices will not accurately sample the full extent of the myocardium. This would be especially misleading in the case of inconsistent choices of slice numbers between stress and redistribution (or resting) cardiac perfusion studies. However, there are circumstances in which using different slice numbers to span the myocardium is appropriate, if the heart is enlarged during the stress portion of the $^{201}$Tl stress test (transient ischemic dilatation), in which case the myocardial shape may truly be different from the situation at rest and can be rather eccentric (43).

A valuable tool available for the technologist who is learning tomographic data processing is standard patient example files, if these are provided by the manufacturer of the computer equipment. A reasonable course of action is for the technologist to analyze these files and then compare the results with processed files supplied by the manufacturer. However, the technologist should not assume that by successfully handling data for a few example patient files that the learning process is complete, but rather should anticipate that it will be necessary to analyze 10 to 20 patients having various pathologies under the supervision of a more experienced user before becoming proficient. It is advisable for technologists to be trained thoroughly in manual processing even though automated algorithms are commercially available, because it sometimes is necessary to manually correct errors produced by automated algorithms. This advice applies to software to reorient tomograms, correct for patient motion, form polar perfusion maps, and compute ejection fractions and related parameters from gated SPECT data.

## ACCEPTANCE TESTING

### Planar Gamma Camera Acceptance Tests

Before a gamma camera can be used for clinical procedures, it must undergo acceptance testing. This is the process whereby the purchaser evaluates newly delivered machinery to ascertain whether it performs according to the manufacturer's specifications and is ready for clinical use. If the machine is not installed properly in the first place, attempting to compensate tomograms via COR and uniformity corrections may prove futile (44). Details as to who will perform the acceptance testing, what it will consist of, criteria for acceptance, etc., must all be negotiated and established in writing prior to purchase of the machinery. We strongly recommend that the tests be conducted by an independent nuclear medicine physicist with experience in testing SPECT devices.

In the process of performing the acceptance tests, the user will become familiar with the properties and limitations of the new equipment before it is put into clinical service. Additionally, it is important to verify that the machinery purchased from the manufacturer really performs as well as the written specifications. The results of these tests provide the baseline for comparison during the coming years as the camera ages and as image quality inevitably worsens. By documenting the equipment's initial imaging characteristics, the extent of deterioration can be quantified. This will facilitate service personnel's understanding and remedying problems the machine will encounter in the future and in helping to decide the point at which it will be necessary to replace the camera. Additionally, information gathered during this process is useful in predicting which new imaging procedures developed after installation can be implemented successfully with the camera.

Acceptance testing begins with inspection of the state of equipment as it is unpacked and assembled. Components to be examined include the gantry, detector housing, multiformat cameras, consoles, computers, collimators, collimator delivery systems, and imaging tables. It is essential to verify immediately that the actual components contracted for have been delivered rather than other equipment. Multiple detector systems should have clearly marked indications as to which collimators correspond to which detectors. The installed gantry should be checked for smooth and reliable rotation of the detector assembly, and all hand controls, emergency stops, and safety features should be tested. The accuracy of light-emitting diode (LED) displays of angles, radius indicators, and clocks should be checked and compared to computer displays of these quantities. Careful scrutiny of the collimators and bare crystal should be undertaken. Intrinsic flood images well below (−20%) and above (+20%) the photopeak should be obtained, showing all of the phototubes, and displaying any abnormalities at the edge of the crystal indicative of the beginnings of hydroscopic damage due to a broken crystal seal. One means of identifying integrity of a collimator's metal foils and collimator hole alignment is by verifying that a point source placed 10 feet from the collimator produces a round shape uncontaminated by any linear features (45). Any damaged articles should be rejected. Also, if unusual procedures are to be attempted, such as the use of F-18 for a SPECT camera, it is necessary to assess prior to clinical use not only the ability of the camera's pulse height analyzers to accommodate these high energies, but also the suitability of any collimator anticipated for use with 511-keV gamma rays (46).

### Intrinsic Spatial Resolution

Electronic testing of SPECT cameras begins with the same procedures specific to ordinary planar gamma cameras, for which the NEMA standards should be followed (3). The device must function well as a planar gamma camera in order for it to be capable of operating properly as a SPECT system. Measurement of intrinsic spatial resolution can be determined with a phantom consisting of a set of 1-mm-wide parallel slits separated from one another by a 30-mm cut into a lead plate (referred to as the "NEMA slit phantom") positioned on or close to the camera's crystal, with an uncollimated $^{99m}$Tc point source producing 10 to 20 kcps as registered by the detector. The point source should be five UFOV diameters or more from the detector. Data are acquired with the usual 20% energy window into a $128^2$ matrix with a zoom factor of 4. Since this provides multiple samples of line spread functions over the entire diameter of the crystal, a single acquisition provides several data sets from which one can derive an accurate average line spread function via count profile generation, so long as each profile peak maximum contains more than 1,000 counts. FWHM values for the average count profile should be measured and recorded, and the data itself should be stored permanently on some suitable storage device.

For purposes of acceptance testing, intrinsic uniformity, sensitivity, and linearity can be measured using the procedures described above (see Camera Quality Control in Single Photon Emission Computed Tomography, above). Extrinsic spatial resolution should be determined during acceptance testing for each collimator, with and without scatter, and for each of the isotopes to be used clinically. The most efficient means of measurement is with a line source, although capillary tubes can be used alternatively.

software supplied by the manufac[...]
whether the delivered software is c[...]
correctly. It is important to verify[...]
and coronal sections are properly[...]
Plexiglas phantoms have been desi[...]
Discrepancies should be resolved[...]
should be tested, including perfu[...]
attenuation corrections, filters, all[...]
interest definition, curve generatic[...]
manual and automatic tomograph[...]

## Multidetector SPECT Sys[...]

For multidetector SPECT system[...]
testing procedures described abov[...]
should be performed for each dete[...]
relevant evaluation parameters (i[...]
intrinsic uniformity, intrinsic sen[...]
temporal resolution, extrinsic uni[...]
sitivity) should agree with one anc[...]
compared among all detector hea[...]
acquisitions, artifacts due to a[...]
nonuniformity, misalignment, inc[...]
energy setting create more con[...]
effects appearing predominantly i[...]
viewed by that detector (56). The[...]
detector separately and of the con[...]
all detectors is important.

### Multidetector Image Regis[...]

Correct registration of multiple d[...]
ated using the Plexiglas line sour[...]
whether the combination of da[...]
results in superior or inferior reso[...]
the individual heads. A full evalu[...]
rate tomographic acquisitions, the[...]
acquisition of the line source for[...]
tion. Data from each of the *N*[...]
structed individually and the *N* F[...]
of each detector's transverse rec[...]
described above (see Quarterly Lin[...]
tion Tests) for single detector SPE[...]
acquisition consists of combining[...]
of the line source acquired for 1/[...]
projection as compared to the[...]
FWHM value is obtained from a[...]
the combined data. Finally, data ar[...]
from all *N* detectors for an angular[...]
and the transverse FWHM value[...]
values from all acquisitions shoul[...]
to within 5%. Deviations greater[...]
that the detectors are not all registe[...]
radiating object in the image mat[...]
to the data being imposed by the[...]

### Intrinsic Energy Resolution

Intrinsic energy resolution can be assessed by acquiring a digitized energy spectrum containing at least 10,000 counts using an uncollimated 100-µCi $^{99m}$Tc point source in air. The point source should provide count rates of 10 to 20 kcps and be situated five UFOV diameters from the uncollimated detector. Each channel of the digitized spectrum should be 1 keV wide and the different energies at which counts are collected must at least range from 130 to 150 keV, but preferably from 0 to 200 keV. If possible, a spectrum using a different isotope such as $^{57}$Co should be stored separately, to verify the photopeak locations corresponding to each energy channel. A plot of counts acquired versus energy channel should be recorded, from which the FWHM of the spectrum may be estimated. The machine's intrinsic energy resolution may then be computed from this FWHM value for a 1-keV energy window used to make the measurements as:

$$(\text{Energy Resolution})^2 = \text{FWHM}^2 - (1 \text{ keV})^2$$

### Camera Count-Rate Characteristics

The NEMA standard that is preferred for measuring dead time uses a decaying source method. The two parameters that are measured and reported are the observed count rate that produces a 20% count loss and the maximum count rate. One means of measuring the maximum count rate of which the detector is capable is by using a $^{99m}$Tc source of sufficient activity (on the order of 5 mCi) to begin to paralyze the detector when close to the crystal. The source is brought toward the uncollimated detector until the point is reached such that moving the source toward or away from the detector results in a drop of the observed count rate. Maximum count rates on the order of 200 to 500 kcps may be expected, depending on the camera (47–49).

To measure the count rate corresponding to a 20% count loss, a source is placed in a lead pig, over top of which are placed 6 mm of copper plates. Sufficient $^{99m}$Tc radioactive source strength (50–200 mCi, depending on the camera) is added until it is obvious that the uncollimated detector is beginning to be paralyzed, by observing that the count rate not only does not rise, but actually declines, as more activity is added. This source is removed and the background count $N_{bkg}$ is measured for 10 minutes. The source is then returned to its position in front of the detector and counted for at least 100,000 counts, recording the initial counts $C1$, the initial time $t1$, and the initial time interval $\Delta t1$ of the measurement. Then subsequent measurements are taken every few hours, each time for 100,000 counts or 10 seconds, whichever is greater. The last collected data point, *n*, should be acquired when the observed count rate drops below 4,000 counts per second (cps). Usually, this will take 2 days to occur following the initial measurement. From these data, the observed count rate (OCR$_i$) for each data point is normalized as:

$$\text{OCR}_i = \frac{(C_i - N_{bkg} * \Delta t_i *) \ \ln(2)}{21672 * (1 - \exp(-\Delta t_i)/21672 * \ln(2)))}$$

where 21,762 seconds is the $^{99m}$Tc half-life. This formula scales each measurement to the beginning time for each data point *i*. From these values are computed the input count rates (ICRs) for each measurement, ICR$_i$, as:

$$\text{ICR}_i = \text{OCR}_n \cdot \exp((t_n - t_i)/21{,}762 \text{ sec} \cdot \ln(2))$$

for last data point, *n*, corresponding to the 4,000-cps rate. The observed count rate for 20% count loss then is seen to be that measurement, *i*, closest to the situation of

$$\text{OCR}_i = 0.8 \cdot \text{ICR}_i$$

A more realistic alternative is to use these sources inside a Plexiglas phantom, to simulate Compton scatter and backscatter. The measurements and calculations described above then are repeated in much the same fashion but with the use of the phantom.

The tests described above are time-consuming and therefore expensive. A more rapid but less accurate means of performing this measurement is with a series of many thin (e.g., 0.5 mm) copper plates (50,51). These are interposed between the uncollimated detector and a collimated 5 mCi $^{99m}$Tc source to attenuate the radiation, thereby providing carefully controlled variable count rate. With all plates in place, the count rate should be below 10 kcps. Then, as plates are removed, the count rate will appear to rise, plateau at saturation, then decline as the electronics become paralyzed. By plotting observed count rates versus the number of attenuating plates on semilog paper, and fitting the last few points to a straight line to compute true count rates, the deviation of observed counts from true counts can be measured, and the input count rate producing a 20% count loss can be estimated.

### Extrinsic Sensitivity

The NEMA standard of extrinsic sensitivity involves the use of a 10-cm-diameter flask or Petri dish with 20 mL of water and enough $^{99m}$Tc (about 1 mCi for a low-energy all-purpose collimator) to provide 10 kcps. The syringe used to convey the $^{99m}$Tc should be assayed before and after delivery of the radioactivity to the vessel and the times noted to enable decay correction of the activity. One-minute count rates of this source may then be used to determine extrinsic sensitivity for each collimator in terms of counts per minute per µCi.

Multiple energy window registration of a multiphotopeak radiation source can be important for some applications, including those involving simultaneous multiple isotope tomography. A collimated source is needed consisting of $^{67}$Ga in a lead pig with a 3-mm hole drilled through the bottom of it. The source is placed carefully at nine predetermined locations on an uncollimated detector, consisting

of the central point, four *x*-
locations. Point source ima
stored separately for at lea
exceeding 10 to 20 kcps, on
photopeaks, each with a 20
tional image should be acqui
with all three energy peaks ac
with energy should be noted
facturer's written specificatio
the specifications must be ad

In conjunction with hig
considerations, acceptance te
should include determination
This is particularly relevant fc
F-18 imaging with SPECT c
uated by placing an unshield
collimated detector, and me
received by the camera, ther
count rates with no sources p

In addition to these NEM
worthwhile in evaluating the
These include the acquisition
10-M counts) of different ene
$^{67}$Ga, $^{111}$In, $^{131}$I) and then usi
correct for all of the other ene
is to subtract one energy floc
sensitivity variations. The eff
flood to correct an extrinsic
investigated. Any systematic
any of these procedures shou
ufacturer.

Constancy with time of t
acquiring 5-M count $^{57}$Co e
period of several days during
then subtracting the initial
floods. The resulting "differ
nized for anomalies and parti
patterns with time. Following
it is advisable to subtract the
subsequent monthly floods to

## SPECT Camera Accep

A useful guide to acceptance
publication issued by the Ar
cists in Medicine (52). The
some of these same tests (3).
as a function of detector posi
using a $^{57}$Co sheet source tap
detector to accumulate 5-M
gantry angles 90 degrees apar
be computed for each flood,
then be used to correct those
The corrected images should
sensitivity variations. Recen

---

## REFERENCES

1. National Committee on Radiation Protection. *Safe handling of radioactive materials.* Recommendations of NCRP, Report 30. National Bureau of Standards Handbook 92, 1964.

2. Garcia EV, Nichols K, Galt J, et al. Instrumentation quality assurance and performance, In Imaging guidelines for nuclear cardiology procedures, part 1. *J Nucl Cardiol* 1996;3:G5–G10.

3. National Electrical Manufacturer's Association. *Performance measurements of scintillation cameras.* Standards publication no. NU1-1994. Washington DC: National Electrical Manufacturer's Association, 1994.

4. Sorensen JA, Phelps ME. *Physics in nuclear medicine.* New York: Grune and Straton, 1987.

5. Rogers WL, Clinthorne NH, Harkness BA, et al. Field-flood requirements for emission computed tomography with an Anger camera. *J Nucl Med* 1982;23:162–168.

6. Gulberg GT. An analytical approach to quantify uniformity artifacts for circular and noncircular detector motion in single photon emission computed tomography imaging. *Med Phys* 1987;14:105–114.

7. O'Connor MK, Vermeersch C. Critical examination of the uniformity requirements for single-photon emission computed tomography. *Med Phys* 1991;18:190–197.

8. Jaszczak R. *SPECT:* Basic considerations for quality control. Society of Nuclear Medicine video tape no. #5280, 1988.

9. Oppenheim BE, Appledorn CR. Uniformity correction for SPECT using a mapped cobalt-57 sheet source. *J Nucl Med* 1985;26:409.

10. Croft BA. *Single-photon emission computed tomography.* Chicago: Year Book Medical, 1986.

11. Blend MJ, Friedman M, O'Dowd T, et al. Improved flood source uniformity using chelation of In-111 in a liquid plexiglass tank. *J Nucl Med* 1996;37:211P.

12. Axelsson B, Israelsson A, Larsson S. Non-uniformity induced artifacts in single-photon emission computed tomography. *Acta Radiol Oncol* 1983;22:215.

13. English RJ, Polak JF, Holman BL. An iterative method for verifying systematic nonuniformities in refillable flood sources. *J Nucl Med Tech* 1984;12:7.

14. Greer KL, Jaszczak RJ, Coleman RE. An overview of a camera-based SPECT system. *Med Phys* 1982;9:455–463.

15. Ficaro EP, Harris AJ. A quality control protocol for transmission-emission tomographic systems. *J Nucl Med* 1997;38:214P.

16. Penney BC, Nagle SK. Quantifying center-of-rotation error using point source acquisitions. *J Nucl Med* 1997;38:219P.

17. Hendee, W. *Medical radiation physics.* Chicago: Year Book Medical, 1979.

18. Gullberg GT, Tung C-H, Zeng GL, et al. Simultaneous transmission and emission computed tomography using a three-detector SPECT system. *J Nucl Med* 1992;33:901P.

19. Tsui BMW, Frey EC, Lalush DS, et al. A fast sequential SPECT/TCT data acquisition method for accurate attenuation compensation in cardiac SPECT. *J Nucl Med* 1995;36:169P.

20. Stone CD, McCormick JW, Gilland DR, et al. Effect of registration errors between transmission and emission scans on a SPECT system using sequential scanning. *J Nucl Med* 1998;39:365–373.

21. DePuey EG, Garcia EV. Optimal specificity of thallium-201 SPECT through recognition of imaging artifacts. *J Nucl Med* 1989;30:441–449.

22. Todd-Pokropek AE, Erbsmann F, Soussaline F. The non-uniformity of imaging devices and its impact in quantitative studies. In: *Medical radionuclide imaging.* Vienna: International Atomic Energy Agency, 1977;1:67–84.

23. Todd-Pokropek AE, Jarritt PH. The noise characteristics of SPECT systems. In: Ell PJ, Holman BL, eds. *Computed emission tomography.* New York: Oxford University Press, 1982:361.

24. Shepp LA, Stein JA. Simulated reconstruction artifacts in computerized x-ray tomography. In: Ter-Pogossian MM, Phelps ME, Brownell GL, et al., eds. *Reconstruction tomography in diagnostic radiology and nuclear medicine.* Baltimore: University Park Press, 1977;33.

25. Todd-Pokropek A, Carlson RA. How to assess tomographic non-uniformity. *J Nucl Med* 1998;39:174P.

26. Farrell TJ, Cradduck TD, Chamberlain RA. The effect of collimators on the center of rotation in SPECT. *J Nucl Med* 1984;25:632–633.

27. Halama JR, Henkin RE. Quality assurance in SPECT imaging. *Appl Radiol* 1987;16(5):41–50.

28. Yang C-K, Orphanoudakis SC, Strohbehn JW, et al. A simulation study of motion artifacts in computed tomography. *Phys Med Biol* 1982;27:51–61.

29. Eisner RL, Noever T, Nowak D, et al. Use of cross-correlation to detect patient motion during SPECT imaging. *J Nucl Med* 1987;28:97–101.

30. Friedman J, Berman DS, Van Train K, et al. Patient motion in thallium-201 myocardial SPECT imaging: an easily identified frequent source of artifactual defect. *Clin Nucl Med* 1988;13:321–324.

31. Friedman J, Van Train K, Maddahi J, et al. "Upward creep" of the heart: a frequent source of false-positive reversible defects during thallium-201 stress-redistribution SPECT. *J Nucl Med* 1989;30:1718–1722.

32. Eisner R, Churchwell A, Never T, et al. Quantitative analysis of the tomographic thallium-201 myocardial bull's-eye display: critical role of correcting for patient motion. *J Nucl Med* 1988;29:91–97.

33. Cooper JA, Neumann PH, McCandless BK. Effect of patient motion on tomographic myocardial perfusion imaging. *J Nucl Med* 1992;33:1566–1571.

34. Eisner RL. Sensitivity of SPECT thallium-201 myocardial perfusion imaging to patient motion. *J Nucl Med* 1992;33:1571–1573.

35. Matsunari I, Boning G, Ziegler SI. Effects of misalignment between transmission and emission scans on attenuation-corrected cardiac SPECT. *J Nucl Med* 1998;39:411–416.

36. Surova-Trojanova H, Barker C, Carrasquillo JA, et al. Influence of improper attenuation/emission registration on the accuracy of SPECT tumor imaging. *J Nucl Med* 1996;37:211P.

37. Geckle WJ, Frank TL, Links JM, et al. Correction for patient motion and organ movement in SPECT: application to exercise thallium-201 cardiac imaging. *J Nucl Med* 1988;29:441–450.

38. Cooper JA, Neumann PH. Visual detection of patient motion during tomographic myocardial perfusion imaging. *Radiology* 1992;185:283.

39. Oppenheim BE, Appledorn CR. Single photon emission computed tomography. In: Gelfand MJ, Thomas SR, eds. *Effective use of computers in nuclear medicine.* New York: McGraw-Hill, 1988:31–74.

40. White MP, Mann A, Saari MA. Gated SPECT imaging 101. *J Nucl Cardiol* 1998;5:523–526.

41. Cullom SJ, Case JA, Bateman TM. Electrocardiographically gated myocardial perfusion SPECT: technical principles and quality control considerations. *J Nucl Cardiol* 1998;5:418–425.

42. Nichols K, Dorbala S, DePuey EG, et al. Influence of arrhythmias on gated SPECT myocardial perfusion and function quantification. *J Nucl Med (in press).*

43. Weiss AT, Berman DS, Lew AS, et al. Transient ischemic dilation of the left ventricle on stress thallium-201 scintigraphy: a marker of severe and extensive coronary artery disease. *J Am Coll Cardiol* 1987;9(4):752.

44. Halama JR, Madsden MT. Is your camera-SPECT system installed and operating optimally? *Appl Radiol* 1992;June:35–41.

45. Malmin RE, Stanley PC, Guth WR. Collimator angulation error and its effect on SPECT. *J Nucl Med* 1990;31:655–659.

46. Laymon CM, Turkington TG, Coleman RE. Effects of collimator septal penetration on 511 keV SPECT images. *J Nucl Med* 1997;38:220P.

47. Lewellen TK, Bice AN, Pollard KR, et al. Evaluation of a clinical scintillation camera with pulse tail extrapolation electronics. *J Nucl Med* 1989;30:1554–1558.

48. Nichols K, DePuey EG, Gooneratne N, et al. First pass ventricular ejection fraction using a single crystal nuclear camera. *J Nucl Med* 1994;35:1292–1300.

49. Plymouth meeting: ECRI, 1996. *Medical Electronic and Equipment News* 1996;36(6).

50. Geldenhuys EM, Lotter MG, Minnaur PC. A new approach to NEMA scintillation camera count rate curve determination. *J Nucl Med* 1988;29:538–541.

51. Breen SL, Cradduck TD. Spectral changes affect intrinsic count rate tests. *J Nucl Med* 1990;31:2074–2075.

52. AAPM SPECT Task Group. *Rotating scintillation camera SPECT acceptance testing and quality control.* AAPM report no. 22. American Institute of Physics (American Association of Physicists in Medicine), 1987.

53. Jahangir SM, Brill AB, Bizais YJC, et al. Count-rate variations with orientation of gamma detector. *J Nucl Med* 1983;24:356.

54. Smith EM, Hopkin K, Chengazi V. SPECT/Coincidence/PET imaging performance (SCIP) phantom—a new SPECT performance phantom. *J Nucl Med* 1998;39:174P.

55. Fahey FA, Harkness BA. Quality control program for a multiheaded, dedicated SPECT camera. *J Nucl Med* 1991;32:1136.

56. Barnes WE, Friedman NC, Shirazi P. Image artifacts in SPECT studies acquired with multiheaded gamma cameras. *J Nucl Med* 1997;38:217P.

57. Areeda J, Chapman D, Van Train K, et al. Methods for characterizing and monitoring rotational gamma camera system performance. In: Esser PD, ed. *Emission computed tomography:* current trends. New York: Society of Nuclear Medicine, 1983:81–90.

58. Graham LS. A rational quality assurance program for SPECT instrumentation. In: Freeman LM, Weissman HS, eds. *Nuclear medicine annual.* New York: Raven Press, 1989:81–108.

59. Harkness BA, Rogers WL, Clithorne NH, et al. SPECT: Quality control procedures and artifact identification. *J Nucl Med Tech* 1983;11:55–60.

60. Greer KL, Coleman RE, Jaszczak RJ. SPECT: a practical guide for users. *J Nucl Med Tech* 1983;11:61–65.

61. Tuscan MJ, Rogers WL, Juni JE, et al. Analysis of gamma camera detector stability and its effect on uniformity correction for SPECT. *J Nucl Med Tech* 1985;13:1–4.

62. Murphy PH. Acceptance testing and quality control of gamma cameras, including SPECT. *J Nucl Med* 1987;28:1221–1227.

63. Graham LS. Acceptance testing of gamma cameras. *J Nucl Med* 1988;29:267.

64. English RJ, Zimmerman RE. Performance and acceptance testing of scintillation cameras for SPECT. *J Nucl Med Tech* 1988;16:132–140.

65. Todd-Pokropek A, Cradduck T. *SPECT quality control—the optimized SPECT system.* Society of Nuclear Medicine slide presentation CEL 164.

66. Graham LS, Erickson J. *Acceptance testing of imaging equipment:* SPECT systems and the scintillation camera. Society of Nuclear Medicine slide presentation CEL 166.

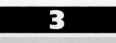

# QUANTITATIVE ANALYSIS OF
# SPECT MYOCARDIAL PERFUSION

**KENNETH F. VAN TRAIN**
**ERNEST V. GARCIA**
**C. DAVID COOKE**
**JOSEPH S. AREEDA**

Quantitative analysis of single photon emission computed tomography (SPECT) myocardial perfusion imaging has undergone moderate changes since the first edition of this book was published. In this edition, the first two sections of this chapter, which are concerned with methods for quantitatively analyzing thallium 201 ($^{201}$Tl) SPECT images, have been condensed. These sections were retained because they offer a historical perspective on the development of the various quantitative techniques and represent the technical foundation on which current methods have been developed. The last section, involving the current quantitative techniques, has been updated to reflect the most recent developments in this area.

Assessment of cardiac performance is markedly enhanced by a quantitative description of the specific physiologic parameters evaluated by scintigraphic images. Quantification enables objective interpersonal comparison and objective assessment of cardiac status in a single patient over time or as a result of intervention. Furthermore, computer algorithms that enhance the images, extract parameters of cardiac performance, and define criteria for normality and abnormality have the potential to be precisely described. These algorithms can then be widely disseminated to promote standardization of image interpretation. More importantly, these algorithms can stand as a foundation from which specific criticisms can be assessed and into which improvements can be readily incorporated.

Cardiovascular nuclear medicine techniques are inherently quantitative. This is because the pixel count value from within a cardiac region is related to some parameter of cardiac performance. In the case of planar equilibrium blood pool studies, in which the radionuclide concentration is assumed to be constant, the pixel count value from a region within the heart is related to chamber volume. In the case of myocardial perfusion imaging, in which the volume is assumed to be constant, the pixel count value from a region is related to the concentration of the radionuclide and thus blood flow. Two standard types of quantification may be applied: absolute quantification, which is the ability to extract from a pixel the number of counts expected from a given radionuclide concentration at the source location, and the true relative quantification, which is the ability to extract from two pixels the ratio of counts expected from a given ratio for radionuclide concentrations at two source locations.

Currently, a clinically accepted method has not been developed for obtaining absolute or true relative quantitative values from the tomographic SPECT data. Therefore, at the present time, the most widely used approaches have used data-based methods of quantification that emulate the physician's method of image interpretation. The concept of data-based quantification involves three major steps: (a) image processing to enhance the image, (b) image analysis to extract pertinent measurements for use in determining abnormality versus normality, and (c) comparison of extracted measurements to a database of results from normal patients to quantify the degree of abnormality. This chapter describes the details of data-based quantification as it applies to myocardial perfusion imaging, and reviews digital image processing techniques developed for quantifying the distribution of myocardial perfusion obtained by SPECT. Many of the techniques illustrated reflect computer methods developed either at Cedars-Sinai Medical Center or Emory University.

## THALLIUM 201 QUANTITATIVE ANALYSIS

Sequential thallium 201 ($^{201}$Tl) scintigraphy is a useful noninvasive method for detecting and evaluating patients with

K. F. Van Train, J. S. Areeda: Department of Nuclear Medicine, Cedars-Sinai Medical Center, Los Angeles, California 90048.
E. V. Garcia, C. D. Cooke: Department of Nuclear Medicine, Emory University School of Medicine, Atlanta, Georgia 30322.

significant coronary artery disease (CAD). Visual interpretation of analog [201]Tl images, even by experienced observers, is subject to substantial variability (1). This approach is further limited by dependence on the quality of the hard-copy output and inability to accurately compensate for background activity or attenuation. Finally, although the regional myocardial washout characteristics of [201]Tl provide important diagnostic information, washout can be difficult to detect by visual inspection.

Several approaches have provided significant contributions to quantitation of the initial distribution and washout of myocardial [201]Tl both from planar (2–5) and tomographic (6–9) scintigraphic projections. This section discusses the steps involved in the quantitation of tomographic stress-redistribution studies with [201]Tl.

Investigations in mid-1985 suggested that rotational myocardial tomography following injection of [201]Tl at peak exercise offered significant improvement over planar scintigraphy for the detection and localization of myocardial ischemia (10,11). Rotational [201]Tl tomography at rest was also reported to be better than planar imaging for the detection and localization of myocardial infarction and for estimating the extent of infarcted myocardium (12,13). Subsequently, several investigators (6,7,14) used extensions of the planar quantitation concept to quantify, from rotational tomograms, the three-dimensional (3D) distribution of myocardial [201]Tl at stress and with its redistribution. These algorithms express the percentage of the myocardium that is involved with perfusion defect, washout abnormality, and/or reversible abnormality.

## Cedars-Sinai Method

Cedars-Sinai Medical Center initially developed a method for quantitatively analyzing the exercise perfusion and washout of [201]Tl from planar myocardial scintigrams (2,15,16). In the 1980s, SPECT became a clinically viable imaging technique and was found to offer greater contrast resolution and 3D information, resulting in better detection and localization capabilities than the planar method (11,17,18). To take full advantage of the improvements offered by the SPECT technique, a comprehensive method was developed that quantifies the 3D distribution of myocardial perfusion following exercise scanning with [201]Tl (6,19,20).

The Cedars-Sinai quantitative approach to SPECT is based on sampling the patient's short- and vertical long-axis myocardial tomograms using maximum count circumferential profiles, and comparing these patient profiles to profiles derived from a database of normal patients. Patient profile points that fall below the normal limits and meet a criterion for abnormality are considered abnormal. The quantitative output of the program includes a polar-map display designating the areas of abnormality, and a report indicating the percentage of abnormal pixels within the total and individual vascular territories. Quantitative methods that involve comparison to a normal database require strict adherence to specific acquisition and processing protocols. The following protocols were developed in 1984 for the Cedars-Sinai quantitative [201]Tl approach.

## Technical Aspects

### Patient Protocol

#### Exercise Protocol

Patients are asked to discontinue beta-blocking medication for 24 to 48 hours prior to the study and long-acting nitrates for 4 hours before the study. Exercise is performed using a standard graded treadmill test (Bruce protocol). Exercise is symptom limited (moderately severe anginal pain, severe dyspnea or severe fatigue), unless one of the following criteria for termination of exercise developed: 4-mm ST segment depression, malignant arrhythmia, or exercise hypotension (greater than 10 mm Hg drop between exercise stages). If the patient has left ventricular hypertrophy (LVH), left bundle-branch block (LBBB), or is taking digoxin, the ST segment response (>4 mm) does not constitute reason for termination. If <85% of the patient's maximal predicted heart rate is achieved, the study is considered submaximal. Exercise is continued for at least 1 minute after injection, and imaging begun 30 minutes after exercise.

At near peak exercise, a dose of 3 to 4 mCi of [201]Tl is injected, and exercise continued for another minute. The amount of [201]Tl injected is adjusted according to the patient's weight with an average of 3.0 mCi administered to a 70-kg patient. Patients are imaged in the supine position, using a rotating tomographic unit, approximately 10 to 15 minutes and 2 to 5 hours after the injection of thallium. The delay of 10 to 15 minutes is employed to reduce the possibility of heart movement or "upward creep," which is related to diaphragmatic relaxation following exercise (21). It is recommended during this delay period that a 5-minute planar anterior-view image be acquired and utilized for the analysis of lung uptake of [201]Tl (22–24), transient ischemic dilatation of the left ventricle (25), and breast attenuation. Thirty or 32 projections (40 seconds/projection) are obtained over a semicircular 180-degree orbit from a 45-degree right anterior oblique (RAO) to a 45-degree left posterior oblique (LPO) position. The scintillation cameras are equipped with a low-energy, all-purpose, parallel-hole collimator. A 20% energy window centered on the 70-keV x-ray peak, and a second 10% energy window centered on the 167-keV x-ray peak of [201]Tl are employed. All projection images are stored on magnetic disks, using a $64 \times 64$-pixel, 16-bit matrix.

### Acquisition and Processing Protocols

Each of the projections is corrected for nonuniformity with a flood source containing $30 \times 10^6$ counts, and the mechan-

## TABLE 3.1. QUANTITATIVE ²⁰¹TL STRESS AND REST PROCESSING PROTOCOL

| Computer | Prefilter | Transaxial Filter | Cutoff (CO)[a] | Order |
|----------|-----------|-------------------|----------------|-------|
| ADAC | No | Yes | 0.15 | 5 |
| Elscint | No | Yes | 0.15 | 5 |
| MDS | 9 pt | No | 0.20 | 5 |
| Medasys | No | Yes | 0.20 | 5 |
| Picker | 0.20 CO | No | Ramp | — |
| Siemens | No | Yes | 0.20 | 5 |
| Sophy | 0.15 CO | Yes | Ramp | — |
| Summit | 0.20 CO | No | Ramp | — |
| Toshiba | 9 pt | No | 0.20 | 5 |

[a]Two-dimensional Butterworth filter.
9 pt (3 x 3 matrix c̄ 4*2*1 weights).

ical center of rotation is determined in order to align the projection data with respect to the reconstruction matrix. Filtering of the data in depth is accomplished using one of two methods. Either the raw data are filtered prior to reconstruction, by applying a nine-point weighted (4-2-1) smoothing algorithm, or the reconstructed transaxial tomograms are filtered using a 1-2-1 filter across slices. Filtered backprojection is then performed using the optimum filter determined for each of the computers. The filters employed for the various computer systems are listed in Table 3.1. Transaxial tomograms are reconstructed encompassing the entire heart. Short-axis, and vertical and horizontal long-axis tomograms are extracted from the filtered transaxial tomograms by performing a coordinate transformation with interpolation (26). All tomograms are reconstructed at a thickness of one pixel per slice, representing 6.4 ± 0.2 mm. Attenuation and scatter correction are not applied to the reconstructed tomograms.

### Selection of Processing Parameters

The operator-interactive steps on the various computers have been developed to comply with a specific processing protocol, and the quantitative outputs are all standardized. In this approach by Cedars, the quantitative method required three operator-interactive steps: tomogram selection, cavity center selection, and profile alignment. These steps have been completely automated in more recent approaches (27).

#### Tomogram Selection

The short-axis tomograms selected are those extending from the subendocardial portion of the apex to the base of the heart. In a normal study, the last basal short-axis slice selected should contain uniform activity around the entire myocardium. The vertical long-axis tomograms selected are those extending from the subendocardial portion of the septum to the subendocardial portion of the lateral wall.

#### Cavity-Center Selection and Radius of Search

For center selection, a cursor is positioned as close as possible to the center of the entire myocardial mass for both the short- and vertical long-axis tomograms. The radius of search is defined by extending the horizontal and vertical lines of the cursor from the center to the outside of the epicardium. The center coordinate will be used as a reference point for sampling the myocardium and generation of the maximum-count circumferential profiles.

#### Profile Alignment

To account for differences in patient heart orientation and potentially offer improved localization of coronary artery disease, a method is implemented for alignment of the profiles. The short-axis profiles are aligned by placing a cursor at the inferior junction of the right with the left ventricle. The current profile angle is calculated from the cursor location, and the profile is shifted, so that it corresponds to the 102-degree angle. The long-axis profiles are aligned by positioning the cursor at the location of the apex, and its profiles will be shifted to the 90-degree angle.

### Myocardial Sampling

Following selection of the processing parameters, the myocardium is sampled by generating maximum-count circumferential profiles for each of the selected short- and vertical long-axis tomograms. Each point in these profiles represents the maximum counts per pixel along a radius extending from the center of the left ventricle to the limit of the radius of search. The profile is constructed by the computer from the values of 60 radii spaced at 6-degree intervals plotted clockwise (Fig. 3.1). Each set of stress and delayed profiles is normalized, so that the maximum pixel value in each slice is set to 100. Since the processing parameters are selected only with the center slice, an important

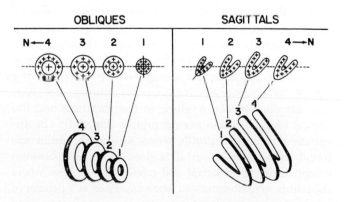

**FIGURE 3.1.** Maximum-count circumferential profiles are generated for each of the short-axis (oblique) and vertical long-axis (sagittal) tomograms. Each profile consists of 60 points and is normalized to 100%.

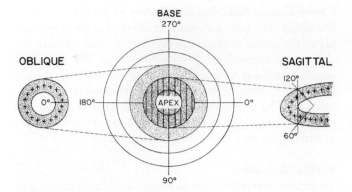

**FIGURE 3.2.** Diagram representing the method for plotting the vertical long-axis (sagittal) profile data and short-axis (oblique) profile data onto the two-dimensional polar maps. (From Garcia EV, Van Train K, Maddahi J, et al. Quantification of rotational thallium-201 myocardial tomography. *J Nucl Med* 1985;26:17–26, with permission.)

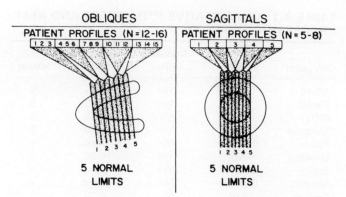

**FIGURE 3.3.** Method for assignment of patient short-axis (oblique) and vertical long-axis (sagittal) profiles to the five short- *(left)* and five vertical long-axis *(right)* anatomic normal limits. This example demonstrates the comparison of 15 short-axis and five long-axis tomographic images from a patient scan. (From Garcia EV, Van Train K, Maddahi J, et al. Quantification of rotational thallium-201 myocardial tomography. *J Nucl Med* 1985;26:17–26, with permission.)

quality control step is to review the processed tomograms and confirm that the maximum-count pixels selected are all located within the myocardium. The count profiles from all of the analyzed short-axis tomograms and the apical portion of the long-axis tomograms are plotted onto a two-dimensional polar map representing the left ventricular myocardium (Fig. 3.2). Because the size of the polar map always remains the same, the size of the left heart is reflected by the number of maximum-count circumferential profiles that are mapped. Thus, in larger hearts, the band representing each slice is thinner relative to that in smaller hearts.

### Gender-Matched Normal Limits

The gender-matched normal limits are derived from 35 patients (20 male and 15 female, age range 30 to 66 years) with a <5% likelihood of having coronary artery disease (low likelihood) based on bayesian analysis of their age, sex, symptoms, and the results of the exercise electrocardiogram (ECG) (28–30). To account for variations in left ventricular size, the ventricle was divided into five regions of equal thickness representing the volume displayed by the short-axis tomograms and five regions of equal thickness representing the volume displayed by the apex, which is derived from the vertical long-axis tomograms. In each of the five regions, representative circumferential profiles were averaged for the patients, resulting in five short-axis and five vertical long-axis mean normal profiles (Fig. 3.3). The distribution of normal profile points around the mean was found to be gaussian in all regions of the myocardium except in the anterolateral and inferoseptal regions, where the points were nongaussian when expressed as a percent of maximal counts. Therefore, among various approaches investigated for the definition of normal-limit profiles, it was determined that constructing profiles by connecting the lowest observed value from the individual normal

patient profiles (range approach) was the optimum method for developing normal-limit profiles (19).

It has been demonstrated that the normal myocardial distribution of $^{201}$Tl in males is different from that in females, most likely due to differing attenuation patterns (31,32). In both genders, the $^{201}$Tl activity is more attenuated in the basal, inferior, and septal regions of the left ventricle. However, in females, additional attenuation of anterolateral wall activity by breast tissue results in a more uniform apparent myocardial distribution of $^{201}$Tl. For these reasons, two separate gender-specific (male and female) normal databases were developed for reference.

### Localization

In addition to detecting CAD, the program localizes disease in individual coronary arteries. This was accomplished through the definition of coronary boundary territories on the quantitative polar maps. These boundaries were derived by examining the defect polar maps of 44 patients with angiographically confirmed coronary artery disease (19,33). This analysis divided the polar maps into multiple segments and determined the segments that had an 80% or greater probability of being affected by a diseased left anterior descending (LAD), left circumflex (LCX), or right coronary artery (RCA). The segments affected by each artery were then grouped to define the vascular territories boundaries (Fig. 3.4). Between each of the boundaries were border zones that represented segments with a less than an 80% probability of being associated with any of the three coronary arteries. Estimates of the extent of a defect (percentage of abnormal pixels) are calculated for the individual coronary territories and for the total territory, which includes any defects located in the border zones.

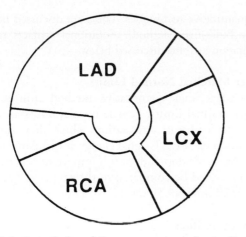

**FIGURE 3.4.** Boundaries of the coronary vascular territories on the quantitative polar map. (From Maddahi J, Van Train KF, Prigent F, et al. Quantitative single photon emission computerized thallium-201 tomography for the evaluation of coronary artery disease: optimization and prospective validation of a new technique. *J Am Coll Cardiol* 1989;14:1689–1699, with permission.)

## Development of Criteria for Disease Detection

This analysis determined the minimum extent of abnormality required for a coronary territory to be called abnormal using this quantitative approach. Using receiver operating characteristics (ROC) curve analysis, various criteria of percent abnormality were assessed to determine those that provided the optimum trade-off in true-positive versus true-negative rates for identifying disease in each of the three coronary vascular territories. The optimum threshold was determined to be 12% for the LAD and LCX, and 8% for the RCA.

## Analysis and Polar Map Display

### Stress Defect Extent and Severity

The patient's stress and rest profiles are compared to the proper gender-matched normal-limit profiles, and the points falling below the limit are considered abnormal. The final display comprises four polar maps, two relative-count maps, and two extent-of-defect maps (Fig. 3.5). The two relative-count maps demonstrate the distribution of counts within the myocardium for both stress and delayed studies. The extent-of-defect maps indicate the location and extent of the patient's abnormal territory for the stress and delayed distribution studies. To derive an indication of the severity of disease, the extent maps are divided into four separate categories (displayed as either four colors or shades of gray). There are two normal categories: normal (>10% above the normal limit) and equivocal (≤10% above the normal limit), and two abnormal categories: abnormal (≤20% below the normal limit) and severely abnormal (>20% below the normal limit). These categories were based on a correlation with the Cedars-Sinai visual interpretation scores of 0, 1, 2, and 3 corresponding to normal, equivocal, abnormal, and severely abnormal in a pilot population.

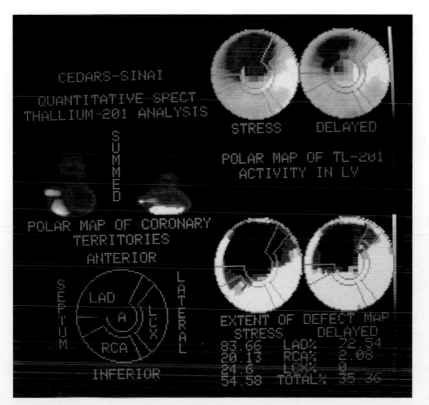

**FIGURE 3.5.** Quantitative thallium 201 ($^{201}$Tl) stress/rest single photon emission computed tomography (SPECT) results from a patient with a prior myocardial infarction. The *lower left* graphic indicates the boundaries defining the coronary artery perfusion on the polar map. The *upper right* graphic demonstrates the relative-count polar maps for stress and rest tomograms. The polar maps in the *lower right* graphic indicate the quantitative results after comparison of the patient's study with the normal limits. The quantitative results indicate anterior and apical stress defects with slight improvement on the rest polar map in this patient, who had single-vessel disease of the proximal left anterior descending coronary artery documented by coronary angiography.

## Validation

The accuracy of the Cedars-Sinai quantitative $^{201}$Tl program was initially established in 138 patients who either underwent coronary arteriography ($n = 110$) or were low likelihood normals ($n = 28$) from Cedars-Sinai (19). This evaluation demonstrated an overall sensitivity, specificity, and low likelihood normalcy rate of 95% (87/92), 56% (10/18) and 86% (24/28), respectively. For patients undergoing coronary arteriography, the sensitivity for localization of disease in the LAD, LCX, and RCA was 78% (60/77), 79% (49/62), and 82% (56/68), respectively, and the specificity was 85% (28/33), 60% (29/48), and 71% (30/42), respectively.

To assess the broad applicability of the program, it was subjected to a larger multicenter trial evaluation (20). This validation involved ten hospitals contributing 318 patients (242 with CAD, based on coronary angiography, having an age range of 24 to 80, and 76 with a low likelihood of CAD, age range 20 to 75). This evaluation demonstrated an overall sensitivity, specificity, and low likelihood normalcy rate of 94% (184/196), 43% (20/46), and 82% (62/76), respectively. For localization of disease in the patients undergoing coronary arteriography, the sensitivity for the LAD, LCX, and RCA was 78% (115/148), 68% (66/97), and 84% (118/141), and the respective specificity was 63% (59/94), 68% (98/145), and 62% (63/101) respectively.

## Artifacts

Myocardial SPECT $^{201}$Tl imaging is potentially a superior method to the planar imaging technique for the detection and localization of CAD. However, the successful implementation of the SPECT technique requires a higher level of technical expertise from both the physician and technologist. Failure to develop and apply this technical expertise will result in the generation of inferior tomographic images, ultimately increasing the number of equivocal, false-positive, and/or false-negative studies.

The quantitative analysis of images containing artifacts generated during either acquisition or reconstruction will tend to correlate with the visual interpretation. In some cases, these artifacts are difficult to identify through quality control at the time of their interpretation, so it is imperative that the technologist apply proper quality control during both the acquisition and processing phase of SPECT imaging. Some of the artifacts occurring during acquisition can be the result of improper peaking, uniformity correction, center-of-rotation (COR) correction, patient motion, and detector alignment. Reconstruction artifacts can be related to improper alignment for oblique angle reconstruction, improper application of filters, and improper orientation. A more in-depth discussion of SPECT acquisition and processing quality control can be found in Chapters 1 and 2, and a discussion of SPECT imaging artifacts can be found in Chapter 12. There are also artifacts related specifically to polar maps or "bull's-

eye" quantitative techniques. These are discussed below (see Emory Bull's-Eye Method). Additional artifacts related to quantitation are also discussed below.

### Gender-Matched Normal Limits

This Cedars-Sinai quantitative method utilizes gender-matched normal limits. Female normal limits are required to account for breast attenuation, which alters the normal distribution of SPECT signal energy as compared to that in the normal male population. It is important that the patient being processed be compared to the proper gender normal limit, or an improper quantitative analysis will result.

### Hot-Spot Artifact

An unsolved difficulty in quantitation of the tomographic studies in cardiac SPECT is in the existence of a "hot spot" in the lateral wall. The cause of this hot spot is unclear but may be related to the normal regional increase in $^{201}$Tl activity due to papillary muscles (34) or to the higher observed counts caused by the weaker attenuation of activity in the lateral myocardial wall of the left ventricle. Since this hot spot also exists in the normal limits, a shift of the hot spot from its usual location at the 2 to 3 o'clock position in a patient's tomogram may produce a false-positive quantitative result in the lateral wall of the patient's study.

## Emory Bull's-Eye Method

### Technical Aspects

#### Patient Protocol

In the original approach implemented at Emory University for the quantification of cardiac SPECT scan findings (7), patients were exercised on the treadmill using a standard Bruce protocol just as described above for the Cedars-Sinai approach. A thallium dose of 3.5 mCi was injected at peak stress. Stress imaging was initiated 7 to 10 minutes after injection or after the patient's breathing returned to normal, to avoid cardiac creep (21). Delayed SPECT was also performed approximately 4 hours after injection. These imaging sequences were the ones used to develop normal data files and criteria for abnormality, and to document the accuracy of the technique. Patients who showed fixed stress perfusion defects by 4 hours were often imaged to evaluate the late reversibility of these defects (35).

Subsequently, the patient protocol was modified to account for the perceived need for reinjection before delayed/resting imaging, as has been suggested (36,37) to make sure there is some $^{201}$Tl in the blood pool during redistribution. In this modified protocol, patients with a chest circumference of less than 44 inches are injected with 3 mCi $^{201}$Tl at stress. The patient is then brought back 3 hours later and reinjected with a 1.5-mCi dose. Importantly, resting/delayed imaging is then started at least a half-hour after this reinjection in order for the thallium to redistribute in regions with resting ischemia. Rare patients with a chest circumference greater than 44 inches are given a 4-mCi stress dose and a 2-mCi reinjection.

## Acquisition and Processing Protocols

The acquisition protocol consists of obtaining 32 projections for 40 seconds each over the 180-degree arc extending from the 45-degree RAO to the 45-degree LAO projection. Each of the 32 projections are corrected for field nonuniformity and for misalignment of the mechanical COR with respect to the reconstruction matrix. The processing protocol for general electric consists of prefiltering each projection prior to backprojection, using a Hanning filter with a cutoff frequency of 0.82 cycles/cm. Filtered backprojection is then performed to reconstruct the transverse axial tomograms (of 6.4 mm each) encompassing the entire heart. Oblique tomograms parallel to the vertical and horizontal long axis and the short axis of the left ventricle are extracted from the filtered transaxial tomograms by performing a coordinate transformation with appropriate interpolation (26). The tomograms are reconstructed without scatter or attenuation correction. These effects are in part compensated by comparison of each patient's thallium distribution to distribution files of normal patients exhibiting similar effects.

## Selection of Processing Parameters

In the Emory bull's-eye approach, only the short-axis slices are used for quantification. The short-axis slices to be quantified are selected by an operator following a strict protocol. Using the long-axis slice with the largest cavity length, the operator selects the short-axis cuts for quantification to extend from the base of the left ventricle (LV) to the apical cap. These selections are made by simultaneously viewing apical and basal cursors superimposed on the long-axis slice and the corresponding short-axis slices as determined from those cursors. Ideally, the selected short-axis apical slice contains the pixel with count reading that matches the maximum counts seen in the apex of the vertical long-axis slice. If the apical short-axis slice appears as a ring, the selection has been made too far into the heart and needs to be moved distally. With ideal selection, the short-axis basal slice appears as a backward "c" (or a crescent) in which the reduction in activity at the septum is due to the reduced myocardium at the valve plane.

On the short-axis slice, falling halfway between the apex and base, the operator then defines the center of the LV cavity and the maximum radius of search (Fig. 3.6, panel 1). Since these same parameters will be used for all slices, it is important that the correct axis of the heart has been

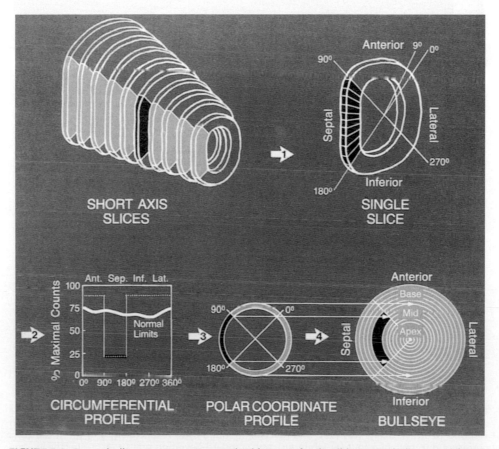

**FIGURE 3.6.** Emory bull's-eye construction method (see text for details). *Arrows* indicate panel number, and each panel is a processing step. (Used by permission of General Electric, Milwaukee, WI.)

selected, in order for these parameters to hold true not only for the most central slice but also for all short-axis slices.

## Myocardial Sampling

The maximal-count circumferential profiles (CPs) for each short-axis slice are then generated automatically from the most apical to the most basal cut, as shown in Fig. 3.6, panel 2.

The actual raw counts are extracted and used without normalization. This procedure is performed for each stress and each delayed tomographic study. Percent washout CPs are also calculated, using the profiles of the corresponding anatomic cut at stress and delayed tomography, respectively.

In Fig. 3.6 (top left panel) alternating short-axis slices of the left ventricle are displayed from base to apex. Approximately 12 slices are obtained from a normal-sized heart. In this example, there is a defect in the septum, which is high-

lighted in the middle slice. In Fig. 3.6, panel 1, this slice has been divided into 40 sectors of 9 degrees each. The septum is represented by the sectors from 90 to 180 degrees. The maximal counts per pixel (mcp) within each sector are determined. In panel 2, these 40 values have been plotted as a maximal-count circumferential profile of the maximal counts per pixel versus angular location. A similar profile is constructed for each slice except for the first two containing the apex, which are represented by a single value representing the mcp within the entire slice. To take into account variations in the number of slices per study, these curves are interpolated to produce a total of 15 profiles. Each of the rectangular-coordinate profiles is translated into a polar coordinate profile (panel 3), which displays the curve as a circle composed of 40 pixels. In panel 4, these data are displayed as a polar map called a bull's-eye plot, which consists of a series of 15 concentric circles with the apex at the cen-

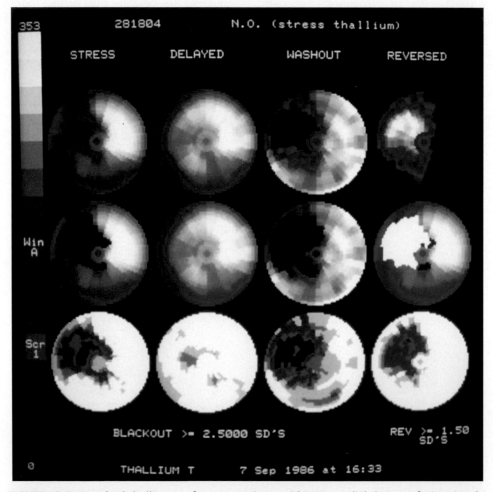

**FIGURE 3.7.** Standard bull's-eyes from a patient with myocardial hypoperfusion in the anteroseptal wall, with marked redistribution and slow washout of tracer. The four columns correspond to stress, delay, washout, and reversibility bull's-eyes, respectively, and the three rows correspond to raw, blackout (or whiteout), and standard-deviation bull's-eyes, respectively.

ter and the base at the periphery. Individual bull's-eyes are constructed for the stress and delayed images as well as for percent washout. Standard bull's-eyes from a patient with myocardial hypoperfusion in the anteroseptal wall, with marked redistribution and slow washout are shown in Fig. 3.7. In this display format, the stress and delay bull's-eyes have been adjusted by multiplying each pixel in the delayed bull's-eye by the ratio of the mcp in the stress bull's-eye to the mcp in the delay bull's-eye.

## Normalization

In the Emory bull's-eye method, normalization occurred only when the profiles were compared with the gender-matched normal files developed from the low probability-of-disease group, in which the mean values and standard deviations (SD) were established from the pooled data for each of the angular locations in each of the 15 profiles (38). This was accomplished by dividing each bull's-eye into four regions of 90 degrees each (anterior, septal, inferior, and lateral), from profiles 4 through 12, and determining the ratio of the average counts per pixel in each region of the patient's bull's-eye to the counts in the same region in the appropriate normal file. The region with the highest ratio was assumed to be normal, and each pixel in the patient's bull's-eye was multiplied by the reciprocal of this ratio before comparison to the normal file.

## Gender-Matched Normal Limits

The commercially released version of the Emory bull's-eye quantification program (on General Electric systems) has a database composed of 36 subjects ranging in age from 27 to 69 years. There were 20 men (mean age 41 years) and 16 women (mean age 39 years). These subjects were determined to have <5% likelihood of having CAD as estimated by bayesian analysis of age, sex, symptom classification,

coronary risk factors, and the results of an ECG stress test (28). All subjects had a normal resting ECG, achieved more than 85% of their age-predicted maximum heart rate, and did not have chest pain or ECG changes during exercise.

The gender-matched normal files were developed from this group by determining the mean values and SDs from the pooled data for each of the 40 angular locations in each of the 15 profiles. The mean normal stress distributions of 201Tl for men and women are displayed as polar maps in Fig. 3.8. In both sexes, the lateral wall demonstrates the highest 201Tl activity. The most significant difference was found in the inferior wall, in which the relative uptake of 201Tl was significantly reduced (*p* <.01) in men as compared with women. The relative uptake in the septum of men is also significantly decreased.

## Localization

A series of guidelines was developed from a pilot group of 45 patients for assigning a perfusion defect to a specific vascular territory. There was, however, significant overlap at the boundaries of these lesions, and defects found primarily in one territory that did not extend significantly over the border of another territory were considered to represent a single lesion. Objective criteria, established from the pilot study, defined the amount of significant overlap that would have to exist to identify multivessel disease from a single contiguous defect. These criteria are shown in Fig. 3.9. This figure also illustrates regions that are assigned as indefinite vascular territories.

Figure 3.10 illustrates how a generic coronary tree would appear superimposed on a perfusion polar map and a 3D perfusion distribution. Note the relationship between the location of the vessels and the diagrams in Figs. 3.9 and 3.10. Note that the regions assigned as indefinite vascular territories can be perfused by multiple vessels. For example, if there is a perfusion defect between 1 o'clock and 3 o'clock, as in the polar map shown in the lower left panel of Fig. 3.9, it is difficult to assess whether the hypoperfusion is caused by a defect in one of the diagonal branches of the LAD or one of the obtuse marginal branches of the LCX.

## *Analysis and Polar Display*

### Stress Defect Extent and Severity

The comparison of each individual patient's bull's-eye to the gender-matched normal files resulted in the conversion of the bull's-eye into an SD map displaying pixels color-coded to the number of SDs below normal (Fig. 3.7). These SD polar maps display the magnitude or severity of the abnormality. The pixels that fell below these limits were submitted to a clustering criteria that prevented pixels without two adjacent abnormal neighbors from being displayed. These quantitative images were then compared with the angiographic data of a pilot group of patients to determine

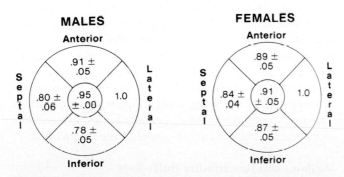

**FIGURE 3.8.** Diagram illustrating the normal distribution of postexercise 201Tl uptake for men and women. The lateral-to-septal wall ratio is greater than 1 for both men and women. The anterior-to-inferior wall ratio is approximately 1 for women but greater than 1 for men because of relatively decreased activity in the inferior wall of men. (From DePasquale E, Nody A, DePuey G, et al. Quantitative rotational thallium-201 tomography for identifying and localizing coronary artery disease. *Circulation* 1988; 77(2):316–327, with permission.)

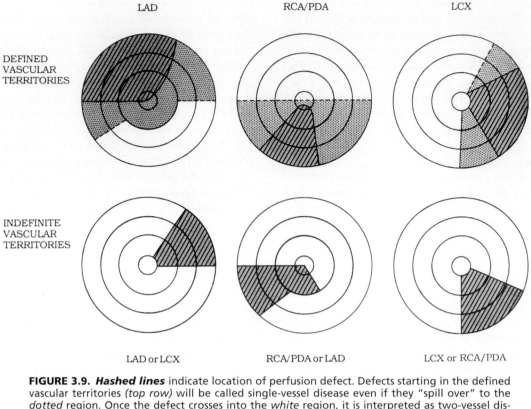

**FIGURE 3.9.** *Hashed lines* indicate location of perfusion defect. Defects starting in the defined vascular territories *(top row)* will be called single-vessel disease even if they "spill over" to the *dotted* region. Once the defect crosses into the *white* region, it is interpreted as two-vessel disease. Defects contained in the indefinite vascular territories *(lower row)* between two defined territories are interpreted as belonging to either one vascular territory or the other.

the best criteria for identifying the presence and location of a significant coronary stenosis. This analysis resulted in establishing profile curves representing 2.5 SD below the mean normal responses as the thresholds for defect detection. The clustered profile points falling below this established normal limit are plotted in a "blackout bull's-eye" in which the black region within the bull's-eye plot defines the extent of the perfusion abnormality. To be significant in male patients, a blackout defect had to contain at least 1.5% of the pixels (nine pixels) in the bull's-eye, while 3% (18 pixels) were required in women. The location, size, and shape of these blackout regions were used in conjunction with heuristic rules developed from a pilot group to identify the stenosed coronary artery associated with specific patterns of perfusion abnormality, as explained in the previous section on localizing CAD.

### Rest Defect Extent and Severity

Bull's-eye polar maps reflecting the same extent ("blackout") and severity of a defect ("standard deviation") were generated for the delayed/resting studies. The same cutoff criteria of 2.5 SD below the mean normal response was used as the threshold for detection of a resting defect. Importantly, these criteria were developed with the intent that they be applied to patients undergoing rest/redistribu-

tion studies, and have never been prospectively evaluated. Moreover, it is strongly discouraged that a reduction in the extent (blackout region) or severity of a defect between the stress and delayed/rest phases of study be used as an indication of myocardial ischemia. This is because delayed/resting studies, owing to the reduction in their count density, are associated with more noise and thus a larger SD. Thus, the lower limit of normal for a resting study is lower than for a stress study. If the same exact count distribution is submitted to both the stress and rest normal limits, it would, because of the differences in these limits, show the same reduction in counts as a smaller defect in the resting study as compared to the stress study, implying redistribution. The appropriate quantitative methods for use in detection of myocardial ischemia are discussed in the next section.

### Washout and Reversibility Bull's-Eyes

As in planar quantification (2,39), washout profiles are determined for each short-axis slice as the percentage of counts changes from stress to delayed imaging. Before comparing the washout profiles with the corresponding normal profiles, the normal curves are adjusted to correspond to the same acquisition interval as the patient's study, by moving the values in the normal curves along a monoexponential curve. Reversibility bull's-eyes are generated by subtracting

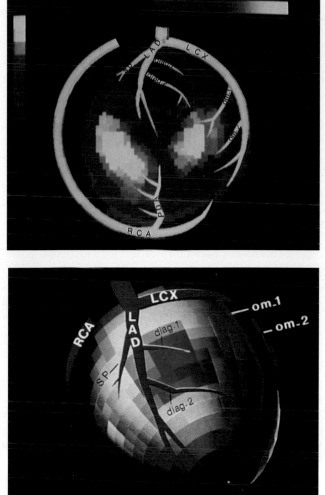

A

B

**FIGURE 3.10.** Generic left and right coronary trees superimposed on polar map **(A)** and on three-dimensional (3D) perfusion distribution **(B)** with a perfusion defect in the anterior wall; diag, diagonal; om, obtuse marginal; PDA, posterior descending artery; SP, septal branch.

the stress profiles from the corresponding delayed profiles after normalizing to a 5- × 5-pixel maximal count reference area in the stress study. In addition to this reversibility bull's-eye polar plot and the reversibility SD bull's-eye, a third polar plot is generated to readily display the application of the best single cutoff criteria determined (1.5 SD above mean normal). This plot duplicates the stress blackout bull's-eye plot but also includes the region that has reversed by the time of delayed imaging as a whiteout region, as determined from the application of normal limits and criteria for reversibility (40,41) (Fig. 3.7).

A numerical report accompanies this reversibility-whiteout bull's-eye map, and includes for each defect the extent (number of pixels) of both the stress perfusion defect (blackout area) and the subregion (whiteout area) within the defect that reverses by 4 hours. A severity score is also

reported, as the sum of the number of SDs from the mean of the pixels in the stress map that have been blacked out and those in the reversibility map that have been whited out. These scores are determined for each defect. A reversal of 15% or more of the original stress defect has been determined to represent significant reversibility (40). A reversal of 5% to 14% of the original stress defect is enough to be associated with what experts might read as a partial redistribution.

### Validation

Applying the Emory bull's-eye quantitative technique to a prospective group of 210 patients (179 with and 31 without CAD) resulted in an overall sensitivity of 95%, specificity of 74%, and an accuracy of 92% for detecting the presence or absence of CAD. The sensitivity for localization of disease for the LAD, LCX, and RCA was 78% (75/96), 65% (51/78), and 89% (93/104), and the specificity was 83% (95/114), 95% (126/132), and 87% (92/106), respectively. The results of this prospective evaluation of the method demonstrate a high sensitivity and specificity for the detection of CAD in patients and in individual coronary stenoses (7). Although these results are encouraging, they are based on the manual measurement of percent diameter stenosis using digital electronic calipers on the coronary arteriogram as a "gold standard," include patients taking antianginal medications, and do not specifically exclude patients with prior myocardial infarction, left ventricular hypertrophy, and coronary collateral vessels, all of which could significantly interfere with the sensitivity and specificity of the procedure. In particular, the use of percent diameter stenosis as a gold standard for assessing the physiologic significance of a coronary obstructive region has been heavily criticized (42).

A prospective multicenter trial was also performed to determine the accuracy of the Emory University quantitative technique and normal limits in detecting and localizing CAD (>50% stenosis). This trial was performed on 124 patients (100 men and 24 women) undergoing coronary angiography and eight patients with low likelihood of disease at five centers independent of Emory University (43). This trial resulted in an overall sensitivity of 95%, specificity of 33%, and normalcy rate of 88%.

Another prospective multicenter trial was performed on 140 patients from four centers to determine the accuracy of quantitative analysis of stress/delayed $^{201}$Tl myocardial tomograms with normal limits in assessing the relative amount of reversibility of stress-induced defects (44). The patients were found to have 85 fixed defects and 124 reversible defects, as determined by visual interpretation. Overall agreement between experts at multicenter sites and reversibility maps was 73% for reversible defects, and 80% of fixed defects. Sensitivity of the method in detecting reversibility was highest for the LCX vascular territory (88%) and lowest for the RCA (60%).

**Artifacts**

A number of important limitations and potential errors of this quantitative method must be emphasized. The reliability of the bull's-eye plot is dependent on an observer's correct selection of the apex and base of the LV from oblique tomographic slices. If the slices extend too far past the actual base or apex, there will be a rim of apparently decreased tracer concentration at the periphery of the bull's-eye, or a localized central defect near the apex, respectively. Recalling that the basal portion of the ventricle is relatively magnified in the bull's-eye plot, and that regions near the apex are minified, basal perfusion abnormalities will appear larger than equivalent defects in the middle and distal portions of the LV. Furthermore, image artifacts resulting in decreased count density, such as attenuation by unusually large breasts or an elevated left hemidiaphragm, patient motion, and errors in the COR will appear as defects in the bull's-eye plot, and will be represented as abnormalities in the thallium score. Alterations in myocardial anatomy and symmetry will also create relative abnormalities in patient data as compared with normal gender-matched files. An artifact of this type is commonly encountered in patients with hypertrophic cardiomyopathy in whom there is a disproportionate increase in thickness of the septum in addition to concentric myocardial hypertrophy. Since the highest count density is in the septum, the remainder of the ventricle will appear relatively decreased in intensity and will be judged to be abnormal when compared with normal files. Relative septal hypertrophy will cause a marked abnormality in the thallium score in all regions of the myocardium, with the exception of the septum. Detailed description of these artifacts are presented in Chapter 12.

With due considerations of the limitations in the quantitative analysis of thallium bull's-eye plots, this method serves as a valuable tool for determining the severity of myocardial ischemia and the amount of myocardium at jeopardy in patients with CAD.

## Other Approaches

Other investigators have also used circumferential profiles to extract the initial myocardial distribution and washout rate of $^{201}$Tl. Tamaki et al. (14) assessed the myocardium by using circumferential profiles from three short-axis sections and one middle vertical long-axis section. The main difference in other approaches has been in how the CPs are normalized. Caldwell et al. (8) scaled the CPs to a percentage of maximal counts in the entire left ventricular region of interest.

## CEQUAL QUANTITATIVE ANALYSIS

In 1990, investigators at Emory University and Cedars-Sinai Medical Center collaborated on the development of a new method for quantitatively analyzing same-day rest-stress SPECT studies done with technetium 99m ($^{99m}$Tc) (45,46).

This program integrated optimal features of the previously described quantitative programs with $^{201}$Tl, along with some new innovative features. These new features included automatic processing, 3D sampling using spherical and cylindrical coordinate searching of the short-axis tomograms, additional two-dimensional polar maps, and new techniques for developing normal limits and establishment of criterion for abnormality. The program is called CEqual, which stands for Cedars and Emory quantitative analysis, representing a sequel to the previously developed programs.

In 1997, investigators at Emory University began development of a comprehensive cardiac imaging package integrating perfusion and function called the Emory Cardiac Toolbox. The CEqual application within the Emory Cardiac Toolbox has been enhanced over the previous version. The enhanced features include an improved automatic processing technique, calculation of transient ischemic dilatation (TID) ratio and estimated myocardial mass of defect extent and viability, interactive normalization techniques, and additional normal-limit databases (rest-redistribution $^{201}$Tl, 2-day $^{99m}$Tc-sestamibi, rest $^{201}$Tl-stress $^{99m}$Tc-sestamibi dual isotope, and $^{99m}$Tc-tetrofosmin same-day). The additional Emory Cardiac Toolbox applications of Emory Gated SPECT (functional analysis), PerSPECTive (3D display of perfusion), and PERFEX (expert system analysis) are discussed in Chapter 4.

Prior to development and implementation of the CEqual technique, the technical aspects associated with SPECT imaging of the myocardium had to be optimized for each of the imaging protocols. This was initially performed for the same-day rest-stress $^{99m}$Tc-sestamibi SPECT protocol (47,48) and then for the other protocols. This included an investigation of the optimal radiopharmaceutical doses, imaging sequences, acquisition parameters, and reconstruction filters. The results of these investigations are discussed below.

## Technical Aspects

### Patient Protocol

The patient protocols for the various normal limits supported by the CEqual program are listed in Table 3.2. The patient exercise protocol is the same used for $^{201}$Tl and can be found above (see Thallium-201 Quantitative Analysis, Technical Aspects, Exercise Protocol). (For further discussion and recommendation of imaging guidelines for nuclear cardiology procedures, see ref. 49.)

### Acquisition and Processing Protocol

Optimization of the image-acquisition parameters for single-detector camera systems was done with phantom studies in which the contrast of simulated defects and uniformity of normal slices were used as parameters for evaluating

**TABLE 3.2. PATIENT PROTOCOLS FOR THE CEQUAL NORMAL LIMITS**

| Protocol | Isotope | Doses[a] (mCi) | | Delay Time Injection Imaging | | Delay Interval Between Studies | |
|---|---|---|---|---|---|---|---|
| | | Stress | Rest | Stress | Rest | Rest-Stress | Stress-Rest |
| Same day (rest/stress) | $^{99m}$Tc-sestamibi | 22–25 | 8–9 | 15 min–1 hour | 1–2 hours | 1–4 hours | |
| Two day | $^{99m}$Tc-sestamibi | 22–25 | 22–25 | 15 min–1 hour | 15 min–1 hour | | 18–24 hours |
| $^{201}$Tl | $^{201}$Tl | 3–4 | NA | 10–15 min | NA | | 4 hours |
| Same day (stress/rest) | $^{99m}$Tc-tetrofosmin | 8–9 | 22–25 | 15 min–1 hour | 1–2 hours | | 1–4 hours |
| Dual isotope | $^{99m}$Tc-sestamibi/$^{201}$Tl | $^{99m}$Tc 22–25 | $^{201}$Tl 2.5 | 15 min–1 hour | 15 min | No Delay | |

[a]Based on 70-kg patient. Doses are adjusted upward for heavier patients ($^{201}$Tl 0.04 mCi/kg and $^{99m}$Tc 0.31 mCi/kg).

imaging characteristics. The optimal acquisition parameters determined for the rest and exercise count-density studies for $^{201}$Tl and $^{99m}$Tc are listed in Table 3.3. The use of the high-resolution collimator for $^{99m}$Tc is particularly important because of its more constant resolution response with depth as compared to an all-purpose collimator. Although the circular 360-degree orbits yielded the best overall uniformity of normal slices, the circular 180-degree orbits were selected because of the shorter acquisition time involved, since the dead time associated with 64 additional steps in step-and-shoot acquisitions was eliminated. Also, the 180-degree orbits exhibited higher contrast of small lesions and higher count density. Elliptical 180-degree orbits yielded unacceptable photopenic artifacts.

Although prone imaging offers some advantages over supine imaging, such as reduced diaphragmatic attenuation, our experience to date is that in prone imaging of normal patients the anterior-wall count is somewhat reduced as compared to that from the other walls owing to attenuation. Since the anterior-wall abnormalities are associated with disease in the LAD artery, the most common type of lesions, this reduction in counts could lead to a reduction in specificity of the test. Thus, our present preference is to image the patient supine. Since minimal redistribution occurs in patients imaged with the $^{99m}$Tc protocols, it is advisable to also obtain a prone SPECT study when using those protocols, especially in patients with increased inferior wall attenuation and those suspected of having RCA disease. The exercise study is ECG-gated using eight frames for the cardiac cycle. We have noted that cine display of the myocardial distribution of $^{99m}$Tc-sestamibi throughout the cardiac cycle has been useful in identifying imaging artifacts. This type of display has also been shown to assist in assessing wall motion and thickening useful in determining myocardial viability (50). Quantification of regional perfusion uses the combined counts from all eight frames.

As with $^{201}$Tl imaging, each of the projections is corrected for nonuniformity with a flood source containing 30 × 10$^6$ counts, and the mechanical center of rotation is determined in order to align the projection data with

**TABLE 3.3. CEQUAL ACQUISITION AND PROCESSING PROTOCOLS**

| | $^{99m}$Tc[a] | $^{201}$Tl |
|---|---|---|
| Energy window | 20% symmetric 140 keV<br>DI: 15% symmetric 140 keV | 30% symmetric 70 keV<br>20% symmetric 167 keV |
| Collimator | High resolution | Low-energy all purpose<br>DI: high resolution |
| Orbit | 180° (45° RAO–45° LPO) | Same |
| Orbit type | Circular or noncircular[b] | Same |
| Pixel size | 6.4 ± 0.2 mm | Same |
| Acquisition type | Continuous or step-and-shoot | Same |
| No. of projections | 64 | Same |
| Matrix | 64 × 64 | Same |
| Time/projection | 20 seconds | Same |

[a]Sestamibi or tetrofosmin.
[b]Prior to using noncircular orbits, an investigation should be conducted to ensure that the noncircular method does not create artifacts.
DI, dual isotope imaging protocol; LPO, left posterior oblique; RAO, right anterior oblique.

respect to the reconstruction matrix. Since camera manufacturers define filters differently, the filter parameters vary for each system. An example of this variation in filter definition is demonstrated in the filter selection for the same-day [99mTc]-sestamibi protocol for two of the manufacturers. For the Siemens MaxDelta system, the filter parameters for the stress study are critical frequency of 0.66% Nyquist, order 2.5, while for the rest study, a critical frequency of 0.50% Nyquist, order 5 is employed. For the General Electric system, the filter parameters for stress are critical frequency of 0.52 cycles/cm, power 5, and for rest, a critical frequency of 0.4 cycles/cm, power 10. The lower the critical frequency and the higher the power of the filter, the more the images will be smoothed. These two filters for each system have a matched response for the lower frequencies that define the myocardium but a different response at the higher frequencies, to allow for the differences in statistical noise between the stress and rest studies. The application of these filters to the stress and rest [99mTc] same-day study will generate tomograms of comparable image texture. The transaxial tomograms are reconstructed one pixel thick (6.4 mm) using a ramp filter. The recommended CEqual filter parameters for the various protocols can be obtained directly from the camera manufacturers.

### Selection of Processing Parameters

Unlike the quantitative [201Tl] methods described above, which require substantial operator interaction, this method incorporates automatic processing to increase the objectivity and reproducibility of the program. The initial automatic processing algorithm was developed at Cedars-Sinai (51) and then improved by investigators at Emory University and Georgia Tech. Four parameters are identified automatically: LV long-axis center, apex, and base, and the radius of a circular region centered about the long axis that encloses the LV in every short-axis slice. The apex and base limit the short-axis extent of myocardial sampling. The long-axis center and radius limit the search range of sampling so that extraneous "hot" structures located outside the myocardial area are not included in the maximum-count CPs. In addition, the LV valve plane is detected as two connected planes: one perpendicular to the LV long-axis in the lateral half of the LV, and one angled plane in the septal half of the LV. All of the automatically selected parameters must be verified and accepted by the user. Manual override of these selected parameters is available in the application. An example of the processing verification page is shown in Fig. 3.11. After automatic processing the following parameters are saved: the apical and basal slice number, the angle of the septal valve plane, the $x, y$ coordinates of the long axis center, and the limiting radius of search for the mcps.

### Myocardial Sampling

In the [201Tl] quantification methods described at the beginning of this chapter, maximal-count CPs are routinely

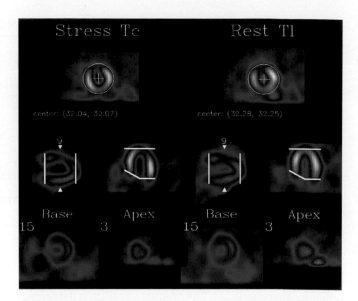

**FIGURE 3.11.** The *top row* shows midventricular short-axis slice images. These are used to illustrate the location of the radial-search boundaries and left ventricular (LV) center. The *middle row* shows both midventricular vertical and horizontal long-axis slice images. The vertical long-axis and horizontal long-axis reference images are used to illustrate the placement of the apical and basal slice selections. The *bottom row* displays short-axis slices, which correspond to the apical and basal slice selections identified in the *middle row*.

extracted from short-axis slices (6,7) and vertical long-axis slices (6) to represent the 3D distribution of myocardial tracer. These approaches are subject to partial-volume effects, particularly in the apical region. The technique developed for CEqual generates count profiles from a hybrid, two-part, 3D sampling scheme of stacked short-axis slices. In this approach the apical third of the myocardium is sampled using spherical coordinates, and the rest of the myocardium is sampled using cylindrical coordinates. This approach promotes a radial sampling that is largely perpendicular to the myocardial wall for all points and thus results in a more accurate representation of the perfusion distribution with minimal partial-volume effects. Following operator verification of the automatically derived features, the 3D maximum-count myocardial distribution is generated from all short-axis tomograms (Fig. 3.12). Maximum-count CPs, each comprising 40 points, are automatically generated from the short-axis slices using this two-part sampling scheme.

### Gender-Matched Normal Limits

As in our quantitative [201Tl] (SPECT) techniques, normal limits were defined from a group of patients with a low likelihood of CAD. Previous studies for [201Tl] (15) and [99mTc]-sestamibi same-day (27) demonstrated a need for gender-matched normal limits based on a difference in the relative uptake of [99mTc]-sestamibi in the inferior wall between the male and female normal populations (27). Therefore, the CEqual normal limits for all of the protocols consist of gen-

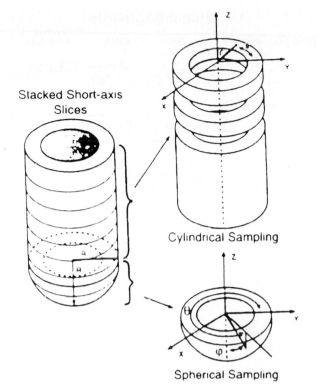

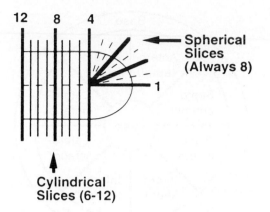

**FIGURE 3.13.** Normal-limit regions of the heart. There are always eight profiles generated from the patient's apical hemisphere, which are compared to normal limits 1 through 4. Usually, there are 6 to 12 profiles generated from the remainder of the myocardium, which are compared to normal limits 5 through 12. (From Van Train KF, Garcia EV, Maddahi J, et al. Multicenter trial validation for quantitative analysis of same-day rest-stress technetium-99m-sestamibi myocardial tomograms. *J Nucl Med* 1994;35:609–618, with permission.)

**FIGURE 3.12.** Three-dimensional sampling scheme used for generation of maximum-count circumferential profiles from $^{99m}$Tc-sestamibi short-axis tomograms. The apical hemisphere is identified as stacked, short-axis slices in which the radius of the top short-axis slice is equal to the depth of the stack. The apical hemisphere is sampled in a spherical coordinate system, as seen in the *bottom right* panel. Each point in the profile represents the maximum counts per pixel encountered along the radius of search for each $\phi$ and $\theta$ angular sample. The remaining portion of the myocardium is relatively cylindrical in shape, and each slice is sampled using a cylindrical coordinate system *(top right)* (From Berman DS, Kiat H, Van Train KF, et al. Technetium 99m sestamibi in the assessment of chronic coronary artery disease. *Semin Nucl Med* 1991;21(3):190–212, with permission.)

der specific normal limits: $^{99m}$Tc-sestamibi same-day (male: 35, female: 25), $^{99m}$Tc-sestamibi 2-day (male: 35, female: 24), stress-redistribution $^{201}$Tl (male: 36, female: 13), $^{99m}$Tc-tetrofosmin same-day (male: 27, female: 22), and dual isotope (male: 35, female: 25).

Normal responses (mean and SD) were determined for the stress and rest distributions of the various $^{99m}$Tc and $^{201}$Tl imaging protocols and for the perfusion distribution difference (reversibility) between stress and rest studies using additional pilot populations consisting of patients with and without CAD. Care was taken not to use patients younger than 35 years old, whose normal distributions might differ from those of older normal subjects. The normal limits consist of a set of 12 different profiles containing a total of 480 points representing the mean and SD for each of the measurements under consideration: stress, rest, and reversibility (Fig. 3.13). The number of patient profiles varies with the size of the patient's heart and the pixel size of the acquired

images. The algorithm assigns each patient profile to one of the 12 normal-limit profiles. The spherical slices are assigned to normal limits 1 to 4. The cylindrical slices are assigned to a specific normal profile by the formula:

$$\text{Cylindrical Normal-Limit Profile} = \text{Patients Cylindrical Slice Number} \times \frac{8}{\text{No. of Patient Cylindrical Slices}}$$

Using this formula, the mean and SD for all 12 normal limits in the male and female with a <5% likelihood of CAD were calculated.

### Profile Normalization

Profile normalization involves determining a scale factor that normalizes the mean of the most normal area of the patient's profiles to the mean of the same area in the normal-patient database. The scaling process is done only on the stress images. It divides the heart into ten regions, as shown in Fig. 3.14. The apical region is represented by normal limits 0 and 1. Eight additional sectors are represented by normal limits 2 through 7 and the basal area by normal limits 8 through 11. Each sector is 45 degrees or five points wide. The mean count values in the eight sectors are calculated for the patient's profile (pt) and the normal database (nl). A ratio for each sector is calculated as pt/nl. The sector with the highest ratio is considered the most normal. The scale factor, used to multiply the patient's stress and rest curves, is the inverse of the ratio chosen. An additional severity assessment is calculated by converting the profiles to SD units by the formula:

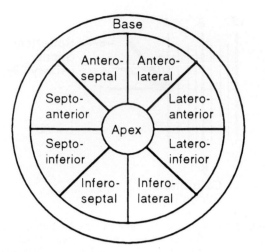

**FIGURE 3.14.** Ten myocardial perfusion territories: the apex, eight sectors, and the base. The patient's profiles are normalized by scaling the most normal of the eight patient sectors to the corresponding sector of the normal database. (From Van Train KF, Garcia EV, Maddahi J, et al. Multicenter trial validation for quantitative analysis of same-day rest-stress technetium-99m-sestamibi myocardial tomograms. *J Nucl Med* 1994;35:609–618, with permission.)

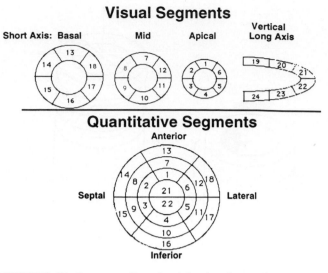

**FIGURE 3.15.** Corresponding visual *(top)* and quantitative *(bottom)* segments used for establishing optimum criteria for detection of perfusion abnormalities. Visual scores of 0 and 1 were considered normal and 2, 3, and 4 were considered abnormal. Each segment's visual score was compared to the quantitative value in the corresponding segment to determine the percent agreement. (From Van Train KF, Garcia EV, Maddahi J, et al. Multicenter trial validation for quantitative analysis of same-day rest-stress technetium-99m-sestamibi myocardial tomograms. *J Nucl Med* 1994;35:609–618, with permission.)

$$s_{pt} = \frac{(pt * scale) - m_{nl}}{s_{nl}}$$

This value represents the degree by which a patient profile point is above or below the mean normal value ($m_{nl}$).

## Generation of Normal-Limit Thresholds and Criteria for Abnormality

The criteria for abnormality was determined by comparing the expert visual reading of the tomographic slices to the output of the quantitative program, and were expressed in terms of the threshold, or the number of SDs from the mean that would best distinguish normal from abnormal myocardial perfusion. Threshold determination was optimized using an automated statistical package that performed ROC curve analysis comparing a database of the visual readings to the program output. The visual and quantitative values were originally determined for 20 corresponding segments as shown in Fig. 3.15. The segments were then grouped into four major regions: anterior (segments 1, 7, and 13), septal (segments 2, 3, 8, and 9), inferior (segments 4, 10, and 16), and lateral (segments 5, 6, 11, 12, 17, and 18). For the $^{99m}$Tc-sestamibi same- and 2-day protocols, normal-limit thresholds were then determined for each of the four myocardial regions. The thresholds for the apex (segments 21 and 22) were extrapolated from the four major myocardial-regions thresholds. For the dual-isotope, $^{99m}$Tc-tetrofosmin same-day, and stress-redistribution $^{201}$Tl protocols, seven myocardial regions were employed (Table 3.4). Multiple SDs were evaluated for each territory. The optimal SDs for the male and female popula-

tions for the various CEqual imaging protocols are shown in Table 3.4. In the evaluation of a patient's study, the patient's profile points are compared to their respective normal-limit values and are considered abnormal if they fall below the normal-limit threshold. After each point is analyzed, a clustering algorithm is employed to eliminate isolated abnormal points. The algorithm looks at each abnormal point and its four surrounding neighbors in the *x* and *y* direction; if the neighbors are all normal, then the point itself is also called normal.

With this approach, four major thresholds for the anterior, septal, inferior, and lateral territories defined the thresholds for the middle location of each territory. In the case of the dual-isotope, same-day $^{99m}$Tc-tetrofosmin and $^{201}$Tl protocols, the septal wall was divided into anteroseptal and inferoseptal segments and the lateral wall was divided into anterolateral and inferolateral segments. The normal-limit threshold values between the midpoints of the segments were assigned by interpolation. These interpolated values were then used for determining if the patient's value in the corresponding location was abnormal. This interpolation was performed on all of the normal-limit threshold values, and allowed for a smooth transition between the major territories of the myocardium.

Previous studies have used the coronary arteriogram as the gold standard for defining criteria for perfusion defects in SPECT studies of myocardial perfusion (7,19,20,43). This study, however, utilized consensus expert visual

**TABLE 3.4. MALE (BLACK) AND FEMALE (RED) NORMAL LIMIT THRESHOLDS FOR THE VARIOUS CEQUAL IMAGING PROTOCOLS**

| Polar Map Territories | Same day[a] Rest/Stress | | Two Day | | [201]Tl | | Same Day[b] Stress/Rest | | Dual | |
|---|---|---|---|---|---|---|---|---|---|---|
| | Str | Rev | Str | Rev | Str | Rev | Str | Rev | Str | Rev |
| Anterior | 3.0 | 1.0 | 3.0 | 1.0 | 2.5 | 2.0 | 2.3 | 2.0 | 2.75 | 1.0 |
| | 2.0 | 1.0 | 2.0 | 1.0 | 2.7 | 0.9 | 2.3 | 1.2 | 2.3 | 1.2 |
| Septal | 2.5 | 1.0 | 2.5 | 1.0 | | | | | | |
| | 2.0 | 1.0 | 2.0 | 1.0 | | | | | | |
| Anteroseptal | | | | | 2.5 | 1.0 | 2.6 | 2.2 | 2.25 | 0.9 |
| | | | | | 2.7 | 0.9 | 2.7 | 1.0 | 2.25 | 1.1 |
| Inferoseptal | | | | | 2.7 | 1.0 | 2.8 | 2.5 | 2.25 | 0.9 |
| | | | | | 2.5 | 0.9 | 3.5 | 1.5 | 2.0 | 1.1 |
| Inferior | 1.75 | 1.0 | 1.75 | 1.0 | 2.3 | 1.0 | 2.1 | 2.3 | 1.75 | 1.0 |
| | 1.75 | 1.0 | 1.75 | 1.0 | 2.4 | 0.9 | 2.8 | 2.0 | 2.3 | 1.0 |
| Lateral | 3.75 | 1.0 | 3.75 | 1.0 | | | | | | |
| | 3.0 | 1.0 | 3.0 | 1.0 | | | | | | |
| Inferolateral | | | | | 2.9 | 1.5 | 3.4 | 1.8 | 2.6 | 1.25 |
| | | | | | 3.3 | 1.1 | 4.4 | 1.3 | 2.8 | 1.25 |
| Anterolateral | | | | | 3.5 | 1.5 | 6.2 | 1.8 | 3.2 | 1.25 |
| | | | | | 3.7 | 1.1 | 6.2 | 1.6 | 2.9 | 1.25 |
| Apical | | | | | 2.1 | 1.0 | 2.2 | 2.0 | 2.3 | 1.0 |
| | | | | | 2.5 | 0.9 | 2.6 | 1.0 | 2.6 | 1.4 |
| Anterior | 2.5 | 1.0 | 2.5 | 1.0 | | | | | | |
| | 2.0 | 1.0 | 2.0 | 1.0 | | | | | | |
| Septal | 2.5 | 1.0 | 2.5 | 1.0 | | | | | | |
| | 2.0 | 1.0 | 2.0 | 1.0 | | | | | | |
| Inferior | 2.0 | 1.0 | 2.0 | 1.0 | | | | | | |
| | 2.0 | 1.0 | 2.0 | 1.0 | | | | | | |
| Lateral | 2.5 | 1.0 | 2.5 | 1.0 | | | | | | |
| | 2.0 | 1.0 | 2.0 | 1.0 | | | | | | |

[a]Same-day [99m]Tc-sestamibi protocol (low-dose rest/high-dose stress).
[b]Same-day [99m]Tc-tetrofosmin protocol (low-dose stress/high-dose rest).
Rev, reversibility; Str, stress.

SPECT interpretation rather than coronary angiographic results for establishing the criterion for perfusion-defect detection. This approach was chosen for several reasons. First, visual analysis by experts is directly correlated with the parameter that is being quantitated—the expected myocardial perfusion distribution. Coronary angiogram offers an accurate estimate of the coronary anatomy but does not necessarily directly correlate with maximal myocardial perfusion. Second, utilization of expert visual scores offered the ability to divide the heart into directly comparable segments, rather than using the indirect assignment of segments to the three territories provided by the coronary angiogram. Also, utilizing expert visual scores allowed more control over the entire process of criterion development. The visual gold standard was obtained using readings that were agreed upon by consensus. In contrast, the angiographic gold standard may result in considering a segment abnormal when a perfusion defect may not be present.

This technique utilized varying SD thresholds for the major territories rather than only one threshold for the entire myocardium. This method was chosen because of the previously observed nongaussian distribution of counts encountered in myocardial perfusion SPECT (19,52). The anterolateral wall routinely contains the highest counts, owing to reduced attenuation and closer camera proximity to the heart, and because the inferoseptal wall routinely contains the lowest counts, owing to increased diaphragmatic attenuation. Thus, the counts in these areas become nongaussian when expressed as a percent of maximal counts. The varying SD thresholds provide a means to account for these nongaussian distributions.

## Feature Extraction and Localization

The feature-extraction algorithm uses the area of the stress abnormality or blackout array to identify the stress defects (53). First, all nonzero pixels are set to 1. Then the array is searched until a defect is found (indicated by a 0). An edge-hugging algorithm is employed to fill the defect with an appropriate defect number (i.e., defect 1 is filled in with 1's, etc.). The defects are then broken down into descriptor territories, comprising three vascular territories (LAD, LCX, and RCA; Fig. 3.4), and ten perfusion territories (eight sectors, the apex, and the base; Fig. 3.14). There is a flag that controls whether stress-defect analysis and/or reversibility analysis is performed. For stress-defect analysis, each defect is described in terms of the total number of SDs and pixels falling within each descriptor territory; these numbers are subsequently stored in a descriptor array. For reversibility analysis, a defect is identified and its corresponding area in the reversibility whiteout array is searched. If reversibility is present, the total number of reversibility SDs and pixels falling within each descriptor territory is calculated and stored in the descriptor array. A report can then be generated using the SDs (severity) and pixels (extent) recorded for each descriptor territory for each defect. Other measures can be used to measure the extent of a defect instead of absolute pixels, such as the percentage of myocardium affected.

The applicability of the polar map of vascular territories made with $^{201}$Tl to imaging with $^{99m}$Tc myocardial perfusion imaging agents was determined in a population of 53 patients (mean age 61.2, range 33 to 83 years) with single-vessel CAD. A similar study as was conducted previously for $^{201}$Tl (19,33) confirmed that the coronary boundaries previously determined for $^{201}$Tl could be applied to the $^{99m}$Tc quantitative polar maps. However, in contrast to the $^{201}$Tl evaluation, this study determined that the percentage of abnormal points required for an abnormality to be significant in each of the territories was slightly different. The percentage of abnormal points for $^{99m}$Tc myocardial perfusion imaging agents was determined to be 10% for left anterior descending and left circumflex coronary artery, and 12% for the right coronary artery.

The present method for localizing CAD only partially accounts for interindividual variations of coronary blood supply. It is possible, for example, that in patients in whom the LAD artery is large and wraps around the apex, and therefore supplies the distal inferior wall, a defect in the territory of the LAD artery could be attributed to both the LAD and posterior descending coronary arteries. Furthermore, in some patients with single-vessel disease involving a large left circumflex or right coronary artery, SPECT perfusion defects imaged with $^{99m}$Tc myocardial perfusion agents may appear to involve the territories of both vessels. These variations of the coronary arterial tree limit the ability to determine, with a very high specificity, disease in individual coronary arteries. A discussion of more accurate techniques, such as integration of artificial intelligence rules into the quantitative interpretation (PERFusion EXpert; PERFEX) and allowing for the superimposition of the coronary arteries onto the perfusion territories, can be found in Chapter 4.

Normal limits provided with CEqual include two same-day protocols one for $^{99m}$Tc-sestamibi (low-dose rest/high-dose stress) and one for $^{99m}$Tc-tetrofosmin (low-dose stress/high-dose rest). Investigators have demonstrated that the same normal reference population may be applicable to both the myocardial perfusion agents (54). This study evaluated a group of patients with CAD who were injected with a high dose of $^{99m}$Tc-sestamibi and $^{99m}$Tc-tetrofosmin 1

week apart and processed with the CEqual same-day $^{99m}$Tc-sestamibi normal limit. The results showed a high correlation for stress extent and reversibility between the two studies, indicating that the high-dose $^{99m}$Tc-sestamibi normal limit can be used to evaluate both of these myocardial perfusion tracers.

## Analysis and Polar Map Display

### Mapping Severity and Reversibility of Abnormalities

The SD maps are polar plots of the number of SD units that each pixel is removed from the mean normal distribution in the patient profile. In the stress and rest maps, only the pixels below the mean are considered. The purpose of the map is to give an impression of the degree of abnormality or how close to abnormal are the patients' profiles. The number of SDs from the mean for each pixel in the severity map is color coded to one of nine colors. In the reversibility maps, only those pixels above the mean are considered. Reversibility is calculated by scaling the rest and stress images to a common value of the most normal region of the stress distribution and subtracting the stress from the rest data. Thus, areas of reversibility with a defect at stress and no defect at rest will contain a high positive number.

### Quantitative Display

In addition to polar maps representing the extent, severity, and reversibility of a defect, the stress and rest raw data count distribution is displayed using both distance- and volume-weighted polar map representations. The distance-weighted polar map is constructed by mapping sequential maximal-count profiles ranging from the apex to the base into successive rings in the polar map. (The apex is mapped into the center and the base is mapped into the periphery.) Each ring within the polar map is assigned the same width in pixels. The width is determined by dividing the radius of the polar map (usually 32 pixels) by the number of sampled segments (spherical rings + cylindrical slices) in the study.

The volume-weighted polar map is constructed in much the same way as the distance-weighted polar map, except that the width of each ring is decreased from apex to base. To determine the width of each ring, the total volume of the myocardium is approximated. The volume of the apical hemisphere is then approximated and its percentage of the total volume is calculated. The apical hemisphere is then mapped in such a way that the area it occupies is the same percentage of the total area of the polar map as the volume of the apical hemisphere is of the total volume. Each ring in the apical hemisphere is equal in width. For those slices outside the apical hemisphere, the percentage of area that each slice occupies in the polar map is proportional to its percentage of the total volume of the myocardium.

The CEqual version in the Emory Cardiac Toolbox provides for the following display options: slices, polar maps, PerSPECTive, and functional analysis. The slices display contains the automatically aligned short-, vertical-, and long-axis tomograms for rest and stress along with the dynamic planar projections and calculated TID ratio (Fig. 3.16). The TID ratio is calculated by dividing the stress (ungated) endocardial volume by the rest endocardial volume, and a value greater than 1.0 may indicate the presence of TID (55). The polar maps display contains information related to raw counts, defect extent, and severity for stress, rest, and reversibility (Fig. 3.17). These displays can be shown in either distance- or volume-weighted configuration with quantitative territory overlays. The severity polar maps show relative perfusion variance compared to the corresponding normal limits. Each SD below the mean is represented by a different color. An appreciation for how severe the defect is within the abnormal area can be obtained from the severity polar maps. The estimated mass display provides myocardial mass estimates, which are obtained by multiplying the myocardial volume, derived from endocardial and epicardial edges within a LV wall thickness of 1 cm, by a density of 1.05 g/mL (Fig. 3.18). The quantitative extent display provides stress defect extent and reversibility as a percent of the total and percent abnormal (area or mass) within the LAD, LCX, and RCA coronary arteries (Fig. 3.19).

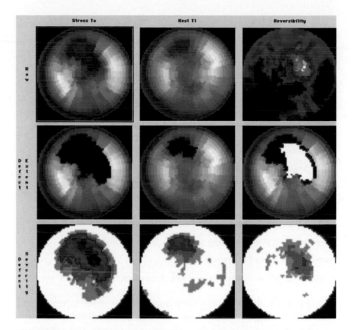

**FIGURE 3.17.** CEqual quantitative output. This example demonstrates abnormal myocardial perfusion in both the stress and rest studies. This is shown in the "blackout" pixels (area below normal limits) in position 4, 5, and 6. Note that the stress polar maps demonstrate more extensive perfusion defects than do the rest images. As shown by the *arrows,* the white pixels in frame 3 and the "whiteout" pixels in frame 6 show the area of potentially ischemic myocardium, which is better perfused at rest than at stress.

## Validation

Initially, the optimum SDs for the various myocardial walls for each of the imaging protocols were determined using pilot populations consisting of normal and abnormal patients (Table 3.4). Then the various normal limits were

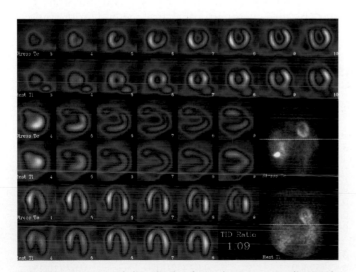

**FIGURE 3.16.** CEqual slice display from the Emory Cardiac Toolbox. The *top two rows* contain short-axis slices, the *middle two rows* contain vertical long-axis (VLA) slices, and the *bottom two rows* contain horizontal long-axis (HLA) slices. The planar projection image sets are displayed *(right).* The calculated transient ischemic dilatation (TID) ratio is displayed at the bottom.

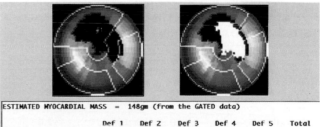

ESTIMATED MYOCARDIAL MASS = 148gm (from the GATED data)

|  | Def 1 | Def 2 | Def 3 | Def 4 | Def 5 | Total |
|---|---|---|---|---|---|---|
| **Stress Defect:** | | | | | | |
| Estimated Mass : | 37gm | 0gm | 0gm | 0gm | 0gm | 37gm |
| Percent of Myo : | 25% | 0% | 0% | 0% | 0% | 25% |
| **Reversibility:** | | | | | | |
| Estimated Mass : | 20gm | 0gm | 0gm | 0gm | 0gm | 20gm |
| Percent of Defect: | 53% | 0% | 0% | 0% | 0% | 54% |
| Percent of Myo : | 13% | 0% | 0% | 0% | 0% | 13% |

Stress Total Severity Score = 772

Probability of Survival: 1 yr: 81% 2 yr: 77% 3 yr: 63% 4 yr: 42%

**FIGURE 3.18.** Illustration of the quantitative mass display and output.

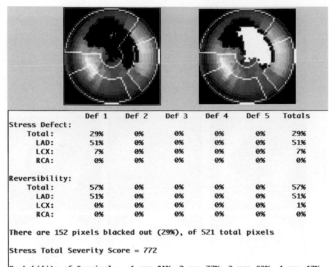

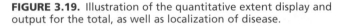

|  | Def 1 | Def 2 | Def 3 | Def 4 | Def 5 | Totals |
|---|---|---|---|---|---|---|
| **Stress Defect:** | | | | | | |
| Total: | 29% | 0% | 0% | 0% | 0% | 29% |
| LAD: | 51% | 0% | 0% | 0% | 0% | 51% |
| LCX: | 7% | 0% | 0% | 0% | 0% | 7% |
| RCA: | 0% | 0% | 0% | 0% | 0% | 0% |
| **Reversibility:** | | | | | | |
| Total: | 57% | 0% | 0% | 0% | 0% | 57% |
| LAD: | 51% | 0% | 0% | 0% | 0% | 51% |
| LCX: | 0% | 0% | 0% | 0% | 0% | 1% |
| RCA: | 0% | 0% | 0% | 0% | 0% | 0% |

There are 152 pixels blacked out (29%), of 521 total pixels

Stress Total Severity Score = 772

Probability of Survival: 1 yr: 81% 2 yr: 77% 3 yr: 63% 4 yr: 42%

**FIGURE 3.19.** Illustration of the quantitative extent display and output for the total, as well as localization of disease.

subjected to an in-house validation. To assess the broad applicability of the program for the various normal limits, they were subjected to prospective multicenter trial evaluations. Results of these prospective multicenter trials using coronary angiography as the gold standard are shown in Table 3.5. The results listed for the [201]Tl protocol are from the previous Cedars-Sinai quantitative [201]Tl method. The CEqual program used the same [201]Tl normal and pilot populations for generation of normal limits and criteria for disease detection. An evaluation of the two techniques obtained similar results within a stress-redistribution [201]Tl patient population for both the previous [201]Tl program and

CEqual using the [201]Tl normal limits. Therefore, the results reported in Table 3.5 for [201]Tl are the results expected if the CEqual [201]Tl normal limits were employed. The results of the pilot and multicenter trial validation for the same-day [99m]Tc-sestamibi protocol was published in the *Journal of Nuclear Medicine* (56,57).

The normal limits were also validated using expert visual interpretation as the gold standard in larger populations. The results of this validation for the same-day [99m]Tc-sestamibi protocol resulted in and overall true-positive rate of 93% (98/105), true-negative rate of 53% (10/19), and normalcy rate in the low-likelihood patients of 86% (30/35). The true-positive/true-negative rates for the LAD, LCX, and RCA were 87% (54/62)/89% (55/62), 77% (41/53)/87% (62/71), and 78% (50/64)/82% (49/60), respectively. For the dual-isotope protocol, the results obtained an overall true-positive rate of 99% (115/116), true-negative rate of 88% (57/65), and normalcy rate in the low-likelihood patients of 91% (21/23). The true-positive/true-negative rates for the LAD, LCX, and RCA were 99% (67/68)/81% (91/113), 95% (41/43)/93% (128/138), and 91% (59/65)/91% (105/116), respectively. For the same-day [99m]Tc-tetrofosmin protocol, the results obtained an overall true-positive rate of 92% (34/37), true-negative rate of 100% (7/7), and normalcy rate in the low-likelihood patients of 88% (15/17). The true-positive/true-negative rates for the LAD, LCX, and RCA were 95% (19/20)/91% (29/32), 87% (13/15)/97% (36/37), and 81% (22/27)/92% (23/25), respectively. The two-day [99m]Tc-sestimibi protocol only had results based on coronary angiography shown in Table 3.5, and the [201]Tl expert visual results can be found in the section on [201]Tl quantitation. These pilot and multicenter trial results demonstrate that this objective quantitative analytical method for the various

**TABLE 3.5. CEQUAL MULTIPLE NORMAL LIMIT DATABASE MULTICENTER TRIAL RESULTS FOR DETECTION OF A STRESS DEFECT; CORONARY ANGIOGRAPHY WAS USED AS THE "GOLD STANDARD" (>50% STENOSIS)**

|  | Same Day[a] (Rest/Stress) | Two Day | [201]Tl | Same Day[b] (Stress/Rest) | Dual Isotope |
|---|---|---|---|---|---|
| Male | 150 | 21 | 276 | 14 | 70 |
| Female | 48 | 10 | 42 | 7 | 19 |
| **Sensitivity** | | | | | |
| Overall | 0.88 (90/102) | 1.0 | 0.94 (184/196) | 0.85 (11/13) | 0.95 (59/62) |
| LAD | 0.67 (52/78) | 0.71 | 0.78 (115/148) | 1.0 (8/8) | 0.77 (37/48) |
| LCX | 0.76 (35/46) | 0.75 | 0.68 (66/97) | 0.83 (5/6) | 0.58 (25/43) |
| RCA | 0.70 (35/50) | 0.88 | 0.84 (118/141) | 0.78 (7/9) | 0.78 (25/32) |
| **Specificity** | | | | | |
| Overall | 0.32 (7/22) | 0.17 | 0.44 (20/46) | — | 0.0 (0/1) |
| LAD | 0.78 (58/74) | 0.82 | 0.63 (59/94) | 0.92 (12/13) | 0.67 (10/15) |
| LCX | 0.77 (44/57) | 0.77 | 0.68 (98/145) | 1.0 (15/15) | 0.70 (14/20) |
| RCA | 0.85 (57/67) | 0.71 | 0.62 (63/105) | 0.92 (11/12) | 0.71 (22/31) |
| Normalcy rate | 0.81 (30/37) | 0.83 | 0.82 (62/76) | 0.75 (6/8) | 0.91 (21/23) |

[a]Same-day [99m]Tc-sestamibi protocol (low-dose rest/high-dose stress).
[b]Same-day [99m]Tc-tetrofosmin protocol (low-dose stress/high-dose rest).
LAD, left anterior descending; LCX, left circumflex; RCA, right coronary artery.

SPECT imaging protocols offers a high correlation with expert visual interpretation and coronary angiography and are clinically applicable for the accurate detection and localization of CAD.

Two recent papers have demonstrated additional clinical parameters provided by the CEqual quantitative analysis program. The first was published by Kang et al. (58) demonstrating that the CEqual values for rest sestamibi SPECT defect extent and severity provided a useful means of assessing infarct size in patients with remote infarction. The CEqual measurements in this paper were correlated with rest left ventricular ejection fraction (LVEF) and semiquantitative expert visual analysis (58). The second paper demonstrated the prognostic value of the CEqual program for the dual-isotope myocardial perfusion imaging protocol (59). In this study, 1,043 consecutive patients with known or suspected CAD were followed for at least 1 year. During the follow-up period, 28 hard events occurred. The study demonstrated that patients with higher defect extent and reversibility by quantitative SPECT defect analysis had a significantly higher hard-event rate compared to patients with a normal scan. These results indicate that the data provided by the CEqual quantitative analysis program can be used to prognostically stratify patients with the same accuracy as that obtained by semiquantitative expert visual analysis.

## Other Database Quantification Techniques

There are several other quantitative techniques currently available for analysis of myocardial perfusion. Three of the techniques (Verani, Tamaki, and O'Connor), which all employ a user-entered threshold value for the normal limit, were evaluated and found to offer comparable results for detection of area at risk (60). Other techniques (O'Connor, Mortelmans, and Liu) have been found to offer accurate methods for infarct sizing and for the quantitative analysis of myocardial perfusion SPECT studies (61–63).

A method developed at the University of Michigan, called 3D-MSPECT (CardiaQ), performs automatic 3D/4D processing and quantification of SPECT, gated SPECT, and attenuation corrected SPECT cardiac images (64,65). Ventricular surfaces are automatically determined and color-coded 3D surface and polar map displays, and corresponding normalized and co-registered multislice displays of orthogonal long-axis and short-axis images including the entire cardiac volume, are formatted for review and interpretation (Fig. 3.20). 3D-MSPECT automatically processes from 1 to 256 files with or without operator intervention. The application includes an integrated database generator that allows individual sites to create their own normal databases. Supplied databases are protocol independent and include attenuation corrected and uncorrected, gated and ungated, stress/redistribution [201]Tl, same-day and 2-day Tc-sestamibi, and dual-isotope rest thallium/

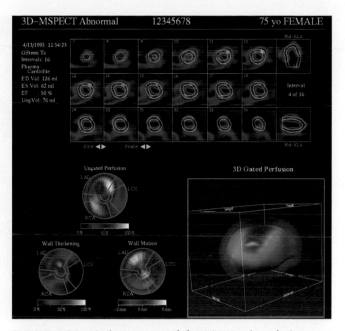

**FIGURE 3.20.** Display output of function and perfusion provided by the 3D-MSPECT quantitative analysis program of a female patient with a lateral wall abnormality.

stress sestamibi databases. Sestamibi databases include ungated, end-diastolic and end-systolic perfusion, wall thickening, and wall motion. From one to four studies may be displayed side by side with or without the corresponding 3D and polar map images. 3D-MSPECT automatically generates displays of attenuation corrected and uncorrected stress/rest or stress/redistribution, etc. studies with normal database limit comparisons.

A method developed by Focus Imaging called CardioMatch provides for the quantitative analysis of myocardial perfusion SPECT images using a 3D image processing and visualization technique. The method utilizes an objective processing technique employing automatic 3D registration of stress and rest images to aligned templates (66). For normal-limit comparisons, the images are normalized for size and shape, and the patient data are registered to a 3D reference using a loss-less transformation. The technique utilizes a single threshold of −2.2 SD for stress compared to the normal population and a threshold of +1.5 SD for the rest images compared to the patients stress images. Perfusion defects are characterized through automatic identification and annotation by color coding and anatomic localization of lesions (67). Multiple reference standards are included, which are used to account for factors such as gender, age, weight, and heart size in the diagnosis of CAD. CardioMatch provides for estimates of defect size, extent, and percentage of left ventricular mass. An additional feature provides for determination of pre- and posttest probabilities incorporating patient history and other noninvasive test information.

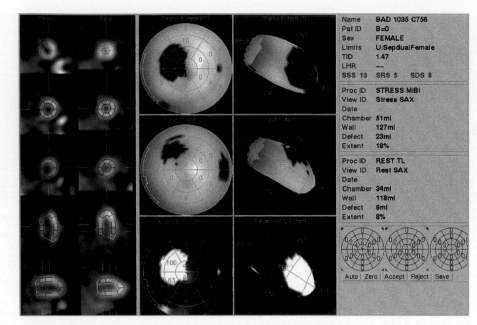

**FIGURE 3.21.** Quantitative display output for the Cedars-Sinai Quantitative Perfusion SPECT (QPS) program. Myocardial contours, percent abnormal for defect extent and reversibility, and automatically generated visual score output are presented.

An additional method has been developed by Germano et al. (68–70) from Cedars-Sinai called Quantitative Perfusion SPECT (QPS). QPS is a completely automatic 3D software approach to quantitative perfusion SPECT. The salient features of the algorithm are the following: (a) the myocardium is sampled based on an ellipsoidal model; (b) the count profiles composed of the endocardial and epicardial surfaces are used, rather than just the maximal counts; (c) the approach is independent of myocardial shape, size, and orientation, resulting in the same number of sampling points for every patient; (d) 20-segment, five-point scores as well as global and regional quantitative perfusion measurements are automatically generated; and (e) normal limits are automatically generated for any given patient population. Figure 3.21 demonstrates the output provided by the QPS method.

## ACKNOWLEDGMENTS

The authors would like to thank Russell Folks and Gerrard Silagan for their technical support. This study was supported in part by grants RO1-HL41628-01 and RO1-HL42052 from the National Institutes of Health, Bethesda, Maryland, by a grant from the American Heart Association, Greater Los Angeles Affiliate, as well as a grant from E.I. du Pont de Nemours & Co., North Billerica, Massachusetts.

## REFERENCES

1. Trobaugh GV, Wackers FJTh, Sokole EB, et al. Thallium-201 myocardial imaging: an interinstitutional study of observer variability. *J Nucl Med* 1978;19:395.

2. Garcia EV, Maddahi J, Berman DS, et al. Space-time quantitation of thallium-201 myocardial scintigraphy. *J Nucl Med* 1981; 22:309–317.

3. Meade RC, Bamrah VS, Horgan JD, et al. Quantitative methods in the evaluation of thallium-201 myocardial perfusion images. *J Nucl Med* 1978;19:1175.

4. Burow RD, Pond M, Schafer AW, et al. Cicumferential profiles: a new method for computer analysis of thallium-201 myocardial perfusion images. *J Nucl Med* 1979;20:771.

5. Watson DD, Campbell NP, Read EK, et al. Spatial and temporal quantitation of plane thallium myocardial images. *J Nucl Med* 1981;22:577–584.

6. Garcia EV, Van Train K, Maddahi J, et al. Quantification of rotational thallium-201 myocardial tomography. *J Nucl Med* 1985; 26:17–26.

7. DePasquale E, Nody A, DePuey G, et al. Quantitative rotational thallium-201 tomography for identifying and localizing coronary artery disease. *Circulation* 1988;77(2):316–327.

8. Caldwell J, Williams D, Harp G, et al. Quantitation of size of relative myocardial perfusion defect by single-photon emission computed tomography. *Circulation* 1984;70:1048–1056.

9. Vogel RA, Kirch DL, LeFree MT, et al. Thallium-201 myocardial perfusion scintigraphy: results of standard and multi-pinhole tomographic techniques. *Am J Cardiol* 1979;43:787.

10. Go RT, Cook SA, MacIntyre WJ, et al. Comparative accuracy of stress and redistribution thallium-201 cardiac single photon emission transaxial tomography and planar imaging in the diagnosis of myocardial ischemia. *J Nucl Med* 1982;23:24–25(abst).

11. Maddahi J, Van Train KF, Wong C, et al. Comparison of thallium-201 SPECT and planar imaging for evaluation of coronary artery disease. *J Nucl Med* 1986;27:999(abst).

12. Tamaki S, Nakajima H, Murakami T, et al. Estimation of infarct size by myocardial emission computed tomography with thallium-201 and its relation to creatine kinase-MB release after myocardial infarction in man. *Circulation* 1982; 66:994–1001.

13. Ritchie JL, Williams DL, Harp G, et al. Transaxial tomography

with thallium-201 for detecting remote myocardial infarction. *Am J Cardiol* 1982;50:1236–1241.

14. Tamaki N, Yonekura Y, Kadaa S, et al. Value of quantitative stress thallium-201 emission CT for localization of coronary artery disease: comparison with qualitative analysis. *J Nucl Med* 1984;25: 61.

15. Maddahi J, Garcia EV, Berman DS, et al. Improved noninvasive assessment of CAD by quantitative analysis of regional stress myocardial distribution and washout of thallium-201. *Circulation* 1981;64:924–935.

16. Van Train K, Berman DS, Garcia E, et al. Quantitative analysis of stress Tl-201 myocardial scintigrams: a multicenter trial validation utilizing standard normal limits. *J Nucl Med* 1986;27: 17–25.

17. Fintel DJ, Links JM, Brinker JA, et al. Improved diagnostic performance of exercise thallium-201 single photo emission computed tomography over planar imaging in the diagnosis of coronary artery disease: a receiver operating characteristic analysis. *J Am Coll Cardiol* 1989;13:600.

18. Iskandrian AS, Heo J, Askenase A, et al. Thallium imaging with single photon emission computed tomography. *Am Heart J* 1987;114:852–865.

19. Maddahi J, Van Train KF, Prigent F, et al. Quantitative single photon emission computerized thallium-201 tomography for the evaluation of coronary artery disease: optimization and prospective validation of a new technique. *J Am Coll Cardiol* 1989;14: 1689–1699.

20. Van Train KF, Maddahi J, Berman DS, et al. Quantitative Analysis of tomographic stress thallium-201 myocardial scintigrams: a multicenter trial. *J Nucl Med* 1990;31:1168–1179.

21. Friedman J, Van Train K, Maddahi J, et al. "Upward creep" of the heart: a frequent source of false positive reversible defects during thallium-201 stress-redistribution SPECT. *J Nucl Med* 1989;30:1718–1722.

22. Boucher CA, Zir LM, Beller GA, et al. Increased lung uptake of thallium-201 during exercise myocardial imaging: clinical, hemodynamic and angiographic implications in patients with coronary artery disease. *Am J Cardiol* 1980;46:189–196.

23. Kushner FG, Okada RD, Kirschenbaum HD, et al. Lung thallium-201 uptake after stress testing in patients with coronary artery disease. *Circulation* 1981;63:341–347.

24. Levy R, Rozanski A, Berman DS, et al. Analysis of the degree of pulmonary thallium washout after exercise in patients with coronary artery disease. *J Am Coll Cardiol* 1983;2(4):719–728.

25. Weiss AT, Berman DS, Lew AS, et al. Transient ischemic dilation of the left ventricle on stress thallium scintigraphy: a marker of severe and extensive coronary artery disease. *J Am Coll Cardiol* 1987;9:752–759.

26. Borrello JA, Clinthorne NH, Rogers WL, et al. Oblique-angle tomography: a restructuring algorithm for transaxial tomographic data. *J Nucl Med* 1981;22:472–473.

27. Van Train, Areeda J, Garcia E, et al. Development and prospective validation of quantitative same-day Tc-99m sestamibi SPECT. *Circulation* 1991;84(4):304(abst).

28. Diamond GA, Forrester JS. Analysis of probability as an aid in the clinical diagnosis of coronary artery disease. *N Engl J Med* 1979;300:1350–1358.

29. Diamond GA, Forrester JS, Hirsch M, et al. Application of conditional probability analysis to the clinical diagnosis of coronary artery disease. *J Clin Invest* 1980;65:1210–1221.

30. Rozanski A, Diamond GA, Forrester JS, et al. Alternative referent standards for cardiac normality. Implications for diagnostic testing. *Ann Intern Med* 1984;101:164–171.

31. Van Train KF, Maddahi J, Wong C, et al. Definition of normal limits in stress Tl-201 myocardial rotational tomography. *J Nucl Med* 1986;27(6):899(abst).

32. Eisner RL, Tamas MJ, Cloninger K, et al. Normal SPECT thallium-201 bull's-eye display: gender differences. *J Nucl Med* 1988; 29:1901–1909.

33. Prigent F, Maddahi J, Berman DS. Quantitative stress-redistribution Tl-201 single-photon emission tomography (SPECT): development of a scheme for localization of coronary artery disease. *J Nucl Med* 1986;27:997(abst).

34. Clausen M, Civelek C, Bice CA, et al. Short axis circumferential profiles of the heart in healthy subjects: comparison of Tl-201 SPECT and two-dimensional echocardiography. *Radiology* 1988; 168:723–726.

35. Cloninger KG, DePuey EG, Garcia EV, et al. Incomplete redistribution in delayed thallium-201 single photon emission tomographic (SPECT) images: an overestimation of myocardial scarring. *J Am Coll Cardiol* 1988;12:955–963.

36. Dilsizian V, Rooco TP, Freedman NM, et al. Enhanced detection of ischemic but viably myocardium by the reinjection of thallium after stress-redistribution imaging. *N Engl J Med* 1990;323(3): 141–146.

37. Dilsizian V, Smetzer WR, Freedman NM, et al. Thallium reinjection after stress-redistribution imaging—does 24-hour delayed imaging after reinjection enhance detection of viable myocardium? *Circulation* 1991;E3(4):1247–1255.

38. Eisner RL, Gober A, Cerqueira M, et al. Quantitative analysis of normal thallium-201 tomographic studies. *J Nucl Med* 1984;26: 49–50 (abst).

39. Wackers FJ, Bales D, Fetterman RC, et al. Nonuniform washout of thallium-201 (within normal range): criterion for improved detection of single vessel coronary disease. *J Nucl Med* 1983;24: 46(abst).

40. Klein JL, Garcia EV, DePuey EG, et al. Reversibility bull's-eye: a new polar bull's-eye map to quantify reversibility of stress induced SPECT-Tl-201 myocardial perfusion defects. *J Nucl Med* 1990;31:1240–1246.

41. Luna E, Klein L, Garcia E, et al. Reversibility bull's-eye polar map: accuracy in detecting myocardial ischemia. *J Nucl Med* 1987;95 (abst)29(5).

42. Marcus ML, Skorton DJ, Johnson MR, et al. Visual estimates of percent diameter coronary stenosis: "a battered gold standard." *J Am Coll Cardiol* 1988;11:882–885.

43. Garcia E, DePuey EG, Brown MN, et al. Quantification of rotational thallium-201 myocardial tomograms: a multicenter trial using Bull's-eye polar maps and standard normal limits. *J Nucl Med* 1987;4:673(abst).

44. Garcia E, DePuey EG, Sonnemaker RE, et al. Quantification of the reversibility of stress induced SPECT thallium-201 myocardial perfusion defects: a multicenter trial using bull's-eye polar maps and standard normal limits. *J Nucl Med* 1990;31:1761–1765.

45. Garcia E, Cooke CD, Van Train KF, et al. Technical aspects of myocardial SPECT imaging with technetium-99m sestamibi. *Am J Cardiol* 1990;66:23E–31E.

46. Berman DS, Kiat H, Van Train KF, et al. Technetium 99m sestamibi in the assessment of chronic coronary artery disease. *Semin Nucl Med* 1991;21(3):190–212.

47. Van Train K, Folks R, Wong C, et al. Optimization of Tc-MIBI SPECT acquisition and processing parameters: collimator, matrix size and filter evaluation. *J Nucl Med* 1989;30:757(abst).

48. Folks R, Van Train K, Wong C, et al. Evaluation of Tc-MIBI SPECT acquisition parameters: circular vs elliptical and 180 degree vs 360 degree orbits. *J Nucl Med* 1989;30:795(abst).

49. Van Train K, Kiat H, Cullom J, et al. Myocardial perfusion SPECT protocols. In: Garcia EV, ed. *Imaging guidelines for nuclear cardiology procedures. J Nucl Cardiol* 1996;May/June: G34–G45.

50. Kahn JK, Henderson EB, Akers AS, et al. Prediction of reversibility of perfusion defects with a single post-exercise technetium-

## Surface Shading

Surface shading refers to methods that display the actual myocardial shape derived directly from image voxels. These methods originated from those used to generate 3D displays of bony surfaces from computed tomography (CT) imaging (6).

Generating a surface-shaded display requires three steps: segmentation, boundary-tracking, and two-dimensional (2D) projection. Segmentation is the process of separating the myocardium from the background and can be accomplished using various methods, such as hand-tracing the myocardium in every slice, or using a thresholding technique in which pixels with values greater than the threshold are assumed to be part of the myocardium, and all other pixels are assumed to be background. The goal of the segmentation process is to produce a binary data set in which myocardial voxels (volume elements) have a value of 1 and background voxels have a value of 0. A boundary-tracking algorithm is then used to identify the surface of the myocardium as the boundary between

1's and 0's. The resultant binary data set is rendered as a shaded surface by rotating it to the desired viewing angle and projecting it onto a two-dimensional image plane. Figure 4.1 shows slices from a technetium 99m ($^{99m}$Tc)-sestamibi myocardial perfusion study. This patient had an infarct in the anteroapical region, with an associated apical aneurysm. Figure 4.2 shows four views of this patient's myocardium, rendered using the threshold technique as implemented by Nowak (7).

The advantage of this kind of display is that it is often fast and easy to implement, and with the proper segmentation can give useful results. The disadvantage of this technique is that most cardiac SPECT studies contain both physiologic and anatomic information. To segment a SPECT study into a binary data set often ignores some of the important physiologic information present in the scan. Another disadvantage is that improper segmentation from incorrect tracing or thresholds can give erroneous results. Unfortunately, since single thresholds are generally used for segmenting the myocardium, improper segmentation is a common finding.

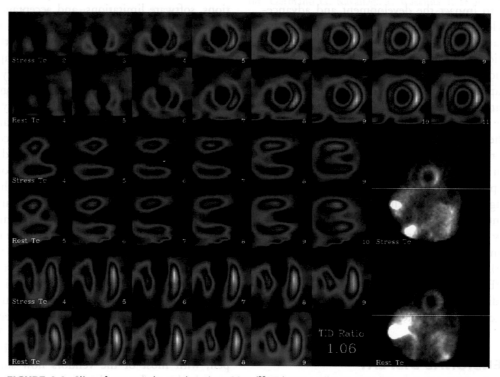

**FIGURE 4.1.** Slices from a 1-day technetium 99m ($^{99m}$Tc)-sestamibi myocardial perfusion study of a patient with large fixed defects in the septum, anterior wall, and apex. The divergence of the myocardial walls toward the apex (best seen in the horizontal and vertical long-axis slices) suggests the presence of an apical aneurysm. The six rows contain, from *top* to *bottom: stress short-axis, rest short-axis, stress vertical long-axis, rest vertical long-axis, stress horizontal long-axis, and rest horizontal long-axis slices. In addition, two representative views of the acquired single photon emission computed tomography (SPECT) projections are shown at the* bottom right (stress is on *top,* rest is on *bottom*), as well as a measurement of transient ischemic dilatation (TID). This TID measurement is the ratio of the stress endocardial chamber volume to the rest endocardial chamber volume, and is within normal limits for this patient.

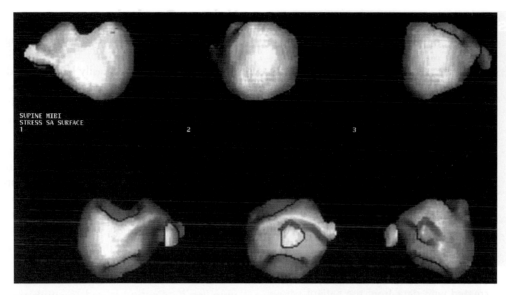

**FIGURE 4.2.** Four views of a three dimensional (3D) shaded surface display of the patient whose stress/rest sestamibi perfusion slices are shown in Fig. 4.1. The orientation is similar to the horizontal long-axis views, with the apex at the top. Note the large apical defect, corresponding to the apical aneurysm.

One study showed that surface-shaded displays of myocardial perfusion were as sensitive as quantitative bull's-eye analysis and standard slice displays, and showed a trend toward higher specificity (2). The authors concluded that surface shading is a valuable tool for determining the presence, extent, and location of coronary artery disease (CAD) and can be a useful first-look tool for referring physicians.

## Surface Modeling

The surface model display differs from the surface-shaded display in that graphics primitives (such as triangles, plates, and patches), instead of the raw voxels, are used to form a model of the surface of the myocardium. The model is generally built from coordinates extracted from the myocardium, or another surface of interest, during a surface detection process.

As an example, the method used in the Emory Cardiac Toolbox for detecting the surface of the myocardium is a maximal-count circumferential profile technique based on a

hybrid-sampling scheme in which the apical portion of the myocardium is sampled in spherical coordinates and the remaining myocardium is sampled in cylindrical coordinates (Fig. 4.3). The coordinates of each sampled point are saved for use in generating the 3D surface models. The model is built by filtering the sampled coordinates and gen-

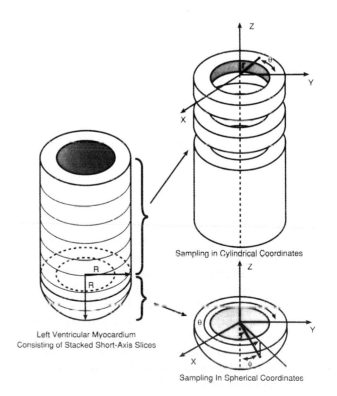

**FIGURE 4.3.** Hybrid sampling scheme in which maximum-count circumferential profiles are automatically generated from a stacked volume of short-axis slices. The apical portion is sampled using a spherical coordinate system *(bottom right)*, and the remaining portion of the myocardium is sampled on a slice-by-slice basis, using a cylindrical coordinate system *(top right)*. Each point in the profile represents the maximum number of counts per pixel encountered along the radius of search for each angular sample. (From Cooke CD, Garcia EV, Folks RD, et al. Visualization of cardiovascular nuclear medicine tomographic perfusion studies. In: *Proceedings of the first conference on visualization in biomedical computing*. Atlanta, GA: IEEE Computer Society Press, 1990:185–190, with permission).

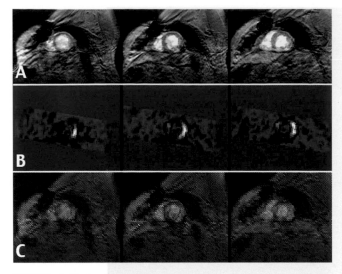

**FIGURE 4.12.** Cardiac SPECT perfusion images registered with anatomic magnetic resonance imaging (MRI) of the same patient. From *top* to *bottom rows* are shown ED short-axis slices of **(A)** MRI, **(B)** registered SPECT, and **(C)** unified MRI and SPECT. This patient had a severe anterior-apical perfusion defect associated with a myocardial infarction.

was validated by calculating the difference between user-identified landmarks in the two images after transformation, using six MRI/PET image pairs and an average of 14 landmarks per pair. The accuracy was determined to be 1.3 ± 1.1 mm for the end-diastolic images and 1.95 ± 1.6 mm for end-systolic images.

## Registration of Echocardiographic and Metabolism Images

Cardiac ultrasound images have also been aligned to PET images of glucose metabolism. In the study described by Savi et al. (38), anatomic landmarks were interactively chosen in both short-axis echocardiograms and short-axis PET images. In particular, the two papillary muscles and the

inferior junction of the right ventricle were identified in short-axis images acquired using both acquisition modalities. The registration was performed in the plane defined by the three landmarks; a least-squares minimization was performed to determine the best rotation, scaling, and translation to transform one set of $(x, y)$ coordinates into the other. This technique was demonstrated on two case studies. While this work is still in a preliminary stage, it is important, given the high availability and utilization of echocardiography. If found to be useful, it could easily be extended to process high-resolution SPECT images, and perhaps be automated to improve its usability and reproducibility.

## Registration of SPECT and Coronary Angiographic Data

Ideally, accurate assessment of the extent and severity of CAD requires the integration of physiologic information derived from SPECT perfusion images and anatomic information derived from coronary angiography. This integration has been performed by explicitly registering a 3D LV model representing myocardial perfusion with the patient's own 3D coronary artery tree, and presenting both in a single unified display. The patient-specific coronary arterial tree is obtained from a 3D geometric reconstruction performed on simultaneously acquired, digital, biplane angiographic projections, or from two single plane projections acquired at different angles (39). The 3D reconstructed arterial tree is approximated by successive conical segments, and scaled and rotated to fit onto the myocardial surface. The left and/or right coronary arteries are registered with the myocardial perfusion surface model by automatically minimizing a cost function that describes the relationships of the coronary artery tree with the interventricular and atrioventricular groove and the surface of the myocardium (40). Figure 4.13 illustrates this unified display. Reports have described preliminary validations of this technique in animal studies (41); human study validations are currently being performed (42).

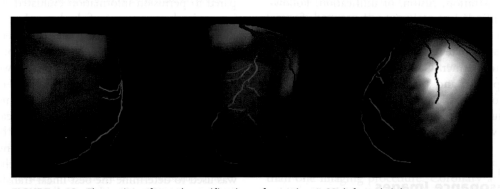

**FIGURE 4.13.** Three views from the unification of a patient's 3D left and right coronary artery trees with the SPECT perfusion images. Perfusion is color-coded onto the LV epicardial surface; the *blacked-out region* indicates an anterior/apical perfusion defect. The *green portion* of the LAD indicates the segment of the artery distal to the stenosis. Note the overlap between the stenosed left anterior descending coronary artery and the perfusion defect.

Similar work has been reported by Krause et al. (43). Three-dimensional models of the LV epicardium were generated from SPECT and aligned with 3D models of the left coronary artery tree created from angiograms. In this work, however, the alignment was performed by using acquisition parameters for SPECT and angiography to determine "patient coordinates" of the two models. Once these coordinates were known, the models could be easily aligned, and a simple translation between the two models was applied, if necessary, to refine the match. A display was generated by reprojecting both 3D models into the desired view angle.

## TELERADIOLOGY

Over the past several years, physicians have become more and more interested in being able to read studies remotely, for a variety of reasons. This section presents an introductory discussion of teleradiology, which is defined as the transfer of medical images beyond the boundaries of a local area network (LAN) for professional interpretation. The purpose of a teleradiology installation can be classified based on the location of the interpreting physician with respect to the imaging center.

### Site-to-Site: The Remote Physician

There are several arrangements in which the most appropriate physician to interpret a study is not on-site. A common example is a small remote clinic that does not have a caseload to justify a full-time NM specialist. Another case is a group of physicians, each located at different clinics and each specializing in a specific class of procedures. These sites have several common features:

- They are at fixed locations, so the use of fixed, high-speed digital lines is possible and usually preferred for their increased speed and reliability.
- There is typically a large amount of data transferred between the locations on a regular basis, reducing the per-study cost of the transmission.
- Response times are usually not critical. If studies are transferred during the day and reports are dictated and returned twice a day, service is considered excellent. Exceptions exist such as emergency studies or special requests.

### Site-to-Remote: On Call/Emergency Readings

On-call reading is a common use of teleradiology. It differs from the site-to-site arrangement because the volume of data transferred is less, the demand is more variable from day to day, and the budget for equipment at the remote site

is lower. Furthermore, the physician is often mobile, which makes it difficult to establish permanent high-speed lines. Some features of on-call reading are the following:

- There can be multiple locations. Usually, the primary location is the physician's home, but the physician is often mobile, or even out of town.
- The volume of data is usually low, averaging only a few studies per day, but the off hours and emergency nature of the studies makes transfer time important.
- Equipment and communications costs are often the personal responsibility of the physician.

### The Occasional Consult

Teleradiology can be used to share data between widely separated sites on an occasional basis, for situations such as expert consultation, rare findings, collection of teaching materials, and publication of manuscripts. The issues with these situations are much different from those cited above. The transfer time and technology is usually unimportant; a disk in overnight mail is often adequate. Because of the diversity of possible equipment and the lack of routine data exchange, the primary concern is the compatibility of media and data formats between the sender and receiver.

### The Sender

The site at which the images originate requires software that provides access to the patient image database, converts the images to a standard format (if needed), and transfers the data to the remote site.

There are two classes of image data servers: push servers and pull servers. If the server originates the transfer, it is referred to as a push server; if the remote site originates the transfer, it is referred to as a pull server. Though there are advantages to both types of servers, the most efficient use of an image data server comes when the person who identifies the need originates the transfer. For example, when a study is identified as a particular physician's responsibility, it can be pushed to his system; if the physician then has a need for additional data or wishes to review additional studies, he can pull the studies without the help of on-site personnel.

Image format and transfer protocols determine compatibility between the image server and the receiving station. Often, data must be converted to a common format on the sending or receiving system:

- American College of Radiology/National Electrical Manufacturers' Association (NEMA) Digital Imaging and Communications in Medicine (DICOM) is the standard for image data exchange between systems. It fully specifies the data formats, network protocols, and necessary display information to allow disparate systems to exchange information. The following network protocols do not specify image format, only the network protocols.

allowing simultaneous acquisition of anterior and posterior images. A double-detector camera with SPECT capability could also increase throughout for 360 degrees SPECT imaging by halving imaging time. This gain in sensitivity may also be traded off to give more precise images by allowing the use of higher resolution collimators.

These improvements, however, may mean very little for cardiac SPECT where a 180-degree orbit is recommended (2). The new technetium cardiac agents may benefit from a 360-degree orbit, in which case an opposed double-detector system may prove useful. The addition of a second detector at 180 degrees does not result in doubled sensitivity for cardiac imaging because counts in posterior planar images are much more severely attenuated than those of the anterior projections. Most manufacturers offer systems where the two detectors are not mounted rigidly opposite each other but may be rotated next to each other (90 degrees) on the gantry, a configuration that is more useful for cardiac imaging (Fig. 5.1).

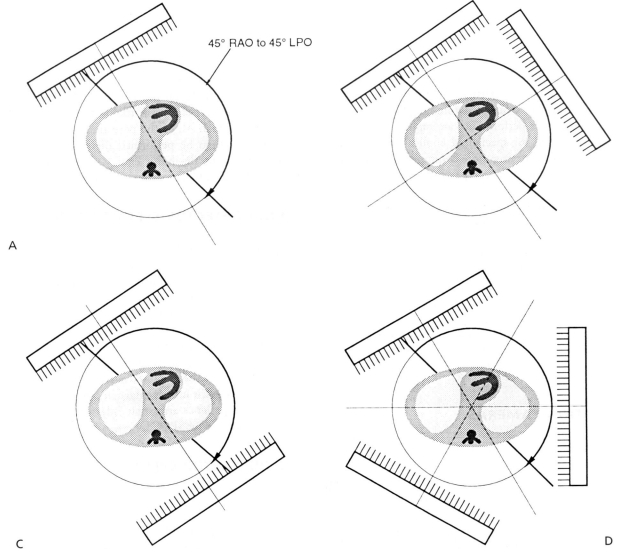

**FIGURE 5.1.** Multidetector SPECT camera configurations. **A:** Standard single-detector camera. One important consideration is that for thallium 201 (²⁰¹Tl) cardiac SPECT, over 66% of the counts will be collected in the 180 degrees between 45 degrees RAO (right anterior oblique) and 45 degrees LPO (left posterior oblique). **B:** Addition of a second detector at 90 degrees doubles the sensitivity for both 180- and 360-degree orbits and is preferred for cardiac imaging. Flexibility may be lost, however, where simultaneous anterior and posterior images are desired. **C:** Addition of a second detector at 180 degrees will double the sensitivity for 360-degree SPECT, but provides no increase in sensitivity if an 180-degree orbit is recommended. **D:** Three detectors, mounted at 60-degree intervals, will increase sensitivity by only 50% for 180 degrees SPECT, but triples the sensitivity for 360-degree orbits.

Drawbacks of double detector cameras include the increase in quality control required by the addition of the second detector and some loss of flexibility. Double-detector systems do not allow the same flexibility of movement that is enjoyed with many single-detector systems. This may prevent them from being easily used for some types of planar imaging (such as gated blood pool) where it is often difficult to position the camera correctly. There is a great deal of variation between manufacturers in the camera movement allowed for planar imaging.

Triple-detector cameras are usually dedicated to SPECT imaging. The three detectors, as discussed for double-detector systems, will result in increased sensitivity that may be used to increase throughput, counts, or resolution. These systems have not had a major impact on cardiac imaging with 180-degree orbits for the reasons discussed above. Triple-detector SPECT systems are best suited for clinics that do a great deal of 360-degree SPECT and can afford to have a camera dedicated solely to that task.

## COLLIMATORS

Low-energy all-purpose (LEAP) and general all-purpose (GAP) collimators were once the workhorse collimators for cardiac nuclear medicine. Development of technetium 99m ($^{99m}$Tc)-based radiopharmaceuticals that result in higher counts has made the use of high-resolution (HRES) collimators routine.

Collimators must be made of material that cannot be easily penetrated by photons of the range used in nuclear medicine (70 to 300 keV). This limits the selection to dense metals such as lead, silver, gold, and tungsten. Most collimators are made of lead, but some tungsten collimators are available at great expense.

### Low-Energy All-Purpose Versus High-Resolution Collimators

Most parallel hole collimators are classified as one of two types—LEAP or HRES. The distinguishing feature of these collimators is usually the hole length or bore. Increasing the length of the hole increases resolution by decreasing the angle subtended by the hole (Fig. 5.2). This increase in resolution comes at the expense of sensitivity. It should be noted that, in general, images with better resolution do not need as many counts to achieve the same image quality. Unless the images are very count poor, or must be acquired very quickly, HRES collimation is generally preferred to LEAP collimation.

### Converging Collimation

Converging collimators allow more of the crystal to be used, increasing sensitivity (Fig. 5.3). Converging collimators require more complex setup procedures than do parallel hole collimators if used for SPECT. Once the projections are acquired, converging collimators require special reconstruction software that may result in much longer reconstruction

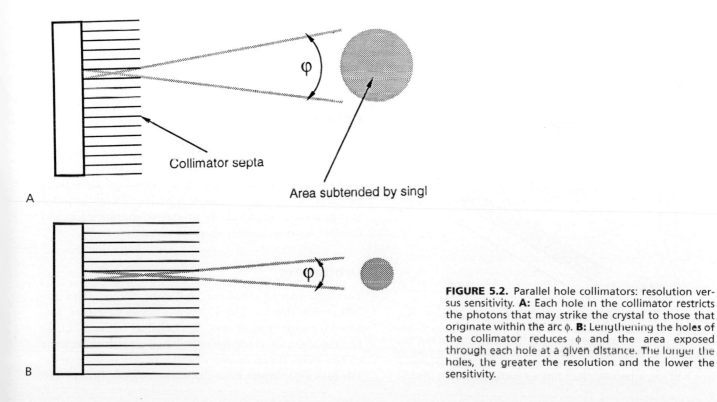

FIGURE 5.2. Parallel hole collimators: resolution versus sensitivity. **A:** Each hole in the collimator restricts the photons that may strike the crystal to those that originate within the arc φ. **B:** Lengthening the holes of the collimator reduces φ and the area exposed through each hole at a given distance. The longer the holes, the greater the resolution and the lower the sensitivity.

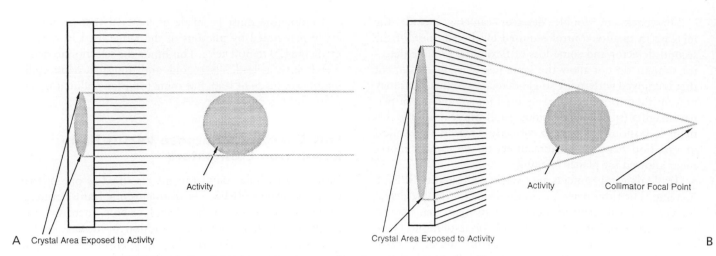

**FIGURE 5.3.** Parallel hole and fan beam collimators. **A:** Parallel hole collimators expose the crystal only to photons that originate directly in front of the collimator (ideally). The image formed will be a projection of the radionuclide distribution the same size as the distribution. **B:** Fan beam collimators have holes that are directed toward a line a fixed distance in front of the collimator (parallel to the imaging table). The projection is magnified, and since more of the crystal is used, sensitivity is increased. Objects at differing distances from the collimator will be magnified by different amounts, resulting in a distorted image. Cone beam collimators are similar but converge to a point instead of a line.

times. The results of SPECT with the converging collimators, however, can be impressive. The problem associated with converging collimators in cardiac SPECT is that, while the heart may remain in the field of view for the entire study, other parts of the body in the same plane as the heart may be clipped and produce reconstruction artifacts (Fig. 5.4).

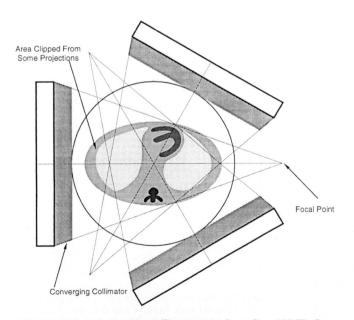

**FIGURE 5.4.** Converging collimators and cardiac SPECT. Converging collimators mounted on a triple-detector system may result in greatly increased sensitivity. The large size of the thorax, however, may make it impossible to avoid clipping parts of the body from other projections. This will result in reconstruction artifacts, especially when filtered backprojection is used.

## Cast Versus Foil Collimators

Collimators are manufactured by two different processes. Cast collimators are cast in one piece, the holes being formed by a mold. Foil collimators are made by joining corrugated strips of metal to form the shape of the holes. Foil collimators may be lighter and less expensive than cast collimators, but they are more likely to have defects. Joints in the metal sometimes separate, forming gaps and inconsistencies in the collimator. Foil collimators are also more likely to have deformed holes and nonuniform angulations. It should be remembered that SPECT is not as forgiving of defects in the collimator as planar imaging.

## CAMERA ORBITS

The traditional orbit used for SPECT imaging has been circular, 360 degrees, with step-and-shoot motion. Advancements in radiopharmaceuticals and technology are making more complicated motions more appealing. Factors included in the camera orbit include the orbital arc, the movement and speed of rotation, and the shape of the camera orbit.

## Orbital Arc

For years, users have had two choices of camera orbital arc: 180 or 360 degrees. The 180-degree orbits have been preferred for some types of imaging (including cardiac SPECT) because of the severe photon attenuation experienced at some camera views. It may make it desirable to exclude less that the full back 180 degrees from the reconstruction. Arcs of 240

**TABLE 5.1. TIME TO COMPLETE A SPECT ACQUISITION
USING STEP-AND-SHOOT AND CONTINUOUS ACQUISITIONS**

| Number of Frames | Seconds/Frame | Acquisition Time in Minutes | | Lost Time |
| --- | --- | --- | --- | --- |
| | | Continuous | Step-and-Shoot[a] | |
| Long acquisition | | | | |
| 16 | 60 | 16.0 | 16.8 | 5% |
| 32 | 30 | 16.0 | 17.6 | 9% |
| 64 | 15 | 16.0 | 19.2 | 17% |
| Short acquisition | | | | |
| 16 | 12 | 3.2 | 4.0 | 20% |
| 32 | 6 | 3.2 | 4.8 | 33% |
| 64 | 3 | 3.2 | 6.4 | 50% |

[a]Lost time per frame due to camera motion: 3 seconds.
SPECT, single photon emission computed tomography.

and 270 degrees require modification of the reconstruction software and are available from a few manufacturers. Flexibility in choosing the arc may be a great advantage in multi-detector cameras, where projections are acquired over 360 degrees, regardless of whether they will be used (3).

## Step-and-Shoot or Continuous Motion

Most scintillation cameras move in a fashion called step-and-shoot as they orbit the patient. The camera moves, stops, acquires an image, moves again, stops, and acquires another image. The optimal number of stops is determined by the system resolution and the pixel size. (The better the resolution and the smaller the pixels, the more stops required.) During the time the camera moves, counts are wasted. This can be very significant since many cameras take 2 to 4 seconds to move.

Continuous-orbit cameras resolve this problem by acquiring counts at all times, even while the camera moves. Traditionally, continuous-motion cameras move slowly and smoothly while counts from designated arcs are collected to form the planar projections. The smaller the arc used for each projection, the less the blurring due to the camera's motion. Many manufactures offer a hybrid motion sometimes called continuous step-and-shoot. The camera duplicates the motion of a step-and-shoot acquisition, but the camera continues to acquire counts while it steps.

Table 5.1 gives the lost time due to step-and-shoot motion for both long (16 minutes, typical of most cardiac SPECT) and short (3- to 5-minute) acquisitions assuming that the lost time per frame is 3 seconds. Most cardiac SPECT studies use 32 or 64 total frames. The 16 frame entry in the table assumes a 90-degree dual-detector SPECT system and an acquisition with 32 total projections (16 per detector).

## Body Contour Orbits

One highly advertised feature of many SPECT systems is the ability to do elliptical or body contour orbits (Fig. 5.5).

These orbits seek to minimize the distance from the camera to the body throughout the tomographic acquisition, maximizing resolution. Some research indicates that body contour orbits may result in unacceptable image artifacts, particularly when 180-degree orbits are used. The use of body contour orbits for cardiac SPECT is a subject of much debate (4–6).

## 18FDG IMAGING WITH SCINTILLATION CAMERAS

Positron emission tomography of fluorine-8 deoxyglucose (18FDG) has proven to be a powerful tool for determining myocardial viability. Interest in the use of this positron-emitting tracer for tumor imaging as well as myocardial viability has driven the search for a more economical way of imaging 18FDG than conventional PET scanners. Two approaches to imaging 18FDG without a PET scanner have been developed: 511-keV SPECT and coincidence imaging with modified dual-detector SPECT cameras. While both approaches have their clinical role, they should not be expected to produce the pristine images of conventional PET, or to duplicate its sensitivity and specificity. Both modalities suffer from poor count sensitivity, compared to PET, and in practice poorer resolution.

## 511-keV SPECT

The 511-keV SPECT requires that a camera optimized for imaging photons at low energies (60 to 400 keV) be adapted to image 511-keV photons produced after a positron/electron annihilation event. This necessitates the addition of a collimator designed for 511 keV photons. Septal thickness must be increased, and the trade-offs of sensitivity versus resolution require that the holes be larger and longer. The resulting collimator may weigh three to six times that of a conventional collimator, which is prohibitively heavy for many systems. In addition,

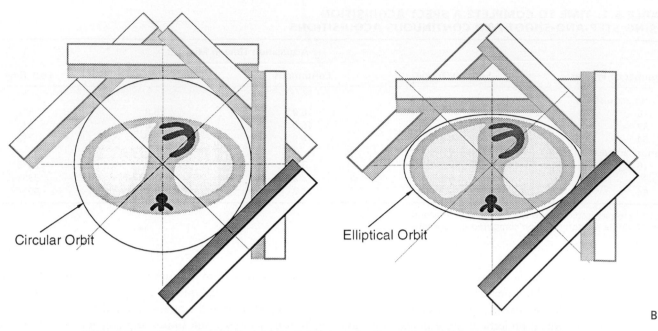

Circular Orbit

Elliptical Orbit

A

B

**FIGURE 5.5.** Circular and elliptical orbits. **A:** When a circular camera orbit is used, the camera is close to the body in some projections but far away in others. **B:** Elliptical and body-contour orbits try to maximize resolution by keeping the camera as close to the body as possible during the entire orbit. The asymmetric position of the heart within the body may lead to a widely varying heart-to-camera distance (and thus resolution) during the orbit, resulting in reconstruction artifacts.

more shielding may be needed in the camera detector to prevent image contamination by 511-keV photons from other parts of the body outside of the camera's field of view (7).

Traditionally, scintillation cameras use ⅜-inch thallium-doped sodium iodide crystals [NaI(Tl)]. Thin crystals are preferred because they produce better resolution for the most frequently used radionuclides. While the ⅜-inch crystal thickness produces a photopeak efficiency of 84% for 140-keV 99mTc photons, the efficiency drops to 13% at 511 keV. Using crystals of ½-, ⅝-, and ¾-inches can increase this efficiency to 17%, 21%, and 24%, respectively (8). Increasing crystal thickness, however, results in a loss of spatial resolution. Manufacturers that offer thicker crystal cameras have indicated that the loss of resolution is small and does not significantly impact the quality of conventional low-energy images.

The combination of poor crystal efficiency and heavy collimators compromises the sensitivity and resolution of these systems. Nevertheless, because high resolution and sensitivity are not requirements of imaging myocardial viability, this high-energy collimation SPECT imaging approach has been found useful in this application. Simultaneous dual-isotope imaging of stress $^{99m}$Tc-sestamibi and rest $^{18}$FDG is possible on some cameras and has been reported to be highly successful in diagnosing coronary artery disease, particularly in assessing myocardial viability (9).

## Coincidence Imaging

Another approach to the imaging of the 511 keV photon pairs produced after a positron/electron annihilation event is the adaptation of state-of-the-art digital dual-detector SPECT systems to function as a PET scanner (10). The collimators are removed, and coincidence circuitry is introduced to perform positron imaging. This type of technology is usually referred to as "coincidence imaging" to contrast with the PET approach.

The spatial resolution of coincidence imaging systems is between 4 and 6 mm, at least as good as conventional PET scanners. The main drawback of coincidence systems compared to conventional PET systems is in the area of sensitivity. NaI(Tl) crystals are not very efficient for the detection of photons at 511 keV (as discussed above for 511-keV SPECT). Geometry is also a factor. In a traditional PET scanner, a 360-degree ring of detectors surrounds the patient. In most coincidence systems, you are limited to the two detectors of a dual-detector SPECT system, leaving the sides open and losing the possibility of imaging photons emitted at these angles.

Attenuation correction is even more of a problem in coincidence imaging (and in PET) than in SPECT because there is attenuation along the entire path of the body between the two camera detectors. In SPECT, the attenuation is only from the point of origin of the photon to the

**TABLE 5.2. PROPERTIES OF SCINTILLATORS**

| Detector | p (g/cm³) | Effective Z | Decay time (ns) | Light output (%) | Hygroscopic |
|---|---|---|---|---|---|
| NaI(Tl) | 3.67 | 50.6 | 230 | 100 | Yes |
| CsI(Tl) | 4.51 | 54.1 | 1,000 | 45 | No |
| CsI(Na) | 4.51 | 54.1 | 630 | 85 | Yes |
| BGO | 7.13 | 74.2 | 350 | 15 | No |
| LSO | 7.40 | 65.5 | 42 | 75 | No |

camera face. Therefore, for a photon originating in the center of the abdomen, attenuation from half the abdomen's girth occurs, while in coincidence, attenuation occurs from the abdomen's center to each detector, 180 degrees apart. Attenuation of the inferior wall of the myocardium makes [18]FDG myocardial viability images difficult to interpret without attenuation correction. Conventional PET performs attenuation correction based on a transmission scan, and similar technology must be incorporated into coincidence scanners before they can be used for imaging of the myocardium (11).

### LSO Hybrid PET/SPECT Coincidence Cameras

An exciting recent development has been the arrival of a new scintillation material lutetium oxyorthosilicate (LSO) (12) that is suitable for high-energy coincidence imaging. LSO has a higher density than BGO (bismuth germanate oxide) (Table 5.2) which when combined with its slightly lower effective atomic number leads to a similar effective attenuation and thus excellent stopping power for 511 keV. LSO can stop a 511-keV photon in about 1.16 cm, BGO in 1.05 cm, and NaI(Tl) in 2.88 cm. Yet LSO has five times the light output of BGO and about one-tenth the decay time, making it an excellent scintillator. One drawback of the LSO crystal is that it produces its own natural radiation.

LSO crystal elements are being used by one manufacturer as one of the key elements of a hybrid PET/SPECT coincidence camera that can perform both SPECT and PET (13). The LSO crystal is waffled with a conventional NaI(Tl) crystal to make up the scintillator element. The NaI(Tl) crystal is used both for SPECT imaging and for detecting and subtracting the background radiation emitted from the LSO crystal. Because of the excellent imaging characteristics of the LSO components, it is predicted that this hybrid system with two opposing flat detectors will have similar PET imaging performance to a low-end conventional PET scanner at reduced cost.

## SOLID-STATE DETECTORS

Solid-state detectors have been developed with the aim of eliminating the complex system of scintillation crystals and photomultiplier tubes used in conventional scintillation cameras. Two approaches to the incorporation of semiconductor electronics have been developed. The first retains the scintillation crystal but replaces the photomultiplier tubes with a solid-state photodiode. The other approach eliminates the need for the scintillation crystal altogether through the use of direct detection of the high-energy photons with a semiconducting detector.

An example of the first approach is the use of an array of 3-mm × 3-mm pixel elements consisting of a thallium-activated cesium iodide [CsI(Tl)] scintillation crystal and a silicon photodiode (14). The benefits of the system include a fixed, high intrinsic spatial resolution at any energy and true digital positioning. Because photomultiplier tubes are not used, these systems can be made significantly smaller, lighter (23 kg), and relatively mobile compared to conventional scintillation cameras that can weight up to 2,300 kg. These detectors can also be built with a sodium-activated cesium iodide crystal [CsI(Na)] for somewhat different properties as described in Table 5.2 (15,16).

In the second approach, a photon emitted from an organ strikes a solid-state crystal, such as cadmium zinc telluride (CdZnTe or CZT), which is a semiconductor that converts the photon directly to a digital electronic signal (17). This is a one-step process rather than the two-step process used in conventional SPECT NaI(Tl) crystals. Moreover, in a semiconductor detector, each location in the detector is a separate digital pixel, and once it is activated by a photon strike, it provides the position of the interaction with high spatial and energy resolution. This is a much more direct detection of the position and energy of the emitted photon than the process used in conventional SPECT detectors. The increase in spatial and energy resolution of these solid-state detectors is translated to higher contrast resolution and improved detection of abnormalities.

mrad (79). For the technologist, additional exposure can result from scattered transmission radiation originating from the patient. Absorbed dose from scattered radiation can be up to an order of magnitude ten times less than from direct exposure to the transmission radiation (37). However, site planning should provide conservative estimates for exposure as part of a radiation safety program. It is possible to be exposed to some of the primary beam radiation for certain positions of the detector although partial collimation of the source is used. With some systems, it is required to load the external source with activity such as $^{99m}$Tc or $^{201}$Tl (34). Additional exposure to the technologist will result from handling of this activity, and guidelines for proper handling should be followed.

The half-lives of the proposed external sources require them to be periodically replaced (see Table 6.1). This requirement is minimized by manufacturing the sources with a filter made out of an attenuating material such as copper that is placed in front of the beam in the housing to harden the beam and reduce its intensity (40). Beam hardening by the filter removes low-energy photons that are less likely to penetrate the patient and therefore increase patient dose with little contribution to image information. When the source decays significantly, the filter can be removed to replenish the source.

## CLINICAL STATUS OF ATTENUATION CORRECTION

The potential clinical ramifications of a fully implemented attenuation correction approach are substantial. This approach should provide enhanced visual and quantitative analyses through an improved count density distribution that approaches homogeneity in the presence of normal perfusion; higher sensitivity for detection of disease, including mild-moderate, single-vessel, and multivessel disease with relative balanced flow reduction; higher specificity due to reduced artifacts from attenuation; and improved delineation of myocardial viability in terms of accuracy of assessment of tracer uptake in dysfunctional areas. Unfortunately, truly clinical studies on the value of currently implemented attenuation correction methods are few, and most of the studies to date are validation studies. It is likely that with recent improvements designed to overcome first-generation hardware/software systems for attenuation correction, these long-awaited investigations will soon appear in the literature.

What has been established is that the various approaches improve the relative uniformity of tracer uptake in low-likelihood subjects for a range of systems, protocols, and transmission sources. Ficaro et al. (42) described the impact of a SPECT transmission-based attenuation correction method on the homogeneity of perfusion in ten normal volunteers with adenosine $^{201}$Tl stress-reinjection using simultaneous emission-transmission imaging with $^{241}$Am as the transmis-

sion source. Using a nine-segment polar map model, lateral-to-posterior and basal-to-apical wall ratios showed statistically significant improvement in homogeneity (relative value equal to 1.0) with attenuation correction compared with uncorrected images. In a later study, as part of an investigation of the diagnostic accuracy of an attenuation correction technique in stress $^{99m}$Tc-sestamibi studies, the same group studied 59 patients (22 males) with ≤5% probability of disease also using a triple-detector system with $^{241}$Am as the transmission source (43). Improved perfusion homogeneity was also demonstrated for males and females compared with uncorrected images. Statistically, this study went on to demonstrate no significant difference between male and female attenuation corrected databases (20 patients each), and therefore a gender-composite polar map for quantitative analysis was formed. Visual normalcy rates were significantly improved from 0.88 to 0.98.

Prvulovich et al. (80) performed a similar analysis to that of Ficaro et al. using pharmacologic stress on 36 $^{201}$Tl studies. This study used a $^{153}$Gd transmission sources and an MLEM-based reconstruction for attenuation correction and FBP-based method for attenuation map reconstruction. Using a 17-segment polar map model, improved tracer homogeneity in both male and female populations, as measured by septal-to-lateral wall ratios, and anterior-basal wall activity were demonstrated to be significantly improved compared with the noncorrected images. Chouraqui et al. (81) showed similar improvement in 42 patients (29 males ≤5% prob. of disease) using a 31-segment model with $^{201}$Tl SPECT and $^{153}$Gd. Scanning line source Matsunari et al. (82) investigated normal perfusion distributions in rest $^{201}$Tl/stress $^{99m}$Tc-sestamibi acquired simultaneously using a similar system to that of Ficaro et al. In this study of 21 low likelihood (≤5%) patients, segmental analysis demonstrated significant differences in attenuation corrected stress and rest images. This finding highlighted differences that can exist with attenuation corrected studies, and that method-specific considerations are required including method-specific attenuation corrected normal databases.

Studies on the diagnostic accuracy of attenuation correction techniques are more varied in their findings compared with low-likelihood populations (42,43,83–87). Ficaro et al. (43) investigated the diagnostic accuracy of attenuation correction compared with uncorrected studies in 60 patients (38 males) with angiographic documented coronary artery disease using a stress $^{99m}$Tc-sestamibi/rest $^{201}$Tl protocol. For detection of coronary artery disease (CAD), sensitivity/specificity values significantly improved from 0.78/0.46 (without correction) to 0.84/0.82 with correction for visual analysis and 0.84/0.46 (NC) to 0.88/0.82 with quantitation analysis using a gender-composite normal database described earlier. ROC analysis demonstrated significantly improved discrimination for right coronary disease, but left circumflex (LCX) discrimination was not improved significantly. Significant improvement in attenuation correction to localize diseased vessels in single-vessel and multivessel disease was also demonstrated. Kluge et al. (84) evaluated attenuation correction with 90-degree dual-detector and $^{153}$Gd scanning line sources comparing attenuation corrected and uncorrected studies in two groups of males and $^{99m}$Tc-tetrofosmin stress imaging (bicycle exercise and pharmacologic) (84). The first group consisted of 25 males with CAD of the right coronary artery (RCA) and/or LCX arteries, all without significant narrowing of the LAD. The second group (also 25 males) had <10% likelihood for the presence of CAD. In this study, diagnostic accuracy was significantly improved in the first group and homogeneity of tracer in group 2 was also significantly improved in this limited study.

## RESULTS

Gallowitsch et al. (85) also investigated the effect of attenuation correction on diagnostic accuracy and the impact on the extent and severity of perfusion abnormalities in 107 patients (69 males) undergoing stress redistribution imaging with exercise (bicycle) or pharmacologic (dipyridamole) stress and dual 90° scanning line source $^{153}$Gd transmission imaging. The patients were assigned to two groups: chest pain ($n$ = 49) with no history of infarction or intervention and known CAD ($n$ = 58) with previous myocardial infarction. Analysis of severity and extent showed. Polar map analysis was performed using a 31-segment model. Overall sensitivity was improved with attenuation correction from 79.2 to 94.3. Specificity improved from 79.6 to 90.7. The authors reported that extent and severity were significantly influenced by attenuation correction, as fewer abnormal and less severe abnormal segments were demonstrated with attenuation correction, consistent with other studies.

Hendel et al. (86) recently presented results from the first prospective multicenter trial evaluating attenuation correction using $^{153}$Gd line sources with stress $^{99m}$Tc-sestamibi imaging obtained from dual-isotope and one day $^{99m}$Tc-sestamibi studies. This technique of attenuation correction employed photopeak scatter and variable spatial resolution compensation. Ninety-six patients with angiographic-demonstrated CAD and 88 with low-likelihood CAD (<5%) were studied. Detection of >50% stenosis was similar with and without correction (0.76 vs. 0.75, nonsignificant). Normalcy rate, however, was significantly improved with correction using visual analysis (86% vs. 96%) and quantitative analysis (86% vs. 97%). There was, however, a reduction in the detection of extensive CAD.

Becker et al. (87) investigated a method that also incorporated a correction technique for patient motion in conjunction with the corrections for scatter, attenuation, and spatial resolution. They investigated 61 normal studies (41 males ≤5% likelihood of disease), 13 patients with high probability

of normal results, and 51 patients with angiographic CAD. This study used a simultaneous dual 90° emission-transmission acquisition on a dual 90-degree detector system with $^{153}$Gd as the transmission source. This preliminary study showed improved diagnostic accuracy when distance-dependent spatial resolution with attenuation correction and correction for patient motion. The incremental value of the motion correction program to the image quality was not clearly delineated but suggests that it is an important part of a comprehensive approach.

The presence of artifacts or complications from enhancement of visceral uptake by attenuation correction is a common limitation cited in clinical studies with attenuation correction. Attenuation correction, without scatter correction, unmasks the presence of scatter artifacts (6). Ficaro et al. (43) reported that with 119 $^{99m}$Tc-seatamibi stress images, liver activity was problematic in six uncorrected studies and 12 corrected studies. Kluge et al. (84) reported that in 50 stress studies, enhanced liver activity was observed in two uncorrected and three attenuation corrected studies. Gallowitsch et al. (85) reported that enhanced gut activity affected the posterior wall in attenuation corrected studies obtained with dipyridamole compared with those studies with bicycle exercise. Most of the clinical studies suggest that scatter correction and/or nonstationary resolution compensation seems to be indicated to further optimize the performance clinically.

Notably absent in the literature is the description of quality control protocols describing minimal hardware performance, including transmission imaging prior to the acquisition of study data. It is highly likely that quality control is more important in assessing clinical studies with new technologies and methods compared with established methods, particularly as we come to understand these new techniques in the absence of industry standards (Table 6.2). In the absence of a quality control knowledge base for attenuation correction, one has to wonder if the inconsistent results of early clinical investigations might not have been affected by suboptimal instrumentation performance or the lack of standards for interpretation. In highly controlled trials or single laboratory studies, there is usually present sophisticated technical support (physics), and results are very positive. It is an important purpose of multicenter evaluations to objectively assess the value of a technique across the range of circumstances affecting clinical operation in diverse laboratories. This points to the need for further prospective multicenter evaluation and the development of quality control and interpretative tools to fully evaluate the potential and limitations of attenuation correction methods.

### SUMMARY

We are very enthusiastic about the future potential of emerging attenuation correction techniques for cardiac perfusion SPECT, especially as current developments respond-

ations of edges are required, it is advisable to repeat the calculation a few times to assess the degree to which any alterations affect outcome for individual studies. Other checks for consistency include ensuring that the reported volumes and ejection fraction values are in the physiologic range, as well as consistent with the visual impression provided by the cinematic playback of tomographic slices.

## Limitations of Gated SPECT Quantitation

Accuracy of the absolute volumes for the smallest volumes, and the highest ejection fractions, should be viewed with some skepticism, given recent studies suggesting that most quantitative gated SPECT algorithms underestimate volumes in this range (68,84). This phenomenon is due to the relatively low resolution of nuclear cardiac images, resulting in the partial or complete obliteration of the LV cavity at end-systole in patients with small ventricles, especially in conjunction with $^{201}$Tl imaging. Underestimating end-systolic volumes can, in turn, cause overestimation of LVEF (85,86). This problem may be obviated through the use of correcting factors (87) or greater acquisition or reconstruction zooms (7). However, it should be stressed that an abnormally high ejection fraction in a patient with normal perfusion and a small heart can be safely reported as being in the normal range. The greater concern is the difficulty that underestimation of small hearts volumes poses for the construction of gated SPECT normal limits. To date, only two publications address the issues of gated SPECT volume and ejection fraction normal limits (88,89). These studies agree to a remarkable extent with regard to gated SPECT values found for large numbers of normal subjects. However, it should be noted that these gated SPECT volume limits are similar to those reported in the echocardiography (90) and MRI (91) literature, but substantially smaller than the normal values found by contrast angiography (92) and cine computed tomography (CT) (93) studies. In contrast, gated SPECT normal limits for LVEF (88,89) are essentially the same as those found for the other imaging modalities just mentioned. Therefore, caution will need to be exercised in applying any approaches that seek to correct the smallest gated SPECT LV volumes (85), as such corrections are likely to require recalibrating gated SPECT normal limits. This remains an active area of investigation.

## CONCLUSION

Gated myocardial perfusion SPECT imaging is an easy and inexpensive way to add global and regional myocardial function assessment to perfusion assessment using nuclear techniques. The perfusion and function data are acquired simultaneously, are intrinsically registered, and can be quantitatively measured in an accurate and reproducible fashion, as demonstrated by a wealth of published reports using a variety of algorithms and validation standards. While the hardware needed to perform gated SPECT imaging is the same as for standard SPECT imaging and the only requirement is that adequate counts be collected, special care must be exercised in the quality control of gated SPECT data. This is especially true with regard to the identification of gating errors when a wide cardiac beat length acceptance window is used. The development of automated quality control tools and the provision for an extra acquisition frame to hold rejected counts is likely to increase the reliability of both the perfusion and the function component of a gated SPECT study and will further promote the diffusion of this already highly successful technique.

## ACKNOWLEDGMENT

We would like to thank James A. Case, Ph.D., Cardiovascular Consultants, P.C., Kansas City, Missouri, for many of the figures used in this manuscript (86).

## REFERENCES

1. Freeman MR, Konstantinou C, Barr A, et al. Clinical comparison of 180-degree and 360-degree data collection of technetium 99m sestamibi SPECT for detection of coronary artery disease. *J Nucl Cardiol* 1998;5(1):14–18.
2. Germano G, Erel J, Kiat H, et al. Quantitative LVEF and qualitative regional function from gated thallium-201 perfusion SPECT. *J Nucl Med* 1997;38(5):749–754.
3. Everaert H, Vanhove C, Hamill JJ, et al. Cardiofocal collimators for gated single-photon emission tomographic myocardial perfusion imaging. *Eur J Nucl Med* 1998;25(1):3–7.
4. Maniawski PJ, Morgan HT, Wackers FJ. Orbit-related variation in spatial resolution as a source of artifactual defects in thallium-201 SPECT (see comments). *J Nucl Med* 1991;32(5):871–875.
5. DePuey EG, Rozanski A. Using gated technetium-99m-sestamibi SPECT to characterize fixed myocardial defects as infarct or artifact. *J Nucl Med* 1995;36(6):952–955.
6. Cullom S, Hendel R, Liu L, et al. Diagnostic accuracy and image quality of a scatter, attenuation and resolution compensation method for Tc-99m cardiac SPECT: preliminary results. *J Nucl Med* 1996;37(5):81P(abst).
7. Schwartz R, Mixon L, Germano G, et al. Gated SPECT reconstruction with zoom and depth dependent filter improves accuracy of volume and LVEF in small hearts. *J Nucl Cardiol* 1999;6(1, pt 2):S17(abst).
8. Bacharach SL, Bonow RO, Green MV. Comparison of fixed and variable temporal resolution methods for creating gated cardiac blood-pool image sequences. *J Nucl Med* 1990;31(1):38–42.
9. Port S. First-pass radionuclide angiography. In: Marcus ML, Braunwald E, eds. *Marcus cardiac imaging: a companion to Braunwald's heart disease.* Philadelphia: WB Saunders, 1996:923–941.
10. American Society of Nuclear Cardiology. Imaging guidelines for nuclear cardiology procedures. Instrumentation quality assurance and performance. *J Nucl Cardiol* 1996;3(3):G5–10.
11. Berman DS, Kiat H, Friedman JD, et al. Separate acquisition rest thallium-201/stress technetium-99m sestamibi dual-isotope myocardial perfusion single-photon emission computed tomography: a clinical validation study. *J Am Coll Cardiol* 1993;22(5):1455–1464.

12. American Society of Nuclear Cardiology. Imaging guidelines for nuclear cardiology procedures. Myocardial perfusion SPECT protocols. *J Nucl Cardiol* 1996;3(3):G34–46.

13. Germano G, Kavanagh PB, Berman DS. Effect of the number of projections collected on quantitative perfusion and left ventricular ejection fraction measurements from gated myocardial perfusion single-photon emission computed tomographic images. *J Nucl Cardiol* 1996;3(5):395–402.

14. Case J, Bateman T, Cullom S, et al. Obtaining optimum and consistent SPEW myocardial counts using an anterior planar view to determine SPECT acquisition times. *J Am Coll Cardiol* 1998;31(2 suppl A):82A–83A(abst).

15. Cooke CD, Garcia EV, Cullom SJ, et al. Determining the accuracy of calculating systolic wall thickening using a fast Fourier transform approximation: a simulation study based on canine and patient data. *J Nucl Med* 1994;35(7):1185–1192.

16. Germano G, Kiat H, Kavanagh PB, et al. Automatic quantification of ejection fraction from gated myocardial perfusion SPECT. *J Nucl Med* 1995;36(11):2138–2147.

17. Berman D, Germano G, Lewin H, et al. Comparison of post-stress ejection fraction and relative left ventricular volumes by automatic analysis of gated myocardial perfusion single-photon emission computed tomography acquired in the supine and prone positions. *J Nucl Cardiol* 1998;5(1):40–47.

18. Friedman J, Van Train K, Maddahi J, et al. "Upward creep" of the heart: a frequent source of false-positive reversible defects during thallium-201 stress-redistribution SPECT. *J Nucl Med* 1989;30(10):1718–1722.

19. Johnson LL, Verdesca SA, Aude WY, et al. Postischemic stunning can affect left ventricular ejection fraction and regional wall motion on post-stress gated sestamibi tomograms (see comments). *J Am Coll Cardiol* 1997;30(7):1641–1648.

20. Sharir T, Bacher-Stier C, Dhar S, et al. Post exercise regional wall motion abnormalities detected by Tc-99m sestamibi gated SPECT: a marker of severe coronary artery disease. *J Nucl Med* 1998;39(5):87P–88P(abst).

21. Sharir T, Lewin H, Germano G, et al. Automatic quantitation of wall motion and thickening by gated SPECT: validation and application in identifying severe coronary artery disease. *J Am Coll Cardiol* 1999;33(2 suppl A):418A–419A(abst).

22. O'Keefe J, Case J, Moutray K, et al. Post-stress drop in ejection fraction on ECG-gated SPECT thallium-201 scintigraphy predicts poor prognosis. *J Am Coll Cardiol* 1999;33(2 suppl A):469A(abst).

23. Shaw LJ, Heinle SK, Borges-Neto S, et al. Prognosis by measurements of left ventricular function during exercise. Duke Noninvasive Research Working Group. *J Nucl Med* 1998;39(1):140–146.

24. Roelants V, Vander Borght T, Walrand S, et al. Impact of attenuation correction on gated Tc-99m MIBI SPECT for wall thickening analysis in the evaluation of myocardial viability. *J Nucl Med* 1998;39(5):74P(abst).

25. Ficaro E, Duvernoy C, Fessler J, et al. End-diastolic vs ungated attenuation corrected myocardial perfusion SPECT for the detection of coronary heart disease. *J Nucl Med* 1998;39(5):74P(abst).

26. Germano G, Kavanagh PB, Kavanagh JT, et al. Repeatability of automatic left ventricular cavity volume measurements from myocardial perfusion SPECT. *J Nucl Cardiol* 1998;5(5):477–483.

27. White HD, Norris RM, Brown MA, et al. Left ventricular end-systolic volume as the major determinant of survival after recovery from myocardial infarction. *Circulation* 1987;76(1):44–51.

28. Nichols K, Dorbala S, DePuey E, et al. Influence of arrhythmias on gated SPECT myocardial perfusion and function quantification. *J Nucl Med* 1999;40:924–936.

29. Nichols K, DePuey E, Dorbala S, et al. Prevalence of gating errors in myocardial perfusion SPECT data. *J Nucl Med* 1998;39(5):45P(abst).

30. Nichols K, DePuey E, Yao S, et al. Clinical impact of gating errors on visual assessment of myocardial perfusion and ventricular function from SPECT data. *J Am Coll Cardiol* 1999;33(2 suppl A):435A(abst).

31. Garcia EV, Cooke CD, Van Train KF, et al. Technical aspects of myocardial SPECT imaging with technetium-99m sestamibi. *Am J Cardiol* 1990;66(13):23E–31E.

32. Galt JR, Cullom SJ, Garcia EV. Attenuation and scatter correction in myocardial perfusion SPECT. *Semin Nucl Med* 1999;24(3):204–220.

33. Dodge H, Sandler H, Ballew D, et al. Use of biplane angiocardiography for the measurement of left ventricular volume in man. *Am Heart J* 1960;60(5):762–776.

34. Williams KA, Taillon LA. Left ventricular function in patients with coronary artery disease assessed by gated tomographic myocardial perfusion images. Comparison with assessment by contrast ventriculography and first-pass radionuclide angiography. *J Am Coll Cardiol* 1996;27(1):173–181.

35. Smith WH, Kastner RJ, Calnon DA, et al. Quantitative gated single photon emission computed tomography imaging: a counts-based method for display and measurement of regional and global ventricular systolic function. *J Nucl Cardiol* 1997;4(6):451–463.

36. Calnon DA, Kastner RJ, Smith WH, et al. Validation of a new counts-based gated single photon emission computed tomography method for quantifying left ventricular systolic function: comparison with equilibrium radionuclide angiography. *J Nucl Cardiol* 1997;4(6):464–471.

37. Schiepers C, Almasi J. Equilibrium gated blood pool imaging at rest and during exercise. In: Gelfand MJ, Thomas SR, eds. *Effective use of computers in nuclear medicine:* practical clinical applications in the imaging laboratory. New York: McGraw-Hill, 1988:136–160.

38. Hoffman EJ, Huang SC, Phelps ME. Quantitation in positron emission computed tomography: 1. Effect of object size. *J Comput Assist Tomogr* 1979;3(3):299–308.

39. Galt JR, Garcia EV, Robbins WL. Effects of myocardial wall thickness on SPECT quantification. *IEEE Trans Med Imaging* 1990;9(2):144–150.

40. DePuey EG, Nichols K, Dobrinsky C. Left ventricular ejection fraction assessed from gated technetium-99m-sestamibi SPECT. *J Nucl Med* 1993;34(11):1871–1876.

41. Nichols K, DePuey EG, Rozanski A. Automation of gated tomographic left ventricular ejection fraction. *J Nucl Cardiol* 1996;3(6 pt 1):475–482.

42. Katz A, Force T, Folland E, et al. Echocardiographic assessment of ventricular systolic function. In: Marcus ML, Braunwald E, eds. *Marcus cardiac imaging:* a companion to Braunwald's heart disease. Philadelphia: WB Saunders, 1996:297–324.

43. Dulce MC, Mostbeck GH, Friese KK, et al. Quantification of the left ventricular volumes and function with cine MR imaging: comparison of geometric models with three-dimensional data. *Radiology* 1993;188(2):371–376.

44. Faber T, Cooke C, Folks R, et al. Left ventricular function and perfusion from gated SPECT perfusion images: an integrated method. *J Nucl Med* 1999;40(4):650–659.

45. Faber TL, Akers MS, Peshock RM, et al. Three-dimensional motion and perfusion quantification in gated single-photon emission computed tomograms. *J Nucl Med* 1991;32(12):2311–2317.

46. Faber TL, Stokely EM, Peshock RM, et al. A model-based four-dimensional left ventricular surface detector. *IEEE Trans Med Imaging* 1991;10(3):321–329.

47. Goris ML, Thompson C, Malone LJ, et al. Modelling the integration of myocardial regional perfusion and function. *Nucl Med Commun* 1994;15(1):9–20.

48. He Z, Mahmarian J, Preslar J, et al. Correlations of left ventricular ejection fractions determined by gated SPECT with thallium and sestamibi and by first-pass radionuclide angiography. *J Nucl Med* 1997;38(5):27P(abst).

49. Inubushi M, Tadamura E, Kudoh T, et al. Simultaneous assessment of myocardial fatty acid utilization and LV function using I-123 BMIPP gated SPECT (GSPECT). *J Nucl Cardiol* 1999; 6(1 pt 2):S66(abst).

50. Moriel M, Germano G, Kiat H, et al. Automatic measurement of left ventricular ejection fraction by gated SPECT Tc-99m sestamibi: a comparison with radionuclide ventriculography. *Circulation* 1993;88(4):I-486(abst).

51. Bateman T, Case J, Saunders M, et al. Gated SPECT LVEF measurements using a dual-detector camera and a weight-adjusted dosage of thallium-201. *J Am Coll Cardiol* 1997;29(2 suppl A): 263A(abst).

52. Carpentier P, Benticha H, Gautier P, et al. Thallium 201 gated SPECT for simultaneous assessment of myocardial perfusion, left ventricular ejection fraction and qualitative regional function. *J Nucl Cardiol* 1999;6(1 pt 2):S39(abst).

53. Everaert H, Bossuyt A, Franken PR. Left ventricular ejection fraction and volumes from gated single photon emission tomographic myocardial perfusion images: comparison between two algorithms working in three-dimensional space. *J Nucl Cardiol* 1997;4(6):472–476.

54. Zanger D, Bhatnagar A, Hausner E, et al. Automated calculation of ejection fraction from gated Tc-99m sestamibi images - comparison to quantitative echocardiography. *J Nucl Cardiol* 1997; 4(1 pt 2):S78(abst).

55. Bateman T, Magalski A, Barnhart C, et al. Global left ventricular function assessment using gated SPECT-201: comparison with echocardiography. *J Am Coll Cardiol* 1998;31(2 suppl A): 441A(abst).

56. Cwajg E, Cwajg J, He Z, et al. Comparison between gated-SPECT and echocardiography for the analysis of global and regional left ventricular function and volumes. *J Am Coll Cardiol* 1998;31(2 suppl A):440A–441A(abst).

57. Mathew D, Zabrodina Y, Mannting F. Volumetric and functional analysis of left ventricle by gated SPECT: a comparison with echocardiographic measurements. *J Am Coll Cardiol* 1998;31(2 suppl A):44A(abst).

58. Di Leo C, Bestetti A, Tagliabue L, et al. 99mTc-tetrofosmin gated-SPECT LVEF: correlation with echocardiography and contrastographic ventriculography. *J Nucl Cardiol* 1997;4(1 pt 2):S56(abst).

59. Akinboboye O, El-Khoury Coffin L, Sciacca R, et al. Accuracy of gated SPECT thallium left ventricular volumes and ejection fractions: comparison with three-dimensional echocardiography. *J Am Coll Cardiol* 1998;31(2 suppl A):85A(abst).

60. Atsma D, Croon C, Dibbets-Schneider P, et al. Good correlation between left ventricular ejection fraction and wall motion score assessed by gated SPECT as compared to left ventricular angiography. *J Am Coll Cardiol* 1999;33(2 suppl A):409A(abst).

61. He Z, Vick G, Vaduganathan P, et al. Comparison of left ventricular volumes and ejection fraction measured by gated SPECT and by cine magnetic resonance imaging. *J Am Coll Cardiol* 1998;31(2 suppl A):44A(abst).

62. Atsma D, Kayser H, Croon C, et al. Good correlation between left ventricular ejection fraction, end-systolic and end-diastolic volume measured by gated SPECT as compared to magnetic resonance imaging. *J Am Coll Cardiol* 1999;33(2 suppl A): 436A(abst).

63. Vaduganathan P, He Z, Vick G, et al. Evaluation of left ventric-ular wall motion, volumes, and ejection fraction by gated myocardial tomography with technetium 99m-labeled tetrofosmin: a comparison with cine magnetic resonance imaging. *J Nucl Cardiol* 1999;6(1 p 1):3–10.

64. Tadamura E, Kudoh T, Motooka M, et al. Assessment of regional and global left ventricular function by reinjection [201]Tl and rest Tc-99m sestamibi ECG-gated SPECT. *J Am Coll Cardiol* 1999; 33(4):991–997.

65. Toba M, Ishida Y, Fukuchi K, et al. Application of ECG-gated Tc-99m sestamibi cardiac imaging to patients with arrhythmogenic right ventricular dysplasia (ARVD). *J Nucl Cardiol* 1999;6(1 part 2):S41(abst).

66. Germano G, VanDecker W, Mintz R, et al. Validation of left ventricular volumes automatically measured with gated myocardial perfusion SPECT. *J Am Coll Cardiol* 1998;31(2 suppl A):43A (abst).

67. Nichols K, DePuey EG, Rozanski A, et al. Image enhancement of severely hypoperfused myocardia for computation of tomographic ejection fraction. *J Nucl Med* 1997;38(9):1411–1417.

68. Nichols K, Tamis J, DePuey EG, et al. Relationship of gated SPECT ventricular function parameters to angiographic measurements. *J Nucl Cardiol* 1998;5(3):295–303.

69. Stollfuss JC, Haas F, Matsunari I, et al. Regional myocardial wall thickening and global ejection fraction in patients with low angiographic left ventricular ejection fraction assessed by visual and quantitative resting ECG-gated 99mTc-tetrofosmin single-photon emission tomography and magnetic resonance imaging. *Eur J Nucl Med* 1998;25(5):522–530.

70. Yang KT, Chen HD. Evaluation of global and regional left ventricular function using technetium-99m sestamibi ECG-gated single-photon emission tomography. *Eur J Nucl Med* 1998;25 (5):515–521.

71. Schwartz R, Thompson C, Mixon L, et al. Gated SPECT analysis with 3-D wall parametrization method: accurate and reproducible evaluation of left ventricular volumes and ejection fraction. *Circulation* 1995;92(8):I-449(abst).

72. Everaert H, Franken PR, Flamen P, et al. Left ventricular ejection fraction from gated SPET myocardial perfusion studies: a method based on the radial distribution of count rate density across the myocardial wall. *Eur J Nucl Med* 1996;23(12): 1628–1633.

73. Schwartz R, Eckdahl J, Thompson C. 3-D wall parametrization method for quantitative LVEF of gated SPECT sestamibi with LV dysfunction and severe perfusion defects. *J Nucl Cardiol* 1995;2(2):S114(abst).

74. Adiseshan P, Corbett J. Quantification of left ventricular function from gated tomographic perfusion imaging: development and testing of a new algorithm. *Circulation* 1994;90(4):I-365 (abst).

75. Cittanti C, Mele D, Colamussi P, et al. Determination of left ventricular volume and ejection fraction by g-SPECT myocardial perfusion scintigraphy. A comparison with quantitative 3-D echocardiography. *J Nucl Cardiol* 1999;6(1 pt 2):S34(abst).

76. Daou D, Helal B, Colin P, et al. Are LV ejection fraction (EF), end diastolic (EDV) and end systolic volumes (ESV) measured with rest [201]Tl gated SPECT accurate? *J Nucl Cardiol* 1999;6(1 pt 2):S31(abst).

77. Iskandrian A, Germano G, VanDecker W, et al. Validation of left ventricular volume measurements by gated SPECT Tc-99m sestamibi imaging. *J Nucl Cardiol* 1998;5(6):574–578.

78. Germano G, Erel J, Lewin H, et al. Automatic quantitation of regional myocardial wall motion and thickening from gated technetium-99m sestamibi myocardial perfusion single-photon emission computed tomography. *J Am Coll Cardiol* 1997;30(5): 1360–1367.

79. Fukuchi K, Uehara T, Morozumi T, et al. Quantification of sys-

tolic count increase in technetium-99m-MIBI gated myocardial SPECT. *J Nucl Med* 1997;38(7):1067–1073.

80. Germano G, Kavanagh PB, Berman DS. An automatic approach to the analysis, quantitation and review of perfusion and function from myocardial perfusion SPECT images. *Int J Cardiol Imaging* 1997;13(4):337–346.

81. Germano G, Kavanagh P, Waechter P, et al. A new automatic approach to myocardial perfusion SPECT quantitation. *J Nucl Med* 1998;39(5):62P(abst).

82. Nichols K, DePuey EG, Krasnow N, et al. Reliability of enhanced gated SPECT in assessing wall motion of severely hypoperfused myocardium: echocardiographic validation. *J Nucl Cardiol* 1998;5(4):387–394.

83. Germano G, Berman D. On the accuracy and reproducibility of quantitative gated myocardial perfusion SPECT. *J Nucl Med* 1999;40(5):810–813.

84. Case J, Cullom S, Bateman T, et al. Overestimation of LVEF by gated MIBI myocardial perfusion SPECT in patients with small hearts. *J Am Coll Cardiol* 1998;31(2 suppl A):43A(abst).

85. Case J, Bateman T, Cullom S, et al. Improved accuracy of SPECT LVEF using numerical modeling of ventricular image blurring for patients with small hearts. *J Am Coll Cardiol* 1999; 33(2 suppl A):436A(abst).

86. Cullom SJ, Case JA, Bateman TM. Electrocardiographically gated myocardial perfusion SPECT: technical principles and quality control considerations. *J Nucl Cardiol* 1998;5(4): 418–425.

87. DePuey EG, Nichols K, Dobrinsky C, et al. Left ventricular ejection fractions from gated Tc-99m SPECT. *J Nucl Med* 1992;33: 927(abst).

88. Nichols K, DePuey EG, Salensky H, et al. Validation of gated tomographic sestamibi left ventricular ejection fractions. *J Nucl Med* 1994;35:154P(abst).

89. Nichols K, DePuey EG, Salensky H, et al. Semi-automated computation of gated tomographic left ventricular ejection fraction. *J Nucl Med* 1995;36:56P(abst).

90. Lefkowitz D, Nichols K, Rozanski A, et al. Echocardiographic validation of left ventricular volume measurements by Tc-99m sestamibi gated SPECT. *J Am Coll Cardiol* 1996;27: 241A(abst).

91. Nichols K, DePuey EG, Salensky H. Reproducibility of ejection fractions from stress versus rest gated perfusion SPECT. *J Nucl Med* 1996;37:115P(abst).

92. Nichols K, DePuey EG, Yao SS, et al. Clinical impact of gating errors on visual assessment of myocardial perfusion and ventricular function from SPECT data. *J Am Coll Cardiol* 1999;33: 435A(abst).

93. Nichols K, DePuey EG, Salensky H, et al. Ventricular volume measured from sestamibi gated tomograms. *J Nucl Med* 1994; 35:70P(abst).

*Cardiac SPECT Imaging*, 2nd ed., edited by E. G. DePuey, E. V. Garcia, and D. S. Berman. Lippincott Williams & Wilkins, Philadelphia © 2001.

# RADIOPHARMACEUTICALS

## RAYMOND TAILLEFER

Radionuclide myocardial perfusion imaging is now a well-established clinical procedure for the diagnosis and evaluation of patients with suspected or known coronary artery disease (CAD). Since its introduction more than two decades ago, myocardial perfusion scintigraphy has significantly evolved. Two major factors have contributed to this evolution: technical improvements in scintigraphic data acquisition and analysis and introduction of new technetium 99m ([99m]Tc)-labeled perfusion imaging radiopharmaceuticals with different properties. This chapter reviews the most important characteristics of the various radionuclide myocardial perfusion imaging agents that are currently commercially available or are likely to be available in the relatively near future: thallium 201 ([201]Tl), [99m]Tc-sestamibi, [99m]Tc-teboroxime, [99m]Tc-tetrofosmin, [99m]Tc-furifosmin, and [99m]TcN-NOEt. Since numerous extensive studies and reviews on [201]Tl imaging have been previously reported, this chapter focuses on [99m]Tc-labeled perfusion imaging agents.

## THALLIUM 201

In the mid-1950s, Sapirstein (1) elaborated the criteria necessary for a radiopharmaceutical to be used to determine regional perfusion. As described by the Sapirstein principle, a given type of radiopharmaceutical will be distributed in proportion to regional perfusion if its extraction by the organ of interest is high and if its clearance from the blood is rapid. One of the first class of radiopharmaceuticals used to image myocardial perfusion was the potassium analogs, a group of monovalent cations of potassium, cesium, rubidium, and thallium, which enter the myocardium by the sodium-potassium adenosine triphosphatase (ATPase) pump mechanism (2). Although different radioisotopes of these cations have been evaluated, [201]Tl was found to have

the best physical and biologic characteristics for imaging in humans. Since the mid-1970s, and for more than two decades, [201]Tl has been the most popular radionuclide myocardial perfusion imaging agent used in noninvasive detection and evaluation of patients with known or suspected CAD.

## Chemistry and Constituents

Thallium 201 is a metallic element in group IIIA of the periodic table with a crystal radius of 1.44 Å (between that of potassium and rubidium). [201]Tl is a cyclotron-produced monovalent cation with a physical half-life of 73.1 hours. It decays by electron capture to mercury ([201]Hg). [201]Tl is a low-energy gamma emitter with principal photopeaks at 135.3 keV (2.7% abundance) and 167.4 keV (10% abundance) and x rays emitted from the mercury daughter at 68 to 80.3 keV (95% abundance). Some contaminants such as [200]Tl (<0.3%), [202]Tl (<1.2%), and [202]Pb (<0.2%) can be contained, but they usually represent less than 2% of the total [201]Tl activity at the time of calibration. In contrast to the [99m]Tc-labeled myocardial perfusion imaging agents, there is no in-house preparation, and no quality control procedure required before injection in humans.

## Physiologic Characteristics

### Basic Characteristics of Myocardial Perfusion Imaging Radiotracers

Although many different classes of radioactive myocardial perfusion imaging agents exist, they should all present a minimum of common basic characteristics (3). The myocardial uptake of the radiotracer must be proportional to the regional myocardial blood flow over a relatively wide range of blood flows. The myocardial uptake should be high enough to allow for detection of regional inhomogeneity by external gamma scintigraphy. The initial myocardial distribution of the radiotracer at the time of injection must remain stable during the acquisition time of the images. The effect of blood flow on myocardial transport of the radiotracer must be predominant to the effect of metabolic

R. Taillefer: Department of Nuclear Medicine, Université de Montreal; Department of Nuclear Medicine, Hôtel-Dieu du C.H.U.M., H2W 1T8 Montreal, Canada.

cellular alterations. Finally, the agent should be labeled to a radionuclide having adequate physical characteristics in order to provide high photon flux and optimal counting statistics.

Information on basic properties of radionuclide myocardial perfusion imaging agents is generally obtained from cultured myocardial cells, isolated perfused hearts, or *in vivo* animal models (4). Precise measurements of cellular or capillary-tissue tracer kinetics are usually obtained from cell cultures and isolated perfused heart models, whereas regional tracer distribution and uptake in other organs are studied in *in vivo* animal models.

The two most important physiologic factors that affect the myocardial uptake of a myocardial perfusion imaging agent are the variations in regional myocardial blood flow and the myocardial extraction of the radiotracer. Three major parameters ($E_{net}$, $E_{max}$, and $PS_{cap}$) can be determined using indicator-dilution techniques and radiolabeled albumin used as an intravascular reference. The difference between the intravascular albumin reference and the radiopharmaceutical that is evaluated (i.e., a diffusible perfusion agent) on a venous dilution curve is used to calculate its instantaneous cardiac extraction. The early peak of the curve, or $E_{max}$, represents the maximum fractional tissue extraction of the diffusible agent. This value is used to calculate the capillary permeability–surface area product ($PS_{cap}$). The net extraction ($E_{net}$) is the integral of the curve and is used as a measure of myocardial radiotracer retention, including both initial extraction and subsequent back-diffusion. A high value for $E_{max}$ and $PS_{cap}$ indicates a rapid blood-tissue exchange and suggests that the diffusible radiotracer will be able to assess high levels of hyperemic flow accurately. The myocardial transmicrovascular transport of

$^{201}$Tl was evaluated by Leppo and Meerdink (5) in a blood-perfused, isolated rabbit heart model. The averaged myocardial extraction ($E_{max}$) of $^{201}$Tl was 0.73 ± 0.10. The net myocardial extraction measured over a 2- to 5-minute period was 0.57 ± 0.13. The mean $PS_{cap}$ of $^{201}$Tl was 1.30 ± 0.45 mL/g/min. Table 8.1 summarizes and compares these values, as a reference, to those of the five $^{99m}$Tc-labeled perfusion imaging agents.

Although considered biologically similar to potassium, the myocardial uptake of $^{201}$Tl is greater than that of potassium. The myocardial extraction fraction of $^{201}$Tl in an *in vivo* model is approximately 87% at normal flow rates (6). Studies of the relationship of myocardial uptake of $^{201}$Tl to regional coronary blood flow as determined by radiolabeled microspheres showed that there is a nearly linear correlation over a wide range of coronary blood flows. However, at high flow rates (approximately 2.5 mL/min/g), there is a diffusion limitation, a fall in tracer extraction fraction, and increased cellular washout, resulting in a plateau in myocardial uptake. This results in an overall underestimation of higher levels of coronary blood flows. Conversely, at very low flow rates (usually less than 10% of the baseline blood flow), there is an increased myocardial extraction fraction of $^{201}$Tl relative to blood flow, resulting in an overestimation of coronary blood flow. This phenomenon has been described with all other $^{99m}$Tc-labeled myocardial perfusion imaging agents, at various degrees.

One of the most clinically important characteristics of $^{201}$Tl is its myocardial redistribution. Myocardial uptake of $^{201}$Tl is not static over time. This property forms the basis of the stress-redistribution imaging protocol currently used to diagnose the presence of CAD with $^{201}$Tl. The redistribution or the filling in of a myocardial perfusion defect

## TABLE 8.1. COMPARATIVE CHARACTERISTICS OF RADIOPHARMACEUTICALS FOR MYOCARDIAL PERFUSION IMAGING

| | $^{201}$Tl | $^{99m}$Tc-Sestamibi | $^{99m}$Tc-Teboroxime | $^{99m}$Tc-Tetrofosmin | $^{99m}$Tc-Furifosmin | $^{99m}$Tc-N-NOEt |
|---|---|---|---|---|---|---|
| Class | Element | Isonitrile | BATO | Diphosphine | Schiff base phosphine | Nitrodo |
| Charge | Cation | Cation | Neutral | Cation | Cation | Neutral |
| $E_{max}$ | 0.73 ± 1.0 | 0.38 ± 0.09 | 0.72 ± 0.09 | 0.32 ± 0.07 | 0.26 ± 0.05 | 0.48 ± 0.10 |
| $E_{net}$ | 0.57 ± 0.13 | 0.41 ± 0.15 | 0.55 ± 0.18 | 0.23 | 0.12 ± 0.05 | 0.24 ± 0.08 |
| $PS_{cap}$ (mL/gr/min) | 1.30 ± 0.45 | 0.44 ± 0.23 | 1.10 ± 0.40 | 0.40 | 0.48 ± 0.16 | 1.02 ± 0.32 |
| Myocardial redistribution | Yes | Partial | Yes | No | No | Yes |
| Myocardial uptake (%ID) | 3.0–4.0 | 1.4 ± 0.3 | 3.0–4.0 | 1.0–1.2 | 2.0–2.2 | 3.0–3.5 |
| Labeling | Ready | 100°C × 10 min | 100°C × 15 min | 15–25°C × 15 min | 100°C × 15 min | 100°C × 15 min |
| IV imaging interval | 5–10 min | 15–60 min | <2 min | 15 min | 15 min | 10–15 min |
| Target organ | Kidney | Upper large intestine | Upper large intestine | Gallbladder wall | Gallbladder wall | Kidneys |

BATO, boronic acid technetium dioxime; $PS_{cap}$, mean capillary permeability surface area product.

occurring shortly (generally between 3 to 5 hours) after the injection of $^{201}$Tl at peak stress is related to two factors: the rate of influx of $^{201}$Tl into the myocardium from whole-body blood pool activity, and the rate of clearance or washout of $^{201}$Tl from the myocardium. A myocardial perfusion defect related to ischemic disease will show a normalization of the $^{201}$Tl uptake at 3 to 4 hours after the injection at stress because of delayed accumulation into the ischemic segment and more rapid washout from normal myocardial segments. Two $^{99m}$Tc-labeled perfusion imaging agents also demonstrate some degree of myocardial redistribution, similar to that of $^{201}$Tl: $^{99m}$Tc-teboroxime and $^{99m}$TcN-NOEt.

## Biodistribution

The greatest concentration of $^{201}$Tl is found in kidneys, heart, and liver. The activity in these organs remains high for a few hours after the injection. The maximal myocardial uptake, which is approximately 3.7% to 4.0% of the injected dose, is achieved by 10 to 15 minutes after the administration of the radiopharmaceutical. $^{201}$Tl myocardial uptake has two components: an early component with a half-life of approximately 4 hours (80%), and a delayed component with a half-life of 40 hours (20%). Disappearance of $^{201}$Tl from the blood compartment is rapid, with two components: 92% of the blood activity disappears with a half-life of 5 minutes, and the other 8% will be cleared from the blood with a half-life of approximately 40 hours. This rapid clearance of $^{201}$Tl from the blood results in a decreased blood pool background when myocardial perfusion imaging is performed.

## Dosimetry

Table 8.2 summarizes the radiation dose estimates for $^{201}$Tl and all other $^{99m}$Tc-labeled myocardial perfusion imaging agents. Data on $^{201}$Tl were obtained in humans (7) assuming a bladder voiding interval of 4.8 hours. Kidneys are the target organs.

**TABLE 8.2. RADIATION DOSE ESTIMATE FOR MYOCARDIAL PERFUSION IMAGING AGENTS (RADS/30 MCI)**

| | $^{99m}$Tc-Sestamibi | | $^{99m}$Tc-Teboroxime | $^{99m}$Tc-Tetrofosmin | | $^{99m}$Tc-Furifosmin | $^{99m}$Tc-N-NOEt | | $^{201}$Tl |
|---|---|---|---|---|---|---|---|---|---|
| | Rest | Stress | Rest | Rest | Stress | Rest | Rest | Stress | Stress (rads/3 mCi) |
| Adrenals | — | — | — | 0.5 | 0.5 | 0.5 | — | — | 0.7 |
| Brain | — | — | 0.4 | 0.2 | 0.3 | 0.1 | — | — | 0.7 |
| Breasts | 0.2 | 0.2 | — | 0.2 | 0.2 | 0.3 | — | — | 0.4 |
| Gallbladder wall | 2.0 | 2.8 | 2.9 | 5.4 | 3.7 | 3.0 | — | — | 0.9 |
| LLI | 3.9 | 3.3 | 2.6 | 2.5 | 1.7 | 2.2 | — | — | 1.6 |
| ULI | 5.4 | 4.5 | 3.7 | 3.4 | 2.2 | 2.9 | 1.9 | 1.4 | 0.8 |
| Small intestine | 3.0 | 2.4 | 2.0 | 1.9 | 1.3 | 1.7 | — | — | 0.2 |
| Stomach | 0.6 | 0.5 | — | 0.5 | 0.5 | 0.5 | — | — | 0.3 |
| Heart wall | 0.5 | 0.5 | 0.6 | 0.4 | 0.5 | 0.7 | 0.7 | 0.8 | 0.3 |
| Kidneys | 2.0 | 1.7 | 0.6 | 1.4 | 1.2 | 1.7 | 1.6 | 2.0 | 5.1 |
| Liver | 0.8 | 0.4 | 1.9 | 0.5 | 0.4 | 0.5 | 1.3 | 1.2 | 1.1 |
| Lungs | 0.3 | 0.3 | 0.8 | 0.2 | 0.2 | 0.4 | 0.5 | 0.6 | 0.5 |
| Muscles | — | — | — | 0.4 | 0.4 | 0.4 | — | — | 0.5 |
| Ovaries | 1.5 | 1.2 | 1.1 | 1.1 | 0.9 | 1.0 | 1.1 | 1.0 | 1.1 |
| Pancreas | — | — | — | 0.5 | 0.6 | 0.6 | — | — | 0.8 |
| Red marrow | 0.5 | 0.5 | 0.5 | 0.4 | 0.5 | 0.5 | 0.4 | 0.4 | 0.6 |
| Bone surface | 0.7 | 0.6 | — | 0.6 | 0.7 | 0.7 | — | — | 1.0 |
| Spleen | — | — | 0.4 | 0.4 | 0.5 | 0.5 | 0.6 | 0.5 | 2.0 |
| Testes | 0.3 | 0.3 | 0.3 | 0.3 | 0.4 | 0.4 | 0.3 | 0.3 | 0.9 |
| Thymus | — | — | — | 0.3 | 0.3 | 0.4 | — | — | 0.5 |
| Thyroid | 0.7 | 0.3 | 0.3 | 0.6 | 0.5 | 0.4 | 0.6 | 0.6 | 3.0 |
| Bladder wall | 2.0 | 1.5 | 0.8 | 2.1 | 1.7 | 1.9 | — | — | 0.6 |
| Uterus | — | — | — | 0.9 | 0.2 | 0.9 | — | — | 1.0 |
| Total body | 0.5 | 0.4 | 0.5 | 0.4 | 0.4 | — | 0.5 | 0.4 | — |
| Effective dose equivalent (rem/30 mCi) | 1.5 | 1.3 | 1.1 | 1.0 | 0.6 | 1.1 | 0.8 | 0.8 | 3.9 (rem/3 mCi) |

LLI, lower large intestine; ULI, upper large intestine.

# 99MTC-SESTAMIBI

Although several hundred studies have demonstrated the clinical value of [201]Tl myocardial perfusion scintigraphy since its first use in 1975, the physical characteristics of this radionuclide are suboptimal for scintillation camera imaging. Therefore, in the late 1970s and early 1980s, many investigators attempted to develop a myocardial perfusion imaging agent labeled with [99m]Tc in order to circumvent the physical limitations of [201]Tl. The potential advantages of a [99m]Tc-labeled agent over [201]Tl are significant and include the following: (a) The 140-keV photon energy of [99m]Tc, which is optimal for standard gamma camera imaging, results in improved resolution due to less Compton scatter and less tissue attenuation in the patient (in comparison to the low photon energy of 68 to 80 keV for [201]Tl). (b) The much shorter physical half-life of [99m]Tc (6 hours vs. 73 hours for [201]Tl) and the better radiation dosimetry permit the administration of a ten times higher dose of a [99m]Tc-labeled compound than [201]Tl. This yields better image quality and images can be performed in a shorter time period. (c) The resulting overall better counting statistics of [99m]Tc allows for the perfusion images to be obtained in a gated mode. Simultaneous assessment of perfusion and function (global and regional wall motion) can thus be obtained. (d) It is possible to perform first-pass function studies (if the initial lung transit is rapid enough) with a [99m]Tc-labeled radiopharmaceutical agent. (e) Since [99m]Tc is constantly available from a molybdenum generator in a nuclear medicine laboratory, special deliveries from a distribution center or a commercial radiopharmacy are not required. A [99m]Tc-labeled myocardial perfusion imaging agent can thus be available almost 24 hours a day.

For all the above-mentioned reasons, and although [201]Tl has excellent physiologic characteristics for myocardial perfusion imaging, it was obvious that a [99m]Tc-labeled agent able to assess myocardial perfusion could be very useful clinically (8–10). Significant developments were finally seen in the early 1980s with the initial article published in 1984 by Jones et al. (11) on a new group of [99m]Tc-labeled myocardial perfusion radiotracers, the [99m]Tc-isonitriles. Initial animal studies showed that the myocardial uptake of [99m]Tc-isonitriles was proportional to the regional myocardial blood flow. The first member of the [99m]Tc-isonitrile family to be evaluated in humans was the hexakis (t-butyl-isonitrile)-technetium (I), also known as [99m]Tc-TBI (12,13). Although the myocardial uptake of [99m]Tc-TBI was proportional to myocardial blood flow and was satisfactory for imaging purposes, its routine clinical use was limited by increased lung uptake and prominent and persistent liver uptake, which frequently masked defects in myocardial walls adjacent to the hepatic parenchyma. The initial lung uptake and subsequent washout of [99m]Tc-TBI from the lungs also created significant imaging problems. Then, a second [99m]Tc-isonitrile compound was synthesized and evaluated in humans: the carboxyisopropyl isonitrile or [99m]Tc-CPI (14). Like [99m]Tc-TBI, [99m]Tc-CPI showed excellent myocardial uptake proportional to blood flow but relatively rapid washout from the myocardium and significant progressive accumulation in the liver over time. A third [99m]Tc-isonitrile compound emerged from this intensive search (15), initially known by the coded name of RP-30A (nonlyophilized form) or RP-30 (lyophilized form), and then as either [99m]Tc-hexakis 2-methoxyisobutyl isonitrile, [99m]Tc-hexakis-2-methoxy-2-methylpropyl-isonitrile, [99m]Tc-hexamibi, or [99m]Tc-MIBI (Table 8.3); DuPont Phar-

## TABLE 8.3. VARIOUS IDENTIFICATIONS OF [99m]TC-LABELED PERFUSION IMAGING AGENTS

| Generic name | Trademark name | Other names |
|---|---|---|
| [99m]Tc-Sestamibi | Cardiolite | RP-30A, RP-30 |
| | | Hexamibi |
| | | Isonitrile |
| | | 2-Methoxy-2-methyl propyl-isonitrile |
| | | Methoxy-isobutyl-isonitrile |
| | | Hexakis-2-methoxy-isobutyl isonitrile |
| [99m]Tc-Teboroxime | Cardiotec | SQ-30.217 |
| | | CDO-MEB |
| | | BATO (boronic acid Tc-dioxime) |
| | | Cyclohexane dione |
| | | Dioxine methyl boronic acid |
| | | Meboroxime |
| [99m]Tc-Tetrofosmin | Myoview | P-53 |
| | | PPN1011 |
| | | 1,2-bis bis 2-ethoxyethyl phospine ethane |
| [99m]Tc-Furifosmin | Technecard | Q-12 |
| | | Tri (3-methoxy-1-propyl) phosphine |
| [99m]Tc-NOEt | | Bis (*N*-ethoxy, *N*-ethyl-dithiocarbonate) nitrido |

maceutical commercially developed $^{99m}$Tc-sestamibi (generic name) or Cardiolite (trademark name). In comparison to its two isonitrile predecessors, $^{99m}$Tc-sestamibi had the most favorable biologic characteristics for clinical applications. Unlike $^{99m}$Tc-TBI and $^{99m}$Tc-CPI, which showed poor myocardial-to-background activity ratio, $^{99m}$Tc-sestamibi showed transient liver uptake and subsequent rapid hepatobiliary excretion. Furthermore, the lung uptake was minimal in comparison to the other two isonitrile agents. Technetium 99-sestamibi was approved by the United States Food and Drug Administration (FDA) in December 1990 for clinical application.

## Chemistry and Constituents

$^{99m}$Tc-sestamibi or hexakis (2-methoxyisobutyl isonitrile) technetium is a monovalent cation with a central Tc (I) core that is octahedrally surrounded by six identical lipophilic ligands coordinated through the isonitrile carbon (Fig. 8.1). A 5-mL vial of $^{99m}$Tc-sestamibi, or Cardiolite, supplied by DuPont Merck Pharmaceutical (Billerica, MA) contains a sterile, nonpyrogenic, lyophilized mixture of the following:

1. 1.0 mg of Tetrakis (2-methoxyisobutyl isonitrile) copper tetrafluoroborate
2. 0.025 mg (minimum) of stannous chloride dihydrate
3. 2.6 mg of sodium citrate dihydrate
4. 0.086 mg (maximum) of total tin

5. 1.0 mg of L-cysteine hydrochloride monohydrate
6. 20 mg of mannitol

The contents of the vial (pH = 5.3–5.9) are lyophilized and stored under nitrogen. After reconstition with oxidant-free sodium pertechnetate $^{99m}$Tc, the pH of the product to be injected is 5.5 (5.0 to 6.0). There is no bacteriostatic preservative. The final structure of the technetium complex is $^{99m}$Tc–2-methoxyisobutyl isonitrile (MIBI)6+. Intravenous injection of $^{99m}$Tc-sestamibi has been associated with very few adverse reactions. According to the product monograph, during clinical trials (phase III study), approximately 5% to 10% of patients have experienced transient parosmia and/or taste perversion (metallic or bitter taste) occurring a few seconds after the injection. Usually, this side effect disappears within 15 to 30 seconds. Parosmia and taste perversion seem to be related to the presence of copper salt in the kit formulation, and its incidence may be related to the concentration of $^{99m}$Tc-sestamibi used.

## Physiologic Characteristics

### Initial Myocardial Uptake of $^{99m}$Tc-Sestamibi

Among the $^{99m}$Tc-labeled myocardial perfusion imaging agents, $^{99m}$Tc-sestamibi has been probably the one most extensively studied using the previously mentioned research models. $^{99m}$Tc-sestamibi is a cationic complex that is taken up by myocytes in proportion to regional myocardial blood

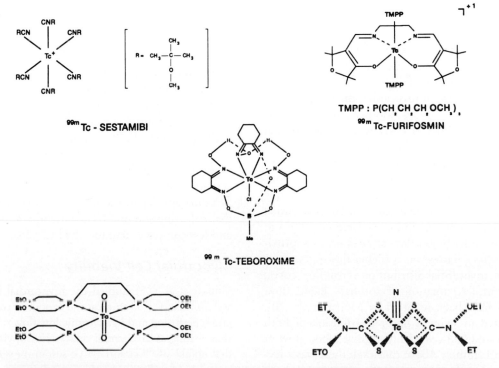

**FIGURE 8.1.** Schematic chemical structures of the five technetium 99m ($^{99m}$Tc)-labeled perfusion imaging agents.

flow. The cationic charge of the compound provides hydrophilic properties, while the six isonitrile groups allow hydrophobic interaction with cell membranes.

The myocardial uptake of $^{99m}$Tc-sestamibi is known to be dependent on mitochondrial-derived membrane electrochemical gradient, cellular pH, and intact energy production pathways. Piwnica-Worms et al. (16) studied the net myocardial uptake and retention of $^{99m}$Tc-sestamibi using cultured chick embryo ventricular myocytes model. They showed that when mitochondrial and plasma membrane potentials are hyperpolarized, there is an increase in cellular uptake and retention of $^{99m}$Tc-sestamibi. Conversely, when mitochondrial and plasma membrane potentials are depolarized, there is inhibition of net myocardial uptake and retention of the radiotracer. $^{99m}$Tc-sestamibi, retained within cells because of the negative charge generated on the mitochondria, has high affinity for the cytoplasm and shows very little extracellular exchange. Thus, metabolic derangements affecting myocytes viability would also result in decreased $^{99m}$Tc-sestamibi uptake, independently of myocardial blood flow. Using aerobic metabolic blockade (with sodium cyanide) and a sarcolemmal detergent (Triton X-100), which directly disrupt the membrane integrity, Beanlands et al. (17) showed that irreversible cellular injury resulted in a marked increase in the $^{99m}$Tc-sestamibi clearance rate. They concluded that the accumulation and clearance kinetics of $^{99m}$Tc-sestamibi were dependent on sarcolemmal integrity and on aerobic metabolism and were significantly affected by cell viability.

Okada et al. (18) investigated the myocardial kinetics of $^{99m}$Tc-sestamibi in dogs undergoing partial occlusion of the left circumflex coronary artery. They showed that $^{99m}$Tc-sestamibi was rapidly taken up by nonischemic and ischemic myocardium at rest in proportion to regional myocardial blood flow. There was a good correlation between the initial myocardial flow at normal resting-flow rates and the $^{99m}$Tc-sestamibi myocardial distribution (linear relationship with $r = 0.92$). Another study from the same group of investigators (19) using the same animal model evaluated the myocardial kinetics of $^{99m}$Tc-sestamibi after pharmacologic vasodilation with dipyridamole. They showed that $^{99m}$Tc-sestamibi was rapidly taken up by nonischemic, mildly to moderately ischemic, and severely ischemic myocardium and that the initial myocardial uptake of $^{99m}$Tc-sestamibi was linearly related ($r = 0.97$) to the regional myocardial blood flow at rates up to approximately 2.0 mL/min/g. However, at higher flow rates, there is a plateau in the myocardial distribution versus flow curve, resulting in an underestimation of coronary blood flow. Similar findings have been reported by Mousa et al. (20), who demonstrated in swine a linear distribution of both $^{201}$Tl and $^{99m}$Tc-sestamibi with myocardial blood flow at rates up to 2.4 mL/min/g. Above this level, there was a leveling off of the distribution versus flow curve for both radiotracers. Furthermore, myocardial uptake of $^{99m}$Tc-ses-

tamibi in low flow regions is higher relative to nonischemic uptake than in the regional blood flow determined with radiolabeled microspheres. This overestimation of myocardial blood flow at low flows (as previously discussed with $^{201}$Tl) is probably related to increased extraction seen with diffusible indicators. Other studies have confirmed that myocardial uptake of $^{99m}$Tc-sestamibi, as with $^{201}$Tl, is proportional to regional myocardial blood flow over the physiologic flow range with decreased extraction at hyperemic flows and increased extraction at low flows (21).

The myocardial transmicrovascular transport of $^{99m}$Tc-sestamibi was evaluated and compared to that of $^{201}$Tl by Leppo and Meerdink (22) in a blood-perfused, isolated rabbit heart model. The averaged myocardial extraction ($E_{max}$) of $^{99m}$Tc-sestamibi ($0.38 \pm 0.09$) was significantly less ($p < .001$) than that of $^{201}$Tl ($0.73 \pm 0.10$). The net myocardial extraction measured over a 2- to 5-minute period was also significantly ($p < .001$) less for $^{99m}$Tc-sestamibi ($0.41 \pm 0.15$) than for $^{201}$Tl ($0.57 \pm 0.13$). Although the mean $PS_{cap}$ of $^{201}$Tl ($1.30 \pm 0.45$ mL/g/min) is significantly greater ($p < .001$) than that of $^{99m}$Tc-sestamibi ($0.44 \pm 0.13$ mL/g/min), the parenchymal cell permeability and volume distribution of $^{99m}$Tc-sestamibi are much greater than that of $^{201}$Tl, resulting in a longer residence time within the myocardium for $^{99m}$Tc-sestamibi. The net result of these differences in myocellular kinetics of the two radiopharmaceuticals is that very little difference is observed in the initial myocardial accumulation when both are imaged *in vivo*.

## Myocardial Redistribution

In contrast to $^{201}$Tl, $^{99m}$Tc-sestamibi shows very slow myocardial clearance after its initial myocardial uptake. Fractional $^{99m}$Tc-sestamibi clearance of 10% to 15% over a period of 4 hours has been measured by Okada et al. (18) in a canine model of partial coronary occlusion. Clearance was similar in the hypoperfused and normal zones. Animal studies have shown that after injection during brief periods (6 to 15 minutes) of coronary occlusion in dogs, the occluded zone shows continued myocardial uptake of $^{99m}$Tc-sestamibi during the reperfusion phase, resulting in a slight increase in the ischemic/normal wall $^{99m}$Tc-sestamibi activity ratio for 2 to 3 hours. Thus, following transient ischemia and reperfusion, there is some degree of myocardial redistribution of $^{99m}$Tc-sestamibi, although it is slower and less complete than for $^{201}$Tl (23,24).

## Myocardial Cell Viability

Sinusas et al. (25) studied the myocardial uptake of $^{99m}$Tc-sestamibi and $^{201}$Tl in a canine model of transient occlusion and reperfusion and in a chronic low flow state. They showed that as long as myocardial cells were still viable, the myocardial uptake of $^{201}$Tl and $^{99m}$Tc-sestamibi was not affected by a degree of ischemia producing profound systolic dysfunction. They did not observe a flow-independent inhibition of

$^{99m}$Tc-sestamibi myocardial uptake in the stunned or in the chronically ischemic myocardial tissue. Thus, data in experimental models of coronary occlusion and reperfusion and studies of isolated, perfused heart models showed that as long as myocyte membrane integrity is intact and blood flow persists, $^{99m}$Tc-sestamibi is extracted by myocardial cells. These data suggest that $^{99m}$Tc-sestamibi can also assess myocardial viability. $^{99m}$Tc-sestamibi uptake is maintained in viable myocardium but reduced in necrotic tissue. Using a dog model with coronary occlusion and reperfusion, Verani et al. (26) demonstrated that the size of the perfusion defect during occlusion as detected by scintigraphic images correlated with the amount of myocardium supplied by the occluded vessel, the area at risk. A smaller perfusion defect was detected on $^{99m}$Tc-sestamibi imaging during reperfusion. This defect correlated with the amount of infarcted myocardium. The area showing an improved perfusion pattern after reflow represented the salvage myocardium.

## Biodistribution

The results of multicenter phase I and phase II studies on blood clearance, biodistribution, dosimetry, and safety of $^{99m}$Tc-sestamibi after injection at rest or during exercise were initially reported by Wackers et al. (15) in 1989. The phase I study involved a total of 17 normal volunteers. Both rest and stress blood clearance curves approximate a dual exponential curve with an initial fast and later slow component. The maximal activity at rest was noted at 1 minute after injection (36% ± 18% of the injected dose), while the maximal activity after injection during exercise was measured at 0.5 minute. At 1 hour after the intravenous injection of $^{99m}$Tc-sestamibi, the blood-pool activity progressively decreased to 1.10% ± 0.01% and 0.7% ± 0.1% of the injected dose at rest and after stress, respectively.

At 60 minutes after the injection of $^{99m}$Tc-sestamibi at rest, the uptake in the heart was 1.0% ± 0.4% of the injected dose. The 24-hour urinary excretion was 29.5% of the injected dose, whereas the 48-hour fecal excretion was 36.9% of the injected dose. The study of the upper-body organ distribution showed that the highest initial $^{99m}$Tc-sestamibi concentration (counts/pixel) is found in the gallbladder and liver followed (in decreasing order) by the heart, spleen, and lungs. The myocardial activity remains relatively stable over time (27% ± 4% of initial activity has cleared from the heart at 3 hours), whereas activity in the spleen and lung decreases gradually. The maximal accumulation in the gallbladder occurs at approximately 60 minutes after the injection.

The uptake in the heart was 1.4% ± 0.3% of the injected dose at 60 minutes after the injection of $^{99m}$Tc-sestamibi during exercise. The 24-hour urinary excretion was 24.1% of the injected dose, whereas the 48-hour fecal excretion was 29.1% of the injected dose. The upper-body organ distribution evaluation showed that immediately after the injection, the highest concentration of $^{99m}$Tc-sestamibi was also found in the gallbladder, followed by the heart, liver, spleen, and lungs. As for the rest study, by 3 hours after injection, 26% ± 12% of initial cardiac activity had cleared.

## Dosimetry

Radiation dose estimates for $^{99m}$Tc-sestamibi have been evaluated from whole-body images obtained in the phase I study (15). The estimated radiation absorbed dose at rest and at stress, assuming a 2.0-hour void, are summarized in Table 8.2. The uptake in the heart is 1.0% ± 0.4% of the injected dose at 60 minutes after injection at rest and 1.4% ± 0.3% at 60 minutes for the stress study. The upper large intestine wall receives the highest dose of radioactivity, both at rest and at stress. To decrease dosimetry to the urinary bladder, increasing voiding frequency should be encouraged. By administering a total dose of 30 mCi of $^{99m}$Tc-sestamibi, no individual organ dose will exceed 5 rad (50 mGy).

Although there is accumulation of $^{99m}$Tc-sestamibi in the mammary glands, there is minimal transfer into milk: approximately 0.01% to 0.03% of the injected $^{99m}$Tc-sestamibi activity can be excreted in human breast milk of a patient who is breast-feeding (27). No interruption of breast-feeding is required following an injection of $^{99m}$Tc-sestamibi due to this very low activity in milk. However, close contact should be restricted.

## Technical Aspects
### Preparation

Preparation of the $^{99m}$Tc-sestamibi from the kit supplied by the manufacturer is relatively simple. Under aseptic and radiation safety conditions, a recommended maximum dose of 150 mCi (5.6 GBq) of additive-free, sterile, nonpyrogenic sodium pertechnetate $^{99m}$Tc in approximately 1 to 3 mL of solution is added into the 5-mL vial in a lead shield. An equal volume (1 to 3 mL) of head space is removed in order to maintain atmospheric pressure within the vial. The contents of the vial are swirled for a few seconds. Then the vial containing $^{99m}$Tc-sestamibi is placed upright in a boiling water bath for 10 minutes. After this time period, the vial is removed from the water bath and placed in a lead shield, and another period of approximately 15 minutes is needed to allow the vial to cool before the intravenous injection. The vial should be visually inspected for particulates and/or discoloration prior to injection. The reconstituted vial should be stored at 15° to 25°C, and $^{99m}$Tc-sestamibi doses should be aseptically withdrawn within 6 hours.

The total preparation, including the recommended quality control step (described in the next section), usually takes between 30 and 40 minutes. Although this type of radiopharmaceutical preparation is not unusual, it may represent a significant drawback in some acute clinical conditions where a dose of $^{99m}$Tc-sestamibi must be rapidly available to permit administration without any delay. This period of 30 to 40 minutes is too long and would limit the availability of [99m]Tc-sestamibi on an emergency basis. Gagnon et al. (28) and Hung et al. (29) have proposed a method of rapid preparation of [99m]Tc-sestamibi using a microwave oven heating method for labeling [99m]Tc-sestamibi instead of the boiling water bath method. The "heating" time was reduced from 10 minutes with the recommended "standard" method to 13 seconds with the microwave oven method. These authors have emphasized that users of the microwave oven method for the labeling of [99m]Tc-sestamibi must follow the specifications that are published; otherwise, the user must test the labeling procedure with his own microwave oven if the technical specifications differ. The technical specifications of any commercial microwave oven used are very important since the power output, microwave frequency, cavity dimensions, and cavity volume may differ, and thus may have a different impact on the labeling procedure. Labeling [99m]Tc-sestamibi with the microwave oven method has been shown to be safe and reliable. Radiochromatographic quality control methods showed that both the boiling water bath and microwave oven methods gave similar values with a very high labeling efficiency of [99m]Tc-sestamibi. However, it is important to note that the use of the microwave oven method is not the one specified in the package insert. Another method for rapid labeling of [99m]Tc-sestamibi has also been described (30).

### Quality Control

The verification of radiochemical purity of [99m]Tc-sestamibi is not always required prior to its administration to a patient. However, it is considered good radiopharmacy practice to inject a radiopharmaceutical of the highest purity, safety, and efficacy. The recommended radiochromatographic procedure for the determination of radiochemical purity of [99m]Tc-sestamibi involves the use of an aluminum oxide–coated (Baker-flex) plastic thin-layer chromatography plate with absolute ethanol as the developing agent. One drop of ethanol is applied at 1.5 cm from the bottom of a dry plate (plates are dried at 100°C for 1 hour and stored in a desiccator) measuring 2.5 × 7.5 cm, without allowing the spot to dry. Two drops of [99m]Tc-sestamibi solution are added on top of the ethanol spot. The plate is then placed in a desiccator and allowed to dry for approximately 15 minutes. The plate will be developed in a covered thin-layer chromatography tank containing ethanol (a depth of 3 to 4 mm). The plate is cut at 4 cm from the bottom in two pieces. The [99m]Tc activity is measured in each piece by an appropriate radiation detector. The percentage of [99m]Tc-sestamibi radiochemical purity is calculated by dividing the number of microcuries in the top piece by the number of microcuries in both pieces. Only the [99m]Tc-sestamibi migrates with ethanol to the solvent front. It is not recommended to use [99m]Tc-sestamibi if the radiochemical purity is less than 90%.

As for the recommended labeling preparation procedure, the recommended quality control is time-consuming and needs to be significantly reduced in order to use [99m]Tc-sestamibi for emergency purposes. Hung et al. (29) proposed the use of a mini-paper chromatography method. They compared the two methods and showed that the average time for drying and developing the aluminum oxide–coated thin-layer chromatography plates was 35 minutes, whereas the average time for developing the mini-paper chromatography strip was 2.3 minutes. The results of the two methods were similar. Using alternative methods (31–33), it is thus possible to rapidly prepare and perform the quality control of [99m]Tc-sestamibi. However, the legal considerations of using these alternative methods should be judged and decided by each institution based on local or federal regulations.

## [99m]Tc-TEBOROXIME

As for [99m]Tc-sestamibi, [99m]Tc-teboroxime became commercially available in December 1990 when it was approved by the FDA. However, [99m]Tc-teboroxime is far less commonly used than [99m]Tc-sestamibi, mainly because the peculiar pharmacokinetic properties of [99m]Tc-teboroxime have challenged the users of this radiopharmaceutical. Despite the technical constraints related to its use, [99m]Tc-teboroxime remains one of the best myocardial blood flow radiotracers available for planar or tomographic perfusion imaging. The unique pharmacodynamic characteristics of [99m]Tc-teboroxime offer an interesting niche with specific potential clinical applications for myocardial perfusion imaging (34–43). Although no longer used clinically because of the technical limitations, it is possible that [99m]Tc-teboroxime might be used again in the future, especially if high-quality ultrafast single photon emission computed tomography (SPECT) acquisition imaging becomes available.

## Chemistry and Constituents

[99m]Tc-teboroxime, a cationic compound, is chemically very different from [99m]Tc-sestamibi and [201]Tl. It has a smaller molecular size than sestamibi but it is larger than thallium. [99m]Tc-teboroxime, a neutral and highly lipophilic compound, is a member of the boronic acid adducts of technetium dioxime complexes (BATO). These complexes are neutral seven-coordinate technetium vicinal dioxime complexes that have a boron group at one end. [99m]Tc-teboroxime is the generic name for [Bis[1,2-cyclohexanedione dioximato (1-)-O]-[1,2-cyclohexane-dione-ioximato (2-)-O] methylborato(2-)-N,N′,N′′,N′′′,N′′′′,N′′′′′]-chloro-technetium, also referred to as SQ30217 (developmental name) or Cardiotec (trademark name, Squibb Diagnostics, Princeton, NJ). CDO-MEB and Mebroxime are other names given to [99m]Tc-teboroxime.

According to the product monograph, a 5-mL vial of $^{99m}$Tc- teboroxime or Cardiotec supplied by Squibb Diagnostics contains a sterile, nonpyrogenic, lyophilized formulation of the following:

1. 2.0 mg of cyclohexanedione dioxime
2. 2.0 mg of methyl boronic acid
3. 2.0 mg of pentetic acid
4. 9.0 mg of citric acid anhydrous
5. 100 mg of sodium chloride
6. 50 mg of gamma cyclodextrin
7. 0.020 mg to 0.058 mg of total tin expressed as stannous chloride ($SnCl_2$)

The contents of the vial are lyophilized after pH adjustment (3.3 to 4.1) and then sealed under nitrogen. There is no bacteriostatic preservative. $^{99m}$Tc-teboroxime differs from other $^{99m}$Tc-labeled radiopharmaceuticals in that the ligand is not present in the vial before addition of $^{99m}$Tc-pertechnetate since it is formed by template synthesis around the technetium atom.

There are no known contraindications to the administration of $^{99m}$Tc-teboroxime and no known pharmacologic action at the recommended doses. Uncommon adverse reactions have been reported in clinical trials. These include a metallic taste in the mouth, hypotension, nausea, burning at the injection site, facial swelling, and numbness of the hand and arm. Since $^{99m}$Tc-teboroxime is excreted in human milk during lactation, formula feedings should be substituted for breast feedings.

## Physiologic Characteristics

### Myocardial Uptake

Because of its neutral, lipophilic properties, $^{99m}$Tc-teboroxime comes close to being a freely diffusable radiotracer similar to xenon 133. The extraction fraction of $^{99m}$Tc-teboroxime is very high over a wide range of blood flow rates (44), higher than $^{99m}$Tc-sestamibi or $^{201}$Tl. Leppo and Meerdink (45,46) studied the transcapillary exchange of $^{99m}$Tc-teboroxime and $^{201}$Tl in isolated, blood perfused rabbit heart model. Using different blood flows varying from 0.15 to 2.44 mL/min/g, the mean peak extraction ($E_{max}$) of $^{99m}$Tc-teboroxime was $0.72 \pm 0.09$, the mean $E_{net}$ was $0.55 + 0.18$, and the mean $PS_{cap}$ was $1.1 \pm 0.4$ mL/min/g. All these values are higher than those obtained with $^{201}$Tl: $0.57 \pm 0.10$ ($p < .03$), $0.46 \pm 0.17$ ($p < .03$), and $0.7 \pm 0.3$ ($p < .001$), respectively. Subsequent studies performed by Marshall et al. (47) using a similar *in vitro* model showed slightly different results with a better extraction for $^{201}$Tl. However, the authors concluded that $^{99m}$Tc-teboroxime and $^{201}$Tl appear to be comparable radiotracers of myocardial perfusion for up to 10 minutes after injection under the single-pass conditions used in their study. The myocardial uptake of $^{99m}$Tc-teboroxime has been shown to be slightly higher than that of $^{201}$Tl in rat heart.

Narra et al. (48) reported that the myocardial uptake at 1 minute postinjection was 3.44% of the injected dose for $^{99m}$Tc-teboroxime and 3.03% of the injected dose for $^{201}$Tl. Other studies showed that myocardial uptake of $^{99m}$Tc-teboroxime parallels myocardial blood flow in a linear fashion, even when blood flow is increased to four times the level of resting blood flow, without the "roll-off" seen at high flow levels with $^{201}$Tl or $^{99m}$Tc-sestamibi (44,49). Beanlands et al. (49) showed that at 1 minute after injection, the relationship of $^{99m}$Tc-teboroxime retention to blood flow was linear over a wide flow range, up to 4.5 mL/min/g. However, after 5 minutes, the retention-flow relationship was linear only to 2.5 mL/min/g. Stewart et al. (50) injected $^{99m}$Tc-teboroxime intracoronarily in open-chest dogs under baseline conditions and after the administration of intravenous dipyridamole. The first-pass myocardial retention fraction averaged $0.90 \pm 0.04$ in this animal model. However, the authors found a rapid clearance of the radiotracer soon after myocardial uptake was complete. Myocardial clearance of the radionuclide occurred in a biexponential manner, suggesting that the kinetics of $^{99m}$Tc-teboroxime represent both blood flow as well as non–flow-related cellular binding. Sixty-seven percent of retained activity cleared with a half-time of $2.3 \pm 0.6$ minutes, while the residual activity demonstrated slow clearance. Myocardial clearance rate determined by dynamic imaging with tomography averaged $21 \pm 4$ minutes and dropped to $13 \pm 4$ minutes following dipyridamole administration.

Pieri et al. (51) studied sequential changes in the regional distribution of $^{99m}$Tc-teboroxime in nine dogs with graded coronary artery stenosis. Coronary blood flow was measured by Doppler, and regional myocardial perfusion was assessed by microspheres. A linear relationship between the $^{99m}$Tc-teboroxime abnormal/normal activity ratio and coronary blood flow ($r = 0.96$) and regional myocardial perfusion ($r = 0.99$) was found. Their results also showed that the myocardial clearance half-times at 100%, 75%, and 50% flow were not significantly different, while clearance half-time at total occlusion was significantly faster ($p < .01$). The effects of metabolic inhibition on the uptake of $^{99m}$Tc-teboroxime, $^{99m}$Tc-sestamibi, and $^{201}$Tl were assessed in cultured myocardial cells by Maublant et al. (52). Overall, $^{99m}$Tc-teboroxime showed the lowest sensitivity to metabolic impairment. The uptake of $^{99m}$Tc-teboroxime was significantly decreased at low temperature (approximately 30% at 0°C), while osmotic lysis or metabolic inhibition with cyanide (a blocker of the mitochondrial respiratory chain), iodoacetate (an inhibitor of the glycolytic pathway), or ouabain (an inhibitor of Na-K sarcolemmal ATPase) had no definite effect. However, the uptake of $^{201}$Tl and $^{99m}$Tc-sestamibi was severely diminished by metabolic impairment or in the presence of dead cells. Since $^{99m}$Tc-teboroxime myocardial uptake is largely independent of the metabolic status of the cells, it should be particularly suitable as a myocardial blood flow imaging agent in situations such as in the postischemic phase, where there is a discrepancy between coronary blood flow and metabolic activity of the myocardial tissue. The differential uptake of [99m]Tc-teboroxime, [99m]Tc-sestamibi, and [201]Tl was assessed in normal, hypoperfused, and border-zone rabbit myocardium by quantitative dual-radioisotope autoradiography. Based on this technique, Weinstein et al. (53) concluded that [99m]Tc-teboroxime, and to a lesser extent [99m]Tc-sestamibi, can better delineate hypoperfused myocardium in comparison to [201]Tl. Since [99m]Tc-teboroxime detected the largest area of hypoperfusion, the authors suggested that [99m]Tc-teboroxime may provide the most accurate assessment of myocardium at risk distal to coronary stenosis.

### Differential Myocardial Washout

Stewart et al. (54) studied the clearance kinetics of [99m]Tc-teboroxime in poststenotic and normal myocardium in response to occlusive, rapid pacing, and pharmacologic stress in the intact preinstrumented canine experimental model. They showed that the [99m]Tc-teboroxime clearance was accelerated in normal myocardium by adenosine and by dipyridamole compared to the control state. The myocardial clearance half-time was $11.9 \pm 1.8$ minutes in the control state and $8.9 \pm 1.1$ minutes and $9.3 \pm 1.9$ minutes after adenosine and dipyridamole, respectively ($p < .05$). Using the adenosine stress test, the poststenotic clearance half-time was significantly prolonged ($11.2 \pm 3.7$ minutes) compared to nonoccluded contralateral perfusion zones ($6.3 \pm 1.5$ minutes, $p < .05$). These results indicate that [99m]Tc-teboroxime myocardial washout is flow-dependent, and that myocardial regions with reduced blood flow exhibit delayed clearance in comparison with regions with enhanced myocardial perfusion. This differential myocardial washout of [99m]Tc-teboroxime was also shown in human studies (55–57). This reflects differences in regional myocardial flow reserve, as well as ongoing differences in regional blood flow during imaging.

While most of the animal studies have reported decreased [99m]Tc-teboroxime clearance from flow-restricted myocardium following either pharmacologic stress test or atrial pacing, [99m]Tc-teboroxime kinetics in flow-restricted myocardium at rest had not been well defined until Johnson et al. (58) studied [99m]Tc-teboroxime clearance kinetics at rest in normal and flow-restricted myocardium over a period of 1 hour in 23 dogs with stenosed circumflex arteries. The first exponential phase of the myocardial clearance (found to be biexponential over 1 hour) was significantly different in the normal zones (half-time = 4.5 minutes) compared to the stenosed territories (10.2 minutes, $p < .05$). However, the half-times of the second exponential phase were not significantly different (160.7 minutes for normal zones and 140.4 minutes for the stenosed zones). These data demonstrated that there is a differential clearance and

redistribution of [99m]Tc-teboroxime in a canine model of resting hypoperfusion, and this can be used to differentiate between normal and hypoperfused myocardium. The same group of authors (59) studied the regional [99m]Tc-teboroxime clearance kinetics in a canine model using dipyridamole to determine if clearance kinetics could be useful in differentiating the severity of coronary artery flow restriction. A significant difference in fractional myocardial clearance between the normal zones (0.69) versus mild-to-moderate stenosis (0.61, $p < .05$) and severe flow-restricted zones (0.57, $p < .05$) was observed over a 1-hour period. After 7 minutes, the myocardial [99m]Tc-teboroxime clearance was significantly different between normal and mild-to-moderate stenosis zones, whereas after 15 minutes the clearance was significantly different between mild-to-moderate and severe stenosis zones. A significant correlation was also found between blood flow and early myocardial [99m]Tc-teboroxime clearance across all zones.

## Biodistribution

Human biodistribution data have been obtained in nine normal volunteers during a phase I clinical trial (48). After intravenous administration at rest, [99m]Tc-teboroxime diffuses rapidly across the phospholipid cell membrane due to its neutral and highly lipophilic characteristics. Blood and lung activity clears within 1 to 2 minutes after the injection. Blood clearance is rapid, with only 9.5% of the dose remaining in the circulation 15 minutes after the injection. The liver, which is the major route of elimination, shows a low activity initially, but the hepatic uptake is increasing over time, with peak activity starting about 5 minutes after injection. The hepatic half-time differs from that of [99m]Tc-sestamibi since it is approximately 1 to 1.5 hours, suggesting that the mechanisms of uptake and excretion may also differ. During the first 4 hours after the injection of [99m]Tc-teboroxime, an average of 8% of the injected dose is excreted in urine, and from 4 to 24 hours 13% is found in the urine. Total urinary excretion averages 22% of the injected dose while total fecal excretion averages 26% of the injected dose. Myocardial uptake of [99m]Tc-teboroxime is rapid, with excellent myocardial visualization at 1 to 2 minutes after injection. The myocardial clearance, however, is also very rapid and biexponential, with half-times of 2 minutes (68%) and 78 minutes (32%).

## Dosimetry

Absorbed radiation doses from a [99m]Tc-teboroxime intravenous injection have been estimated from human biodistribution data obtained in a phase I clinical trial involving nine normal volunteers (48). The estimated absorbed radiation doses are given in Table 8.2. These numbers were calculated for an intravenous injection of [99m]Tc-teboroxime at rest and are based on the following assumptions: 6-hour gallbladder emptying interval, 2-hour urinary bladder voiding interval, two-thirds of the activity leaving the liver goes directly into the small intestine and the remaining one-third is stored in the gallbladder prior to excretion, and all the activity in the liver is excreted in the feces. The results show that the upper large intestine and the gallbladder are the target organs. Clearly, a significant change in liver and gastrointestinal function can lead to a major change in dose estimations.

## Technical Aspects

### Preparation

Preparation of $^{99m}$Tc-teboroxime from the kit supplied by the manufacturer is relatively simple. Under aseptic and radiation safety conditions, a recommended maximum dose of 100 mCi (3.7 GBq) of sterile, additive-free, nonpyrogenic sodium pertechnetate $^{99m}$Tc in approximately 1 mL of solution is added into the 5-mL vial in a lead shield. Air should not be introduced during reconstitution in order to maintain a nitrogen atmosphere. Sodium pertechnetate $^{99m}$Tc containing oxidants should not be employed since the $^{99m}$Tc-labeling reactions involved in preparing $^{99m}$Tc-teboroxime depend on maintaining the stannous ion in the reduced state.

The contents of the vial are swirled for a few seconds. Then, the vial containing $^{99m}$Tc-teboroxime is placed upright in a boiling water bath or in a heating block for 15 minutes (100°C). After this time period, the vial is removed from the water bath and placed in a lead shield, and another period of approximately 10 to 15 minutes is needed to allow the vial to cool before administration to the patient. The vial should be visually inspected for particulate matter and/or discoloration prior to injection. The reconstituted vial should be stored at room temperature, and $^{99m}$Tc-teboroxime doses should be aseptically withdrawn within 6 hours of preparation.

As for $^{99m}$Tc-sestamibi, the total preparation for $^{99m}$Tc-teboroxime usually takes at least 30 minutes, including the time required to heat the water to boiling or to heat the heating block and the time for the agent to be heated. Since this period of time may be considered relatively too long in some circumstances and may limit the availability of $^{99m}$Tc-teboroxime on an emergency basis, another method for fast labeling and quality control procedure has been described, similar to a procedure previously reported for $^{99m}$Tc-sestamibi preparation. Wilson and Hung (60) described a microwave oven method for fast labeling (20 seconds) of $^{99m}$Tc-teboroxime. As for $^{99m}$Tc-sestamibi preparation with the microwave oven method, there are several technical precautions to be considered when using a microwave oven for preparing $^{99m}$Tc-teboroxime.

### Quality Control

The method for evaluating the radiochemical purity of $^{99m}$Tc-teboroxime involves a two-strip paper chromatography: one to evaluate the percent of reduced hydrolyzed $^{99m}$Tc and the other to evaluate the percent of soluble $^{99m}$Tc contaminants.

#### Reduced Hydrolyzed $^{99m}$Tc

Approximately 5 µL (one drop from a 25- to 27-gauge needle) of $^{99m}$Tc-teboroxime is placed at the origin of a Whatman 31 ET Chrom chromatography paper strip (stationary phase). The strip is then immediately developed in a tank containing a solution of 0.9% NaCl/acetone (1:1 volume ratio), used as the mobile phase. After the solvent front has migrated to a preestablished finish point, the strip is then removed and allowed to dry. The paper strip is cut into two pieces and each piece is counted in an appropriate radiation detector. The percent of reduced hydrolyzed $^{99m}$Tc is calculated by dividing the amount of radioactivity of the bottom segment of the strip (multiplied by 100) by the amount of radioactivity of both the top and bottom segments of the strip.

#### Soluble $^{99m}$Tc Contaminants

One drop of $^{99m}$Tc-teboroxime is placed at the origin of a Whatman 31 ET Chrom chromatography paper strip. The strip is immediately developed in a chromatography chamber containing a 0.9% NaCl solution only. The strip is then removed and allowed to dry. The percent of soluble $^{99m}$Tc contaminants is calculated by dividing the amount of radioactivity of the top segment of the strip (multiplied by 100) by the amount of radioactivity of both the top and the bottom segments of the strip. The percent of radiochemical purity of the final product is calculated from the following equation: 100 − (percent of reduced hydrolyzed $^{99m}$Tc + percent of soluble $^{99m}$Tc contaminants).

As for the recommended labeling preparation procedure, the recommended quality control is time-consuming (10 to 13 minutes) and needs to be significantly reduced in order to use $^{99m}$Tc-teboroxime for emergency purposes or to improve laboratory efficiency. Wilson et al. (60) described a one-strip paper chromatographic procedure offering a faster (2 to 3 minutes instead of 10 to 13 minutes) and more convenient method for determining radiochemical purity of $^{99m}$Tc-teboroxime.

## $^{99M}$Tc-TETROFOSMIN

$^{99m}$Tc-tetrofosmin, a new diphosphine complex of $^{99m}$Tc, was the third $^{99m}$Tc-labeled myocardial perfusion imaging agent to be approved and made commercially available, following $^{99m}$Tc-teboroxime and $^{99m}$Tc-sestamibi. $^{99m}$Tc-tetrofosmin shows myocardial uptake, retention, and blood clearance kinetics that are similar to those of $^{99m}$Tc-ses-tamibi. However, the clearance of $^{99m}$Tc-tetrofosmin from both the liver and the lung is faster than that of $^{99m}$Tc-ses-tamibi. These characteristics can have an impact on the injection and imaging protocols. Furthermore, the preparation of $^{99m}$Tc-tetrofosmin does not require a heating period.

## Chemistry and Constituents

Tetrofosmin is a ligand that forms a lipophilic, cationic complex with $^{99m}$Tc. $^{99m}$Tc-tetrofosmin is the generic name for 1,2,-bis [bis(2-ethoxyethyl) phosphino] ethane, also referred to as P53 (developmental name) or Myoview (trademark name from Medi-Physics, Amersham Health-care, Arlington Heights, IL). PPN1011 was another term used to describe tetrofosmin. Tetrofosmin has a molecular weight of 382, and an empirical formula of $C_{18}H_{40}O_4P_2$. The functionalized diphosphine complex of $^{99m}$Tc has a molecular weight of 895 and a formula of [$TcO_2$ (tetrofos-min)$_2$]+.

According to the product monograph, a 10-mL vial of tetrofosmin or Myoview supplied by Amersham International contains a predispensed, nonpyrogenic, sterile, lyophilized mixture of the following ingredients sealed under a nitrogen atmosphere with a rubber closure:

1. 0.23 mg of tetrofosmin or [6,9-bis(2-ethoxyethyl)-3, 12-dioxa-6,9-diphospha-tetradecane]
2. 0.03 mg of stannous chloride dihydrate (minimum stannous tin 5.0 µg, maximum total stannous and stannic tin 15.8 µg
3. 1.0 mg of sodium D-gluconate
4. 1.8 mg of sodium hydrogen carbonate
5. 0.32 mg of disodium sulphosalicylate

There is no bacteriostatic preservative. The lyophilisate is reconstituted with oxidant-free, sterile, nonpyrogenic $^{99m}$Tc-sodium pertechnetate. The pH of the reconstituted product varies for 7.5 to 9.0. There are no known contraindications to the intravenous administration.

## Physiologic Characteristics

### Assessment of Myocardial Blood Flow

Using an intact canine model of ischemia, Sinusas et al. (61) tested the hypothesis that $^{99m}$Tc-tetrofosmin was a reliable coronary blood flow tracer over a pathophysiologic range of flows seen in ischemia or infarction conditions. Six open-chest mongrel dogs had a complete occlusion of the left anterior descending coronary artery. Dogs were injected with 30 mCi of $^{99m}$Tc-tetrofosmin during peak pharmacologic stress performed with either adenosine or dipyridamole. Radiolabeled microspheres were also injected into the left atrium at baseline, coronary artery occlusion, and

peak pharmacologic stress to measure the regional myocardial blood flow. Dynamic planar imaging and arterial sampling were performed during the radiotracer injection and up to 15 minutes after the administration. The hearts were then rapidly excised at 15 minutes for well counting of myocardial $^{99m}$Tc-tetrofosmin activity and flow. Myocardial $^{99m}$Tc-tetrofosmin activity at 15 minutes after the injection correlated linearly with radiolabeled microsphere flow during peak stress in each dog. The correlation coefficients ranged from 0.71 to 0.94 with an average of 0.84. Myocardial $^{99m}$Tc-tetrofosmin activity appeared to underestimate flow at flows exceeding 1.5 to 2.0 mL/min/g. The plot of $^{99m}$Tc-tetrofosmin activity versus blood flow achieved a plateau at approximately 2.0 mL/min/g. On the other hand, as with $^{99m}$Tc-sestamibi and $^{201}$Tl, $^{99m}$Tc-tetrofosmin activity overestimated coronary blood flow in low flow ranges, at less than 0.2 mL/min/g. $^{99m}$Tc-tetrofosmin activity cleared rapidly from the blood with 2.8% and 0.8% of peak activity remaining in the blood at 5 and 15 minutes, respectively. During this study, the authors also assessed heart, liver, and lung clearance. The myocardial clearance between 3 and 15 minutes was similar in both ischemic and nonischemic regions. The myocardial activity cleared 18% ± 11% in the ischemic region. Lung activity remained lower than myocardial activity, and the liver activity remained elevated over the initial 15-minute period following injection.

### Mechanisms of Myocardial Uptake

Mechanisms of $^{99m}$Tc-tetrofosmin myocardial uptake have been studied by some authors using different experimental models. Dahlberg and Leppo (62) evaluated the effect of coronary blood flow on the uptake of $^{99m}$Tc-tetrofosmin in the isolated rabbit heart model. The $E_{max}$ of 0.37 for $^{99m}$Tc-tetrofosmin suggests a $PS_{cap}$ similar to that of $^{99m}$Tc-ses-tamibi. In comparison, the $E_{max}$ for $^{201}$Tl is 0.73, for $^{99m}$Tc-teboroxime 0.81, and for $^{99m}$Tc-sestamibi 0.39. However, $^{99m}$Tc-tetrofosmin has the lowest $E_{net}$, 0.23, among the four compounds; $^{201}$Tl has 0.57, $^{99m}$Tc-sestamibi 0.41, and $^{99m}$Tc-teboroxime 0.67. This lower value of $E_{net}$ for $^{99m}$Tc-tetrofosmin in rabbits suggests myocardial washout of this compound. However, studies in humans have shown a stable myocardial retention of $^{99m}$Tc-tetrofosmin, at least up to 4 hours after its intravenous injection (63). This difference between animal and human data is not really surprising, considering that similar interspecies variability has been previously observed for the kinetics of other $^{99m}$Tc-labeled phosphine compounds, especially for $^{99m}$Tc-dimethyl phosphinoethane (DMPE) (64). Unfortunately, extrapolation of data from animal or *in vivo* experiment results to humans may be difficult due to species differences.

Platts et al. (65) studied the mechanism of $^{99m}$Tc-tetrofosmin uptake in isolated adult rat myocytes. They also evaluated the subcellular localization in *ex vivo* myocardial tissue. They found that the uptake of $^{99m}$Tc-tetrofosmin into rat myocytes was rapid, temperature dependent (an approximately fourfold decrease in uptake was observed when the incubation temperature was reduced from 37° to 22°C), and independent of extracellular $^{99m}$Tc-tetrofosmin concentration. Metabolic inhibitors such as iodoacetic acid and 2,4-dinitrophenol inhibited $^{99m}$Tc-tetrofosmin uptake at 30 minutes by approximately 50% depending on the dosage that was used. However, the cellular uptake was not affected by cation channel inhibitors such as ouabain, amiloride, bumetanide, and nifedipine. The lack of effect of ion channel inhibitors on $^{99m}$Tc-tetrofosmin uptake is similar to that on uptake of other cations such as $^{99m}$Tc-sestamibi. Thus, $^{99m}$Tc-tetrofosmin differs from $^{201}$Tl in that it does not appear to act as a potassium analog. Based on studies performed on tissue homogenate, it seems that mitochondrial membrane potential plays a major role in the myocardial uptake and retention of $^{99m}$Tc-tetrofosmin, as seen with $^{99m}$Tc-sestamibi.

Younes et al. (66) studied the mechanism of $^{99m}$Tc-tetrofosmin uptake into isolated rat heart mitochondria. The conclusion of their work was that the most probable mechanism of uptake of $^{99m}$Tc-tetrofosmin into myocytes is by potential-driven transport of the lipophilic cation. Their results did not predict the mechanism of uptake at the sarcolemmal membrane. They postulated that the myocardial uptake *in vivo* was related to the metabolic status of the myocytes, in particular the mitochondrial membrane and the plasma membrane potentials.

## Biodistribution

Human biodistribution, dosimetry, and safety of $^{99m}$Tc-tetrofosmin administration at rest and during exercise were studied in 12 male volunteers by Higley et al. (67). Every volunteer was injected with 3.7 to 4.7 mCi of $^{99m}$Tc-tetrofosmin both at rest and at stress within 7 to 14 days. Blood, urinary, fecal, and whole-body clearances were calculated. The blood clearance was rapid for all volunteers. By 10 minutes after the injection, there was less than 5% of the injected dose in the whole blood volume and less than 3.5% of the injected dose in the total plasma volume. The blood clearance was initially faster following exercise. At 2 hours after injection, the urinary clearance was 13.1% ± 2.1% in the resting study and 8.9% ± 1.7% in the exercise study (*p* <.001). At 48 hours postinjection, the rate of urinary clearance was almost identical for both physiologic conditions: 39.0% ± 3.7% at rest and 40.0% ± 3.7% at exercise. The 48-hour cumulative fecal clearance was 34.2% ± 4.3% at rest and 25.2% ± 5.6% after exercise. The whole-body clearance at 48 hours was 67% ± 6% after exercise and 72% ± 6% at rest.

Analysis of whole-body images showed that good-quality images of the heart can be obtained as early as 5 minutes

after the injection of $^{99m}$Tc-tetrofosmin and that this uptake persisted for several hours. Myocardial background clearance resulting from activity in the blood, liver, and lung was rapid. After exercise, there was less $^{99m}$Tc-tetrofosmin activity in certain organs, mainly liver, urinary bladder, and salivary glands in comparison to the rest study. As with $^{99m}$Tc-sestamibi, this relative reduced liver uptake at stress can be explained by an enhanced retention in peripheral muscles as a result of the increased blood flow induced by physical exercise.

After a stress injection, the myocardial uptake of $^{99m}$Tc-tetrofosmin, although relatively stable over time, slightly decreases from 1.3% of the injected dose at 5 minutes to 1.0% at 2 hours after the injection. From 5 minutes to 120 minutes postinjection, liver uptake decreases from 3.2% to 0.5% and lung uptake decreases from 1.2% to 0.2%, while gallbladder activity increases from 0.5% to 3.2% and the gastrointestinal tract activity increases from 2.0% to 8.7%. From 5 minutes to 60 minutes after $^{99m}$Tc-tetrofosmin injection, the heart-to-lung ratio increases from 4.0 ± 1.1 to 5.9 ± 1.3 and the heart-to-liver ratio increases from 0.8 ± 0.3 to 3.1 ± 3.0. After a rest injection, the myocardial activity of $^{99m}$Tc-tetrofosmin remains relatively constant over time, with an uptake of 1.2% of the injected dose at 5 minutes and 1.0% at 2 hours after the injection. From 5 minutes to 120 minutes postinjection, liver uptake decreases from 7.5% to 0.9% and lung uptake decreases from 1.7% to 0.3%, while gallbladder activity increases from 0.8% to 5.3% and the gastrointestinal tract activity increases from 2.9% to 13.8%. From 5 minutes to 60 minutes after $^{99m}$Tc-tetrofosmin injection, the heart-to-lung ratio increases from 3.1 ± 1.8 to 7.3 ± 4.4 and the heart-to-liver ratio increases from 0.4 ± 0.1 to 1.2 ± 0.8.

Sridhara et al. (68) compared $^{99m}$Tc-tetrofosmin and $^{201}$Tl myocardial imaging in patients with documented CAD. Planar imaging was performed at six time points: 5, 30, 60, 90, 120, and 240 minutes. The authors found that there was no significant $^{99m}$Tc-tetrofosmin myocardial redistribution with a slow myocardial washout of approximately 4% to 5% per hour after exercise and 0.4% to 0.6% per hour after a rest injection.

## Dosimetry

Absorbed radiation doses from a $^{99m}$Tc-tetrofosmin intravenous injection have been estimated from human biodistribution data obtained in a phase II clinical trial involving 12 normal male volunteers. The estimated absorbed radiation doses at rest and at stress are given in Table 8.2. These numbers were calculated assuming a 3.5-hour bladder voiding period. The results show that, both at rest and at stress, the gallbladder wall is the target organ followed by the other excretory organs such as upper large intestine, lower large intestine, bladder wall, and small intestine. Overall, the radiation dose to most organs is significantly reduced during exercise in comparison to rest.

## Technical Aspects

### Preparation

The 10-mL glass vial containing the lyophilized mixture for preparation of tetrofosmin is sealed under an inert nitrogen atmosphere with a rubber closure and should be stored at 2° to 8°C. The preparation of [99m]Tc-tetrofosmin from the kit supplied by the manufacturer is simpler than [99m]Tc-sestamibi or [99m]Tc-teboroxime preparation since radiolabeling of tetrofosmin does not require heating. Under standard aseptic and radiation safety conditions, the vial is reconstituted with 4 to 8 mL of a sterile, additive-free, nonpyrogenic sodium pertechnetate [99m]Tc solution. The radioactive concentration of the diluted [99m]Tc generator eluate should not exceed 1.1 GBq/mL when added to the vial. The [99m]Tc-tetrofosmin vial, placed in a lead shield, is then shaken gently to ensure complete dissolution of the lyophilized powder, and the vial is allowed to stand at room temperature (15° to 25°C) for approximately 15 minutes. Different strategies to decrease the preparation time (although faster than [99m]Tc-sestamibi or [99m]Tc-teboroxime) have not been successful thus far. The reconstituted injectate must be used within 8 hours and stored at 2° to 25°C.

### Quality Control

As with other [99m]Tc-labeled radiotracers, radiochemical purity determination should be carried out before use. The method for evaluating the radiochemical purity of [99m]Tc-tetrofosmin involves a single-strip paper chromatography (69). Using a 1-mL syringe with a 22- to 25-gauge needle, a test sample of 10 to 20 μL of [99m]Tc-tetrofosmin solution is applied onto the origin position of a Gelman instant thin-layer chromatography–silica gel (ITLC-SG) strip measuring 2.0 × 20.0 cm. This should give rise to a spot diameter of 7 to 10 mm. Since smaller samples have been shown to give rise to unrepresentative radiochemical purity values, it is important to correctly perform this technical procedure.

The strip is then immediately placed in a prepared ascending chromatography chamber containing a fresh solution (1 cm depth) of 35:65 acetone/dichloromethane. The strip should be removed once the solvent has eluted to the solvent front line, and cut into three pieces: the bottom (from the origin to Rf = 0.2), the middle (from Rf = 0.2 to Rf = 0.8), and the distal piece (from Rf = 0.8 to the top, including the solvent front). Each piece is then counted in an appropriate radiation detector. Free [99m]Tc-pertechnetate runs to the top of the strip, [99m]Tc-tetrofosmin complex runs to the middle portion, and reduced hydrolyzed [99m]Tc and other hydrophilic complexes will remain at the origin of the strip. The percent of [99m]Tc-tetrofosmin radiochemi-cal purity is calculated as the activity in the middle portion multiplied by 100 and divided by the total activity of all three pieces. As with other [99m]Tc-labeled myocardial perfusion imaging agents, the percentage of [99m]Tc-tetrofosmin radiochemical purity should be more than 90% before use.

The manufacturer-recommended chromatography system for [99m]Tc-tetrofosmin radiochemical purity assessment generally requires almost 30 minutes for completion. This time period added to the preparation time may represent a relative drawback for [99m]Tc-tetrofosmin in clinical practice. Geyer et al. (70) investigated the possibility of using an alternative technique to obtain a more rapid assessment of radiochemical purity of [99m]Tc-tetrofosmin preparations without altering the overall accuracy of the procedure. They used a miniaturized chromatographic system that resulted in a significant reduction in the time required to perform the procedure. The parameters of the miniaturized system are the same as those used in the standard system with the exception of the paper strip size and the [99m]Tc-tetrofosmin spot size: the ITLC-SG paper strip measured 10 cm (instead of 20 cm in the standard system) and the spot measured 5 μL (instead of 10 to 20 μL with the standard system). The miniaturized chromatography system was compared to the standard chromatography system by evaluating the radiochemical purity of 112 [99m]Tc-tetrofosmin preparations. Radiochemical purity results were similar with a mean difference in purity of 1.3% ± 1.5%. Differences of radiochemical purity were less than 2% in 92 of 112 paired samples. In all instances, determinations of acceptable radiochemical purity (>90%) were concordant between the miniaturized and standard chromatography systems. The average time required to develop the standard strip was 28 minutes, while the time needed for the miniaturized strip was approximately 4 minutes. This represents a more than sixfold reduction in developing time, related to the use of miniaturized paper strips.

## [99M]Tc-FURIFOSMIN

The first [99m]Tc-labeled cationic radiopharmaceutical to be evaluated as a myocardial perfusion imaging agent in humans was the Tc(III) complex [99m]Tc-DMPE. Although animal studies were very promising, unsatisfactory images were observed in humans (64,71–73) because of the rapid myocardial washout and intense liver uptake that were the results of an *in vivo* reduction of the Tc(III) complex to the neutral Tc(II) analog (which is more lipophilic). In 1987, Deutsch et al. (74) reported the synthesis of a new class of nonreducible Tc(III) cationic complexes for myocardial perfusion imaging that were designated as the Q complexes. Two compounds from this series of Q complexes were more extensively studied in humans: [99m]Tc-Q3 and [99m]Tc-Q12. Since the latter has been identified as the agent of the Q class with the most optimal imaging characteristics in humans, this chapter focuses on the properties and clinical results of [99m]Tc-Q12, or [99m]Tc-furifosmin. This radiopharmaceutical is the fourth [99m]Tc-labeled agent to be more extensively studied for myocardial perfusion imaging in humans (75).

## Chemistry and Constituents

[99m]Tc-furifosmin, a cationic compound, is structurally different from [99m]Tc-tetrofosmin (diphosphine complex) because it contains two monodentate phosphine ligands and a distinct tetradentate Schiff base ligand (Fig. 8.1). This agent is a nonreducible cationic, lipophilic, mixed-ligand technetium complex that possesses the same monophosphine ligand (TMPP) as [99m]Tc-Q3, with an additional pair of furan rings in the Schiff base ligand (76). [99m]Tc-furifosmin is the generic name for {trans-(1,2-bis-(dihydro-2,2,5,5-tetramethyl-3(2H) furonato-4-methyleneamino) ethane) bis [tris (3-methoxy-1-propyl) phosphine] technetium(III)-99m}, also referred to as [99m]Tc-Q12 (developmental name) or Technecard (trademark name from Malinckrodt Medical, St. Louis, MO). The electrochemically inert core of Tc(III) of the octahedral coordination sphere of [99m]Tc-furifosmin prevents its reduction *in vivo*.

A vial of [99m]Tc-furifosmin or Technecard supplied by Malinckrodt Medical contains a sterile, nonpyrogenic, lyophilized formulation of the following:

1. 20 mg MP-1549 (Schiff-base ligand)
2. 1.5 mg MP-1515 (TMPP ligand-tris(3-methoxy-1-propylphosphine)); TMPP acts both as ligand and as a reducing agent
3. 50 mg gamma cyclodextrin (phosphine stabilizer)
4. 1.5 mg sodium carbonate (for pH adjustment)
5. 2.0 mg sodium ascorbate (antioxidant)

In contrast to the other [99m]Tc-labeled myocardial perfusion imaging agents, the kit for the preparation of [99m]Tc-furifosmin does not contain stannous ion. It seems that stannous ion is not necessary since the phosphine ligand sufficiently reduces the [99m]Tc-pertechnetate to the desired Tc(III) product. Furthermore, the absence of tin reduces the potential for formation of any reduced/hydrolyzed [99m]Tc within the vial. Cyclodextrin stabilizes the lyophilized formulation more than 100-fold over formulations without a cyclodextrin stabilizing agent. The formulation containing gamma-cyclodextrin has been shown to provide the best overall stability during product storage (77). The pH during labeling is approximately 9.5. The proposed formulation is $C_{44}H_{84}O_{10}N_2P_2$ Tc with a nuclidic mass of 961.6.

## Physiologic Characteristics

### Cellular Uptake

Cationic compounds such as [99m]Tc-furifosmin, [99m]Tc-sestamibi, and [99m]Tc-tetrofosmin are known to partition across sarcolemmal and mitochondrial membranes in response to their negative membrane potentials. The handling of [99m]Tc-furifosmin by isolated rat cardiac myocytes and mitochondria has been studied by Roszell et al. (78). They demonstrated that the uptake and retention mechanism of [99m]Tc-furifosmin in cardiac tissue was essentially identical to the uptake and retention mechanism of [99m]Tc-sestamibi and [99m]Tc-tetrofosmin in heart tissue. All these agents accumulate in cardiac tissue by crossing the myocyte membrane in a nonspecific manner dependent on lipophilicity but driven by transmembrane potential. [99m]Tc-furifosmin, as with the other two agents, is sequestered by the mitochondria, which have a greater transmembrane potential than the sarcolemmal membrane. The cellular uptake of [99m]Tc-furifosmin is greatly modified by perturbing the negative membrane potential with trifluorocarbonyl cyanide phenylhydrazone.

### Myocardial Uptake Versus Coronary Blood Flow

Kinetic properties of [99m]Tc-furifosmin have been studied by Gerson et al. (79) in an animal model. Twenty-one open-chest mongrel dogs with occlusion on the left circumflex coronary artery were studied with dipyridamole and [99m]Tc-furifosmin. Blood disappearance of [99m]Tc-furifosmin was biexponential with an initial half-time of $1.8 \pm 0.01$ minutes and a delayed half-time of $69.0 \pm 8.2$ minutes. The overall blood clearance was $1.83 \pm 0.13$ mL/kg/min. The myocardial uptake of [99m]Tc-furifosmin was related to myocardial blood flow over a range of flows from 0.3 to 2.0 mL/min/g. For blood flows superior to 2 mL/min/g the activity of [99m]Tc-furifosmin showed a plateau and thus underestimated blood flow, while at myocardial blood flows inferior to 0.3 mL/min/g [99m]Tc-furifosmin uptake overestimated myocardial blood flow. As with other myocardial perfusion imaging agents, the myocardial uptake of [99m]Tc-furifosmin is relatively linearly related to myocardial blood flows corresponding to physiologic resting conditions, mild-to-moderate ischemia, and moderate hyperemic conditions observed with dynamic exercise. This study also showed that there was no myocardial redistribution of [99m]Tc-furifosmin over a period of 4 hours.

Meerdink et al. (80) estimated the transcapillary exchange of [99m]Tc-furifosmin in isolated perfused rabbit hearts. The $E_{max}$ was $0.26 \pm 0.05$ (0.71 for [201]Tl), $PS_{cap}$ was $0.48 \pm 0.16$ (1.94 for [201]Tl), and $F_{net}$ was $0.12 \pm 0.05$ (0.57 for [201]Tl). Their data also showed that cardiac transcapillary exchange of [99m]Tc-furifosmin was linear with perfusion over a relatively wide flow range, although less than [201]Tl.

### Comparative Studies

Plasma clearances of [99m]Tc-furifosmin and [99m]Tc-sestamibi were compared in 26 patients by Richter et al. (81). The plasma clearance of both radiopharmaceuticals was biexponential with a half-life of the fast and slow clearance component of $^{99m}$Tc-furifosmin of $2.0 \pm 0.8$ minutes and $129 \pm 24$ minutes, respectively. For $^{99m}$Tc-sestamibi, these values were $1.6 \pm 0.5$ minutes ($p$ = ns) and $86 \pm 21$ minutes ($p$ <.001), respectively, for the fast and slow clearance component. Pharmacokinetic constants for cellular influx were comparable for both radiotracers: $0.31 \pm 0.11$/min for $^{99m}$Tc-furifosmin and $0.25 \pm 0.08$/min for $^{99m}$Tc-sestamibi ($p$ = ns).

Extraction and retention of $^{99m}$Tc-furifosmin, $^{99m}$Tc-sestamibi, and $^{201}$Tl were studied and compared in isolated rat hearts during acidemia by McGoron et al. (82). $E_{max}$ for controls were $70.1 \pm 3.6$, $29.5 \pm 3.1$, and $25.6 \pm 0.7$ for $^{201}$Tl, $^{99m}$Tc-furifosmin, and $^{99m}$Tc-sestamibi, respectively, whereas these values were $64.6 \pm 3.3$, $27.7 \pm 2.6$, and $23.4 \pm 0.6$ under acidemia. $E_{net}$ for controls at 10 minutes were $16.3 \pm 2.4$, $13.7 \pm 3.4$, and $19.4 \pm 1.1$ for $^{201}$Tl, $^{99m}$Tc-furifosmin, and $^{99m}$Tc-sestamibi, while under acidemia, these values were $9.6 \pm 2.0$, $13.8 \pm 3.1$, and $18.2 \pm 0.5$, respectively. Therefore, moderate coronary acidemia (an important physiologic feature of prolonged ischemia) reduced $E_{max}$ and $E_{net}$ for $^{201}$Tl but not significantly for $^{99m}$Tc-furifosmin and $^{99m}$Tc-sestamibi, which are preferentially retained over $^{201}$Tl. In isolated rat hearts, the uptake and retention of $^{99m}$Tc-sestamibi and $^{99m}$Tc-furifosmin appear to be less sensitive to pH than is $^{201}$Tl.

## Biodistribution

Human biodistribution of $^{99m}$Tc-furifosmin was studied by Rossetti et al. (76) in ten normal volunteers (nine males and one female). Seven subjects were studied at rest and the other three were studied by injecting $^{99m}$Tc-furifosmin under exercise conditions. A group of 70 patients with suspected or proven CAD were also studied. Eleven out of the total group of 80 patients/volunteers (14%) reported a transient metallic taste occurring immediately after the injection of the radiotracer, similar to what has been reported for the previously discussed $^{99m}$Tc-labeled myocardial perfusion imaging agents.

After an injection of $^{99m}$Tc-furifosmin at stress and at rest, the activity in the gallbladder peaks at 35 minutes and remains relatively constant. The myocardial uptake is higher than that previously reported for other perfusion imaging agents—2.2% of the injected dose at 1 hour after a rest injection and 2.4% of the injected dose after the stress injection. The myocardial uptake remains substantially constant with time, with no evidence of washout or redistribution over 5 hours. After the injection of $^{99m}$Tc-furifosmin under stress conditions, the biodistribution pattern is relatively similar to that seen at rest. The blood clearance in humans shows a dual exponential function. The whole-blood pool activity at rest is approximately 40% of the injected dose at 2 minutes postinjection, 10% at 10 minutes, and less than 5% at 20 minutes postinjection. The blood pool activity remains negligible from 20 minutes to 24 hours after the injection. The blood pool activity at stress follows a similar pattern. The amount of $^{99m}$Tc-furifosmin excreted in the urine at 1 hour after the injection was $14.6\% \pm 4.1\%$ at rest and $10.2\% \pm 2.4\%$ at stress, and at 24 hours after injection the excreted activity was 26% at rest and 23% at stress.

## Dosimetry

Radiation dose estimates for $^{99m}$Tc-furifosmin have been evaluated from data obtained in seven normal volunteers who were injected with 5 to 7 mCi at rest and 20 to 23 mCi at stress (83). The principal target organs are the gallbladder, large and small intestines, kidneys, and urinary bladder. No individual organ dose exceeds 3 rad (30 mGy), with an administration of 30 mCi (1,110 Mbq) of $^{99m}$Tc-furifosmin. For the combined rest and stress administration of 30 mCi of $^{99m}$Tc-tetrofosmin, the effective dose equivalent is 0.9 rem (11 mSv) or 10 µSv/MBq (38 mrem/mCi). Table 8.2 summarizes the estimated radiation dose for various organs from $^{99m}$Tc-furifosmin intravenous injection in humans.

## Technical Aspects

### Preparation

Preparation of $^{99m}$Tc-furifosmin from the kit supplied by the manufacturer is relatively simple. Under aseptic and radiation safety conditions, 2 to 3 mL of additive-free, sterile, nonpyrogenic sodium pertechnetate $^{99m}$Tc is added into the vial of furifosmin in a lead shield. The contents of the vial are swirled for a few seconds. Then, the vial containing $^{99m}$Tc-furifosmin is placed upright in a boiling water bath or in a heating block for 15 minutes (100°C). After this time period, the vial is removed from the water bath and placed in a lead shield, and another period of approximately 10 to 15 minutes is needed to allow the vial to cool before administration to the patient. The vial should be visually inspected for particulate matter and/or discoloration prior to injection. The reconstituted vial should be stored at room temperature, and $^{99m}$Tc-furifosmin doses should be aseptically withdrawn within 6 hours of preparation.

As with $^{99m}$Tc-sestamibi and $^{99m}$Tc-teboroxime, two $^{99m}$Tc-labeled myocardial perfusion imaging agents necessitating a boiling period for preparation, the total preparation for $^{99m}$Tc-furifosmin usually takes approximately 30 minutes, including the time required to heat the water to boiling or to heat the heating block and the time for the agent to be heated. Preparation of $^{99m}$Tc-furifosmin using a microwave oven has also been evaluated. However, since the manufacturer of $^{99m}$Tc-furifosmin recommends a 15-minute heating period, which is 50% longer than that required for compounding $^{99m}$Tc-sestamibi, Coupal et al. (84) have modified their standard microwave oven method (with specific technical characteristics) usually performed for $^{99m}$Tc-sestamibi labeling. The parameters used to label $^{99m}$Tc-sestamibi (a 12-second heating of the $^{99m}$Tc-sestamibi vial within the microwave oven used in their laboratory followed by a 10-minute cool-down period) resulted in unacceptable radiochemical purity of less than 90% when applied to $^{99m}$Tc-furifosmin. However, by increasing both the microwave oven heating time to 18 seconds (by a factor of 50%) and the cool-down time to 15 minutes, $^{99m}$Tc-furifosmin radiochemical purity was more than 90% both initially and throughout its shelf life of 6 hours. The increased preparation time with the microwave oven seems to be necessary for sufficient chelate formation.

## Quality Control

The method for evaluating the radiochemical purity of $^{99m}$Tc-furifosmin involves the use of a C18 Sep-Pak cartridge. The cartridge is prepared by pushing 10 mL of absolute ethanol through the Sep-Pak, followed by 5 mL of air. The sample is then analyzed by applying 0.1 mL of $^{99m}$Tc-furifosmin to the head of the cartridge (85). Slowly, 10 mL of absolute ethanol are introduced through the Sep-Pak cartridge and the eluate is collected. This represents the first fraction. Subsequently, the cartridge is eluted to obtain the second fraction, but this time 10 mL of 0.9% saline solution is introduced in the cartridge followed by 5 mL of air. A second fraction is then collected separately. The first elution performed with ethanol is counted in an appropriate radiation counter device. This fraction contains the $^{99m}$Tc-furifosmin complex. The second elution performed with the saline solution and containing the elutable impurities is also counted. Finally, the activity in the Sep-Pak cartridge must also be monitored since it contains the nonelutable impurities.

The radiochemical percent purity of $^{99m}$Tc-furifosmin is calculated by dividing the activity recorded in the first fraction (with ethanol) by the total activity of all three fractions (ethanol + saline + Sep-Pak) multiplied by 100. As for other radiopharmaceuticals, the minimum radiochemical purity accepted for clinical administration is 90%.

## $^{99m}$TcN-NOEt

$^{99m}$Tc-labeled bis (*N*-ethoxy, *N*-ethyl dithiocarbamato) nitrido technetium (II) or $^{99m}$TcN-NOEt is another new $^{99m}$Tc-labeled myocardial perfusion imaging agent that is currently undergoing phase II and III clinical evaluation (86). Since this is the newest of the $^{99m}$Tc-labeled agent that can be used for myocardial perfusion imaging, published data are more limited than those already available for $^{99m}$Tc-sestamibi, $^{99m}$Tc-teboroxime, $^{99m}$Tc-tetrofosmin, and even $^{99m}$Tc-furifosmin. However, the biologic characteristics of $^{99m}$TcN-NOEt are very interesting, and differ from those of the other myocardial perfusion radiopharmaceuticals.

Like $^{99m}$Tc-teboroxime (and contrary to the other $^{99m}$Tc-labeled agents), $^{99m}$TcN-NOEt is a neutral $^{99m}$Tc complex. However, in contrast to $^{99m}$Tc-teboroxime, $^{99m}$TcN-NOEt

is the first reported neutral $^{99m}$Tc complex showing long retention times in normal myocardial tissue. Furthermore, unlike $^{99m}$Tc-sestamibi, $^{99m}$Tc-tetrofosmin, and $^{99m}$Tc-furifosmin, $^{99m}$TcN-NOEt shows a significant myocardial redistribution over time. Therefore, $^{99m}$TcN-NOEt is the first $^{99m}$Tc-labeled myocardial perfusion imaging agent that demonstrates characteristics similar to those of $^{201}$Tl.

## Chemistry and Preparation

$^{99m}$TcN-NOEt is a member of a class of neutral myocardial imaging agents named $^{99m}$Tc-nitrido dithiocarbamates that are characterized by the presence of a triple-bond core [Tc = N] 2+ (87,88). It is a neutral and highly lipophilic compound with a octanol/water partition coefficient of approximately 3,100 (89).

$^{99m}$TcN-NOEt has not yet been approved for clinical use in humans. However, the kit for the preparation of $^{99m}$TcN-NOEt supplied by Cis Bio International (Gif sur Yvette, France) for animal and human research purposes can be available either in a liquid or in a freeze-dried formulation. So far, the radiotracer is obtained through a two-step reaction. The constituents of a vial of $^{99m}$TcN-NOEt depend on the type of radiolabeling procedure.

## Liquid Formulation

In the first step of $^{99m}$TcN-NOEt preparation using the liquid formulation, $^{99m}$Tc-pertechnetate (600 to 1,800 Mbq) is added to an intermediate vial containing the following:

1. 1.0 mg DTCZ (*S*-methyl, *N*-methyl dithiocarbazate) or [$H_2NN(CH_3) C(=S)SCH_3$]
2. 3.0 mg TPPS (tris(m-sulfophenyl) phosphine sodium salt) or [$P(m-C_6H_4SO_3)_3$] Na$_3$,

which are dissolved in 1.0 mL Hcl (0.10 M). This resulting mixture is heated at 100°C for 15 minutes and then cooled at room temperature; 1 mL sodium phosphate buffer (0.20 M) is added to obtain a pH = 8.0. Then, 1 mL of an aqueous solution containing 10 mg of the sodium salt of *N*-ethoxy, *N*-ethyl dithiocarbamate ([Et(OEt) NCS$_2$] Na) is added to the vial at room temperature. The final compound is formed almost instantaneously at room temperature and completed within 5 minutes. To avoid adsorption of $^{99m}$TcN-NOEt into the vial walls or into the walls of the syringe (due to the high lipophilicity and lack of charge of the radiotracer), 20 mg of gamma-cyclodextrin is added to the final solution (89).

## Lyophilized Formulation

For the preparation of $^{99m}$TcN-NOEt with the lyophilized formulation, $^{99m}$Tc-pertechnetate (600 to 1,800 Mbq) is added to a vial containing the following components in a freeze-dried form:

1. 1.0 mg DTCZ (*S*-methyl, *N*-methyl dithiocarbazate)
2. 0.1 mg $SnCl_2\text{-}2H_2O$
3. 10 mg DTPA (1,2-diaminopropane-*N*.*N*.*N'*, *N'*-tetra-acetic acid)

The resultant mixture is heated at 100°C for 15 minutes and then cooled to room temperature. As for the liquid formulation, 10 mg of the sodium salt of *N*-ethoxy, *N*-ethyl dithiocarbamate dissolved in 1 mL of water is added to the reaction vial. The final solution stands for 5 minutes at room temperature, and 20 mg of gamma-cyclodextrin (which serves as a surfactant and solubilizing agent) is added.

## Quality Control

As with the other $^{99m}$Tc-labeled myocardial perfusion imaging agents, labeling efficiency of $^{99m}$TcN-NOEt is obtained with thin-layer chromatography. The quality control procedure is performed with a Scheicher and Schull silicagel strip measuring 2.5 × 15 cm, which is eluted using ascending chromatography with dichloromethane. In this system, free $^{99m}$Tc-pertechnetate and any unreacted $^{99m}$TcN-intermediate species remain at the origin of the strip. $^{99m}$TcN-NOEt complex will migrate in the middle to the upper part of the strip with an Rf of approximately 0.7 to 0.8. The product remains stable for at least 6 hours after reconstitution.

## Physiologic Characteristics

### Myocardial Uptake Versus Blood Flow

Ghezzi et al. (90) compared myocardial distribution of $^{99m}$TcN-NOEt and regional myocardial blood flow in dogs after permanent and temporary partial coronary occlusion of the left anterior descending artery and dipyridamole infusion in 15 mongrel dogs. Comparative blood clearances of $^{99m}$TcN-NOEt and $^{99m}$Tc-sestamibi and first-pass extraction fraction were evaluated. As with other $^{99m}$Tc-labeled myocardial perfusion imaging agents, $^{99m}$TcN-NOEt tended to overestimate coronary blood flow in the low-flow range and to underestimate flow in the high-flow range at 15 minutes after its injection, under basal conditions and with dipyridamole. The ischemic-to-nonischemic zone activity ratio was always higher with $^{99m}$TcN-NOEt than that determined with blood flow data. The first-pass extraction fraction of $^{99m}$TcN-NOEt was 75% ± 4% under basal conditions and 85% ± 2% under hyperemic conditions. This high extraction fraction is similar to that of $^{99m}$Tc-teboroxime (although slightly less). The lipophilic properties and consequently the large permeability/surface area product explain the high extraction fraction of both radiopharmaceuticals.

Despite the persistent significant linear correlation between $^{99m}$TcN-NOEt activity and regional myocardial blood flow for 90 minutes after the injection when partial coronary occlusion was maintained, there was an increase in myocardial $^{99m}$TcN-NOEt activity relative to the blood flow as measured by microspheres in the 0% to 20% flow range and a decrease in the 80% to 100% flow range. These data suggest a continuous and slow myocardial redistribution of $^{99m}$TcN-NOEt 15 to 90 minutes after the injection. Some of the data from this study also indirectly showed that there was an early myocardial redistribution of $^{99m}$TcN-NOEt within the first 15 minutes following its administration.

The blood clearance of $^{99m}$TcN-NOEt and $^{99m}$Tc-sestamibi was also evaluated by Ghezzi et al. (90) using the same experimental model. The blood activity at 30, 90, and 240 minutes after the injection of $^{99m}$TcN-NOEt was 20%, 19%, and 14%, respectively, of that measured at 2 minutes after the injection. In contrast, $^{99m}$Tc-sestamibi blood activity decreased much faster with 10% and 4.5% (of the level measured at 2 minutes) at 30 minutes and 90 minutes postinjection, respectively. The blood clearance of $^{99m}$TcN-NOEt was biexponential with an initial half-life of 4.7 minutes and a late half-life of 674 minutes, while the initial blood half-life of $^{99m}$Tc-sestamibi was 1.7 minutes and the late half-life was 55 minutes. No metabolite of $^{99m}$TcN-NOEt has been detected in the blood at 2 or 60 minutes postinjection. With this animal model, *in vivo* imaging showed that the myocardial uptake of $^{99m}$TcN-NOEt at 60 minutes postinjection had decreased by 43% of that measured at 5 minutes. The lung uptake was initially high but decreased faster than cardiac uptake with a heart-to-lung ratio of 1.04 at 5 minutes and 1.84 at 60 minutes postinjection. The liver uptake remained constant over time.

Glover et al. (91) studied the myocardial uptake of $^{99m}$TcN-NOEt in nine dogs with either critical or mild left anterior descending coronary artery stenoses during adenosine infusion. Five minutes after the injection, the *in vitro* $^{99m}$TcN-NOEt uptake was higher than $^{201}$Tl over a wide range of flow. Although myocardial uptake of both agents underestimated the level of flow disparity, $^{99m}$TcN-NOEt uptake more closely matched coronary blood flow than did $^{201}$Tl. The authors concluded that $^{99m}$TcN-NOEt is the first $^{99m}$Tc-labeled myocardial perfusion imaging agent with cardiac retention higher than that of $^{201}$Tl at 5 minutes postinjection.

The same group of authors (92) assessed the first-pass myocardial extraction fraction of $^{99m}$TcN-NOEt in animal model. The mean $^{99m}$TcN-NOEt extraction fraction was 87% ± 1% (range: 81–90%) at normal coronary flow rate and 82% ± 1% with adenosine infusion. This extraction fraction is similar to the one reported for $^{201}$Tl using a similar experimental model (82–87%).

### Subcellular Distribution of $^{99m}$TcN-NOEt

The subcellular distribution of $^{99m}$TcN-NOEt was determined by Uccelli et al. (93) in Sprague-Dawley rat hearts using standard differential centrifugation techniques. Subcellular distribution of $^{99m}$Tc-sestamibi was also assessed using the same procedures performed for $^{99m}$TcN-NOEt. These authors showed that $^{99m}$TcN-NOEt can diffuse and localize in the hydrophobic components of myocardial cells with no evidence of specific association of activity with the mitochondrial and cytosolic components.

Structural membrane integrity was found to be important in the myocardial retention of $^{99m}$TcN-NOEt. After induction of severe cell membrane and organelle disruption, there was no release of $^{99m}$TcN-NOEt activity in the cytosol, while approximately 70% of $^{99m}$Tc-sestamibi activity was released into the cytosolic fraction as a result of the disruption of mitochondria, as previously reported. These observations strongly support the hypothesis that $^{99m}$TcN-NOEt, a neutral and lipophilic radiotracer, remains tightly bound to the hydrophobic components of the cell and that the cell membranes are the most probable subcellular localization site of $^{99m}$TcN-NOEt. These results are also in agreement with those reported by Maublant et al. (94) in cell cultures from newborn rat myocytes where relatively high wash in rates and long half-times for washout have been found.

The concept that $^{99m}$TcN-NOEt is localized predominantly in or on cell membranes was also validated in a study performed by Johnson et al. (95). Using a perfused rat heart model with Triton X-100 (causing membrane disruption), the clearance of $^{99m}$TcN-NOEt was increased markedly in conditions of membrane disruption.

## Myocardial Kinetics

The myocardial extraction of $^{99m}$TcN-NOEt was determined by Dahlberg et al. (96) in isolated rabbit hearts using multiple indicator-dilution methods over a wide range of coronary blood flows. The $F_{max}$ was $0.48 \pm 0.10$, the $E_{net}$ at 5 minutes was $0.24 \pm 0.08$, and the $PS_{cap}$ was $1.02 \pm 0.32$. These values were $0.75 \pm 0.06$, $0.57 \pm 0.10$, and $2.30 \pm 1.02$, respectively, for $^{201}$Tl. These results show that after a moderate initial extraction, there is a significant myocardial clearance of $^{99m}$TcN-NOEt. Another study (97) also showed that initial $^{99m}$TcN-NOEt extraction and retention were moderately reduced by severe ischemic injury but unaffected after brief ischemia, demonstrating that the cardiac transport of $^{99m}$TcN-NOEt is less sensitive than $^{201}$Tl to ischemic injury.

Uptake and release kinetics of $^{99m}$TcN-NOEt were examined in cultures of beating myocardial cells of newborn rats (98). The myocardial uptake appeared to be independent of extracellular $^{99m}$TcN-NOEt concentration. Metabolic inhibition (induced by Rotenone or iodoacetic acid) and amiloride, ouabain, and bumetanide had no effect on the 1-minute or 30-minute $^{99m}$TcN-NOEt uptake. However, verapamil and diltiazem significantly reduced the uptake of $^{99m}$TcN-NOEt. Furthermore, BayK 8644, a calcium channel activator, increased the uptake, suggesting that $^{99m}$TcN-NOEt uptake might be, at least partially, mediated through an interaction with calcium channels.

## Myocardial Redistribution and Viability

*In vitro* experiments and studies performed in animals and in humans have demonstrated myocardial redistribution of $^{99m}$TcN-NOEt with a similar behavior to that of $^{201}$Tl. Ghezzi et al. (99) studied the myocardial distribution of $^{99m}$TcN-NOEt and $^{201}$Tl under conditions of low-flow ischemia (30-minute duration) in open-chest dogs with partial occlusion of the left anterior descending artery. Myocardial uptake of $^{99m}$TcN-NOEt and $^{201}$Tl were determined by *in vitro* counting and correlated with radiolabeled microspheres data. Their results clearly demonstrated that $^{99m}$TcN-NOEt myocardial redistribution was comparable to that of $^{201}$Tl.

Vanzetto et al. (100) also compared $^{201}$Tl and $^{99m}$TcN-NOEt myocardial uptake in open-chest dogs with partial occlusion of the left anterior descending coronary artery with a 50% flow reduction. In their model of sustained low coronary blood flow with severe regional left ventricular dysfunction, the myocardial uptake and kinetics of $^{99m}$TcN-NOEt were comparable to those of $^{201}$Tl. They showed a trend toward resolution of the $^{99m}$TcN-NOEt perfusion defect over time consistent with redistribution at rest. The count ratio of left anterior descending-to-left circumflex artery improved from $66\% \pm 4\%$ at 15 minutes postinjection to $72\% \pm 2\%$ at 120 minutes.

The same group of authors (101) compared myocardial uptake of $^{99m}$TcN-NOEt and $^{201}$Tl in a canine model of acutely infarcted reperfused myocardium. Dogs were injected after 3 hours of total occlusion of the left anterior descending artery and 1 hour of reperfusion. The infarct-to-normal wall activity ratio was $0.32 \pm 0.07$ for $^{201}$Tl (reflecting the extent of necrosis) and $0.74 \pm 0.12$ for $^{99m}$TcN-NOEt ($p < .01$, reflecting reperfusion flow). The authors concluded that in the setting of acutely infarcted reperfused myocardium, $^{99m}$TcN-NOEt uptake was a good marker of reperfused flow, whereas $^{201}$Tl uptake appeared to be a better marker of viability.

Johnson et al. (102) investigated the effects of moderate to severe stenosis on $^{99m}$TcN-NOEt kinetics at rest using an animal model (dogs) with a 90% reduction in the left circumflex flow. This study showed that resting ischemia caused by a stenosis can be detected by planar $^{99m}$TcN-NOEt imaging. Furthermore, quantification of both *ex vivo* and *in vivo* scintigraphic data confirmed the presence of significant $^{99m}$TcN-NOEt myocardial redistribution that was nearly complete within 90 to 120 minutes. The apparent rest-redistribution of $^{99m}$TcN-NOEt was mainly explained by differential clearance of the radiotracer where the clearance from the normally perfused myocardial region is more rapid than clearance from the ischemic zone. Although a smaller component of delayed uptake in the underperfused myocardial regions was not totally excluded in their study, it is likely that [99m]TcN-NOEt does not exhibit a true redistribution (like [201]Tl does) but rather a differential clearance. However, the final scintigraphic result will remain the same, that is, resolution of the myocardial perfusion defect on delayed study. Although there is a myocardial redistribution of [99m]TcN-NOEt over time, the clinical relationship of redistribution to myocardial viability assessment is still unknown at the present time.

The apparent discordance between extremely high myocardial retention of [99m]TcN-NOEt reported in isolated myocytes and perfused hearts (94,95,103) and data from canine and human studies showing washout (92,98, 104–106) seems to be related to interactions with blood elements. Although species-specific differences may explain the discordance, Johnson et al. (107) showed that [99m]TcN-NOEt has significant affinities for binding to both albumin and red blood cells. They demonstrated a bidirectional transfer of [99m]TcN-NOEt between red blood cells and the myocardium. This finding can partially explain the phenomenon of [99m]TcN-NOEt myocardial redistribution.

## Biodistribution

Biodistribution of [99m]TcN-NOEt in humans was initially studied by Giganti et al. (106) in three patients with CAD and by Fagret et al. (108) in ten normal healthy volunteers (four males, six females). Although there are some discrepancies between the two studies that can be explained by the small number of observations, the different type of patient populations, or the methodology, these two preliminary studies showed that the myocardial uptake of [99m]TcN-NOEt is rapid, high, and stable in time, and it is rapidly cleared from the circulating blood. Although the myocardial uptake of [99m]TcN-NOEt is higher than the uptake of other [99m]Tc-labeled myocardial perfusion imaging agents, the lung uptake is also higher, with approximately 20% of the injected dose in the lungs 5 minutes after the injection at rest with a lung half-life of 50 minutes at rest and 77 minutes at stress. Giganti et al. (106) also reported an initial lung uptake of [99m]TcN-NOEt of 24% at 30 minutes after the injection with a lung half-life of 11 minutes. This increased lung uptake is thought to be related to the presence of cyclodextrin in the kit preparation. Cyclodextrin, as previously mentioned, is used to avoid significant adsorption of [99m]TcN-NOEt on the vial, plastic syringes, and catheters due to the lipophilic character and the neutral charge of [99m]TcN-NOEt. Ongoing studies are being performed to find an alternative dispersant to decrease the lung uptake.

Besides the lung uptake of 24% of the injected dose at 30 minutes, Giganti et al. (106) also reported that the liver uptake was 21% of injected dose at 30 minutes, 27% at 2

hours, and 20% at 4 hours. The myocardial uptake of 5.2% of the injected dose at 30 minutes and 4.8% at 4 hours was slightly higher than the one previously reported.

## Dosimetry

Only preliminary data on radiodosimetric estimation of [99m]TcN-NOEt in normal human are currently available and published in an abstract form (108,109). Two teams of investigators have reported their radiation dose estimates— in a group of ten normal volunteers (four males, six females) with a mean age of $36 \pm 11$ years (108), and in a group of three fasted patients with CAD (109). Table 8.2 summarizes the results of the two sets of data. Radiation dose estimates vary most significantly for the liver and ovaries. Further data will be needed to complete these estimates and to compare radiodosimetry of [99m]TcN-NOEt to that of the other [99m]Tc-labeled myocardial perfusion imaging agents.

## IMAGING PROTOCOLS
### Thallium 201

Several different imaging protocols have been described for [201]Tl myocardial scintigraphy, especially for myocardial viability assessment. Since it is not the purpose of this chapter to review these protocols, only imaging protocols using both [201]Tl and [99m]Tc-labeled perfusion imaging agents (dual radionuclide imaging) will be briefly described.

Although both 2-day and 1-day [99m]Tc-sestamibi imaging protocols have their respective advantages, they also present some disadvantages. To avoid these limitations (mainly the relatively long time necessary to complete both rest and stress studies) and to allow for optimal assessment of perfusion and myocardial viability in a single study, Berman et al. (110) introduced a dual-radionuclide imaging protocol. This protocol consists of an injection of 3.0 to 3.5 mCi of [201]Tl at rest and an injection of 25 to 30 mCi of [99m]Tc-sestamibi at stress. SPECT imaging starts 10 to 15 minutes after the initial injection of [201]Tl at rest. Immediately following [201]Tl imaging, the patient performs an exercise. At near-maximal exercise, a dose of 25 to 30 mCi of [99m]Tc-sestamibi is injected. SPECT imaging starts 15 to 30 minutes later. The separate-acquisition dual-radionuclide imaging procedure can be completed in approximately 2 hours. Due to the small contribution of [201]Tl photons into the [99m]Tc energy window, this separate-acquisition approach does not require any specific physical correction, contrary to the initial procedure that was suggested in which a single imaging period with multiple energy windows to simultaneously detect both [201]Tl (corresponding to rest study) and [99m]Tc (corresponding to the stress study) was used. This approach of a single acquisition is very attractive in clinical practice because it requires only one image acquisition (111), it may significantly improve patient throughput, and there is a perfect alignment of both rest and stress images since they are simultaneously acquired. However, a simple and validated method to correct for the spillover of both radionuclides does not exist at the present time.

The dual-radionuclide [201]Tl/[99m]Tc-sestamibi imaging approach (with two separate acquisitions) was popularized and extensively validated by the investigators at Cedars-Sinai Medical Center (112–114) and by other groups (115,116). Their results demonstrated a high diagnostic accuracy with good correlation with coronary angiography and standard [99m]Tc-sestamibi imaging. The dual-radionuclide study was also compared to rest-stress [99m]Tc-sestamibi imaging to evaluate the degree of defect reversibility. In segments with no prior myocardial infarction, the segmental agreement between rest [201]Tl and rest [99m]Tc-sestamibi was 97% (kappa: 0.79, $p$ <.001), whereas in segments with myocardial infarction, the segmental agreement was 98% (kappa: 0.93, $p$ <.001). The agreement for defect reversibility pattern (normal, transient, or fixed) was 95% (kappa: 0.89, $p$ <.001).

The dual-radionuclide imaging protocol is considerably shorter than a 1-day [99m]Tc-sestamibi protocol and thus can be used to increase patient throughput. It also has the advantage of combining the use of the optimal radionuclide for exercise imaging ([99m]Tc-sestamibi) and the optimal radiotracer for myocardial viability assessment ([201]Tl). However, this protocol presents some disadvantages. The physical characteristics of the two radionuclides involved are quite different, resulting in a different count density (related to the difference in the injected doses and in the characteristics of emitted photons). This may affect the evaluation of the degree of defect reversibility, especially in patients with prior myocardial infarction and an abnormal [201]Tl rest study (117,118). Furthermore, the quality of the rest [201]Tl studies is sometimes suboptimal. Financial impact must also be taken into consideration since two different radionuclides are involved. Depending on the availability and the cost of the radiotracers, the dual-radionuclide protocol may be more expensive. Nevertheless, this protocol has been shown to be as accurate as rest-stress [99m]Tc-sestamibi imaging protocol.

The dual-radionuclide imaging protocol can also be modified (Fig. 8.2), according to clinical indications. It has

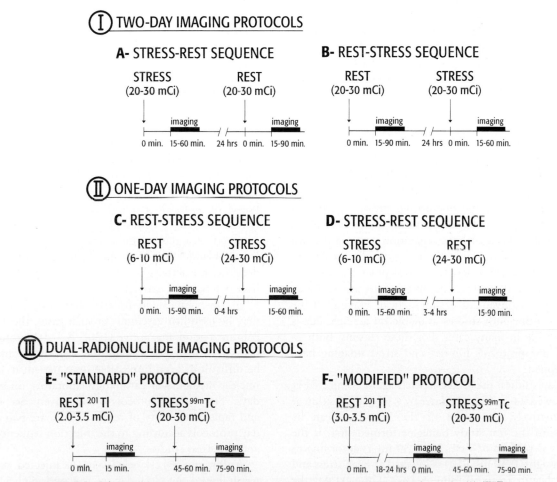

**FIGURE 8.2.** Schematic representation of the most common imaging protocols used with [99m]Tc-labeled myocardial perfusion imaging agents, including dual-radionuclide imaging protocols.

been shown that a 15-minute delay between the injection of $^{201}$Tl at rest and the imaging may sometimes be insufficient to accurately assess myocardial viability in patients with resting hypoperfusion (119). This modification consists of an injection of 3.0 to 3.5 mCi of $^{201}$Tl at rest the day (usually the evening) before the stress study. The next day, an 18- to 24-hour $^{201}$Tl redistribution image is performed. In the standard protocol, $^{99m}$Tc-sestamibi is injected at stress immediately after $^{201}$Tl rest imaging. This delay of 18 to 24 hours following the $^{201}$Tl injection at rest permits a more complete redistribution in viable myocardium. The main disadvantages are that this protocol is lengthy (at least 24 hours) and requires modifications of laboratory logistics (injection of $^{201}$Tl in the evening before the stress test), and the quality of the 18- to 24-hour $^{201}$Tl images is frequently suboptimal. However, it is an attractive approach for both detection of CAD and assessment of myocardial viability. Finally, it offers another approach to cardiac investigation with radionuclide techniques.

## $^{99m}$Tc-Sestamibi, $^{99m}$Tc-Tetrofosmin, and $^{99m}$Tc-Furifosmin

Unlike $^{201}$Tl, $^{99m}$Tc-sestamibi, $^{99m}$Tc-tetrofosmin, and $^{99m}$Tc-furifosmin do not significantly redistribute in the myocardium after their injection. This characteristic offers interesting advantages in clinical practice: (a) Imaging after the stress injection is much more flexible than with $^{201}$Tl. (b) Image acquisition can be repeated if there is significant patient motion or instrument malfunction. (c) It is likely that the image will not be degraded by increased respiratory movements, "upward creep" movement of the heart, or rapid myocardial redistribution as seen when imaging is performed rapidly after an injection of $^{201}$Tl.

Because of the absence of significant myocardial redistribution, two separate injections of these three agents, one with the patient at rest and one during stress, are required to differentiate ischemia from scar. Given the 6-hour physical half-life of $^{99m}$Tc, a 24-hour separation between the two injections is optimal to minimize background radioactivity for the second set of images. In clinical practice, however, having patients undergo imaging on two separate days may sometimes be inconvenient or impractical. Having all the information from both studies available on a single day is highly desirable in many cases. For these reasons, both 2-day and 1-day protocols for rest and stress imaging have been developed.

For 2-day studies, the $^{99m}$Tc-labeled agent is injected at stress, followed 24 or 48 hours later by a second injection at rest. Alternatively, the order of the injections can be reversed, with the rest study being performed first. If the stress study is performed first, 20 to 30 mCi (according to the body weight, 0.30 mCi/kg) is injected at peak stress and imaging is begun 15 to 60 minutes later. The next day the patient is injected with 20 to 30 mCi at rest, and image

acquisition is begun 60 to 90 minutes later with $^{99m}$Tc-sestamibi and 15 to 45 minutes later with $^{99m}$Tc-tetrofosmin and $^{99m}$Tc-furifosmin. If the rest study is done first, 20 to 30 mCi is injected at rest, and imaging is begun 60 to 90 minutes later for $^{99m}$Tc-sestamibi and earlier with the other two agents. The next day the patient is injected with 20 to 30 mCi at peak stress, and imaging is started 15 to 60 minutes later.

The advantages of the 2-day protocol are the following: the 2-day stress-rest protocol has been suggested to be best for novice users of these agents. It is the ideal one based on the physical half-life of $^{99m}$Tc. The 2-day protocol also provides scheduling flexibility in that a patient need only be scheduled for a single study on a given day. The 2-day stress-rest protocol offers also the possibility of eliminating the rest study in cases when the stress study is strictly normal (120). However, as with $^{201}$Tl, the ability to judge a single $^{99m}$Tc-labeled agent image as strictly normal requires a good deal of experience.

Initial studies with $^{99m}$Tc-sestamibi showed that 1 hour after stress injection appeared to be a favorable time for image acquisition because the liver activity has significantly decreased (121,122). Using the higher contrast imaging afforded with SPECT, some investigators have further shortened the injection-to-imaging time to 15 minutes for exercise studies (123). Thus, after a stress injection of $^{99m}$Tc-sestamibi, the liver clearance is rapid enough to permit image acquisition as early as 15 minutes. However, after a rest injection or injection after pharmacologic intervention such as dipyridamole or adenosine, the best compromise is achieved between 60 and 90 minutes after $^{99m}$Tc-sestamibi injection. However, earlier imaging can be performed with $^{99m}$Tc-tetrofosmin and $^{99m}$Tc-furifosmin. Imaging beyond 2 hours after injection is not recommended unless previous images showed a persistent significantly increased subdiaphragmatic activity from small bowel or stomach activity secondary to an enterogastric reflux (124,125). Although initial reports had suggested using either a glass of milk or a small fatty meal to stimulate gallbladder emptying and decrease liver uptake, feeding decreases the activity in the gallbladder but has no effect on liver parenchyma activity.

In some clinical circumstances, making a rapid diagnosis may be useful or essential. In such cases, the 1-day protocols are a good alternative (126). A 1-day protocol may be necessary for practical reasons as well. For example, it may be difficult or even impossible for a patient to come to the nuclear medicine or cardiology laboratory on two separate days. The 1-day protocols offer convenience for patients and rapid availability of results. There are two different 1-day protocols according to the injection sequence of the rest and the stress studies.

A dose of $^{99m}$Tc-labeled agent is injected at stress or at rest followed the same day by a second, higher dose at rest or at stress irrespectively. The initial 1-day protocol has been suggested by Taillefer et al. (127), who have used a rest-stress sequence. The $^{99m}$Tc-sestamibi doses of 8 to 10 mCi at rest and 25 to 30 mCi at stress were empirically chosen based on preliminary data obtained in their laboratory. The rest-stress dose ratio of approximately 1:3 was also empirically determined, taking into consideration the time interval of 2 hours between the doses used for the rest-stress injection sequence. A lower ratio can be used, but doing so necessitates increasing the time interval between the two injections. Rest-stress and stress-rest injection sequences for 1-day $^{99m}$Tc-sestamibi studies have been compared. Taillefer et al. concluded that a rest-stress sequence is preferable when using a 1-day protocol with a short time interval (less than 2 hours) between the two $^{99m}$Tc-sestamibi injections, because the rest image performed initially represents a true rest study. This is not necessarily the case with the stress-rest sequence due to crosstalk from the stress study present in the rest images. In the rest-stress protocol, there is no contamination on the rest study from previous $^{99m}$Tc-sestamibi injection. If the stress-rest sequence is used with a longer time interval or with a higher dose at rest, it is likely that results will improve (128).

Heo et al. (129) compared a rest-stress and a stress-rest protocol for $^{99m}$Tc-sestamibi SPECT imaging in 32 patients. They also showed that the rest-stress protocol provided better image contrast and an increased ability to detect reversibility of perfusion defects. However, the investigators reported that the images obtained using either of the two 1-day protocols were of high quality, and diagnostic results were equivalent (34). The 1-day stress-rest protocol offers advantages that must be taken into consideration: it allows for elimination of the rest study if the stress study is found to be normal, and it offers scheduling similar to that of $^{201}$Tl imaging, which may be more convenient for the nuclear medicine or cardiology staff.

## $^{99m}$Tc-Teboroxime

The peculiar pharmacokinetic properties of $^{99m}$Tc-teboroxime, which are markedly different from those of $^{201}$Tl and other $^{99m}$Tc-labeled agents, have challenged investigators to find a clinically useful and optimal imaging protocol (117,130). Since it takes between 1 and 2 minutes for the $^{99m}$Tc-teboroxime blood pool activity to clear, the hepatic uptake peaks at about 5 to 6 minutes after the injection, and the myocardial washout is very rapid, there is a narrow time window for optimal myocardial perfusion imaging with $^{99m}$Tc-teboroxime. Scattered activity from hepatic uptake up into the heart may cause impaired visualization of the inferior left ventricular wall, especially in obese patients or those with high diaphragms. Because of the $^{99m}$Tc-teboroxime characteristics, initial studies have been mostly performed with planar imaging. However, $^{99m}$Tc-teboroxime SPECT imaging was also shown to be feasible, especially when performed with multidetector SPECT systems. Requisites for all $^{99m}$Tc-teboroxime imaging protocols must include a less than 2-minute time interval between administration and onset of image acquisition and a short total acquisition time, with completion by 8 to 9 minutes after the injection.

A 1-day $^{99m}$Tc-teboroxime imaging protocol can be quickly performed. Because of the rapid myocardial washout, the second injection of $^{99m}$Tc-teboroxime can be performed soon after the first one, within 60 to 90 minutes. Furthermore, the sequence of injections of $^{99m}$Tc-teboroxime in a 1-day protocol (rest-stress or stress-rest) and the time interval between the two injections are not critical as with other $^{99m}$Tc-labeled agents since at 1 hour after the first injection the myocardial background activity is negligible. The initial $^{99m}$Tc-teboroxime stress imaging protocol for detection of CAD was based on the conventional $^{201}$Tl imaging protocol. At peak stress or after the injection of dipyridamole, a dose of 12 to 20 mCi of $^{99m}$Tc-teboroxime is intravenously injected as a bolus. The patient is then immediately positioned supine or upright in front of the gamma camera. Ideally, imaging should begin within 2 minutes of injection. After an interval of few hours (usually 2 hours), a second dose of $^{99m}$Tc-teboroxime (15 to 20 mCi) is injected at rest, and imaging is repeated immediately thereafter.

While most of the initial clinical $^{99m}$Tc-teboroxime imaging studies have been performed using planar acquisition, SPECT imaging has been utilized and shown to be feasible, especially when some modifications in the imaging protocol are adopted and when possible artifacts are taken into consideration (131–135). Unless a continuous acquisition is performed instead of a "step and shoot" one, it may be difficult with a single-headed SPECT gamma camera to acquire images in sufficient time before $^{99m}$Tc-teboroxime myocardial washout affects defect visualization. A triple-headed SPECT gamma camera, which can complete image acquisition within 3 to 5 minutes, is better suited for SPECT $^{99m}$Tc-teboroxime imaging than double- or single-detector cameras.

Since $^{99m}$Tc-teboroxime shows a rapid myocardial clearance and differential washout, it is possible to obtain delayed imaging soon after a single injection at stress, similar to $^{201}$Tl imaging but within few minutes of the stress injection. Hendel et al. (55), using planar $^{99m}$Tc-teboroxime imaging, showed that radiotracer redistribution was seen on the images obtained 5 to 10 minutes after exercise in approximately 50% of the patients who had ischemic defects on the stress images obtained 2 to 5 minutes after the injection. A study performed by Henzlova and Machac (136) in 56 patients with a single-headed SPECT gamma camera showed that $^{99m}$Tc-teboroxime adenosine washout myocardial perfusion imaging can be quickly accomplished and that the detected reversibility of the perfusion defects did not significantly differ from the reversibility observed on the rest images.

Pharmacologic vasodilation with either dipyridamole or adenosine is probably the best stress modality to use with $^{99m}$Tc-teboroxime imaging for clinical and technical reasons. While the myocardial extraction fraction of other perfusion agents and their subsequent uptake fall off at high coronary blood flows induced by dipyridamole or adenosine, resulting in an underestimation of flow, $^{99m}$Tc-teboroxime shows a more linear relationship with myocardial blood flow over a wide range of flows. $^{99m}$Tc-teboroxime, being an excellent flow tracer even at very high flows, is thus suitable for the detection of coronary reserve during pharmacologic stress and it should be able to detect milder degrees of coronary stenosis (137–139). Because of the high myocardial blood flows achieved with adenosine, the myocardial washout of $^{99m}$Tc-teboroxime is even faster. The time interval between the two injections of $^{99m}$Tc-teboroxime can be shortened because there is less residual activity from the first injection. Pharmacologic vasodilation is also very useful for practical considerations. When performing treadmill stress test with $^{99m}$Tc-teboroxime, the gamma camera (especially SPECT camera) must be ready to acquire images before stress begins. Furthermore, the patient must be moved quickly from the treadmill to the camera after completion of exercise. With dipyridamole or adenosine, the protocol is simpler because the pharmacologic stressor can be infused while the patient is positioned under the camera. Furthermore, since acquisition must start within a few minutes after the injection of $^{99m}$Tc-teboroxime during the treadmill stress test, imaging artifacts due to upward creep movement of the heart, patient motion, or cardiac motion secondary to increased respiratory depth (immediately following exercise) may occur, whereas this is not seen with dipyridamole or adenosine administration.

### $^{99m}$TcN-NOEt

At the present time, the number of reported clinical imaging protocols is very limited. Since $^{99m}$TcN-NOEt demonstrates some degree of myocardial redistribution, similar to $^{201}$Tl, Fagret et al. (104) have used at stress-redistribution imaging protocol with $^{99m}$TcN-NOEt. They showed a similar diagnostic accuracy between the two agents with such imaging protocol. More comparative data will be needed, but it is likely that if these results are confirmed by other studies, imaging protocols similar to those used for $^{201}$Tl could be applicable to $^{99m}$TcN-NOEt myocardial perfusion imaging.

## CLINICAL RESULTS

The diagnostic accuracy of radionuclide myocardial perfusion imaging depends on several technical factors and patient population characteristics. These include the radio-pharmaceutical, type of data acquisition (planar, SPECT, gated, attenuation corrected imaging), type of data analysis (qualitative, semiquantitative, quantitative), type of stress testing, level of stress, end points (treadmill, pharmacologic vasodilation, or pharmacologic stress test), criteria to define significant CAD, the number of diseased vessels, the severity of stenosis, inclusion or exclusion of patients having previous known myocardial infarction, and the referral bias. Given all these major factors, it is not surprising to see significantly different results from one study to another. Therefore, it is important to evaluate and consider these variables before ascertaining the real sensitivity and specificity of a specific radionuclide imaging procedure. The following data mostly summarize the clinical results obtained with the various radionuclide myocardial perfusion imaging agents in the detection of chronic CAD, and thus utilization of these scintigraphic procedures is subject to this limitation.

## Thallium 201

In a recent extensive review of the medical literature, Maddahi et al. (140) discussed some of the impact of the above-mentioned factors on the diagnostic accuracy of $^{201}$Tl imaging in detection of CAD. The overall sensitivity and specificity of exercise-redistribution planar $^{201}$Tl imaging for detection of CAD using qualitative (visual) analysis was 82% and 88%, respectively, in a total of 4,678 patients regrouped in 48 studies performed between 1977 and 1985. The sensitivity increases from 79% for detection of single-vessel disease to 88% and 92% for double- and triple-vessel disease, respectively. Detrano et al. (141) reported that the mean sensitivity was 79% in patients without myocardial infarction and 96% in patients with myocardial infarction. Quantitative analysis of planar $^{201}$Tl imaging did not show a significantly increased diagnostic accuracy, with a sensitivity of 89%, a specificity of 68%, and a normalcy rate of 88%. However, quantitative analysis of planar scintigraphy has been shown to reduce interobserver and intraobserver variability.

The overall sensitivity and specificity of SPECT $^{201}$Tl scintigraphy with qualitative analysis in five large studies was 90% and 77%, respectively. Data from seven studies showed that quantitative analysis had the same sensitivity (90%) and a slightly decreased specificity (70%) in comparison to qualitative analysis. As for planar imaging, the extent of disease has an impact on the accuracy of SPECT study. In five studies, the overall sensitivity increased from 83% for single-vessel disease to 93% for double-vessel and to 95% for triple-vessel disease.

Results obtained from pharmacologic vasodilation are similar to those reported with treadmill stress test $^{201}$Tl scintigraphy, with an overall sensitivity of 87% and a specificity of 81%. In five studies directly comparing treadmill and dipyridamole $^{201}$Tl scintigraphy performed in the same patient population, both treadmill and dipyridamole had the same sensitivity (79%) with a specificity of 92% and 95%, respectively (142).

## $^{99m}$Tc-Sestamibi

Several studies have compared $^{201}$Tl and $^{99m}$Tc-sestamibi planar and SPECT imaging for detecting angiographically significant CAD in the same patient population (143). Sensitivity, specificity, and normalcy rate have been determined for the overall detection of CAD and the detection of disease in individual coronary arteries. Initial studies with $^{99m}$Tc-sestamibi mainly used planar imaging, whereas more recent studies were performed with SPECT imaging. Although both radiotracers show a similar sensitivity, the specificity and the normalcy rates of $^{99m}$Tc-sestamibi are slightly better than with $^{201}$Tl. However, it is important to emphasize that all the numbers on the specificity and normalcy rate have been obtained in a very limited number of patients, and thus cannot demonstrate a statistically significant difference. The overall sensitivity varies between 73% and 98% for $^{201}$Tl and between 73% and 96% for $^{99m}$Tc-sestamibi. The specificity and the normalcy rate varies between 50% and 100% for $^{201}$Tl and between 75% and 100% for $^{99m}$Tc-sestamibi. Several studies confirmed a very high degree of concordance between the two radiotracers in detecting CAD.

Thus, although $^{201}$Tl and $^{99m}$Tc-sestamibi have different biologic and physical characteristics, the overall diagnostic sensitivities and specificities for both planar and SPECT imagings are similar. Of note, however, some authors have found that, although there is usually good agreement between the two radiotracers, the defect size at stress is sometimes smaller on $^{99m}$Tc-sestamibi imaging than on $^{201}$Tl studies (143). Although this observation does not seem to affect the diagnostic sensitivity of $^{99m}$Tc-sestamibi imaging, it is hypothesized that differences in the physical characteristics, in myocardial extraction, and in technical acquisition may account for this slight discrepancy between the two radiopharmaceuticals.

Several radionuclide imaging procedures have been used or are still used in the detection and localization of myocardial infarction (144). Myocardial perfusion imaging with an injection of $^{201}$Tl at rest also has been used for that purpose. Since $^{201}$Tl presents some physical and physiologic disadvantages as mentioned above, $^{99m}$Tc-sestamibi has been studied in a multicenter phase III clinical trial to evaluate the efficacy of this radiopharmaceutical in detecting, localizing, and sizing myocardial infarction (145,146). A total of 122 patients and 24 normal volunteers were involved in the study reported by Boucher (145). Planar imaging was performed 1 to 4 hours after a rest injection of $^{99m}$Tc-sestamibi. The results of the $^{99m}$Tc-sestamibi perfusion study were compared to those of rest electrocardiogram and $^{99m}$Tc-red blood cells gated cardiac blood pool study. Of the

122 patients, 115 had Q waves on the electrocardiogram. $^{99m}$Tc-sestamibi study was abnormal in 113 (98%) of these individuals. Of 115 patients with a wall motion abnormality, 108 (94%) had an abnormal $^{99m}$Tc-sestamibi study. In contrast, $^{99m}$Tc-sestamibi imaging was normal in 22 (92%) of 24 normal volunteers.

Dilsizian et al. (147) performed quantitative analysis of $^{99m}$Tc-sestamibi uptake at rest in 38 patients with myocardial infarction and known coronary anatomy. They correlated the myocardial uptake in each vascular territory with the percent of coronary stenosis. The mean $^{99m}$Tc-sestamibi uptake in the vascular territories supplied by occluded arteries with good collaterals was 61% ± 23%, whereas the uptake in territories with normal vessels or stenoses <50% was 87% ± 10% ($p$ <.001). Using quantitative evaluation, they have defined an abnormal vascular territory as a segment showing less than 67% (> 2 standard deviations) of the peak myocardial $^{99m}$Tc-sestamibi activity. The accuracy of quantitative analysis of $^{99m}$Tc-sestamibi uptake at rest was 91% in differentiating myocardial regions with occluded vessels and poor collateral blood flow from those with normal coronary anatomy. Other studies showed that $^{99m}$Tc-sestamibi imaging was able to provide a very accurate measurement of the area at risk during acute myocardial infarction, as compared to coronary angiography (148). Furthermore, $^{99m}$Tc-sestamibi perfusion defect size has been found to be closely related with regional wall motion and values of left ventricular ejection fraction in patients with myocardial infarction (149). The size of the $^{99m}$Tc-sestamibi perfusion defect at rest also closely correlates with that of $^{201}$Tl defect size on the redistribution imaging.

The lack of significant myocardial redistribution of $^{99m}$Tc-sestamibi for a few hours after its administration offers a unique opportunity for radionuclide myocardial perfusion imaging to be used in acute clinical settings. A dose of $^{99m}$Tc-sestamibi can be administered immediately before therapy is initiated, and imaging can be postponed until the patient's condition is stabilized. Two new acute indications for myocardial perfusion imaging have emerged since the clinical introduction of $^{99m}$Tc-sestamibi: evaluation of thrombolytic therapy in patients with acute myocardial infarction, and detection of myocardial ischemia in patients with spontaneous chest pain (150). Several studies have shown that $^{99m}$Tc-sestamibi imaging can be used to predict reperfusion of the infarct-related artery in patients who have received thrombolytic therapy for acute myocardial infarction (142). Serial $^{99m}$Tc-sestamibi imaging is performed as follows: a patient with an acute myocardial infarction, and who is candidate for thrombolytic therapy, is injected with $^{99m}$Tc-sestamibi (at rest) before treatment starts. Imaging is performed when it is clinically safe for the patient and technically convenient for the nurse and technical staff. Since $^{99m}$Tc-sestamibi has been injected before thrombolytic therapy has been administered, the first $^{99m}$Tc-sestamibi images will reflect the hypoperfused myocardium at risk. Then, a second $^{99m}$Tc-sestamibi injection is performed a few hours or a few days after thrombolytic therapy. The resultant images will reflect the hypoperfused myocardium with the completed infarction. The difference in the size and severity of $^{99m}$Tc-sestamibi myocardial defect between the pre- and postthrombolytic therapy $^{99m}$Tc-sestamibi images will correspond to the myocardium that was salvaged by thrombolysis.

$^{99m}$Tc-sestamibi imaging can also be useful in detecting or ruling out myocardial ischemia in patients with spontaneous chest pain (151). This symptomatology represents a diagnostic challenge since 12-lead electrocardiogram and serial cardiac enzyme determination may be falsely negative. $^{99m}$Tc-sestamibi can be administered during a chest pain episode. The patient can be treated, if necessary, and planar or SPECT myocardial perfusion imaging is performed a few hours later. A normal study will strongly suggest that the chest pain is not related to CAD. However, if myocardial perfusion defects are detected, then a second injection of $^{99m}$Tc-sestamibi is administered when the patient is pain free, either on the same day or the day after (depending on the dose initially injected). If the second study shows a decrease in the perfusion defect size compared to the one seen on the initial study, then it is likely that the spontaneous chest pain is related to transient myocardial ischemia.

One of the major advantages of $^{99m}$Tc-sestamibi over $^{201}$Tl imaging is its ability to assess both myocardial perfusion and ventricular function simultaneously with a single radiotracer injection (first-pass study). The injected dose of $^{99m}$Tc-sestamibi (up to 30 mCi) and its high counting statistics permit the determination of the left ventricular ejection fraction and the regional and global ventricular function (both at rest and during peak exercise). Using this approach, it is now possible to obtain information similar to that formerly requiring two separate studies—myocardial perfusion study and radionuclide angiocardiography.

Due to the high counting statistics of $^{99m}$Tc-sestamibi myocardial perfusion studies, acquisition of planar or SPECT gated images synchronized to the patient's electrocardiogram can be performed, similar to a radionuclide gated blood pool imaging. In addition to the perfusion imaging, it is also possible to simultaneously assess ventricular function in a different fashion than with $^{99m}$Tc-sestamibi first-pass radionuclide ventriculography. With gated $^{99m}$Tc-sestamibi studies, especially gated SPECT, many different parameters such as regional wall motion and wall thickening, in addition to left ventricular ejection fraction and end-diastolic images, can be obtained (142). Although gated planar $^{99m}$Tc-sestamibi imaging is relatively easy to perform, recent advances in dedicated software have led to widespread use of gated $^{99m}$Tc-sestamibi SPECT. Contrary to first-pass $^{99m}$Tc-sestamibi studies, gated SPECT studies do not require specially dedicated imaging devices and thus can be performed easily.

Several clinically relevant applications of gated SPECT $^{99m}$Tc-sestamibi studies have been described (152–157).

The availability of dedicated software and significantly increased computer capability have contributed to a more extensive clinical use of these studies. Because it is relatively simple to perform and because of the clinical usefulness of the provided information, it is expected that this procedure will expand and that all perfusion SPECT $^{99m}$Tc-sestamibi studies will be acquired in the gated mode. The major clinical applications of gated SPECT $^{99m}$Tc-sestamibi studies are as follows:

1. Differentiation of myocardial infarction from soft tissue attenuation artifact.
2. Improved detection of CAD with end-diastolic images.
3. Evaluation of patients with myocardial infarction.
4. Use of only a single study in detection of CAD.
5. Evaluation of patients in whom functional impairment can be greater than perfusion abnormalities (small vessel disease, diabetes, cardiomyopathy).

These applications are described in Chapter 11.

## $^{99m}$Tc-Teboroxime

Although $^{99m}$Tc-teboroxime has been approved for clinical use for many years now, there are few reports in the literature on its clinical value in large patient populations. Most of the reported data are based on studies performed in 20 to 50 patients, including two multicenter trials. Nevertheless, investigators agree that the diagnostic accuracy of $^{99m}$Tc-teboroxime is similar to that of $^{201}$Tl scintigraphy in detection of CAD. Furthermore, the unique biologic characteristics of $^{99m}$Tc-teboroxime can be used for more specific clinical applications.

The initial studies involving $^{99m}$Tc-teboroxime administration in patients with CAD were published in late 1980s. Good agreement between $^{99m}$Tc-teboroxime and $^{201}$Tl for the detection of perfusion abnormalities (abnormal vs. normal), patient diagnosis, and myocardial segmental analysis, and for the identification of diseased vascular territories has been reported in several clinical studies performed with both exercise and dipyridamole stress test, using either planar or SPECT imaging. The sensitivity and specificity of the two radiopharmaceuticals are also similar in detection of CAD. A higher diagnostic accuracy of $^{99m}$Tc-teboroxime has been reported in studies using a shorter imaging protocol compared with other studies using a longer time interval between $^{99m}$Tc-teboroxime injection and imaging.

Seldin et al. (158) found a good correlation between $^{99m}$Tc-teboroxime and $^{201}$Tl for detection of coronary lesions, but the hepatic uptake of $^{99m}$Tc-teboroxime obscured inferoapical segments in some planar views in 14 out of 20 patients without interfering with abnormal vessel identification. Although these authors have found a good correlation between the two agents, the high liver uptake was responsible for 68% of nonevaluable inferior segments on $^{99m}$Tc-teboroxime images. Fleming et al. (159), using an automated quantitative coronary arteriography, found no difference between $^{99m}$Tc-teboroxime and $^{201}$Tl in detecting CAD. These authors used a $^{99m}$Tc-teboroxime imaging protocol that was completed within 60 to 90 minutes for both rest and stress studies.

Taking into consideration the rapid myocardial clearance of $^{99m}$Tc-teboroxime and the potential problems in relation to the inferior wall of the left ventricle because of extensive hepatic uptake and resultant scatter, Hendel et al. (55) used a novel patient positioning technique (seated) and a rapid dynamic data acquisition protocol (40 to 80 seconds per view) to compare planar $^{99m}$Tc-teboroxime and $^{201}$Tl imaging; postexercise studies were completed in an average time of less than 5 minutes. They found a high diagnostic agreement in 28 of the 30 patients. They also compared early imaging to delayed postexercise images obtained 5 to 10 minutes after exercise. They were the first authors to describe the rapid differential washout of $^{99m}$Tc-teboroxime, resulting in a rapid disappearance of exercise-induced perfusion defects noted on the initial postexercise views.

The results of three multicenter clinical trials on planar and SPECT $^{99m}$Tc-teboroxime imaging were reported in the early 1990s (160). Stress and rest $^{99m}$Tc-teboroxime studies were completed within 3 hours. Sensitivity and specificity of $^{99m}$Tc-teboroxime imaging in 155 subjects evaluable for efficacy analysis were 83.2% and 92.1%, respectively. $^{99m}$Tc-teboroxime imaging agreed with $^{201}$Tl in 90.4% of the cases and coronary angiography agreed with $^{99m}$Tc-teboroxime and $^{201}$Tl in 76.2% and 80.3% of the cases, respectively. Results of the Canadian multicenter trial on SPECT $^{99m}$Tc-teboroxime imaging were reported by Burns et al. (161). Treadmill stress $^{99m}$Tc-teboroxime SPECT studies performed with single-head gamma cameras were compared to $^{201}$Tl SPECT imaging in 50 patients. There was a concordance between the two agents in 80% (360/450) of the myocardial segments. Taillefer et al. (162) reported the results of the Canadian multicenter clinical trial of $^{99m}$Tc-teboroxime planar imaging performed in ten centers. Forty-seven patients with significant disease on coronary angiography (>50% stenosis) and seven patients with normal angiography took part in two planar imaging studies, one with $^{99m}$Tc-teboroxime and the other with $^{201}$Tl. The sensitivity for detection of CAD was 85% for $^{201}$Tl and 83% for $^{99m}$Tc-teboroxime.

Correlative studies also have been performed with other radionuclide myocardial perfusion imaging agents. A study from our institution (163) compared $^{201}$Tl, $^{99m}$Tc-sestamibi, and $^{99m}$Tc-teboroxime in 18 patients with significant CAD. The patients were subjected to three treadmill stress tests and imaged with the three radiopharmaceuticals separately. Segmental comparison showed agreement in 85% of the segments between $^{201}$Tl and $^{99m}$Tc-teboroxime, in 92% between $^{201}$Tl and $^{99m}$Tc-sestamibi, and in 84% between $^{99m}$Tc-sestamibi and $^{99m}$Tc-teboroxime. Abnormal $^{201}$Tl, $^{99m}$Tc-sestamibi, and $^{99m}$Tc-teboroxime studies were

seen in 89%, 89%, and 83% of patients, respectively, detecting 77, 75, and 65 abnormal segments. Ischemic-to-normal wall ratios were 0.75 ± 0.06, 0.73 + 0.08, and 0.78 ± 0.08 for $^{201}$Tl, $^{99m}$Tc-sestamibi, and $^{99m}$Tc-teboroxime, respectively. Therefore, although the biologic characteristics of these agents are different, this study showed in a high pretest likelihood population a good correlation between them in detection of significant CAD.

As for $^{99m}$Tc-sestamibi, because of the high count statistics related to the $^{99m}$Tc labeling, $^{99m}$Tc-teboroxime imaging may provide the opportunity for the first-pass evaluation of left and right ventricle at rest and at stress in conjunction with myocardial perfusion study. Williams et al. (164) compared $^{99m}$Tc-teboroxime, $^{99m}$Tc-sestamibi, and $^{99m}$Tc-DTPA as radiotracers used for first-pass radionuclide angiographic studies to determine left ventricular function in 25 patients with clinically normal left ventricular function. These authors did not find significant differences between the observed clinical results of first-pass tracer kinetics of $^{99m}$Tc-sestamibi and $^{99m}$Tc-DTPA. However, although $^{99m}$Tc-teboroxime is also a $^{99m}$Tc-labeled radiotracer, there was a significantly greater first-pass pulmonary extraction of $^{99m}$Tc-teboroxime compared with $^{99m}$Tc-sestamibi or $^{99m}$Tc-DTPA. This increased initial pulmonary uptake results in clinically important differences: the pulmonary background during the levophase of the tracer transit is greater, the measured mean pulmonary transit time is prolonged, the raw and final ejection fractions are lower, the image quality and details are poorer (which may compromise functional image and regional wall motion interpretation), and left ventricular border definition is obscured, resulting in larger geometrically derived left ventricular volumes. The results of this study suggest that, unless sophisticated and dedicated software or other methods are developed to specifically correct for $^{99m}$Tc-teboroxime high initial pulmonary background, first-pass radionuclide studies with $^{99m}$Tc-teboroxime are not optimal. Stable myocardial uptake during the acquisition and high-count statistics are prerequisites for optimal gated planar or SPECT imaging. Although myocardial images obtained after $^{99m}$Tc-teboroxime injection transiently show high counts, the rapid myocardial washout of the radiotracer limits the possibility of acquiring good-quality ECG-gated studies, especially gated SPECT studies, in contrast to $^{99m}$Tc-sestamibi.

## $^{99m}$Tc-Tetrofosmin

Initial clinical studies, especially multicenter trials performed in different countries, involved the comparison of $^{99m}$Tc-tetrofosmin and $^{201}$Tl in patients undergoing coronary angiography (165–171). Three types of data have been correlated: detection of CAD (sensitivity and specificity), detection of stenosed coronary arteries, and comparison of myocardial segments and final patients diagnosis. The sensitivity in detection of significant CAD is similar for both radiopharmaceuticals, varying from 77% to 100% for 99mTc-tetrofosmin and 78% to 95% for 201Tl. The specificity is also similar, but the number of patients is relatively limited and may be not necessarily representative. The sensitivity and the specificity for detection of stenosed coronary arteries is also similar. Studies comparing myocardial segments and final patients diagnosis show a high level of concordance (with an average of 85%) between 99mTc-tetrofosmin and 201Tl. These numbers are similar to those obtained in comparing 99mTc-sestamibi and 201Tl.

Although 99mTc-tetrofosmin shows an overall diagnostic accuracy similar to 201Tl in detection of CAD, there are some differences between the two agents, as also seen with 99mTc-sestamibi. Many authors have confirmed that the quality of stress and rest 99mTc-tetrofosmin SPECT images was superior to those of 201Tl tomographic images, despite a shorter acquisition time. Greater photon flux and count density with higher photon energy resulting in a decrease in soft tissue attenuation improve the final image quality and should translate into a more consistent reading. Reduced variability of image readings should lead to more uniform

diagnostic interpretation between different laboratories. Hendel et al. (172) performed a study to determine the relative image quality and the interobserver variability among four experienced readers of 99mTc-tetrofosmin and 201Tl scintigraphies. The data were obtained in 212 patients enrolled in the Phase III Multicenter Tetrofosmin Trial, an international study comparing 99mTc-tetrofosmin with 201Tl planar imaging and performed in Europe and the United States. All studies were sent to a central laboratory and processed in a uniform manner. The readers blindly interpreted each stress/rest image set and graded subjectively the image quality. More images were categorized as "excellent" with 99mTc-tetrofosmin images (52%) than 201Tl (28%, $p$ <.05). The kappa value, used as a measure of agreement between the four observers, was generally higher for 99mTc-tetrofosmin than for 201Tl studies for each type of perfusion defect: 0.62 vs. 0.56 for infarction, 0.54 vs. 0.47 for ischemia, 0.65 vs. 0.62 for mixed defects, and 0.36 vs. 0.29 for the total diagnostic agreement.

Although most of the studies have been performed with 201Tl as a comparator, it is important to compare two 99mTc-labeled perfusion imaging agents, since they are now

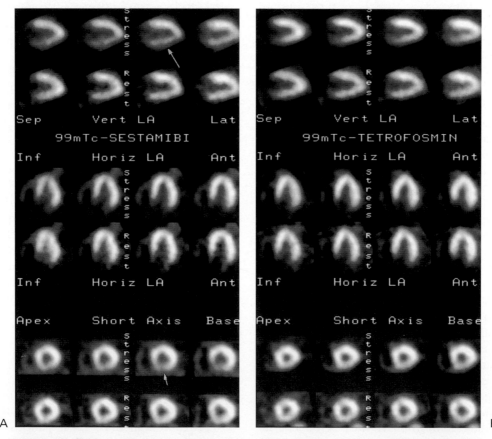

**FIGURE 8.3.** Patient with a 90% stenosis of the right coronary artery and 75% stenosis of the left anterior descending artery. **A:** 99mTc-sestamibi study performed after dipyridamole injection (stress) shows a significant ischemic defect of all the inferior wall *(arrow)* and transient dilatation of the left ventricle. **B:** The perfusion defect is significantly less intense on the 99mTc-tetrofosmin study performed 2 days after 99mTc-sestamibi imaging.

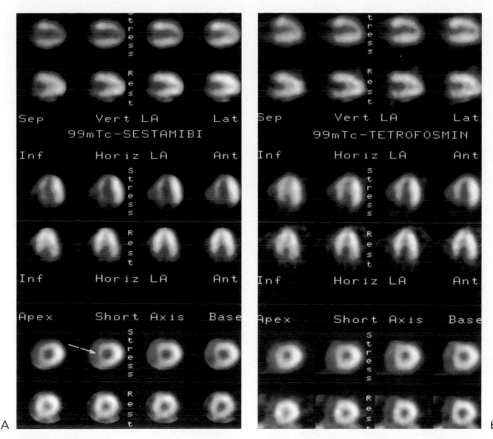

**FIGURE 8.4.** [99m]Tc-sestamibi **(A)**, and [99m]Tc-tetrofosmin **(B)** studies performed in the same patient with a 90% stenosis of the left anterior descending artery. Dipyridamole was used as the stress agent. The septal ischemic defect is more obvious on the [99m]Tc-sestamibi study *(arrow).*

widely used. Few studies have compared [99m]Tc-sestamibi to [99m]Tc-tetrofosmin myocardial perfusion imaging in the same patient population (173–176). Most of the data published so far showed that the results obtained with the two agents are very similar in patients undergoing treadmill stress. However, two studies comparing [99m]Tc-sestamibi and [99m]Tc-tetrofosmin imaging using pharmacologic vasodilation with dipyridamole showed that there were some differences between the two agents, suggesting that [99m]Tc-sestamibi imaging demonstrates better visualization of the intensity and extension of ischemic defects (177,178). Based on experimental data showing that myocardial extraction of [99m]Tc-sestamibi is higher than that of [99m]Tc-tetrofosmin and that the roll-off in the coronary blood flow versus myocardial uptake curve occurs at lower flow rate with [99m]Tc-tetrofosmin, a prospective study was conducted to compare [99m]Tc-sestamibi and [99m]Tc-tetrofosmin imaging performed with pharmacologic vasodilation in the same population of patients (178). A group of 88 patients without previous myocardial infarction and with recent evidence of mild to moderate CAD defined as 50% to 90% stenosis in one or two epicardial arteries were submitted within a week to two studies, one with [99m]Tc-sestamibi and one with [99m]Tc-tetrofosmin in random order.

SPECT imaging was performed 60 minutes after the injection of the radiotracers for both the rest and the dipyridamole studies. All images were interpreted by two blinded observers. The coronary angiogram was normal in one patient, and 45 patients had single-vessel and 36 had double-vessel disease. Six normal volunteers were also studied. Changes in heart rate and blood pressure were similar for both agents. The segmental analysis showed an agreement between the two agents of 86.3% (1,291/1,496 segments). [99m]Tc-Sestamibi and [99m]Tc-tetrofosmin detected 363 and 285 ischemic segments, respectively ($p$ <.001). The sensitivity of [99m]Tc-sestamibi was 63% (51/81) and 58% (47/81) for [99m]Tc-tetrofosmin ($p$ = ns). The ischemic to normal wall ratio was 0.73 ± 0.16 for [99m]Tc-sestamibi and 0.78 ± 0.17 for [99m]Tc-tetrofosmin ($p$ <.01). The extent of the perfusion defect was 15.8% ± 12.3% for [99m]Tc-sestamibi and 12.3% ± 11.4% for [99m]Tc-tetrofosmin ($p$ <.01). Therefore, although the overall sensitivity was similar, more ischemic myocardial segments were identified with [99m]Tc-sestamibi than with [99m]Tc-tetrofosmin, and the extent and the severity of the perfusion defects were greater with [99m]Tc-sestamibi imaging (Figs. 8.3 and 8.4). These results suggest a better visualization of ischemia with [99m]Tc-sestamibi following dipyridamole administration and are similar to those previously reported comparing $^{201}$Tl and $^{99m}$Tc-tetrofosmin SPECT imaging (179). Such differences may be clinically significant, especially for prognosis where the extent and severity of the ischemic perfusion defects are relevant. More comparative studies between these two agents and also with other $^{99m}$Tc-labeled perfusion imaging agents are necessary.

## $^{99m}$Tc-Furifosmin

Human experience with $^{99m}$Tc-furifosmin has been limited to phase II and III multicenter clinical trials because at the present time it is not approved for clinical use. However, the results so far are very promising and quite similar to those reported for $^{99m}$Tc-sestamibi and $^{99m}$Tc-tetrofosmin. Rossetti et al. (76) published the results of a study performed in ten normal volunteers and in 70 patients with suspected or proven CAD who were subjected to a 1-day rest/stress (10 and 30 mCi) $^{99m}$Tc-furifosmin imaging protocol. The major purpose of this preliminary study was to evaluate the optimal time between the $^{99m}$Tc-furifosmin injection and imaging, not to evaluate the diagnostic accuracy of $^{99m}$Tc-furifosmin in detection of CAD. However, the authors reported that myocardial perfusion defects were detected in 46 out of 47 patients with angiographically proven CAD. Furthermore, all studies were considered to be of good quality by three independent observers, with an adequate diagnostic value not related to the time of acquisition (from 15 minutes to 60 minutes after the injection of $^{99m}$Tc-furifosmin) or the fasting conditions (fast vs. nonfast).

Gerson et al. (180) studied 20 patients with proven CAD and ten normal subjects using $^{201}$Tl SPECT imaging and a 1-day rest-stress SPECT imaging protocol after the injection of $^{99m}$Tc-furifosmin. The rest-stress $^{99m}$Tc-furifosmin imaging protocol was designed to permit completion of the entire test sequence within 100 minutes. Patients were injected at rest with 5 to 7 mCi of $^{99m}$Tc-furifosmin, and tomographic imaging was started 15 minutes later. On completion of rest imaging, the patients were injected at peak stress with 20 to 23 mCi of $^{99m}$Tc-furifosmin. Imaging started 15 minutes after tracer injection so that both studies were completed within 100 minutes. Although background lung and liver activity were greater for $^{99m}$Tc-furifosmin compared with $^{201}$Tl, it did not interfere with interpretation of myocardial images. Segmental agreement between the two radiotracers was seen in 89% of the segments (kappa = 0.88). Blinded reading showed regional perfusion abnormalities on $^{99m}$Tc-furifosmin imaging in 85% of patients with corresponding documented CAD and in 90% of patients on $^{201}$Tl imaging. Eight of the ten normal subjects (80%) had a normal $^{99m}$Tc-furifosmin study, and nine (90%) had a normal $^{201}$Tl scintigraphy. These differences between the two radiotracers were not statistically significant, but the number of observations was relatively limited. The interobserver agreement in the interpretation

of myocardial segments was 87% for both agents. However, the agreement between $^{99m}$Tc-furifosmin and $^{201}$Tl for reversibility of segmental perfusion defects was poor, with a kappa value of 0.38 (16 ischemic defects on $^{201}$Tl versus nine ischemic defects for $^{99m}$Tc-furifosmin). Nevertheless, results of this study were similar to results of some studies comparing other $^{99m}$Tc-labeled myocardial perfusion imaging agents to $^{201}$Tl.

Hendel et al. (181) reported the results of a phase III multicenter trial comparing $^{99m}$Tc-furifosmin and $^{201}$Tl SPECT myocardial perfusion imaging. A total of 150 evaluable patients with an unequivocally positive $^{201}$Tl scintigraphy (performed within 2 weeks before the $^{99m}$Tc-furifosmin study) or a clinically high pretest likelihood for CAD were enrolled in this study from seven sites. Furthermore, 39 volunteers with a low likelihood of CAD based on clinical criteria stress test parameters were included in this study to define the normalcy rate of $^{99m}$Tc-furifosmin imaging. An initial dose of 10 mCi of $^{99m}$Tc-furifosmin was injected at peak stress and SPECT imaging was started 15 to 30 minutes later. A rest dose of approximately 30 mCi of $^{99m}$Tc-furifosmin was administered 3 to 4 hours after exercise and imaging was repeated 1 hour later. All patients underwent symptom-limited exercise treadmill testing, and all images were interpreted by a consensus of three blinded readers. Subjective assessment of the quality of images showed that more $^{99m}$Tc-furifosmin studies (34%) were of excellent quality than the corresponding $^{201}$Tl images (25%, $p$ = .006). Agreement for the presence of a perfusion abnormality was seen in 86% of patient studies with a kappa value of 0.67, while the exact concordance for the diagnostic categories was 67.3%. The concordance between $^{99m}$Tc-furifosmin and $^{201}$Tl was 94.9% in patients with a history of a prior myocardial infarction (kappa = 0.75) and 76.1% in patients without a previous infarction (kappa = 0.52). The normalcy rate of both radiotracers was 100% since all of the volunteer studies were interpreted as having normal perfusion. All these agreement values are comparable to those previously reported between $^{201}$Tl and other $^{99m}$Tc-labeled perfusion imaging agents.

The imaging properties of $^{99m}$Tc-furifosmin ($^{99m}$Tc-Q12) and $^{99m}$Tc-Q3 were also compared in humans by Gerson et al. (182). As previously mentioned, $^{99m}$Tc-furifosmin and $^{99m}$Tc-Q3 have identical monophosphine ligands, but the Schiff base ligand of $^{99m}$Tc-furifosmin contains an additional pair of furan rings. The authors studied ten patients with known coronary artery anatomy and in whom both $^{99m}$Tc-furifosmin and $^{99m}$Tc-Q3 were administered. The same imaging protocol was used with the two agents. A dose of 5 to 7 mCi of the radiotracer was injected at rest, and SPECT imaging started 15 minutes later. On completion of rest imaging, patients were submitted to a treadmill stress test and 20 to 23 mCi of the radiotracer was injected at peak stress. The imaging was started 15 minutes later. Nine patients had a significant CAD and one had no disease. The overall presence or absence of CAD was accurately determined in nine of ten patients with $^{99m}$Tc-Q3 (90%) and in ten of ten patients with $^{99m}$Tc-furifosmin (100%). Correct determination of the presence or absence of significant (i.e., greater than 50%) stenosis in individual coronary arteries occurred in 27 of 30 vessels (90%) with $^{99m}$Tc-Q3 and 26 of 30 vessels (87%, $p$ = ns) with $^{99m}$Tc-furifosmin. The overall agreement between the two radiotracers for detection of a perfusion defect was 80% (40 of 50 myocardial segments) with a kappa value of 0.60. The concordance for the presence of normal segmental perfusion versus ischemia versus fixed defect was seen in 32 of 50 (64%) myocardial segments. The authors also studied the heart-to-organ ratios of the two agents at 20 minutes after the injection. The heart-to-liver ratio at rest was 0.78 ± 0.14 for $^{99m}$Tc-furifosmin and 0.54 ± 0.16 for $^{99m}$Tc-Q3 ($p$ <.01), and at stress 0.95 ± 0.15 and 0.77 ± 0.18, respectively. The heart-to-lung ratio at rest was 1.50 ± 0.24 for $^{99m}$Tc-furifosmin and 1.93 ± 0.47 for $^{99m}$Tc-Q3 ($p$ <.01), and at stress 1.54 ± 0.28 and 1.95 ± 0.33, respectively. Therefore, relative to myocardial activity, lower liver activity is observed 20 minutes after stress or rest injection of $^{99m}$Tc-furifosmin in comparison to $^{99m}$Tc-Q3 (183,184). This should help to avoid hepatic overlap with the inferior wall of the heart. However, $^{99m}$Tc-Q3 yielded lower background lung activity in comparison to $^{99m}$Tc-furifosmin. This can theoretically result in improved myocardial visualization with $^{99m}$Tc-Q3. No definite conclusions can be made due to the very limited size of this study, but it seems that the two agents have similar diagnostic accuracy. Because of the lower hepatic uptake associated with $^{99m}$Tc-furifosmin, however, this radiotracer appears to be more favorable.

## $^{99m}$TcN-NOEt

So far, the most extensive experience with $^{99m}$Tc-N-NOEt in humans has been reported by Fagret et al. (104), who studied 25 patients undergoing cardiac catheterization (19 patients with significant CAD and six patients with normal coronary arteries) who also were evaluated with both $^{201}$Tl and $^{99m}$Tc-N-NOEt myocardial scintigraphy. Patients underwent stress-redistribution (4 hours later) and reinjection (15 minutes later) $^{201}$Tl imaging protocol. Within a few days of the $^{201}$Tl study, patients were injected at peak stress with 15 mCi (555 Mbq) of $^{99m}$TcN-NOEt. SPECT images were obtained at 30 minutes, and 2, 4, and 6 hours after the injection of $^{99m}$TcN-NOEt (stress-delayed imaging protocol). Within a 24-hour interval of the stress study, the patients also received 15 mCi (555 MBq) of $^{99m}$TcN-NOEt injected at rest. SPECT imaging was performed at 30 minutes and 4 hours after the injection (rest-delayed protocol).

The quality of $^{201}$Tl and $^{99m}$TcN-NOEt images was compared. No images were of poor quality. Following exercise, the score of the image quality was lower for $^{99m}$TcN-

NOEt (1.76 ± 0.44) than for $^{201}$Tl (1.94 ± 0.22, $p$ <.05). Good-quality images were seen in 19/25 patients with $^{99m}$TcN-NOEt and 24/25 with $^{201}$Tl. However, 4 hours after the injection, the score did not differ between $^{99m}$TcN-NOEt (1.58 ± 0.63) and $^{201}$Tl (1.65 ± 0.48, $p$ = ns). The difference in the image quality between $^{201}$Tl and $^{99m}$TcN-NOEt seems to be related to the persistent $^{99m}$TcN-NOEt lung activity, even on the images obtained 30 minutes after the injection at stress. There was no correlation between the increased lung uptake and the severity of coronary lesions. The authors suggested that increasing the injected dose to 30 mCi and searching for a new dispersant to use in the preparation of $^{99m}$TcN-NOEt could improve the overall quality of $^{99m}$TcN-NOEt images. However, despite differences in image quality, both agents gave comparable diagnostic information.

Using a threshold of 50% or more reduction in luminal diameter, stress $^{99m}$TcN-NOEt and $^{201}$Tl imaging were concordant in 22/25 patients (88%, kappa = 0.76). The concordance in patients with prior myocardial infarction was 89% (8/9). The sensitivity for the detection of CAD was 74% (14/19) for $^{99m}$TcN-NOEt and 68% (13/19) for $^{201}$Tl ($p$ = ns). The specificity was 100% (6/6) for both radiotracers. Using a threshold of 70% reduction in luminal diameter to define significant CAD, both tracers had a sensitivity of 79% (11/14); the specificity was 73% (8/11) for $^{99m}$TcN-NOEt and 82% (9/11) for $^{201}$Tl ($p$ = ns). The concordance between $^{99m}$TcN-NOEt and $^{201}$Tl for the presence of disease in individual coronary arteries was 96% (72/75, kappa = 0.92) with an identical sensitivity of 59% (17/29) and specificity of 93% (43/46). The overall agreement in segmental analysis was 94% (211/225 segments). However, $^{99m}$TcN-NOEt showed a lower defect contrast with a mean score of defect severity of 2.0 ± 1.2 in comparison to 2.5 ± 0.7 for $^{201}$Tl ($p$ <.01).

The concordance between $^{99m}$TcN-NOEt perfusion defect normalization and $^{201}$Tl segmental redistribution on images obtained 4 hours after injection was 100%, whereas $^{99m}$TcN-NOEt defect normalization was incomplete 2 hours after the injection. Therefore, these data demonstrate similarity in the apparent myocardial kinetics of both radiotracers and suggest that $^{99m}$TcN-NOEt can be used as a potential marker of myocardial viability. However, much more data are necessary to evaluate the role of $^{99m}$TcN-NOEt in myocardial viability assessment.

## CONCLUSION

Many radionuclide myocardial perfusion imaging agents are now commercially available and others should be in the near future. Although many of their characteristics differ, they all share the same utility in the diagnosis and evaluation of patients with CAD. Moreover, we are still learning how to obtain the best diagnostic results from $^{201}$Tl and

$^{99m}$Tc-sestamibi myocardial perfusion scintigraphy. It is likely that with new agents and constantly evolving technology in data acquisition and analysis, our knowledge will improve further, and all these agents will be able to fulfill a more specific role in clinical practice.

## REFERENCES

1. Sapirstein LA. Regional blood flow by fractional distribution of indicators. *Am J Physiol* 1958;193:161–166.
2. Zimmer L, McCall D, D'Addabbo L, et al. Kinetics and characteristics of thallium exchange in cultured cells. *Circulation* 1979;59:138–143.
3. Beller GA, Watson DD. Physiological basis of myocardial perfusion imaging with the technetium99m agents. *Semin Nucl Med* 1991;12:173–181.
4. Dahlberg ST, Leppo JA. Myocardial kinetics of radiolabeled perfusion agents: basis for perfusion imaging. *J Nucl Cardiol* 1994;1:189–197.
5. Leppo JA, Meerdink DJ. Comparison of the myocardial uptake of a technetium-labeled isonitrile analogue and thallium. *Circ Res* 1989;65:632–639.
6. Weich HF, Strauss HW, Pitt B. The extraction of Tl-201 by the myocardium. *Circulation* 1977;56:188–192.
7. Krahwinkel W, Herzog H, Feinendegen LE. Pharmacokinetics of thallium-201 in normal individuals after routine myocardial scintigraphy. *J Nucl Med* 1988;29:1582–1586.
8. Deutsch E, Bushong W, Glavan KA, et al. Heart imaging with cationic complexes of technetium. *Science* 1981;214:85–86.
9. Dudczak R, Angelberger P, Homan R, et al. Evaluation of $^{99m}$Tc-dichloro bis (1,2-dimethylphosphino)ethane ($^{99m}$Tc-DMPE) for myocardial scintigraphy in man. *Eur J Nucl Med* 1983;8:513–515.
10. Gerson MC, Deutsch EA, Libson KF, et al. Myocardial scintigraphy with $^{99m}$Tc-Tris-DMPE in man. *Eur J Nucl Med* 1984;9:403–407.
11. Jones AG, Davison A, Abram S, et al. Biological studies of a new class of technetium complexes: the hexakis (alkylisonitrile) technetium (I) cations. *Int J Nucl Med Biol* 1984;11:225–234.
12. Holman BL, Jones AG, Lister-James J, et al. A new Tc-99m-labelled imaging agent, hexakis (T-butyl-isonitrile)-technetium (I) (Tc-99m-TBI): initial experience in the human. *J Nucl Med* 1984;25:1350–1355.
13. Sia STB, Holman BL, McKusick K, et al. The utilization of Tc99m TBI as a myocardial perfusion agent in exercise studies. Comparison with Tl201 thallous chloride and examination of its biodistribution in humans. *Eur J Nucl Med* 1986;12:333–336.
14. Sia STB, Holman BL, Campbell S, et al. The utilization of technetium-99m CPI as a myocardial perfusion imaging agent in exercise studies. *Clin Nucl Med* 1987;12:681–687.
15. Wackers FJ, Berman DS, Maddahi J, et al. Technetium-99m hexakis-2-methoxyisobutyl isonitrile: human biodistribution, dosimetry, safety and preliminary comparison to thallium-201 for myocardial perfusion imaging. *J Nucl Med* 1989;30:310–311.
16. Piwnica-Worms D, Kronauge JF, Chiu ML. Uptake and retention of hexakis (2-methoxyisobutyl-isonitrile) technetium (I) in cultured chick myocardial cells. Mitochondrial and plasma membrane potential dependence. *Circulation* 1990;82:1826–1838.
17. Beanlands RSB, Dawood F, Wen WH, et al. Are the kinetics of technetium-99m methoxyisobutyl isonitrile affected by cell metabolism and viability? *Circulation* 1990;82:1802–1814.
18. Okada RD, Glover D, Gaffney T, et al. Myocardial kinetics of technetium-99m-hexakis-2-methoxy-2-methylpropyl-isonitrile. *Circulation* 1988;77:491–498.
19. Glover DK, Okada RD. Myocardial kinetics of Tc-MIBI in canine myocardium after dipyridamole. *Circulation* 1990;81:628–636.
20. Mousa SA, Cooney JM, Williams SJ. Relationship between regional myocardial blood flow and the distribution of $^{99m}$Tc-sestamibi in the presence of total coronary artery occlusion. *Am Heart J* 1990;119:842–847.
21. Canby RC, Silber S, Pohost GM. Relations of the myocardial imaging agents Tc-99m mibi and Tl-201 to myocardial blood flow in a canine model of myocardial ischemic insult. *Circulation* 1990;81:289–296.
22. Leppo JA, Meerdink DJ. Comparison of the myocardial uptake of a technetium-labeled isonitrile analogue and thallium. *Circ Res* 1989;65:632–639.
23. Li QS, Solot G, Frank TL, et al. Myocardial redistribution of technetium-99m-methoxyisobutyl isonitrile (sestamibi). *J Nucl Med* 1990;31:1069–1076.
24. Sinusas AJ, Beller GA, Smith WH, et al. Quantitative planar imaging with technetium-99m methoxy isobutyl isonitrile: comparison of uptake patterns with thallium-201. *J Nucl Med* 1989;30:1456–1463.
25. Sinusas AJ, Bergin JD, Edwards NC, et al. Redistribution of $^{99m}$Tc-sestamibi and 201Tl in the presence of a severe coronary artery stenosis. *Circulation* 1994;89:2332–2341.
26. Verani MS, Jeroudi MO, Mahmarian JJ, et al. Quantification of myocardial infarction during coronary occlusion and myocardial salvage after reperfusion using cardiac imaging with technetium-99m hexakis 2–methoxyisobutyl isonitrile. *J Am Coll Cardiol* 1988;12:1573–1581.
27. Rubow S, Klopper J, Wasserman H, et al. The excretion of radiopharmaceuticals in human breast milk: additional data and dosimetry. *Eur J Nucl Med* 1994;21:144–153.
28. Gagnon A, Taillefer R, Bavaria G, et al. Fast labeling of technetium-99m-sestamibi with microwave oven heating. *J Nucl Med Tech* 1991;19:90–93.
29. Hung JC, Wilson ME, Brown ML, et al. Rapid preparation and quality control method for technetium-99m-2-methoxy isobutyl isonitrile (technetium-99m-sestamibi). *J Nucl Med* 1991;32:2162–2168.
30. Porter WC, Karvelis KC. Microwave versus recon-o-stat for preparation of technetium-99m sestamibi: a comparison of hand exposure, radiochemical purity and image quality. *J Nucl Med Tech* 1995;23:279–281.
31. Hung JC, Wilson ME, Brown ML, et al. Comparison of four alternative radiochemical purity testing methods for $^{99m}$Tc-sestamibi. *Nucl Med Commun* 1995;16:99–104.
32. Patel M, Sadek S, Jahan S, et al. A miniaturized rapid paper chromatographic procedure for quality control of technetium-99m sestamibi. *Eur J Nucl Med* 1995;22:1416–1419.
33. Reilly RM, So M, Polihronis J, et al. Rapid quality control of $^{99m}$Tc-sestamibi. *Nucl Med Commun* 1992;13:664–666.
34. Beller GA, Watson DD. Physiological basis of myocardial perfusion imaging with the technetium agents. *Semin Nucl Med* 1991;21:173–181.
35. Berman DS, Kiat H, Van Train KF, et al. Comparison of SPECT using technetium-99m agents and thallium-201 and PET for the assessment of myocardial perfusion and viability. *Am J Cardiol* 1990;66:72E–79E.
36. Johnson LL, Seldin DW. Clinical experience with technetium-99m teboroxime, a neutral, lipophilic myocardial perfusion imaging agent. *Am J Cardiol* 1990;66:63E––67E.
37. Johnson LL. Clinical experience with technetium-99m teboroxime. *Semin Nucl Med* 1991;21:182–189.

38. Johnson LL. Myocardial perfusion imaging with technetium-99m-teboroxime. *J Nucl Med* 1994;35:689–692.

39. Leppo JA, DePuey EG, Johnson LL. A review of cardiac imaging with sestamibi and teboroxime. *J Nucl Med* 1991;32:2012–2022.

40. Narra RK, Nunn AD, Kuczynski BL, et al. A neutral technetium-99m complex for myocardial imaging. *J Nucl Med* 1989;30:130–137.

41. Nunn AD. Radiopharmaceuticals for imaging myocardial perfusion. *Semin Nucl Med* 1990;20:111–118.

42. Taillefer R. New agents labelled with technetium 99m for myocardial perfusion imaging. *Can Assoc Radiol J* 1992;43:258–266.

43. Taillefer R. Technetium-99m teboroxime. In: Taillefer R, Tamaki N, eds. *New radiotracers in cardiac imaging: principles and applications.* Stamford, CT: Appleton Lange, 1999:49–74.

44. Di Rocco RJ, Rumsey WL, Kuczynski BL, et al. Measurement of myocardial blood flow using a co-injection technique for technetium-99m-teboroxime, technetium-96-sestamibi and thallium-201. *J Nucl Med* 1992;33:1152–1159.

45. Leppo JA, Meerdink DJ. Comparative myocardial extraction of two technetium-labeled BATO derivatives (SQ30217, SQ32014) and thallium. *J Nucl Med* 1990;31:67–74.

46. Meerdink DJ, Leppo JA. Experimental studies of the physiologic properties of technetium-99m agents: myocardial transport of perfusion imaging agents. *Am J Cardiol* 1990;66:9E–15E.

47. Marshall RC, Leidholdt EM, Zhang DY, et al. The effect of flow on technetium-99m-teboroxime (SQ30217) and thallium-201 extraction and retention in rabbit heart. *J Nucl Med* 1991;32:1979–1988.

48. Narra RK, Feld T, Nunn AD. Absorbed radiation dose to humans from technetium-99m-teboroxime. *J Nucl Med* 1992;33:88–93.

49. Beanlands R, Muzik O, Nguyen N, et al. The relationship between myocardial retention of technetium-99m teboroxime and myocardial blood flow. *J Am Coll Cardiol* 1992;20:712–719.

50. Stewart RE, Schwaiger M, Hutchins GD, et al. Myocardial clearance kinetics of technetium-99m-SQ30217: a marker of regional myocardial blood flow. *J Nucl Med* 1990;31:1183–1190.

51. Pieri P, Yasuda T, Fischman AJ, et al. Myocardial accumulation and clearance of technetium 99m teboroxime at 100%, 75%, 50% and zero coronary blood flow in dogs. *Eur J Nucl Med* 1991;18:725–731.

52. Maublant JC, Moins N, Gachon P, et al. Uptake of technetium-99m-teboroxime in cultured myocardial cells: comparison with thallium-201 and technetium-99m-sestamibi. *J Nucl Med* 1993;34:255–259.

53. Weinstein H, Reinhardt CP, Leppo JA. Teboroxime, sestamibi and thallium-201 as markers of myocardial hypoperfusion: comparison by quantitative dual-isotope autoradiography in rabbits. *J Nucl Med* 1993;34:1510–1517.

54. Stewart RE, Heyl B, O'Rourke RA, et al. Demonstration of differential post-stenotic myocardial technetium-99m teboroxime clearance kinetics after experimental ischemia and hyperemic stress. *J Nucl Med* 1991;32:2000–2008.

55. Hendel RC, McSherry B, Karimeddini M, et al. Diagnostic value of a new myocardial perfusion agent, teboroxime (SQ 30,217), utilizing a rapid planar imaging protocol: preliminary results. *J Am Coll Cardiol* 1990;16:855–861.

56. Weinstein H, Dahlberg ST, McSherry B, et al. Rapid redistribution of teboroxime. *Am J Cardiol* 1993;71:848–852.

57. Yamagami H, Ishida Y, Morozumi T, et al. Detection of coronary artery disease by dynamic planar and single photon emission tomographic imaging with technetium-99m teboroxime. *Eur J Nucl Med* 1994;21:27–36.

58. Johnson G, Glover DK, Hebert CB, et al. Early myocardial clearance kinetics of technetium 99m-teboroxime differentiate normal and flow-restricted canine myocardium at rest. *J Nucl Med* 1993;34:630–636.

59. Johnson G, Glover DK, Hebert CB, et al. Myocardial clearance kinetics of technetium-99m-teboroxime following dipyridamole: differentiation of stenosis severity in canine myocardium. *J Nucl Med* 1995;36:111–119.

60. Wilson ME, Hung JC. Microwave preparation of and one-strip paper chromatography for technetium Tc 99m teboroxime. *Am J Hosp Pharmacol* 1993;50:2376–2379.

61. Sinusas AJ, Shi QX, Saltzberg MT, et al. Technetium-99m-tetrofosmin to assess myocardial blood flow: experimental validation in an intact canine model of ischemia. *J Nucl Med* 1994;35:664–671.

62. Dahlberg ST, Leppo JA. Myocardial kinetics of radiolabeled perfusion agents: basis for perfusion imaging. *J Nucl Cardiol* 1994;1:189–197.

63. Sridhara BS, Braat S, Rigo P, et al. Comparison of myocardial perfusion imaging with technetium-99m tetrofosmin versus thallium-201 in coronary artery disease. *Am J Cardiol* 1993;72:1015–1019.

64. Deutsch E, Ketring AR, Libson K, et al. The Noah's ark experiment: species dependent biodistributions of cationic ⁹⁹ᵐTc complexes. *Nucl Med Biol* 1989;16:191–232.

65. Platts EA, North TL, Pickett RD, et al. Mechanism of uptake of technetium-tetrofosmin. I: uptake into isolated adult rat ventricular myocytes and subcellular localization. *J Nucl Cardiol* 1995;2:317–326.

66. Younes A, Songadele JA, Maublant J, et al. Mechanism of uptake of technetium-tetrofosmin. II: uptake into isolated adult rat heart mitochondria. *J Nucl Cardiol* 1995;2:327–333.

67. Higley B, Smith FW, Smith T, et al. Technetium-99m-1,2-bis[bis(2-Ethoxyethyl) Phosphino]ethane: human biodistribution, dosimetry and safety of a new myocardial perfusion imaging agent. *J Nucl Med* 1993;34:30–38.

68. Sridhara B, Sochor H, Rigo P, et al. Myocardial single-photon emission computed tomographic imaging with technetium-99m tetrofosmin: stress-rest imaging with same-day and separate-day rest imaging. *J Nucl Cardiol* 1994;1:138–143.

69. Jones S, Hendel RC. Technetium-99m tetrofosmin: a new myocardial perfusion agent. *J Nucl Med Tech* 1993;21:191–195.

70. Geyer MC, Zimmer AM, Spies WG, et al. Rapid quality control of technetium-99m-tetrofosmin: comparison of miniaturized and standard chromatography systems. *J Nucl Med Tech* 1995;23:186–189.

71. Gerson MC, Deutsch EA, Nishiyama H, et al. Myocardial perfusion imaging with ⁹⁹ᵐTc-DMPE in man. *Eur J Nucl Med* 1983;8:513–515.

72. Jurisson SS, Dancey K, McPartlin M, et al. Synthesis, characterization, and electrochemical properties of technetium complexes containing both tetradentate Schiff base and monodentate tertiary phosphine ligands: single-crystal structure of trans-(N,N'-ethylenebis(acetylacetone iminato)) bis (triphenylphosphine) technetium (III) hexafluorophosphate. *Inorg Chem* 1984;23:4743–4749.

73. Kronauge JF, Noska MA, Davison A, et al. Interspecies variation in biodistribution of technetium (2-carbomethoxy-2-isocyanopropane)6+. *J Nucl Med* 1992;33:1357–1365.

74. Deutsch E, Vanderheyden JL, Gerundini P, et al. Development of nonreducible technetium-99m(III) cations as myocardial perfusion imaging agents: initial experience in humans. *J Nucl Med* 1987;28:1870–1880.

75. Taillefer R. Technetium-99m furifosmin. In: Taillefer R, Tamaki

N, eds. *New radiotracers in cardiac imaging: principles and applications.* Stamford, CT: Appleton Lange, 1999:101–111.

76. Rossetti C, Vanoli G, Paganelli G, et al. Human biodistribution, dosimetry and clinical use of technetium (III)-99m-Q12. *J Nucl Med* 1994;35:1571–1580.

77. Bugaj JE, De Rosch MA, Marmion ME, et al. Novel chemistry used in the cyclodextrin-stabilized technescan (r) Q12 kit. *J Nucl Med* 1994;35:139(abst).

78. Roszell NJ, McGoron AJ, Biniakiewicz DS, et al. [99m]Tc-Q12 handling by isolated rat cardiac myocytes and mitochondria. *Circulation* 1995;92:I-181(abst).

79. Gerson MC, Lukes J, Deutsch E, et al. Comparison of imaging properties of technetium 99m Q12 and technetium 99m Q3 in humans. *J Nucl Cardiol* 1995;2:224–230.

80. Meerdink DJ, Dahlberg ST, Gilmore M, et al. Transcapillary exchange of Q12 and Thallium-201 in isolated rabbit hearts. *Circulation* 1993;88:I-249(abst).

81. Richter WS, Aurisch R, Fischer S, et al. Comparison of plasma clearances of Tc-99m Q12 (furifosmin) and Tc-99m sestamibi. *J Nucl Med* 1997;38:99(abst).

82. McGoron AJ, Biniakiewicz DS, Roszell NJ, et al. Extraction and retention of [99m]Tc Q12, [99m]Tc-sestamibi and 201Tl imaging agents in isolated rat heart during acidemia. *Circulation* 1995;92:I-180–181(abst).

83. Gerson MC, Lukes J, Deutsch E, et al. Comparison of technetium 99m Q12 and thallium 201 for detection of angiographically documented coronary artery disease in humans. *J Nucl Cardiol* 1994;1:499–508.

84. Coupal JJ, Hackett MT, Marmion-Dyszlewski ME, et al. Prolonged microwave-oven heating is needed for compounding of Tc-99m furifosmin: preliminary findings. *J Nucl Med* 1997;38:178–179(abst).

85. Hendel RC, Verani MS, Miller DD, et al. Diagnostic utility of tomographic myocardial perfusion imaging with technetium 99m furifosmin (Q12) compared with thallium 201: results of a phase III multicenter trial. *J Nucl Cardiol* 1996;3:291–300.

86. Taillefer R. Technetium-99m-N-NOEt. In: Taillefer R, Tamaki N, eds. *New radiotracers in cardiac imaging: principles and applications.* Stamford, CT: Appleton Lange, 1999:113–124.

87. Pasqualini R, Comazzi V, Bellande E, et al. A new efficient method for the preparation of [99m]Tc-radiopharmaceuticals containing the Tc≡N multiple bond. *Appl Radiat Isot* 1992;43:1329–1333.

88. Pasqualini R, Duatti A, Bellande E, et al. Bis (dithiocarbamato) nitrido technetium-99m radiopharmaceuticals: a class of neutral myocardial imaging agents. *J Nucl Med* 1994;35:334–341.

89. Bellande E, Hoffschir D, Comazzi V, et al. Interaction of the myocardial imaging agent TcN-NOET with cyclodextrins: influence of the stability of the inclusion complex on the biological properties. *J Nucl Med* 1994;35:261(abst).

90. Ghezzi C, Fagret D, Arvieux CC, et al. Myocardial kinetics of TcN-NOET: a neutral lipophilic complex tracer of regional myocardial blood flow. *J Nucl Med* 1995;36:1069–1077.

91. Glover DK, Ruiz M, Calnon DA, et al. Favorable first-pass myocardial extraction fraction for technetium-99m-N-NOET: implications for pharmacologic stress imaging. *J Nucl Med* 1997;38:65(abst).

92. Glover DK, Vanzetto G, Calnon DA, et al. Kinetics of bis (N-ethoxy, N-ethyl dithiocarbamato) nitrido 99m-Tc (NOET) in a canine model of transient coronary artery occlusion: comparison with Tl-201. *Circulation* 1996;94:I-302(abst).

93. Uccelli L, Giganti M, Duatti A, et al. Subcellular distribution of technetium-99m-N-NOEt in rat myocardium. *J Nucl Med* 1995;36:2075–2079.

94. Maublant J, Zhang Z, Ollier M, et al. Uptake and release of bis(N-ethoxy, N-ethyl dithiocarbamato) nitrido [99m]Tc(V) in cultured myocardial cells: comparison with Tl-201, MIBI, and teboroxime. *Eur J Nucl Med* 1992;19:597(abst).

95. Johnson G, Allton IL, Nguyen KN, et al. Clearance of technetium 99m N-NOET in normal, ischemic-reperfused, and membrane-disrupted myocardium. *J Nucl Cardiol* 1996;3:42–54.

96. Dahlberg ST, Gilmore MP, Flood M, et al. Extraction of technetium-99m-N-NOET in the isolated rabbit heart. *Circulation* 1994;90:I-368(abst).

97. Guillaud C, Comazzi V, Joubert F, et al. Metabolite analysis of the neutral technetium-99m nitrido dithiocarbamate complex TcN-NOET after injection in rats. *J Nucl Med* 1996;37:188–189(abst).

98. Ghezzi C, Fagret D, Mouton O, et al. In vitro uptake kinetics of bis(N-ethoxy, N-ethyl dithiocarbamato) nitrido technetium-99m (V), a myocardial perfusion imaging agent: a study in cultured cardiac cells. *Circulation* 1996;90:I-301(abst).

99. Ghezzi C, Fagret D, Brichon PY, et al. Redistribution of bis(N-ethoxy, N-ethyl dithiocarbamato) nitrido technetium-99m-(V), a new myocardial perfusion imaging agent: comparison with [201]Tl redistribution. *Circulation* 1996;94:I-302(abst).

100. Vanzetto G, Calnon DA, Ruiz M, et al. Tc-99m-N-NOET uptake in dogs with a severe coronary artery stenosis: comparison to thallium-201 and regional blood flow. *Circulation* 1996;94:I-301(abst).

101. Vanzetto G, Calnon DA, Ruiz M, et al. Myocardial uptake of 99Tc-NOET in dogs with reperfused acute myocardial infarction: comparison to Tl-201. *J Nucl Cardiol* 1997;4:S21(abst).

102. Johnson G, Nguyen KN, Liu Z, et al. Planar imaging of [99m]Tc-labeled (bis(N-ethoxy, N-ethyl dithiocarbamato) nitrido technetium (V)) can detect resting ischemia. *J Nucl Cardiol* 1997;4:217–225.

103. Pasqualini R, Comazzi V, Bellande E, et al. A new efficient method for the preparation of [99m]Tc-radiopharmaceuticals containing the Tc≡N multiple bond. *Appl Radiat Isot* 1992;43:1329–1333.

104. Fagret D, Marie PY, Brunotte F, et al. Myocardial perfusion imaging with technetium-99m-Tc NOET: comparison with thallium-201 and coronary angiography. *J Nucl Med* 1995;36:936–943.

105. Glover DK, Ruiz M, Vanzetto G, et al. Myocardial uptake of Tc-99m-NOET during adenosine hyperemia in dogs with mild to moderate coronary stenoses. *J Nucl Cardiol* 1997;4:S65(abst).

106. Giganti M, Cittanti C, Colamussi P, et al. Biodistribution in man of bis [(N-ethyl, N-ethoxy) dithiocarbamate] nitrido technetium (V), a promising new tracer for myocardial perfusion imaging. *J Nucl Med* 1994;35:155(abst).

107. Johnson G, Nguyen KN, Pasqualini R, et al. Interaction of technetium-99m-N-NOET with blood elements: potential mechanism of myocardial redistribution. *J Nucl Med* 1997;38:138–143.

108. Fagret D, Vanzetto G, Mathieu JP, et al. Biodistribution and dosimetry of [99m]TcN-NOET in normal human. *J Nucl Med* 1996;37:229(abst).

109. Giganti M, Uccelli L, Cittanti C, et al. Dosimetric estimations in man of bis [(N-ehtyl, N-ethoxy) dithiocarbamate] nitrido technetium (V). *J Nucl Cardiol* 1997;4:S46(abst).

110. Berman DS, Kiat H, Friedman JD, et al. Separate acquisition rest thallium-201/stress technetium-99m sestamibi dual-isotope myocardial perfusion single-photon emission computed tomography: a clinical validation study. *J Am Coll Cardiol* 1993;22:1455–1464.

111. Yang DC, Ragasa E, Gould L, et al. Radionuclide simultaneous dual-isotope stress myocardial perfusion study using the "three window technique." *Clin Nucl Med* 1993;18:852–857.

112. Berman D, Friedman J, Kiat J, et al. Separate acquisition dual isotope myocardial perfusion SPECT: results of a large clinical trial. *J Am Coll Cardiol* 1992;19:202A(abst).

113. Kiat H, Germano G, Friedman J, et al. Comparative feasibility of separate or simultaneous rest thallium-201/stress technetium-99m-sestamibi dual-isotope perfusion SPECT. *J Nucl Med* 1994;35:542–548.

114. Kiat H, Germano G, VanTrain K, et al. Quantitative assessment of photon spillover in simultaneous rest Tl-201/stress Tc-sestamibi dual isotope myocardial perfusion SPECT. *J Nucl Med* 1992;33:854–855.

115. Heo J, Wolmer I, Kegel J, et al. Sequential dual-isotope SPECT imaging with thallium-201 and technetium-99m-sestamibi. *J Nucl Med* 1994;35:549–553.

116. Weinmann P, Foult JM, LeGuludec M, et al. Dual-isotope myocardial imaging: feasibility, advantages and limitations. Preliminary report on 231 consecutive patients. *Eur J Nucl Med* 1994;21:212–215.

117. Wackers FJT. The maze of myocardial perfusion imaging protocols in 1994. *J Nucl Cardiol* 1994;1:180–188.

118. Siebelink HMJ, Natale D, Sinusas AJ, et al. Quantitative comparison of single-isotope and dual-isotope stress-rest single-photon emission computed tomographic imaging for reversibility of defects. *J Nucl Cardiol* 1996;3:483–493.

119. Dilsizian V, Rocco TP, Freedman NMT, et al. Enhanced detection of ischemic but viable myocardium by the reinjection of thallium after stress-redistribution imaging. *N Engl J Med* 1990;323:141–146.

120. Worsley DF, Fung AY, Coupland DB, et al. Comparison of stress-only vs. Stress-rest technetium-99m methoxyisobutylisonitrile myocardial perfusion imaging. *Eur J Nucl Med* 1992;19:441–444.

121. Taillefer R, Dupras G, Sporn V, et al. Myocardial perfusion imaging with a new radiotracer, technetium-99m-hexamibi (methoxy isobutyl isonitrile): comparison with thallium-201 imaging. *Clin Nucl Med* 1989;14;89–96.

122. Taillefer R, Lambert R, Dupras G, et al. Clinical comparison between thallium-201 and Tc 99m methoxy isobutyl isonitrile (hexamibi) myocardial perfusion imaging for detection of coronary artery disease. *Eur J Nucl Med* 1989;15:280–286.

123. Taillefer R, Lambert R, Bisson G, et al. Myocardial technetium-99m-labeled sestamibi single-photon emission computed tomographic imaging in the detection of coronary artery disease: comparison between early (15 minutes) and delayed (60 minutes) imaging. *J Nucl Cardiol* 1994;1:441–448.

124. Hassan IM, Mohammad MMJ, Constantinides C, et al. Problems of duodenogastric reflux in Tc-99m hexa MIBI planar, tomographic and bull's eye display. *Clin Nucl Med* 1989;14:286–289.

125. Middleton GW, Williams JH. Significant gastric reflux of technetium-99m MIBI in SPECT myocardial imaging. *J Nucl Med* 1994;35:619–620.

126. Taillefer R. Technetium-99m sestamibi myocardial imaging: same-day rest-stress studies and dipyridamole. *Am J Cardiol* 1990;66:80–84E.

127. Taillefer R, Gagnon A, Laflamme L, et al. Same day injections of Tc-99m methoxy isobutyl isonitrile (hexamibi) for myocardial tomographic imaging: comparison between rest-stress and stress-rest injection sequences. *Eur J Nucl Med* 1989;15:113–117.

128. Picard M, Franceschi M, Sia BST, et al. Tc-99m-methoxyisobutyl isonitrile (MIBI): comparing a one. and two-day protocol for the assessment of transient ischemia. *J Nucl Med* 1988;29:851(abst).

129. Heo J, Kegel J, Iskandrian AS, et al. Comparison of same-day protocols using technetium-99m-sestamibi myocardial imaging. *J Nucl Med* 1992;33:186–191.

130. McSherry BA. Technetium-99m-teboroxime: a new agent for myocardial perfusion imaging. *J Nucl Med Tech* 1991;19:22–26.

131. Germano G, Chua T, Kavanagh PB, et al. Detection and correction of patient motion in dynamic and static myocardial SPECT using a multi-detector camera. *J Nucl Med* 1993;34:1349–1355.

132. Heo J, Iskandrian B, Cave V, et al. Single photon emission computed tomographic teboroxime imaging with a preprocessing masking technique. *Am Heart J* 1992;124:1603–1608.

133. Iskandrian AS, Heo J, Nguyen T, et al. Myocardial imaging with Tc-99m teboroxime: technique and initial results. *Am Heart J* 1991;121:889–894.

134. Nuyts J, Dupont P, Van Den Maegdenbergh V, et al. A study of the liver-heart artifact in emission tomography. *J Nucl Med* 1995;36:133–139.

135. O'Connor MK, Cho DS. Rapid radiotracer washout from the heart: effect on image quality in SPECT performed with a single-headed gamma camera system. *J Nucl Med* 1992;33:1146–1151.

136. Henzlova M, Machac J. Clinical utility of technetium-99m. teboroxime myocardial washout imaging. *J Nucl Med* 1994;35:575–579.

137. Chua T, Kiat H, Germano G, et al. Rapid back to back adenosine stress/rest technetium-99m teboroxime myocardial perfusion SPECT using a triple-detector camera. *J Nucl Med* 1993;34:1485–1493.

138. Glover DK, Ruiz M, Bergmann EE, et al. Myocardial technetium-99m-teboroxime uptake during adenosine-induced hyperemia in dogs with either a critical or mild coronary stenosis: comparison to thallium-201 and regional blood flow. *J Nucl Med* 1995;36:476–483.

139. Li QS, Solot G, Frank TL, et al. Tomographic myocardial perfusion imaging with technetium-99m-teboroxime at rest and after dipyridamole. *J Nucl Med* 1991;32:1968–1976.

140. Maddahi J, Rodrigues E, Berman DS, Kiat H. State-of-the-art myocardial perfusion imaging. *Cardiol Clin* 1994;12:199–222.

141. Detrano R, Janosi A, Lyons KP, et al. Factors affecting sensitivity and specificity of a diagnostic test: the exercise thallium scintigram. *Am J Med* 1988;84:699–705.

142. Taillefer R. Technetium-99m-sestamibi. In: Taillefer R, Tamaki N, eds. *New radiotracers in cardiac imaging: principles and applications.* Stamford, CT: Appleton Lange, 1999:3–48.

143. Maublant JC, Marcaggi X, Lusson JR, et al. Comparison between thallium-201 and technetium-99m methoxyisobutyl isonitrile defect size in single-photon emission computed tomography at rest, exercise and redistribution in coronary artery disease. *Am J Cardiol* 1992;69:183–187.

144. Taillefer R. Detection of myocardial necrosis and inflammation by nuclear cardiac imaging. *Cardiol Clin* 1994;12:289–302.

145. Boucher CA. Detection and location of myocardial infarction using technetium-99m sestamibi imaging at rest. *Am J Cardiol* 1990;66:32–35E.

146. Boucher CA, Wackers FJT, Zaret BL, et al. Technetium-99m sestamibi myocardial imaging at rest for assessment of myocardial infarction and first-pass ejection fraction. *Am J Cardiol* 1992;69:22–67.

147. Dilsizian V, Rocco RP, Strauss HW, et al. Technetium-99m isonitrile myocardial uptake at rest. I. Relation to severity of coronary artery stenosis. *J Am Coll Cardiol* 1989;14:1673–1677.

148. Huber KC, Bresnahan JF, Bresnahan DR, et al. Measurements of myocardium at risk by technetium-99m sestamibi: correlation with coronary angiography. *J Am Coll Cardiol* 1992;19:67–73.

149. Gibbons RJ, Verani MS, Behrenbeck T, et al. Feasibility of tomographic $^{99m}$Tc-hexakis-2-methoxy-2-methylpropyl-isoni-

trile imaging for the assessment of myocardial at risk and the effect of treatment in acute myocardial infarction. *Circulation* 1989;80:1277–1286.

150. Wackers FJT. Thrombolytic therapy for myocardial infarction: assessment of efficacy by myocardial perfusion imaging with technetium-99m sestamibi. *Am J Cardiol* 1990;66:36–41E.

151. Grégoire J, Théroux P. Detection and assessment of unstable angina using myocardial perfusion imaging: comparison between technetium-99m sestamibi SPECT and 12-lead electrocardiogram. *Am J Cardiol* 1990;66:42–47E.

152. DePuey EG. How to detect and avoid myocardial perfusion SPECT artifacts. *J Nucl Med* 1994;35:699–702.

153. DePuey EG, Jones ME, Garcia EV. Evaluation of right ventricular regional perfusion with technetium-99m-sestamibi SPECT. *J Nucl Med* 1991;32:1199–1205.

154. DePuey EG, Nichols KJ, Dobrinsky C. Left ventricular ejection fraction assessment from gated technetium-99m-sestamibi SPECT. *J Nucl Med* 1993;34:1871–1876.

155. DePuey EG, Rozanski A. Using gated technetium-99m-sestamibi SPECT to characterize fixed myocardial defects as infarct or artifact. *J Nucl Med* 1995;36:952–955.

156. Taillefer R, DePuey EG, Udelson JE, et al. [99m]Tc-sestamibi gated SPECT perfusion study in detection of coronary artery disease in women: comparison between the end-diastolic images and the summed images. *J Nucl Cardiol* 1999;6:169–176.

157. Taillefer R, DePuey EG, Udelson JE, et al. Comparative diagnostic accuracy of thallium-201 and Tc-99m-sestamibi SPECT imaging (perfusion and ECG-gated SPECT) in detecting coronary artery disease in women. *J Am Coll Cardiol* 1997;29:69–77.

158. Seldin DW, Johnson LL, Blood DK, et al. Myocardial perfusion imaging with technetium-99m SQ30217: comparison with thallium-201 and coronary anatomy. *J Nucl Med* 1989;30:312–319.

159. Fleming RM, Kirkeeide RL, Taegtmeyer H, et al. Comparison of technetium-99m teboroxime tomography with automated quantitative coronary arteriography and thallium-201 tomographic imaging. *J Am Coll Cardiol* 1991;17:1297–1302.

160. Zielonka JS, Cannon P, Johnson LL, et al. Multicenter trial of Tc-99m teboroxime (cardiotec) a new myocardial perfusion agent. *J Nucl Med* 1990;31:827.

161. Burns RJ, Lalonde L, Hong Tai Eng F. Exercise Tc99m-teboroxime cardiac SPECT: results of a Canadian multicentre trial. *J Nucl Med* 1991;32:919.

162. Taillefer R, Freeman M, Greenberg D, et al. Detection of coronary artery disease: comparison between [99m]Tc-teboroxime and 201thallium planar myocardial perfusion imaging (Canadian multicenter clinical trial). *J Nucl Med* 1991;32:919.

163. Taillefer R, Lambert R, Essiambre R, et al. Comparison between thallium-201, technetium-99m-sestamibi and technetium-99m-teboroxime planar myocardial perfusion imaging in detection of coronary artery disease. *J Nucl Med* 1992;33:1091–1098.

164. Williams KA, Taillon LA, Draho JM, et al. First-pass radionuclide angiographic studies of left ventricular function with technetium-99m-teboroxime, technetium-99m-sestamibi and technetium-99m-DTPA. *J Nucl Med* 1993;34:394–399.

165. Takahashi N, Tamaki N, Tadamura E, et al. Combined assessment of regional perfusion and wall motion in patients with coronary artery disease with technetium 99m tetrofosmin. *J Nucl Cardiol* 1994;1:29–38.

166. Tamaki N, Takahashi N, Kawamoto M, et al. Myocardial tomography using technetium-99m-tetrofosmin to evaluate coronary artery disease. *J Nucl Med* 1994;35:594–600.

167. Rigo P, Leclercq B, Itti R, et al. Technetium-99m-tetrofosmin myocardial imaging: a comparison with thallium-201 and angiography. *J Nucl Med* 1994;35:587–593.

168. Zaret BL, Rigo P, Wackers FJT, et al. Myocardial perfusion imaging with [99m]Tc-tetrofosmin: comparison to 201Tl imaging and coronary angiography in a phase III multicenter trial. *Circulation* 1995;91:313–319.

169. Nakajima K, Taki J, Shuke N, et al. Myocardial perfusion imaging and dynamic analysis with technetium-99m tetrofosmin. *J Nucl Med* 1993;34:1478–1484.

170. Matsunari I, Fujino S, Taki J, et al. Comparison of defect size between thallium-201 and technetium-99m tetrofosmin myocardial single-photon emission computed tomography in patients with single-vessel coronary artery disease. *Am J Cardiol* 1996;77:350–354.

171. Heo J, Cave V, Wasserleben V, et al. Planar and tomographic imaging with technetium 99m-labeled tetrofosmin: correlation with thallium 201 and coronary angiography. *J Nucl Cardiol* 1994;1:317–324.

172. Hendel RC, Parker MA, Wackers FJT, et al. Reduced variability of interpretation and improved image quality with a technetium 99m myocardial perfusion agent: comparison of thallium 201 and technetium 99m-labeled tetrofosmin. *J Nucl Cardiol* 1994;1:509–514.

173. Flamen P, Bossuyt A, Franken PR. Technetium-99m tetrofosmin in dipyridamole stress myocardial SPECT imaging: intraindividual comparison with technetium-99m-sestamibi. *J Nucl Med* 1995;36:2009–2015.

174. Munch G, Neverve J, Matsunari I, et al. Myocardial technetium-99m tetrofosmin and technetium-99m-sestamibi kinetics in normal subjects and patients with coronary artery disease. *J Nucl Med* 1997;38:426–432.

175. Gremillet E, Champallier A. Comparative myocardial uptake of Tc-99m sestamibi and Tc-99m tetrofosmin one hour after stress injection. *Eur J Nucl Med* 1998;25:1502–1510.

176. Acampa W, Cuocolo A, Sullo P, et al. Direct comparison of technetium-99m-sestamibi and technetium-99m-tetrofosmin cardiac single photon emission computed tomography in patients with coronary artery disease. *J Nucl Cardiol* 1998;5:265–274.

177. Taillefer R, Bernier H, Lambert R, et al. Comparison between Tc-99m-sestamibi and Tc-99m-tetrofosmin SPECT imaging with dipyridamole in detection of coronary artery disease. *J Nucl Med* 1998;39:17P.

178. Soman P, Taillefer R, DePuey EG, et al. Assessment od coronary artery disease by dipyridamole SPECT: superiority of [99m]Tc-sestamibi over [99m]Tc-tetrofosmin. *J Am Coll Cardiol (in press)*.

179. Shanoudy H, Raggi P, Beller GA, et al. Comparison of technetium-99m tetrofosmin and thallium-201 single-photon emission computed tomographic imaging for detection of myocardial perfusion defects in patients with coronary artery disease. *J Am Coll Cardiol* 1998;31:331–337.

180. Gerson MC, Lukes J, Deutsch E, et al. Comparison of technetium 99m Q12 and thallium 201 for detection of angiographically documented coronary artery disease in humans. *J Nucl Cardiol* 1994;1:499–508.

181. Hendel RC, Verani MS, Miller DD, et al. Diagnostic utility of tomographic myocardial perfusion imaging with technetium 99m furifosmin (Q12) compared with thallium 201: results of a phase III multicenter trial. *J Nucl Cardiol* 1996;3:291–300.

182. Gerson MC, Lukes J, Deutsch E, et al. Comparison of imaging properties of technetium 99m Q12 and technetium 99m Q3 in humans. *J Nucl Cardiol* 1995;2:224–230.

183. Gerson MC, Millard RW, McGoron AJ, et al. Myocardial uptake and kinetic properties of Tc-99m Q3 in dogs. *J Nucl Med* 1994;35:1698–1706.

184. Gerson MC, Lukes J, Deutsch EA, et al. Comparison of Tc-99m Q3 and Tl-201 for detection of coronary artery disease in man. *J Nucl Med* 1994;35:580–586.

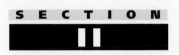

# CLINICAL CONSIDERATIONS

# 9

# DETECTION, EVALUATION, AND RISK STRATIFICATION OF CORONARY ARTERY DISEASE BY THALLIUM-201 MYOCARDIAL PERFUSION SCINTIGRAPHY

## JAMSHID MADDAHI
## DANIEL S. BERMAN

Thallium-201 ($^{201}$Tl) was introduced for clinical application in 1973 by Lebowitz and colleagues (1) and has since been applied extensively in the clinical evaluation of patients with or suspected of having coronary artery disease (CAD). This chapter provides an overview of the technical and clinical aspects of $^{201}$Tl imaging. The discussion of the technical aspects deals primarily with the myocardial kinetics of $^{201}$Tl, planar and single photon emission computed tomography (SPECT) acquisition protocols, quantitative analysis of images, and pharmacologic stress testing. The review of the clinical applications of myocardial $^{201}$Tl imaging includes the detection, localization, and identification of CAD, and risk stratification in suspected or known CAD. Applications of $^{201}$Tl imaging to the evaluation of myocardial viability is presented elsewhere in this book.

## TECHNICAL CONSIDERATIONS

### Myocardial Kinetics of $^{201}$Tl

Thallium is a metallic element in group IIIA of the periodic table, with biologic properties similar but not identical to those of potassium. The ionic radii of these two elements are

closely similar, and as with potassium, the distribution of the thallous ion following its intravenous administration is primarily intracellular (2,3). Transport of thallium across the cell membrane has been reported to occur partly via an ouabain-inhibitable mechanism, presumed to be the sodium-potassium adenosine triphosphatase (ATPase) pump (4).

The myocardial kinetics of $^{201}$Tl following its intravenous injection can be divided into two overlapping phases: initial distribution and redistribution. The initial distribution of $^{201}$Tl in the myocardium is determined by the product of regional blood flow and the extraction fraction (ability of the myocardium to extract the tracer from blood), which is 87% (5) at normal flow rates. Regional myocardial uptake of $^{201}$Tl in the experimental animal has been shown to be linearly related to regional myocardial blood flow (6,7). At exceedingly low flow rates (<10% of baseline), $^{201}$Tl uptake increases relative to blood flow because of an increase in the myocardial extraction fraction. Conversely, at high flow rates (exceeding twice the control level), the myocardial extraction fraction for $^{201}$Tl decreases, resulting in a "roll-off" of the relationship between myocardial uptake of $^{201}$Tl and increasing flow (8,9). Overall, initial defects in myocardial $^{201}$Tl images, whether injection is made at rest, during exercise, or following the administration of a coronary vasodilator, are produced predominantly by regional deficits in myocardial blood-flow distribution. In clinical situations, the additional role played by myocardial ischemia or drugs in producing image defects (by altering the extraction fraction) is unclear but does not appear to be significant.

J. Maddahi: University of California–Los Angeles School of Medicine, Los Angeles, California 90024.

D. S. Berman: Department of Imaging, Cedars-Sinai Medical Center, Los Angeles, California 90048.

The distribution of [201]Tl in the myocardium is not static but changes as a function of time. This change is referred to as redistribution. Pohost and colleagues (6) demonstrated that following the injection of [201]Tl into patients with exercise-induced ischemia but without infarction, delayed imaging revealed the disappearance of initial perfusion defects. Redistribution of [201]Tl also has been observed after its injection at rest into patients with severe fixed coronary stenosis without infarction (10). This finding has been confirmed in experimental studies (11,12). The disappearance with time of defects initially observed during exercise imaging with [201]Tl generally results from slower clearance of [201]Tl from the underperfused zones as compared to the normal zones (12,13). The normal net myocardial clearance half-life of [201]Tl following its injection is approximately 4 hours if the injection is made during exercise (14), and longer if the injection is made at a submaximal exercise heart rate (15–17) or at rest (18). Although changes in myocardial blood flow following the intravenous administration of [201]Tl do not substantially alter myocardial [201]Tl clearance (19,20), the rate of disappear-ance of [201]Tl from the blood affects the myocardial clearance of [201]Tl (18,21), which in turn may influence the time course of [201]Tl reversibility. Budinger and colleagues (22,23) showed that rapid blood clearance of [201]Tl prevented perfusion defect reversibility in viable myocardial regions for up to 24 hours after [201]Tl administration. Angello and colleagues (24) found that poststress glucose loading resulted in a decreased blood [201]Tl concentration in the initial 2 hours after [201]Tl injection, resulting in a high frequency of nonreversible defects in regions that demonstrated reversibility at 4 hours when [201]Tl imaging was performed without glucose loading. Thus, fasting is recommended to patients on the day of and for the interval between sequential sessions of [201]Tl imaging.

Clinically, [201]Tl defects may be categorized as reversible, partially reversible, nonreversible, or as exhibiting reverse redistribution, based on the change from the initial to the redistribution phase of the scintigraphic study. As mentioned before, the time period for redistribution may vary. Complete redistribution may require 24 hours or more (25,26). This phenomenon of late redistribution has impor-

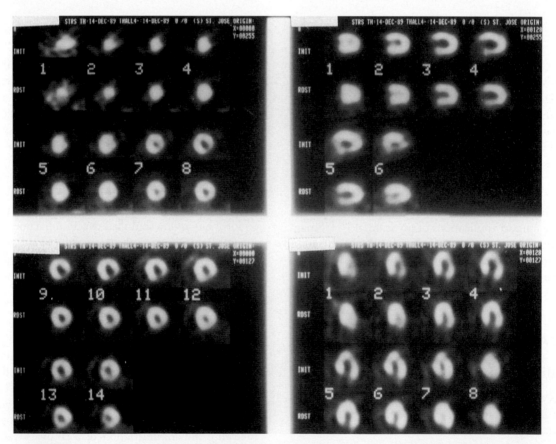

**FIGURE 9.1**. Example of exercise-redistribution myocardial perfusion [201]Tl single photon emission computed tomography (SPECT) images in a patient with reversible defects involving the proximal and midinferolateral regions of the left ventricle. The left upper and lower quadrants display short axis slices of the left ventricle, from apex to the base, numbered 1 through 14. The right upper quadrant displays vertical long-axis slices of the left ventricle expanding from septal (1) to lateral (5) left ventricular regions. The right lower quadrant displays horizontal long-axis slices of the left ventricle expanding from inferior (1) to anterior (8) portions of the left ventricle, Init, initial post exercise images; RDST, redistribution images.

tant implications with respect to the differentiation of viable from nonviable myocardium. The following categorization of type of reversibility assumes that adequate time has been allowed for the ultimate redistribution pattern to be established. In reversible defects (Fig. 9.1), the net myocardial washout rate of $^{201}$Tl is slower in the defect region than in normal areas. This ultimately leads to equalization of the concentration of $^{201}$Tl in normal and abnormal regions. The reversible process, whether following resting or exercise injection, reflects the presence of viable myocardium. In partially reversible defects (Fig. 9.2), the concentrations of $^{201}$Tl in the normal and defect regions become closer to one another during the redistribution phase, but do not equalize. This pattern is believed to occur in myocardial regions that contain a mixture of nonviable and viable but ischemic myocardium. In nonreversible defects, the initial ratio of $^{201}$Tl concentration between the abnormal and normal regions is maintained over time because of similar net clearance of $^{201}$Tl in the normal and abnormal zones. Nonreversible defects are generally associated with myocardial scar. The apparently normal net washout rate of $^{201}$Tl in the region of the scar may well be secondary to washout in normal areas superimposed on or mixed with the abnormal zone. In defects that show reverse redistribution, the ratio of the $^{201}$Tl concentration in the defect to that in the normal region decreases over time because of faster than normal $^{201}$Tl washout from the defect zone (27). This pattern has been observed in the setting of nontransmural myocardial infarction associated with a patent infarct-related coronary artery (27) and may result from higher than normal blood flow to the residual viable myocardium in the partially infarcted zone.

## Acquisition Protocols

### Planar Imaging

For planar imaging, a standard or a large field-of-view (FOV) camera, equipped with a sodium iodide crystal $^{1}/_{4}$- or $^{3}/_{8}$-inch thick, is used. A medium-resolution (all purpose) or high-resolution, parallel hole collimator is generally employed. The recommended energy windows are 20% centered on the 69- to 83-keV peak and 10% centered on the 167-keV peak. Patients are imaged in three orientations:

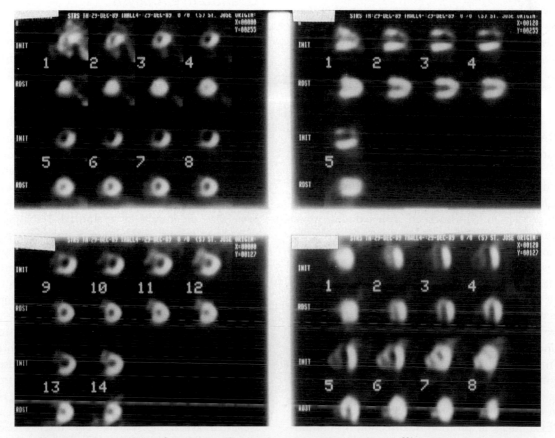

**FIGURE 9.2.** Example of exercise-redistribution myocardial perfusion $^{201}$Tl SPECT study in a patient with reversible and partially reversible defects. Orientation of slices is according to Figure 1 format. Reversible defects involve the distal and midanterior, anteroseptal, and apical regions of the left ventricle. The partially reversible defects involve the mid and basal interoseptal regions of the left ventricle, best seen in the horizontal long-axis slices numbered 2 and 3.

anterior, "best septal" left anterior oblique (LAO), and steep LAO or left lateral views. For the first two views, the patient lies supine on the imaging table, but for the steep LAO or left lateral view, the patient is positioned in the right lateral decubitus position with the left side of the chest against the collimator. Imaging is begun 6 minutes after injection of $^{201}$Tl, and each image is acquired for a preset time of 10 minutes per view. The recommended acquisition matrix for planar imaging is $128 \times 128 \times 8$ bits.

## SPECT Imaging

The planar imaging method appears to be inherently suboptimal for assessing myocardial perfusion, because frequent overlap of normally and abnormally perfused myocardial regions limits its ability to accurately detect, localize, and size myocardial perfusion defects. SPECT, which has a higher contrast resolution and allows the discrimination of overlapping myocardial regions, has overcome these limitations of planar imaging. Since its introduction, SPECT imaging has been extensively evaluated for optimal image acquisition and processing. As with planar $^{201}$Tl imaging, SPECT is generally used in conjunction with stress testing. The patient is injected with 3 to 4 mCi of $^{201}$Tl at least 1 minute before the termination of exercise or pharmacologic stress. For imaging, a large FOV camera, especially designed to rotate around the patient, is used. The most common imaging protocol includes the use of an all-purpose, parallel hole collimator and a $64 \times 64 \times 16$-bit matrix. The patient lies on the imaging table in the supine position, and images are obtained over a semicircular 180-degree arc extending from the 45-degree right anterior oblique (RAO) to the 45-degree left posterior oblique (LPO) position, imaging 32 projections, each for 40 seconds. SPECT imaging in the prone position has been advocated for reducing the inferoseptal attenuation artifact (28). Prone imaging, however, frequently causes an anterior wall attenuation artifact and is associated with reduced overall image count density due to photon attenuation by the imaging table (28,29). SPECT imaging does not begin until at least 10 minutes after the injection of $^{201}$Tl, to diminish the frequency of the upward creep artifact (30). During this 10-minute waiting period, a single 5-minute anterior view planar image may be acquired to assess the lung uptake of $^{201}$Tl, transient ischemic dilation of the left ventricle, and the breast attenuation artifact.

Owing to the length of image acquisition and the nature of the equipment, SPECT imaging is technically very demanding and requires more attention to quality control than planar imaging. An important step in the quality control for SPECT image acquisition is correction for nonuniformity. For this purpose, a $30 \times 10^6$ count image is obtained weekly from a uniform cobalt 57 ($^{57}$Co) flood source. This image is then used to correct each of the projection images for nonuniformity. Another important step prior to image acquisition is the determination of the mechanical center of rotation (COR). The COR is then used to align the detector data with respect to the reconstruction matrix. Failure to correct for the COR can cause misregistration of pixels during the reconstruction process, which leads to artifactual myocardial perfusion defects. Since patient motion during SPECT imaging is a frequent cause of image artifacts, patients should be instructed to lie still during the entire acquisition process, and projection images should be displayed at the end of acquisition in a cine loop format to evaluate the occurrence of patient motion. Several studies have shown that the conventional 4-hour redistribution imaging protocol is suboptimal for detection of defect reversibility and assessment of regional myocardial viability because approximately 65% of nonreversible 4-hour redistribution defects have evidence of myocardial viability (31). To minimize this problem, various $^{201}$Tl late redistribution and reinjection protocols have been developed. For detailed discussion of this topic and the role of $^{201}$Tl imaging for assessment of myocardial viability, see Chapter 10.

## Quantitative Analysis

Several methods have been developed and successfully applied clinically for objective, quantitative analysis of the initial myocardial count distribution and washout rate of $^{201}$Tl on planar (13,14,31–40) and SPECT (41–45) images. Overall, these quantitative approaches to $^{201}$Tl image analysis have provided several advantages over qualitative (visual) analysis of images by (a) reducing inter- and intraobserver variability, (b) aiding recognition of normal variant patterns because image results are compared to a normal database, (c) providing a better estimate of size and severity of perfusion defects, and (d) assessing defect reversibility more accurately. It is important to note, however, that the results of quantitative analysis should be viewed as a second expert opinion and do not replace physician interpretation of the images. In this chapter, SPECT image processing and quantitation are presented in some detail. Other publications and other chapters of this book discuss the technical details of image processing and quantitation.

SPECT image processing involves several steps. Each of the projections is first corrected for nonuniformity with a 30-million count flood collected with the use of a $^{57}$Co source. The mechanical COR is determined from the projection data to align detector data with respect to the reconstruction matrix. Raw data are smoothed with a nine-point weighted averaging system. The filtered backprojection technique is used to reconstruct images. A Butterworth filter with a cutoff frequency of 0.2 cycles per pixel and order 5, which has the highest efficiency, is used for filtering of the images prior to reconstruction (42). However, with different camera-computer systems, different filters may be optimal. Images are reoriented into planes that are perpendicular to the long axis (short axis) and parallel to the long axis of the left ventricle (vertical and horizontal long axes). In all three planes, each tomographic slice is one pixel thick, representing a thickness of approximately 6.2 mm. Several methods have been developed and are available for quantitation of relative myocardial count distribution on SPECT images (41–43,45,46). The technique described by Maddahi and associates (42) is briefly presented here to outline the various steps involved in quantitation and display of $^{201}$Tl SPECT images. In contrast to planar image quantitation, assessment of myocardial percent washout of $^{201}$Tl with the SPECT technique does not contribute to detection of disease in individual coronary arteries and is therefore not quantitated.

Detection and localization of coronary disease by SPECT imaging relies on quantitative analysis of exercise images for the presence and location of perfusion defects. Myocardial $^{201}$Tl activity of the apex is analyzed from the apical portion of the vertical long-axis slices, and the myocardial activity of the remaining portions of the left ventricle is analyzed from the short-axis slices. The choice of vertical long-axis slices for analysis of the apex is made, because the apex is subject to partial volume effect on the short-axis slices. For myocardial sampling, the center of the left ventricle and the radius of search on each slice are defined by the operator, and 60 equidistant radii (6 degrees apart) are then automatically generated. Along each radius, the computer searches and selects the maximal count value. The values are then normalized to the highest value found in each slice and are plotted for each angular location on the myocardial periphery, generating a circumferential count profile. For proper comparison of stress and redistribution images with the normal profiles and with one another, an anatomic landmark is defined at the inferior junction of the right and left ventricles on the short-axis cuts, to which the 102-degree angle is assigned. On the vertical long-axis cuts, the most apical point is used for alignment, and the 90-degree angle is assigned to it. As with planar imaging, development of a normal reference database is essential for objective analysis of results in patients. In males, normal myocardial count distribution on SPECT images is different from that in females, because of gender-related differences in soft tissue attenuation patterns. Thus, for each gender, a different set of normal values is used. To develop normal reference circumferential profiles, mean circumferential profiles are generated for five left ventricular anatomic regions from pooled data of patients who had a low pre-$^{201}$Tl SPECT likelihood of CAD. From these mean normal circumferential profiles, lower limits of normal have been derived.

The most common format for display of myocardial counts with SPECT imaging is the "polar-map" or "bull's-eye" approach, in which the left ventricular myocardium is represented two-dimensionally, with the center of display corresponding to the apex and the periphery corresponding to the atrioventricular junction. Different portions of the left ventricular myocardium represent territories of various coronary arteries and their major branches. In a patient with a proximal left anterior descending (LAD) coronary stenosis, defects are noted in the anterior wall, the apex, the anteroseptal wall, and the anterolateral region. In a patient with a distal LAD stenosis, the anteroseptal and anterolateral regions, representing the septal perforator and diagonal branch territories, are not involved, and the defect is limited to the distal anterior wall and apex. In patients with disease in the diagonal branch of the LAD, perfusion defects are limited to the proximal and middle anterior-anterolateral left ventricular regions. The territory of a nondominant left circumflex (LCX) coronary artery is represented by the proximal, middle, and distal anterolateral and inferolateral left ventricular regions. The territory of a dominant LCX coronary artery includes the inferior and inferoseptal regions of the left ventricular myocardium, in addition to the territory of a nondominant LCX territory. In a patient with disease in a dominant right coronary artery (RCA), the inferior and inferoseptal regions of the left ventricular myocardium are involved.

## Pharmacologic Stress Testing

Treadmill and bicycle exercise are the most common types of stress used in conjunction with myocardial perfusion imaging. A significant proportion of patients, however, are unable to exercise because of peripheral vascular, musculoskeletal, or neurologic diseases, or cannot achieve an adequate exercise heart rate due to lack of motivation, poor physical condition, or β-blocking or calcium-channel–blocking medications. In these patients, pharmacologic stress testing may be used effectively as a substitute for exercise in conjunction with myocardial perfusion imaging.

### Mechanism of Action

Two of the three commonly used pharmacologic stress-testing agents, dipyridamole and adenosine, are coronary vasodilators that increase myocardial blood flow three to five times the resting level in myocardial regions that are supplied by normal coronary arteries (47–49). Adenosine is a direct coronary vasodilator and activates the adenosine A$_2$ receptors in the coronary arterial wall. This activation leads to an increase in adenosine cyclase and cyclic 3′, 5′-adenosine monophosphate levels, decreased transmembrane calcium uptake, and, ultimately, coronary vasodilation. Dipyridamole exerts its effect by raising endogenous adenosine blood levels through blocking of cell membrane transport and reuptake of endogenous adenosine. In myocardial regions that are supplied by diseased coronary arteries, the hyperemic response to these agents is attenuated. Not infrequently, after administration of coronary vasodilators, myocardial perfusion may actually decrease below the resting level in regions supplied by diseased coronary arteries, the result of a true "coronary steal" (50–56). Therefore, in patients with CAD, infusion of dipyridamole or adenosine induces a disparity in regional myocardial perfusion similar to that achieved with exercise testing. Because xanthines directly block the action of dipyridamole and adenosine, prior to pharmacologic vasodilation testing, patients should avoid caffeine (coffee, tea, some soft drinks, and medications) for 24 hours and stop all xanthine-containing medications (e.g., aminophylline) for at least 36 hours. Contraindications to coronary vasodilator infusion include unstable angina, acute phase of myocardial infarction, critical aortic stenosis, and hypertrophic cardiomyopathy. Furthermore, these agents are contraindicated in patients with hypotension (systolic blood pressure <90 mm Hg) because they lower systolic and diastolic blood pressures. Coronary vasodilators are also contraindicated in patients with asthma because they may exacerbate bronchospasm. Unlike exercise testing, however, coronary vasodilators can be used in patients with a high resting blood pressure. The third pharmacologic stress agent, dobutamine, is predominantly a $\beta_1$-agonist that increases heart rate, myocardial contractility, and systolic blood pressure. To meet the increased myocardial oxygen demand, normal coronary arteries dilate, whereas stenotic arteries do not dilate at all or dilate insufficiently. Thus, the coronary vasodilatory effect of dobutamine is similar to that of physiologic exercise and is unlike that of dipyridamole and adenosine, which are direct coronary vasodilators. In the study of Hays and co-workers (57), dobutamine infusion increased heart rate and systolic blood pressure, while diastolic blood pressure decreased because of peripheral ($\beta_2$) dilator effect. Krivokapich and associates (58) showed that the increase in blood flow is significantly related to heart rate and suggested that the increase in coronary flow seen with dobutamine is due to increased oxygen demand.

## Pharmacologic Stress Testing with Dipyridamole

Dipyridamole is infused intravenously in a dose of 0.56 to 0.84 mg/kg over a 4-minute period. Three minutes after termination of infusion, at the time of maximal hyperemic effect (47,48), [201]Tl is injected intravenously. Should severe ischemia develop, as evidenced by ST-segment depression or angina pectoris, the effects of dipyridamole may be reversed quickly, usually within 45 seconds, by intravenous administration of aminophylline (50 to 100 mg). Whenever possible, administration of aminophylline should be delayed until at least 1 minute after injection of the [201]Tl so that myocardial hyperemia is not abolished before substan-

tial [201]Tl uptake by the myocardium has occurred. Several variations in this protocol have been proposed, including the use of handgrip exercise (2 minutes after termination of dipyridamole infusion for a period of 3 to 4 minutes), the routine administration of aminophylline 1 to 2 minutes after [201]Tl injection, and low-level treadmill testing before [201]Tl injection, but the effect on the overall efficacy of dipyridamole [201]Tl scintigraphy for diagnosis of coronary disease is uncertain. The side effects of dipyridamole infusion may be categorized into three groups (59,60): The first group is related to systemic vasodilation—dizziness, headache, hypotension, and flushing. The second group is related to the development of myocardial ischemia in the form of angina pectoris or ST-segment depression, or both. The third group relates to gastrointestinal effects in the form of nausea and an "uneasy feeling" in the abdomen. The combined major adverse events among 73,806 patients who were evaluated with dipyridamole [201]Tl testing (60) included cardiac death (0.95 per 10,000), nonfatal myocardial infarction (1.76 per 10,000), nonfatal sustained ventricular arrhythmias (0.81 per 10,000), transient cerebral ischemic attacks (1.22 per 10,000), and severe bronchospasm (1.22 per 10,000). It is generally believed that the risk of serious events is similar to that seen with exercise. Such risks may be diminished by careful screening of patients who are referred for dipyridamole stress testing and by proper attention to the aforementioned contraindications of dipyridamole testing. Physician monitoring of patients undergoing dipyridamole studies is clearly as important as it is in the case of exercise studies. Additionally, because the effects of dipyridamole can last longer than those of aminophylline, any patient requiring aminophylline to reverse the side effects of dipyridamole should have physician monitoring for approximately 20 to 30 minutes after administration of aminophylline.

## Pharmacologic Stress Testing with Adenosine

Adenosine is standardly infused at the rate of 140 µg/kg per minute for 6 minutes. Adenosine has a very short half-life (several seconds) and reaches its peak effect within 1 to 2 minutes after the start of infusion (61,62). The myocardial perfusion imaging agent is injected after 3 minutes of infusion. After termination of infusion, the effects generally dissipate within 1 to 2 minutes (disappearance half-life of 37 seconds). Because of the short duration of effects after termination of infusion, aminophylline is rarely needed to terminate the side effects. Another advantage of the short half-life of adenosine is the feasibility of increasing or decreasing the dose when necessary. The safety of adenosine pharmacologic stress testing has been evaluated in 5,552 patients in the Phase III Multicenter Trial (63) and was updated in 9,256 patients (64). In general, the side effects of adenosine are similar to those of dipyridamole but are more frequent. In addition, adenosine slows atrioventricular conduction, and different types of heart block may result from its infusion, such as first-degree (2.7%), second-degree (4%), or third-degree (0.7%) block (64).

## Pharmacologic Stress Testing with Dobutamine

Candidates for pharmacologic stress testing with dobutamine are patients who cannot undergo stress testing with dipyridamole or adenosine because of a history of asthma. Infusion begins with 5 µg/kg per minute for 3 minutes and is then increased to 10 µg/kg per minute for another 3 minutes and is increased every 3 minutes by 10 µg/kg per minute until a maximum of 40 µg/kg per minute is achieved. Myocardial perfusion tracer is injected 1 minute after the maximal tolerable dose, and infusion is continued for at least 1 minute, or preferably 2 minutes, after injection. The most common adverse effects of dobutamine infusion are palpitations and chest pain. Less common adverse effects are headache, flushing, and dyspnea. The majority of these adverse effects are transient and last only a few minutes after cessation of infusion because of the 2-minute biologic half-life of dobutamine. More serious adverse effects of dobutamine infusion are the development of premature ventricular depolarizations and, occasionally, ventricular tachycardia (which is usually not sustained) or atrial fibrillation (57). Therefore, patients with underlying cardiac arrhythmias must be observed closely for development of these side effects. The adverse effects of dobutamine may be neutralized by esmolol, which is a rapidly acting β-blocker.

## CLINICAL APPLICATIONS

### Diagnostic Accuracy of 201Tl Imaging

As with other tests applied for the detection of CAD, the diagnostic accuracy of the exercise 201Tl study is expressed by its sensitivity and specificity. These indices depend on several technical factors, such as planar versus tomographic imaging, visual versus quantitative analysis, and exercise versus pharmacologic stress testing. In addition, several characteristics of the patient population under study may affect the sensitivity and specificity of 201Tl testing, such as the presence or absence of myocardial infarction, threshold for defining significant CAD, referral bias, level of exercise, and severity (percentage stenosis) and extent (number of diseased vessels) of CAD in the referred population.

### Qualitative Analysis of Planar Images

By far, the most extensive literature available to date in the field of imaging 201Tl is on the use of exercise redistribution imaging by planar acquisition and qualitative analysis. The combined reported sensitivity and specificity of this technique are shown in Fig. 9.3. The overall sensitivity and specificity of the technique in a total of 4,678 patients reported in the literature (13,40,65–109) are 82% and 88%, respectively. Differing reports from center to center are most likely due to the characteristics of the patient population under study. Detrano and colleagues (110), in an analysis of factors affecting the sensitivity and specificity of exercise 201Tl testing in 56 published reports, demonstrated that in patients without myocardial infarction, the sensitivity of the technique was

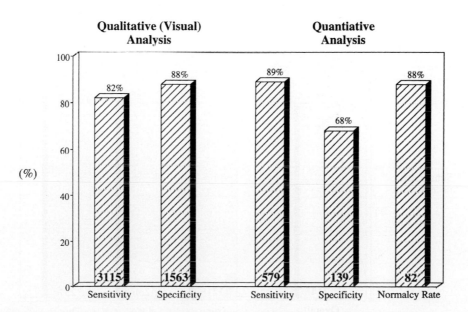

**FIGURE 9.3.** Combined reported sensitivity and specificity of qualitative (visual) and quantitative analyses of stress-redistribution 201Tl myocardial perfusion imaging using the planar imaging technique. The results summarize literature reports as referenced in the text.

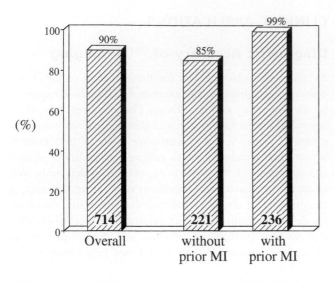

**FIGURE 9.4.** Pooled literature results of sensitivity for stress-redistribution ²⁰¹Tl myocardial perfusion SPECT in subgroups of patients with and without prior myocardial infarction (MI).

## Quantitative Analysis of Planar Images

The interobserver variability in the qualitative analysis of ²⁰¹Tl images has been shown to range from 3% to 16%, and the intraobserver variability from 4% to 11% (66,111–113). To overcome the subjectivity of interpretation inherent in the qualitative visual analysis of ²⁰¹Tl images, several methods for semiquantitative analysis of planar ²⁰¹Tl images have been reported. The initial methods involved visual analysis of processed ²⁰¹Tl images (94,114,115). However, the subsequent quantitative techniques used objective criteria for detecting perfusion defects based on comparison of image data with results from a normal database (13,34,37,116,117). Although quantitative analysis of ²⁰¹Tl scintigrams reduces inter- and intraobserver variability, its effect on the overall sensitivity and specificity of ²⁰¹Tl testing has not been major. This is well demonstrated by the results of reports comparing visual and quantitative analysis in the same patient population (13). If the effect of quantitation of images on the sensitivity and specificity of ²⁰¹Tl testing is assessed by comparing mean literature results obtained in two different patient populations, there appears to be a trend toward increased sensitivity and decreased specificity. The mean sensitivity and specificity in the literature for quantitative planar ²⁰¹Tl imaging (13,34,116,118) in a total of 800 patients are 89% and 68%, respectively (Fig. 9.3). The lower specificity and higher sensitivity, however, are most likely due to other confounding factors encountered in the comparison of results from two different patient populations. More specifically, it is likely that the increased referral bias (described below) encountered in more recently reported studies, which used quantitative analysis, explains the observed differences. In fact, the mean literature normalcy rate for planar quantitative image analysis with ²⁰¹Tl has been 88% (13,118).

79%, or lower than that of patients with prior myocardial infarction, for which the sensitivity was 96% (Fig. 9.4). The sensitivity of exercise ²⁰¹Tl testing is also affected by the threshold of percentage narrowing that is used for the definition of angiographic disease, by how severe the stenoses are in a given population, and by the number of diseased coronary arteries. The effect of the latter is summarized in Fig. 9.5, which presents the published reports from 11 planar studies that specified the effect of extent of disease on test sensitivity (65,66,68,69,71,73,74,80,89,90,99). The mean sensitivity of the planar method increased from 79% for single-vessel disease to 88% for double-vessel disease and 92% for triple-vessel disease.

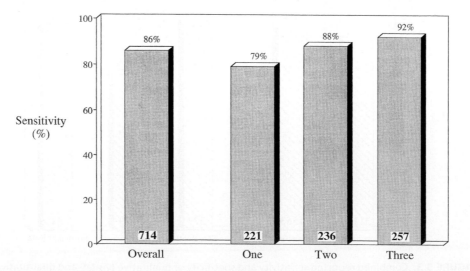

**FIGURE 9.5.** Pooled literature sensitivity of stress-redistribution planar ²⁰¹Tl myocardial perfusion imaging in relation to the number of diseased coronary arteries.

## Effect of Referral Bias on Sensitivity and Specificity

An important factor influencing the sensitivity and specificity of a test after its widespread clinical acceptance is the preferential selection of patients for coronary arteriography based on a positive [201]Tl imaging study result, and the refraining from catheterization of patients with a negative test result (referral bias). This results in an apparent increase in sensitivity and an apparent decrease in specificity of [201]Tl imaging. This effect has been clearly shown by Rozanski and colleagues (119), who noted a decrease in the apparent specificity of exercise radionuclide ventriculography over the years, which was attributed to referral bias. When the full impact of referral bias is in effect and only patients with a positive test are catheterized, clinical bias can have a dramatic effect on test specificity, which, by definition, would fall to zero. Detrano and colleagues (110) found a significant negative relationship between referral bias and test specificity. In their study, the effect on sensitivity was not significant. They showed that studies that attempted to reduce referral bias by not allowing the result of an exercise [201]Tl study to influence the decision to do a coronary angiogram had significantly higher specificities than studies that did not (84% versus 78%). Therefore, the actual specificity of exercise planar [201]Tl imaging may be higher than that reported by many investigators. In an attempt to determine a more representative specificity of [201]Tl testing, we introduced the use of the "normalcy rate," which is observed in patients with a low likelihood of angiographically significant CAD based on an analysis of age, sex, symptoms, and the results of exercise electrocardiography (ECG) (13,118). This approach provides a proxy for specificity that can be used when the referral bias is operational, and it offers the advantage over studying healthy normal volunteers of studying a patient population that is closer in demographics to the patient population in question.

## Qualitative and Quantitative SPECT [201]Tl Imaging

Table 9.1 summarizes the results of the SPECT [201]Tl imaging technique. For the visual analysis, in a total of 706 patients reported (43,44,120,121), the sensitivity and specificity were 92% and 77%, respectively. It is of note that the specificity of the test appeared to be lower in the study of De Pasquale and colleagues (43) reported in 1988 than in the study of Tamaki and colleagues (120) reported in 1984. A similar trend is also noted for the quantitative SPECT method, with a decrease in specificity from 91% to 43% from 1984 to 1990 despite a sensitivity of 98% versus 94%, during the same period. The decline of specificity with time is likely to be due in part to an increase in referral bias in the more recent studies. Although the true, unbiased specificity of the SPECT technique has not been determined, it may be implied from the normalcy rate of 89% in a total of 235 low-likelihood patients (42,45,122). It is therefore likely that the true specificity of the SPECT technique is slightly lower than that of the planar imaging method, which may be due to the fact that SPECT imaging is technically more demanding and has many more sources of artifacts during image acquisition and processing. The literature results for the quantitative SPECT method are also shown in Table 9.1. In a total of 1,527 patients reported (42–45,120–122), the sensitivity, specificity, and normalcy rates were 90%, 70%, and 89%, respectively. In a total of 983 patients reported in the literature (123) that specified sensitivity with respect to presence or absence of prior myocardial infarction, the overall sensitivity was 90%, which is higher (99%) in the subgroup of 324 patients with prior myocardial infarction and is lower (85%) in the subgroup of 659 without prior myocardial infarction (Fig. 9.4). In six SPECT studies that specified the effect of extent of disease on test sensitivity (42–45,48,122), the mean sensitivity of the SPECT

## TABLE 9.1 SENSITIVITY AND SPECIFICITY OF SPECT [201]TI SCINTIGRAPHY

| Year | Lead Author | Sensitivity | | Specificity | | Normalcy rate | |
|---|---|---|---|---|---|---|---|
| Quantitative analysis | | | | | | | |
| 1984 | Tamaki (120) | 76/82 | (93%) | 20/22 | (91%) | | |
| 1988 | De Pasquale (43) | 173/179 | (97%) | 21/31 | (68%) | | |
| 1989 | Fintel (121) | 88/96 | (92%) | — | | | |
| 1990 | Mahmarian (44) | 193/221 | (87%) | 57/75 | (76%) | | |
| Overall | | 530/578 | (92%) | 98/128 | (77%) | | |
| Quantitative analysis | | | | | | | |
| 1984 | Tamaki (120) | 80/82 | (98%) | 20/22 | (91%) | — | |
| 1988 | De Pasquale (43) | 170/179 | (95%) | 23/31 | (74%) | — | |
| 1989 | Maddahi (42) | 88/92 | (96%) | 10/18 | (56%) | 24/28 | (86%) |
| 1989 | Iskandrian (45) | 224/272 | (82%) | 36/58 | (62%) | 123/131 | (94%) |
| 1990 | Van Train (122) | 185/196 | (94%) | 20/46 | (43%) | 62/76 | (82%) |
| 1990 | Mahmarian (44) | 192/221 | (87%) | 65/75 | (87%) | — | |
| Overall | | 939/1,042 | (90%) | 174/250 | (70%) | 209/235 | (89%) |

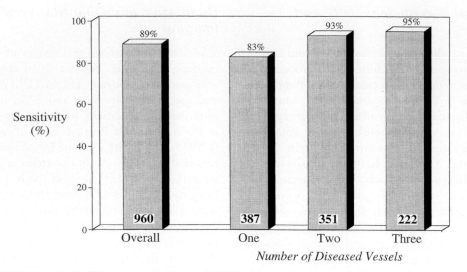

**FIGURE 9.6.** Pooled literature sensitivity of SPECTs stress-redistribution [201]Tl myocardial perfusion imaging in relation to the number of diseased vessel.

method increased from 83% for single vessel disease to 93% for double-vessel disease and 95% for triple-vessel disease (Fig. 9.6). Sensitivity of SPECT [201]Tl imaging in patients without prior myocardial infarction has also been reported in relation to the extent of disease (123). In a population of 135 patients, sensitivities for single-, double-, and triple-vessel coronary disease were 75%, 89%, and 96%, respectively. Sensitivity of SPECT imaging in relation to the degree of underlying coronary narrowing has also been evaluated. In a total of 704 patients reported in the literature (123), the sensitivity of [201]Tl SPECT for detecting moderate coronary stenosis (50% to 70% narrowing) was 63%, and for those with severe coronary narrowing (75% to 100%) it was 88%. Fintel and colleagues (121) compared the visual diagnostic performance of planar and tomographic imaging methods in 136 patients. In a subgroup analysis, they found that [201]Tl tomography was superior in males and in patients with milder disease, such as those with no prior myocardial infarction or with single-vessel disease, or in patients with 50% to 69% coronary stenosis.

### Pharmacologic Versus Exercise Stress Testing

The mean sensitivity and specificity for dipyridamole [201]Tl scintigraphy in 18 published reports covering a total of 1,272 patients (113,123–139) were 87% and 81%, respectively. These results are similar to those noted with exercise [201]Tl scintigraphy. This observation has been confirmed by analysis of the results of five reports (113,126–129) in which exercise and dipyridamole [201]Tl scintigraphy were compared in a single population totaling 207 patients. The sensitivities of dipyridamole and exercise [201]Tl testing were 79% and the specificities were 95% and 92%, respectively (Fig. 9.7).

### Detection of Coronary Artery Disease in Asymptomatic Patients

A large percentage of patients with coronary events (sudden death or myocardial infarction) are totally asymptomatic. It is proposed that in such patients CAD is silent and may be detected by use of noninvasive testing. The appropriateness of noninvasive testing in asymptomatic patients, however, should be viewed in light of Bayes' theorem, which expresses the posttest likelihood of disease as a function of sensitivity and specificity of the test and the prevalence of disease in the population that is being tested. Stated differently, when the sensitivity and specificity of a test and the prevalence of disease in the population under study are known, one can calculate the likelihood of coronary disease being present on the basis of a normal or an abnormal test result. After an extensive literature search, Diamond and Forrester (140) have reported

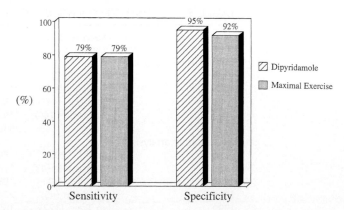

**FIGURE 9.7.** Pooled literature sensitivities and specificities of stress-redistribution [201]Tl myocardial perfusion imaging, comparing dipyridamole pharmacologic stress with maximal exercise.

the prevalence of CAD, based on age, sex, and symptom classification. Literature reports of 28,948 patients were reviewed. For the prevalence of disease in symptomatic patients the angiographic literature of 4,952 patients was surveyed. With respect to symptoms, patients were classified into asymptomatic, nonanginal chest pain, atypical angina, and typical angina categories, using three major characteristics of chest pain (i.e., substernal location, provocation by exercise, and relief gained from rest or nitroglycerin within 10 minutes). For classification into the typical angina category, the patient is required to manifest all three characteristics. When any two of three characteristics of chest pain are present, the pain is classified as atypical angina. When one or none of the characteristics is present chest pain is classified as nonanginal chest pain. Based on their results, the likelihood of CAD, prior to exercise ECG and nuclear imaging testing, may be determined based on the patient's age, sex, and symptoms. These results demonstrate that the prevalence of CAD in the asymptomatic population ranges from 0% to 20% and therefore is low.

The predictive accuracy of exercise [201]Tl myocardial perfusion imaging in a hypothetical population of 1,000 asymptomatic patients (with approximately 10% prevalence of CAD) may be calculated, based on known sensitivity and specificity for exercise planar [201]Tl imaging (80% and 90%, respectively). Of the 100 patients with CAD, 80% (80 patients) would have true-positive tests. Of the 900 patients without CAD, 10% (90 patients) would have false-positive tests. Therefore, of a total of 170 positive tests in this population, only 80 showed results that were correctly positive, resulting in a positive predictive accuracy of only 47%. The posttest likelihood of CAD in asymptomatic patients with negative exercise [201]Tl testing, however, is very low (2% in the above example). This suggests that a positive exercise [201]Tl test in asymptomatic patients does not establish the presence of CAD, while a negative test effectively rules out the presence of CAD. These observations are also applicable to positive and negative exercise treadmill test results (sensitivity and specificity of approximately 70%) in asymptomatic patients. In these patients, the posttest likelihood of CAD after a positive exercise treadmill test is 20%, and the posttest likelihood of CAD after a negative treadmill test is 4.5%. It is of note, however, that when [201]Tl testing is applied to asymptomatic patients with positive exercise treadmill test results (20% likelihood of CAD), a positive [201]Tl test increases the CAD likelihood to 67%, and a negative [201]Tl test decreases the likelihood to less than 5%. Using the bayesian analysis concept, therefore, it becomes apparent that only the subgroup of asymptomatic patients who have a low intermediate likelihood of CAD will benefit from exercise [201]Tl testing, that is, asymptomatic patients with a positive treadmill exercise test or asymptomatic patients with multiple risk factors increasing their likelihood of disease to a low intermediate range.

Several studies support this theoretical conclusion. Uhl and co-workers (141) demonstrated that of 130 asymptomatic United States Air Force pilots who were referred for cardiac catheterization because of a positive stress ECG or coronary risk factors, 22 (17%) had CAD. Of note, the [201]Tl study was abnormal in all 22 who had CAD. In another study, Uhl and co-workers (90) performed exercise [201]Tl imaging in 191 U.S. Air Force crew members who had an abnormal ST-segment response to exercise and underwent both exercise [201]Tl imaging and coronary angiography. Of 135 patients with normal coronary arteries, 131 (97%) had normal [201]Tl studies. Of the 41 patients with CAD, 39 had abnormal exercise [201]Tl studies. Of the remaining 15 with insignificant coronary lesions, ten had abnormal, and five had normal exercise [201]Tl studies. In this population, the positive predictive accuracy of an abnormal ST-segment response to exercise was 21%, and exercise [201]Tl study increased the positive predictive accuracy to 91%. If both an abnormal ST-segment response and an abnormal [201]Tl study had been required before angiography was performed, 136 patients who were found to be free from significant CAD would not have undergone the risk of cardiac catheterization. On the other hand, five patients with insignificant disease and two patients with coronary narrowing of 50% or more would have gone undetected.

## Detection of Coronary Artery Disease in Symptomatic Patients

Bayes' theorem also helps define the appropriateness of stress [201]Tl testing for detection of CAD in symptomatic patients (79,140,142,143). Figure 9.8 demonstrates the posttest like-

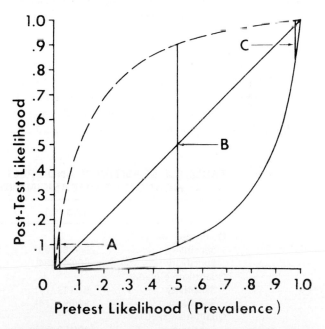

**FIGURE 9.8.** Effect of positive and negative stress-redistribution [201]Tl myocardial perfusion test results on posttest likelihood of coronary artery disease. Results are highlighted for three patients with different pretest likelihoods of coronary artery disease: A, a patient with a low pretest likelihood of coronary artery disease; B, a patient with an intermediate pretest likelihood of coronary artery disease; and C, a patient with a high pretest likelihood of coronary artery disease.

lihood of CAD according to negative and positive $^{201}$Tl test results in patients with differing pretest likelihood of CAD. A sensitivity of 85% and a specificity of 85% have been chosen for $^{201}$Tl imaging. The center line, the line of identity, represents a test with sensitivity and specificity of 50%. At all points along the center line, the posttest likelihood is equal to the pretest likelihood; therefore, a test with these characteristics would have no diagnostic value. The degree to which the upper and lower curves representing abnormal and normal test results deviate from the line of identity can be viewed as a measure of the diagnostic value of the test; the greater the difference between the curves, the more valuable the test. It is evident that at the extremes of pretest likelihood or prevalence, the abnormal and normal test results have very little effect on posttest likelihood of CAD. However, in a patient with an intermediate likelihood of CAD (50%), a positive $^{201}$Tl test increases the likelihood to more than 85%, and a negative test decreases the likelihood to less than 15%.

The application of the bayesian analysis approach to proper utilization of nuclear cardiology procedures has also been demonstrated by several investigators. In a study of 135 women without prior myocardial infarction, Melin and co-workers (92) found that the use of $^{201}$Tl scintigraphy in patients with an intermediate (10% to 90%) probability of CAD resulted in a marked increase in the proportion of patients with a high (>90%) or low (<10%) probability of CAD. They noted that this shift was appropriate, based on the angiographic findings, and they demonstrated that $^{201}$Tl scintigraphy could be used to reduce unnecessary diagnostic catheterization without loss of diagnostic accuracy. In a separate study, Melin and co-workers (103) evaluated another 62 patients with a low intermediate (average of 18%) pretest probability of disease. All six patients who had concordantly positive ECG and $^{201}$Tl test had angiographically significant CAD. However, when the $^{201}$Tl study failed to confirm the electrocardiographic results, the probability of CAD was low, with only 1 of 14 such patients angiographically documented

as having CAD. Christopher and associates (144) also demonstrated the diagnostic usefulness of exercise radionuclide ventriculography, using a bayesian approach. Among 250 patients undergoing exercise radionuclide ventriculography, posttest disease probability moved correctly downward in 85% of the 43 normal patients and upward in 72% of the 207 CAD patients. Failure to increase posttest probability in 28% of the CAD patients occurred most frequently in the groups of patients with anatomically mild CAD. None of the patients with left main CAD, and only 18% of the patients with triple-vessel disease, had a posttest probability less than their pretest probability. Currie and colleagues (145) confirmed the diagnostic usefulness of exercise radionuclide ventriculography in patients with an intermediate probability of CAD. Examples of symptomatic patients with an intermediate pretest likelihood of CAD are those with (a) nonanginal chest pain and a positive or nondiagnostic exercise ECC; (b) atypical angina (unless ECG is markedly abnormal or is normal in a very young patient); and (c) typical angina and a negative exercise ECG (especially in young females).

## Detection of Disease in Individual Coronary Arteries

The coronary arteries and their branches supply different regions of the left ventricular myocardium. Based on the known anatomic relationship between coronary arteries and various myocardial regions and the study of patients with single-vessel and multivessel CAD and with $^{201}$Tl myocardial perfusion studies, general guidelines have been developed for assignment of various myocardial regions to specific coronary arteries. Therefore, it is possible to infer disease of a given coronary artery by noting the location of perfusion defects on planar or tomographic myocardial images. Table 9.2 summarizes the sensitivity and specificity of the visually analyzed defects on planar $^{201}$Tl imaging studies for identification of disease in the LAD, LCX, and RCA. As noted, the mean lit-

**TABLE 9.2 SENSITIVITY AND SPECIFICITY OF $^{201}$TI IMAGING FOR IDENTIFICATION OF DISEASE IN INDIVIDUAL CORONARY ARTERIES**

|  | LAD (%) | LCX (%) | RCA (%) | All vessels (%) |
|---|---|---|---|---|
| Qualitative planar |  |  |  |  |
|   Sensitivity | 264/381 (69) | 98/267 (37) | 190/293 (65) | 552/941 (59) |
|   Specificity | 60/64 (94) | 23/97 (95) | 82/98 (85) | 234/258 (91) |
| Quantitative planar |  |  |  |  |
|   Sensitivity | 87/113 (77) | 42/84 (50) | 83/92 (91) | 212/288 (74) |
|   Specificity | 51/69 (74) | 83/98 (85) | 54/91 (59) | 188/258 (73) |
| Qualitative SPECT |  |  |  |  |
|   Sensitivity | 119/159 (75) | 59/110 (54) | 135/153 (88) | 313/422 (74) |
|   Specificity | 132/155 (85) | 198/204 (97) | 135/161 (84) | 465/520 (89) |
| Quantitative SPECT |  |  |  |  |
|   Sensitivity | 384/482 (80) | 251/347 (72) | 415/499 (83) | 1,050/1,328 (79) |
|   Specificity | 352/424 (83) | 499/593 (84) | 381/151 (84) | 1,232/1,468 (84) |

LAD, left anterior descending; LCX, left circumflex; RCA, right coronary artery; SPECT, single photon emission computed tomography.

erature sensitivities were 69%, 37%, and 65%, respectively, and the mean literature specificities were 94%, 95%, and 85%, respectively (65,66,69,89,146,147). The mean sensitivity and specificity for detection of disease in any coronary artery are 59% and 91%, respectively. It is of note that the sensitivity for detection of individual coronary stenosis is lower than the sensitivity of $^{201}$Tl for detection of individual disease in patients with single-vessel disease and the sensitivity of overall detection of CAD. This relatively lower sensitivity of $^{201}$Tl for detection of disease in individual coronary arteries may be explained by one or more of the following factors. First, in patients with multivessel disease who have multiple adjacent areas of hypoperfusion, only the more hypoperfused regions may appear abnormal because of the relative nature of myocardial $^{201}$Tl perfusion defect analysis. Second, it is possible that in patients with multivessel disease, exercise may be terminated because of development of limiting ischemia in one region before another region becomes ischemic. Third, the assignment of myocardial regions to coronary arteries is not perfect because of significant interindividual variability. Fourth, it is possible that coronary narrowings of 50% that are considered significant by angiography are not hemodynamically significant. Thus, myocardial regions subtended by these vessels do not become ischemic during exercise. Fifth, the role of collateral circulation in preventing ischemia in the distribution of a significant coronary region is variable and unpredictable. Sixth, the overlap of various myocardial regions that is inherent in the planar imaging technique may obscure small defects in a given coronary territory and thus lower the regional sensitivity. This factor may be particularly responsible for the lower sensitivity of $^{201}$Tl testing for the detection of the circumflex CAD. The territory of the LCX coronary artery is observed in only one view represented by the posterolateral wall in the 45-degree LAO view with significant overlap of proximal and distal portions.

Quantitative analysis of planar $^{201}$Tl images has improved identification of disease in individual coronary arteries. As shown in Table 9.2, the mean literature sensitivities and specificities are, respectively, 77% and 74% for the LAD, 50% and 85% for the LCX, and 91% and 59% for the RCA (13,118). Overall, the sensitivity and specificity of the quantitatively analyzed planar images for identification of disease in any coronary artery are 74% and 73%, respectively. This improved sensitivity has been attributed to two factors. First, the slow regional washout rate of $^{201}$Tl is used as an additional index of myocardial hypoperfusion. This index is spatially nonrelative and may demonstrate the presence of hypoperfusion in a relatively less hypoperfused myocardial region in patients with multivessel coronary disease and multiple adjacent regions of ischemia. Second, the use of background subtraction that is inherent in all quantitative methods may enhance $^{201}$Tl perfusion defects that would otherwise be considered negative or equivocal by visual analysis of unsubtracted images.

There have been reports of further improvement of sensitivity for the detection of disease in individual coronary arteries with the use of the SPECT technique. The mean literature sensitivities and specificities of the visually analyzed SPECT images (Table 9.2) are, respectively, 74% and 86% for the LAD, 57% and 94% for the LCX, 88% and 83% for the RCA, with values of 75% and 88% for any coronary artery (43,120). The mean literature sensitivities and specificities of the quantitatively analyzed SPECT $^{201}$Tl images (Table 9.2) are, respectively, 80% and 83% for the LAD, 72% and 85% for the LCX, 83% and 85% for the RCA, and 79% and 84% for any coronary artery (42–44,120,122). By tomographic imaging, improved sensitivity is noted, particularly for detection of disease in the LCX coronary artery, as shown by pooled literature results and direct comparison of SPECT and planar quantitative imaging methods in the same patient population. This improved sensitivity may be related to improved defect contrast and decreased overlap between myocardial regions that result from SPECT imaging.

## Identification of Diagnostic Patients at Low Risk for Coronary Events

During the last decade, clinical application of myocardial perfusion imaging has evolved from diagnosis to risk stratification of CAD. The prognostic application of myocardial perfusion imaging plays an important role in patient management; the decision between using myocardial revascularization and medical therapy depends on the risk of coronary events with medical therapy versus the risk pertaining to myocardial revascularization procedure. In 1983, Brown and colleagues (96) demonstrated that among 61 patients with suspected CAD who had a negative exercise myocardial perfusion study, none died during an average of 46 months of follow-up, and three developed myocardial infarction during this period (0.85% event rate per year). These initial results were subsequently confirmed by several studies. In 13 publications, 2,825 patients without myocardial infarction and with a normal $^{201}$Tl exercise myocardial perfusion planar study have been reported (148). In these studies, the follow-up period has ranged from 12 to 56 months, with an average of 33.3 months. The weighted average incidence of cardiac death per year is 0.24%, ranging from 0% to 0.7%. Furthermore, the average incidence of developing myocardial infarction is 0.53% per year, ranging from 0% to 1.4%. These results suggest that a normal exercise myocardial perfusion study in patients without prior myocardial infarction is associated with a very low likelihood of coronary events during the subsequent year. The observed coronary event rates in this population are very similar to those of patients with normal coronary arteries, which suggests that further cardiac catheterization or intervention is not justified in these patients. An association between a normal stress myocardial perfusion study and a low coronary event rate has also been reported, in rather small groups of patients, using [201]Tl SPECT, technetium 99m-sestamibi SPECT, atrial pacing planar [201]Tl stress testing, and dipyridamole stress planar [201]Tl imaging. An implication of excellent prognosis in patients with normal stress myocardial perfusion study is that the subgroup with coronary disease and normal perfusion studies also had good prognosis. The question as to whether normal [201]Tl studies would have the same benign predictive value for patients with angiographically significant CAD has been addressed in a study by Brown and Rowen (149). These investigators demonstrated that of 75 patients with significant CAD who had normal exercise planar [201]Tl myocardial perfusion studies, one patient developed nonfatal myocardial infarction 28 months after the [201]Tl study, yielding an annual event rate of 7% per year. In comparison, two of the 101 patients with normal exercise planar [201]Tl studies who had either normal coronary arteries (14 patients) or a low likelihood of CAD developed hard events (nonfatal myocardial infarction at 28 months and cardiac death at 23 months), yielding an annual event rate of 1% per year. These results imply that a normal exercise [201]Tl myocardial perfusion study, even in the presence of significant CAD, carries a very benign prognosis with a very low rate of hard cardiac events.

## Identification of Extensive and High-Risk Coronary Artery Disease

An important goal of noninvasive methods currently used to assess patients with CAD is the correct identification of those with extensive coronary disease. Information regarding the extent of coronary disease may be derived from stress redistribution [201]Tl studies by assessing (a) the number of diseased vessels, as suggested by the number of coronary territories with perfusion defects or washout abnormalities; (b) diffuse slow washout rate of [201]Tl, as an index of extensive myocardial ischemia; (c) increased pulmonary capillary wedge pressure, as evidenced by increased lung uptake of [201]Tl; and (d) transient postexercise ischemic dilation of the left ventricle.

### Identification of Left Main and Triple-Vessel Disease

Using the previously described schemes for assigning myocardial perfusion abnormalities to individual coronary arteries, it is possible to determine whether abnormalities involve the distribution of all three coronary arteries or of the left main coronary artery (combined territories of LAD and LCX). Several reports, however, have demonstrated that with this approach the sensitivity of conventional visual analysis of planar [201]Tl images for correct identification of extensive coronary disease is low (67,69,147,150,151). This low sensitivity has been attrib-

uted to the limitation of relative perfusion defect analysis in revealing all hypoperfused myocardial regions in patients with multivessel coronary disease. It has been observed that use of the combined criteria of exercise defect and abnormal regional washout of [201]Tl on planar images improved the sensitivity of visual [201]Tl analysis for correct identification of patients with left main and triple-vessel coronary disease (from 16% to 63%) without significant loss of specificity (150). Sixty-four percent of the patients, who were misclassified by visual analysis as having less extensive disease, were correctly classified as having extensive disease by virtue of quantitative analysis of regional myocardial [201]Tl washout. When the results of quantitative [201]Tl analysis were combined with those of blood pressure and electrocardiographic response to exercise (150), the sensitivity and specificity for identification of patients with left main and triple main coronary disease were 86% and 76%, respectively, and the highest overall accuracy (82%) was obtained. When CAD is extensive and is of relatively uniform severity, regional myocardial hypoperfusion may be balanced during stress, precluding the development of spatially relative perfusion defects. The assessment of myocardial [201]Tl washout rate on planar [201]Tl images may provide diagnostic assistance in these cases (152).

Bateman and colleagues (153) demonstrated that with imaging studies, 13 patients (1%) had the pattern of diffuse slow [201]Tl washout rate in the absence of a regional perfusion defect. Diffuse slow washout was defined as the presence of washout abnormalities in the distribution of all three major coronary arteries but not uniformly in all. Of these 13 patients, nine (69%) were found to have left main or triple-vessel coronary disease. In practice, it is important to keep in mind that the incidence of the diffuse [201]Tl slow washout pattern, indicating extensive disease, is low (approximately 1%). It should be noted that several factors, such as a low exercise heart rate, subcutaneous infiltration of the dose, arm vein uptake, low-count rate studies, inappropriate data acquisition, and imaging protocol deviations, may cause diffuse [201]Tl slow washout in the absence of coronary disease. With the SPECT imaging technique, sensitivity and specificity for correct identification of extensive disease, even without the use of regional washout rate of [201]Tl, is higher than the planar imaging method. The pooled literature results demonstrated that 69% of patients (291 of 423) with three-vessel CAD were correctly identified as such by the SPECT imaging method (43–45,120).

### Size of Infarcted and Jeopardized Myocardium

The extent of myocardial ischemia may not always be inferred by the number of diseased coronary arteries because the size of myocardial ischemia is influenced by the size of the supplying coronary artery; the location, severity, and number of coronary narrowings; and the status of collateral blood flow. On stress myocardial perfusion studies, the magnitude of myocardial hypoperfusion may be expressed by the number of myocardial segments with a defect, the actual percentage of total left ventricular myocardium with perfusion defects, and the severity of hypoperfusion (reflecting the severity of underlying CAD). These defects can be further categorized to reflect infarcted myocardium (if they are nonreversible) or viable but jeopardized myocardium (if they are reversible). Several investigators have evaluated the relationship between the size of myocardial hypoperfusion and subsequent coronary events. Brown and co-workers (96) showed by stepwise logistic regression analysis that in 100 patients without prior myocardial infarction, potential predictors of cardiac death or myocardial infarction were the number of transient $^{201}$Tl defects, the total number of $^{201}$Tl defects, and the number of diseased vessels by angiography. Importantly, after the number of transient $^{201}$Tl defects (which had the highest significant chi-square value) was included in the logistic regression model, no other predictor was found to be significant. In the study of Ladenheim and associates (154) involving 1,689 patients without prior myocardial infarction, stepwise logistic regression identified only three independent predictors of annual coronary events: the number of myocardial regions with reversible hypoperfusion, the magnitude of hypoperfusion, and achieved heart rate.

## Increased Pulmonary Uptake of Thallium-201

An increase in pulmonary $^{201}$Tl activity may be noted on anterior view images in patients with CAD. Both experimental studies and clinical evidence suggest that this increased pulmonary $^{201}$Tl activity is related to the development of left ventricular dysfunction with exercise (85,155,156). To objectify assessment of pulmonary uptake of $^{201}$Tl, two methods have been developed. In the method developed by Kushner and colleagues (157), the degree of pulmonary $^{201}$Tl activity is expressed as the quantitative fraction of the myocardial value. Another approach described by Levy and colleagues (158) quantifies the percentage of pulmonary $^{201}$Tl washout from immediate postexercise to 4-hour redistribution anterior view images. With both techniques, abnormal values have been observed in patients with extensive coronary disease. In the study of Levy and colleagues (158), abnormal pulmonary $^{201}$Tl washout was related to both the anatomic extent and the functional severity of disease; it occurred with greater frequency in patients with multivessel coronary disease and in those with exercise-induced left ventricular dysfunction. It should be noted that increased pulmonary uptake of $^{201}$Tl reflects increased pulmonary capillary wedge pressure, which may be caused by factors other than extensive and severe coronary disease, such as mitral valve regurgitation, mitral stenosis, decreased left ventricular compliance, and nonischemic cardiomyopathy with left ventricular dysfunc-

tion. Therefore, it is important to exercise caution in interpreting increased pulmonary uptake of $^{201}$Tl as an index of extensive coronary disease when it occurs in isolation (without myocardial perfusion defects) or in patients with one or more of the aforementioned conditions.

## Transient Ischemic Dilation of the Left Ventricle

The authors' group (159) and others (160) have noted that some patients with CAD have a pattern of transient dilation of the left ventricle on the immediate poststress images, as compared with the 4-hour redistribution images. Because this dilation must be present for at least 10 to 15 minutes after exercise to be visualized on the postexercise anterior image, this pattern most likely represents severe and extensive CAD, causing transient ischemic dilation of the left ventricle after exercise. Transient dilation of the left ventricle was shown to have a sensitivity of 60% and a specificity of 95% for identifying patients with multivessel critical stenoses, and this phenomenon was more specific than other known markers of severe and extensive coronary disease, such as the presence of multiple perfusion defects or washout abnormalities or both (159). In routine practice, this phenomenon can be estimated by visual inspection of the immediate postinjection and 4-hour anterior views. This phenomenon may also be noted on SPECT images. When transient dilation is observed, it should be interpreted as strong evidence of severe and extensive myocardial ischemia. The significance of transient dilation of the left ventricle after pharmacologic stress testing is similar to that of exercise testing (161).

## Incremental Prognostic Power of Thallium-201 Imaging

The incremental prognostic power of $^{201}$Tl imaging, in comparison with other parameters, such as clinical variables, exercise treadmill results, and coronary angiography, has been extensively evaluated. Four of the reported studies have addressed the incremental value of exercise $^{201}$Tl imaging over and above clinical, exercise ECG, and angiographic variables. As previously mentioned, in the study of Brown and co-workers (96), multivariate regression analysis showed that the number of transient $^{201}$Tl defects was a better predictor of future cardiac events than clinical, ECG, and angiographic data. Kaul and associates (162) evaluated two large patient populations at two different institutions. In 293 patients who were studied at Massachusetts General Hospital, Cox regression analysis showed that the quantitatively assessed lung-to-heart ratio of $^{201}$Tl activity was the most important predictor of a future cardiac event. Other significant predictors were the number of diseased vessels, patient gender, and change in heart rate from rest to exercise. Although the number of diseased vessels was an important independent predictor of cardiac events, it did not add significantly to the overall ability of the exercise $^{201}$Tl test to predict events. Furthermore, information obtained from $^{201}$Tl imaging alone was marginally superior to that obtained from cardiac catheterization alone and significantly superior to that obtained from exercise testing alone in determining the occurrence of events. In addition, unlike the exercise $^{201}$Tl test, which could predict the occurrence of all categories of events, catheterization data were not able to predict the occurrence of all categories of events or the occurrence of nonfatal myocardial infarction. These data suggested that exercise $^{201}$Tl imaging is superior to data from both exercise testing alone and cardiac catheterization data alone for predicting future events in patients with chronic CAD who have undergone both exercise $^{201}$Tl imaging and catheterization for the evaluation of chest pain.

In a subsequent study, Kaul and colleagues (163) evaluated the prognostic utility of $^{201}$Tl stress testing, compared to that of other parameters, in 382 patients from the University of Virginia who were followed up for a mean of 4.6 years. When all clinical, exercise, $^{201}$Tl, and catheterization variables were analyzed by Cox regression analysis, the number of diseased vessels was the single most important predictor of future events, followed by the number of segments demonstrating redistribution on delayed $^{201}$Tl images, except in the case of nonfatal myocardial infarction, for which redistribution was the most important predictor of future events. When CAD was defined as demonstrating 70% or greater luminal diameter narrowing, the number of diseased vessels significantly lost its power to predict events. In this study, when exercise $^{201}$Tl stress test results were considered as a whole (in conjunction with a change in heart rate from rest to exercise, ST-segment depression on the ECG, and ventricular premature beats on exercise), they were as powerful as cardiac catheterization data. Of note, the combination of both catheterization and exercise $^{201}$Tl data was superior to either alone in determining future events. In a more recent study by Pollack and associates (164) from the same group of investigators, the incremental prognostic value of data obtained in succession (clinical, exercise stress test, $^{201}$Tl imaging, and coronary angiography) in patients with suspected CAD was evaluated. $^{201}$Tl imaging provided significant additional prognostic information compared with that provided by clinical and exercise stress test data. In a subgroup of patients in whom lung-to-heart $^{201}$Tl ratio had been analyzed, coronary angiography did not provide additional prognostic information. In this subgroup of patients, the combination of clinical and exercise $^{201}$Tl variables provided greater prognostic information than the combination of clinical and angiographic data. In the remaining subgroup of patients in whom the lung-to-heart ratio had not been analyzed, coronary angiography provided incremental prognostic information compared with clinical and exercise $^{201}$Tl data alone.

## Risk Stratification After Myocardial Infarction

In survivors of myocardial infarction, many high-risk clinical and laboratory variables have been identified. These variables include recurrent angina, left ventricular failure, shock, conduction abnormalities, malignant arrhythmia, and decreased left ventricular ejection fraction. In a subset of patients with uncomplicated myocardial infarction (asymptomatic and without evidence of severe left ventricular dysfunction), 1-year mortality ranges from 2% to 7.5% (165). The aim of noninvasive testing prior to discharge of uncomplicated myocardial infarction patients, therefore, is the identification of those who are at relatively lower or higher risk for subsequent death or recurrent infarction on the basis of residual ischemic myocardium, either adjacent to or remote from the infarction. In 1983, Gibson and associates (166) compared the predictive value of predischarge of maximal exercise $^{201}$Tl imaging with clinical, exercise treadmill, and coronary angiographic data. They demonstrated that the presence of reversible $^{201}$Tl defects involving multiple vascular territories and increased lung uptake of $^{201}$Tl were significant prognostic indicators in these patients. The combination of these $^{201}$Tl variables had significantly greater sensitivity for predicting future cardiac events than that with exercise treadmill and coronary angiographic data.

With wide application of thrombolytic therapy in the acute phase of myocardial infarction, the role of myocardial perfusion imaging for risk stratification of patients after myocardial infarction has changed (167). In patients treated with thrombolytic therapy, $^{201}$Tl redistribution is still more prevalent than ST-segment depression (48% versus 14%), but the prevalence of inducible ischemia is less than that observed in the prethrombolytic era (59% for $^{201}$Tl redistribution and 32% for ST-segment depression) (167). Therefore, although fewer ischemic responses are observed in patients who undergo reperfusion therapy, detection of ischemia is better achieved with exercise perfusion imaging than with exercise ECG alone. Another important prognostic variable in patients surviving uncomplicated acute myocardial infarction is presence of multivessel CAD. Haber and colleagues (168) demonstrated that the sensitivity of ST-segment depression, remote $^{201}$Tl redistribution, and either of the two findings were 29%, 35%, and 58%, respectively. The respective specificities were 96%, 87%, and 78% for detection of multivessel CAD in patients with thrombolytic therapy for acute myocardial infarction. Table 9.3 summarizes the results of four studies that have assessed the usefulness of exercise $^{201}$Tl myocardial perfusion imaging for risk stratification after myocardial infarction (166,169–171). In a total of 537 patients reported with exercise myocardial perfusion studies, the positive and negative predictive accuracies of myocardial perfusion imaging for prediction of future cardiac events have been 40% and 93%, respectively.

**TABLE 9.3 SUMMARY OF STUDIES THAT HAVE EMPLOYED PHARMACOLOGIC CORONARY VASODILATION FOR RISK ASSESSMENT AFTER MYOCARDIAL INFARCTION**

| Studypatients | No. of (Mos.) | Follow-up accuracy (%) | Positive predictive accuracy (%) | Negative predictive |
|---|---|---|---|---|
| Exercise | | | | |
| Wilson (171) | 97 | 39 | 42 | 77 |
| Brown (170) | 59 | 37 | 28 | 100 |
| Gibson (166) | 140 | 15 | 59 | 94 |
| Gibson (169) | 241 | 27 | 31 | 97 |
| Overall | 537 | | | |
| Dipyridamole | | | | |
| Gimple (174) | 36 | 6 | 26(42) | 88 |
| Younis (173) | 68 | 12 | 22 | 94 |
| Leppo (172) | 51 | 19 | 33 | 94 |
| Brown (175) | 50 | 12 | 45 | 100 |
| Overall | 205 | | | |
| Adenosine | | | | |
| Mahmarian (176) | 92 | 15 | 50 | 97 |

The availability of pharmacologic coronary vasodilation with dipyridamole and adenosine has provided a unique opportunity for early post–myocardial infarction risk stratification, using myocardial perfusion imaging. With pharmacologic vasodilation, maximal hyperemia may be achieved without the undesired effects of maximal exercise testing, such as increase of myocardial oxygen consumption, due to significant increase in heart rhythm blood pressure, and increase in intraventricular pressure and possible adverse effects on ventricular remodeling due to increase in systolic and mean blood pressure during exercise. Table 9.3 also summarizes studies that have employed pharmacologic coronary vasodilation for risk assessment after myocardial infarction (172–176). A total of four studies are available that have used dipyridamole pharmacologic coronary vasodilation and [201]Tl imaging early after uncomplicated myocardial infarction in a total of 205 patients. The positive and negative predictive accuracies have been 30% and 94%, respectively (172–175). Of note, in a study by Mahmarian and co-workers (176), adenosine coronary vasodilation and [201]Tl imaging were used to predict cardiac death, myocardial infarction, unstable angina, and congestive heart failure in a total of 92 patients during 1.5 months of follow-up after uncomplicated myocardial infarction. The presence of reversible defect involving 5% of the left ventricle was 50% sensitive and 97% specific for predicting subsequent coronary events.

## Risk Stratification of Patients Undergoing Noncardiac Surgery

Coronary artery disease is common among patients with peripheral vascular disease. Hertzer and co-workers (177) have shown that among 1,000 consecutive patients with peripheral vascular disease who underwent coronary angiography, and had no clinical suspicion for CAD prior to angiography, 37% had one or more 70% coronary stenosis and 15% had CAD significant enough to warrant percutaneous transluminal coronary angioplasty or coronary artery bypass surgery. Mangano and associates (178) have demonstrated that approximately 50% of all deaths associated with elective noncardiac surgery in the United States are related to cardiac deaths. [201]Tl myocardial perfusion imaging has been extensively investigated for its application to the identification of patients who are at high risk for developing cardiac complications during noncardiac surgery.

In 1985, Boucher and colleagues (179) applied pharmacologic stress testing in conjunction with [201]Tl myocardial perfusion planar scintigraphy to assess the perioperative risk of coronary events in 48 patients with peripheral vascular disease. They demonstrated that in 16 patients with reversible defects, three developed hard events (myocardial infarction or death), and five developed unstable angina perioperatively, while among 32 patients with normal or fixed defects, none had perioperative events. Subsequently, several investigators used the technique of dipyridamole stress [201]Tl planar imaging for risk stratification of patients prior to elective noncardiac surgery (172,180–189). In a total of 2,020 reported patients (148), 21% (194 of 905) of patients who had reversible defects developed perioperative cardiac events, in contrast to 2% (20 of 1,115) of those who had normal studies or had fixed defects. These results suggest that lack of reversible defects of dipyridamole stress-redistribution of [201]Tl planar imaging defectively identifies a group of patients who are at very low risk for developing cardiac events during elective noncardiac surgery. However, the positive predictive accuracy is only 20%; that is, only one of five patients with reversible defects develop events. This low figure suggests that other factors influence the development of perioperative cardiac events in these patients.

## ACKNOWLEDGMENTS

We are grateful to Pooneh Hendi, Sepehr Rokhsar, and Eric Stevenson for their assistance in the review of the literature and to Diane Martin for preparation of the figures.

## REFERENCES

1. Leibowitz E, Greene M, Bradley-Moore P, et al. Tl-201 for medical use. *J Nucl Med* 1973;14:421.
2. Mullins L, Moore R. The movement of thallium ions in muscle. *J Gen Physiol* 1960;43:759.
3. Gehring PJ, Hammond PB. The interrelationship between thallium and potassium in animals. *J Pharmacol Exp Ther* 1967; 155(1):187–201.
4. Zimmer L, McCall D, D'Abbado L. Kinetics and characteristics of thallium exchange in cultured cells. *Circulation* 1979;59:138.
5. Weich HF, Strauss HW, Pitt B. The extraction of thallium-201 by the myocardium. *Circulation* 1977;56(2):188–191.
6. Pohost GM, Zir LM, Moore RH, et al. Differentiation of transiently ischemic from infarcted myocardium by serial imaging after a single dose of thallium-201. *Circulation* 1977;55(2): 294–302.
7. Nielsen AP, Morris KG, Murdock R, et al. Linear relationship between the distribution of thallium-201 and blood flow in ischemic and nonischemic myocardium during exercise. *Circulation* 1980;61(4):797–801.
8. Strauss HW, Pitt B. Noninvasive detection of subcritical coronary arterial narrowings with a coronary vasodilator and myocardial perfusion imaging. *Am J Cardiol* 1977;39(3):403–406.
9. Gould KL, Schelbert HR, Phelps ME, et al. Noninvasive assessment of coronary stenoses with myocardial perfusion imaging during pharmacologic coronary vasodilatation. V. Detection of 47 percent diameter coronary stenosis with intravenous nitrogen-13 ammonia and emission-computed tomography in intact dogs. *Am J Cardiol* 1979;43(2):200–208.
10. Berger B, Watson D, Sipes J, et al. Redistribution of thallium at rest in patients with coronary artery disease. *J Nucl Med* 1978; 19:680.
11. Pohost G, O'Keefe D, Gerwirtz H, et al. Thallium redistribution in the presence of severe fixed coronary stenosis. *J Nucl Med* 1978;19:680.
12. Beller G, Pohost G. Mechanism for Tl-201 redistribution after transient myocardial ischemia. *Circulation* 1977;56:1–14.
13. Maddahi J, Garcia EV, Berman DS, et al. Improved noninvasive assessment of coronary artery disease by quantitative analysis of regional stress myocardial distribution and washout of thallium-201. *Circulation* 1981;64(5):924–935.
14. Garcia E, Maddahi J, Berman D, et al. Space/time quantitation of thallium-201 myocardial scintigraphy. *J Nucl Med* 1981; 22(4):309–317.
15. Massie BM, Wisneski J, Kramer B, et al. Comparison of myocardial thallium-201 clearance after maximal and submaximal exercise: implications for diagnosis of coronary disease: concise communication. *J Nucl Med* 1982;23(5):381–5.
16. Maddahi J, Don Michael T, Gurewirz J, et al. Significance of slow myocardial washout of Tl-201 at submaximal exercise heart rate. *J Nucl Med* 1986;27(6):381.
17. Kaul S, Chesler DA, Pohost GM, et al. Influence of peak exercise heart rate on normal thallium-201 myocardial clearance. *J Nucl Med* 1986;27(1):26–30.
18. Maddahi J, Van Train K, Don Michael T, et al. Normal initial myocardial distribution and washout of Tl-201 at rest vs. exercise. *Clin Nucl Med* 1985;10:11.
19. Gewirtz H, Maksad AK, Most AS, et al. The effect of transient ischemia with reperfusion on thallium clearance from the myocardium. *Circulation* 1980;61(6):1091–1097.
20. Okada R, Pohost G. Effect of decreased blood flow and ischemia on myocardial thallium clearance. *J Am Coll Cardiol* 1984;3(3):744.
21. Sklar J, Kirch D, Johnson T, et al. Slow late myocardial clearance of thallium: a characteristic phenomenon in coronary artery disease. *Circulation* 1982;65(7):1504–1510.
22. Budinger T, Knittel B. Cardaic thallium redistribution and model. *J Nucl Med* 1987;28:588(abst).
23. Budinger T, Pohost G, Bichoff P. Tl-201 integral blood concentration over 2 hours explains persistent defects in patients with no evidence of MI by ECG. *Circulation* 1987;76:64(abst).
24. Angello DA, Wilson RA, Palac RT. Effect of eating on thallium-201 myocardial redistribution after myocardial ischemia. *Am J Cardiol* 1987;60(7):528–533.
25. Gutman J, Berman DS, Freeman M, et al. Time to completed redistribution of thallium-201 in exercise myocardial scintigraphy: relationship to the degree of coronary artery stenosis. *Am Heart J* 1983;106(5 pt 1):989–995.
26. Kiat H, Berman DS, Maddahi J, et al. Late reversibility of tomographic myocardial thallium-201 defects: an accurate marker of myocardial viability. *J Am Coll Cardiol* 1988;12(6): 1456–1463.
27. Weiss AT, Maddahi J, Lew AS, et al. Reverse redistribution of thallium-201: a sign of nontransmural myocardial infarction with patency of the infarct-related coronary artery. *J Am Coll Cardiol* 1986;7(1):61–67.
28. Segall GM, Davis MJ. Prone versus supine thallium myocardial SPECT: a method to decrease artifactual inferior wall defects(see comments). *J Nucl Med* 1989;30(4):548–555.
29. Kiat H, Van Train KF, Friedman JD, et al. Quantitative stress-redistribution thallium-201 SPECT using prone imaging: methodologic development and validation. *J Nucl Med* 1992; 33(8):1509–1515.
30. Friedman J, Van Train K, Maddahi J, et al. "Upward creep" of the heart: a frequent source of false-positive reversible defects during thallium-201 stress-redistribution SPECT. *J Nucl Med* 1989;30(10):1718–1722.
31. Maddahi J. Optimizing assessment of myocardial viability with thallium-201. *J Nucl Med* 1994.
32. Maddahi J, Schelbert H, Brunken R, et al. Role of thallium-201 and PET imaging in evaluation of myocardial viability and management of patients with coronary artery disease and left ventricular dysfunction. *J Nucl Med* 1994;35(4):707–715.
33. Watson DD, Campbell NP, Read EK, et al. Spatial and temporal quantitation of plane thallium myocardial images. *J Nucl Med* 1981;22(7):577–584.
34. Berger BC, Watson DD, Taylor GJ, et al. Quantitative thallium-201 exercise scintigraphy for detection of coronary artery disease. *J Nucl Med* 1981;22(7):585–593.
35. Kaul S, Chesler DA, Boucher CA, et al. Quantitative aspects of myocardial perfusion imaging. *Semin Nucl Med* 1987;17(2): 131–144.
36. Wackers F, Bales D, Feterman R, et al. Non-uniform washout of Tl-201( within normal range):criterion for improved detection of of single -vessel coronary artery disease. *J Nucl Med* 1983;24(5):P46(abst).
37. Massie BM, Hollenberg M, Wisneski JA, et al. Scintigraphic quantification of myocardial ischemia: a new approach. *Circulation* 1983;68(4):747–755.
38. Goris ML, Daspit SG, McLaughlin P, et al. Interpolative background subtraction. *J Nucl Med* 1976;17(8):744–747.
39. Watson D, Beller G, Berger B, et al. Notes on the quantitation of sequential Tl-201 images. *Software* 1979;6(4):10.

40. Vogel RA, Kirch DL, LeFree MT, et al. Thallium-201 myocardial perfusion scintigraphy: results of standard and multi-pinhole tomographic techniques. *Am J Cardiol* 1979;43(4):787–793.

41. Garcia EV, Van Train K, Maddahi J, et al. Quantification of rotational thallium-201 myocardial tomography. *J Nucl Med* 1985;26(1):17–26.

42. Maddahi J, Van Train K, Prigent F, et al. Quantitative single photon emission computed thallium-201 tomography for detection and localization of coronary artery disease: optimization and prospective validation of a new technique(see comments). *J Am Coll Cardiol* 1989;14(7):1689–1699.

43. De Pasquale EE, Nody AC, DePuey EG, et al. Quantitative rotational thallium-201 tomography for identifying and localizing coronary artery disease. *Circulation* 1988;77(2):316–327.

44. Mahmarian JJ, Boyce TM, Goldberg RK, et al. Quantitative exercise thallium-201 single photon emission computed tomography for the enhanced diagnosis of ischemic heart disease (see comments). *J Am Coll Cardiol* 1990;15(2):318–329.

45. Iskandrian AS, Heo J, Kong B, et al. Effect of exercise level on the ability of thallium-201 tomographic imaging in detecting coronary artery disease: analysis of 461 patients (see comments). *J Am Coll Cardiol* 1989;14(6):1477–1486.

46. Mahmarian JJ, Verani MS. Exercise thallium-201 perfusion scintigraphy in the assessment of coronary artery disease. *Am J Cardiol* 1991;67(14):2D–11D.

47. Gould K, Westcott R, Albro P, et al. Noninvasive assessment of coronary stenosis by myocardial imaging during pharmacologic coronary vasodilation. II. Clinical methodology and feasibility. *Am J Cardiol* 1978;41:279.

48. Brown B, Josephson M, Peterson R, et al. Intravenous dipyridamole combined with isometric handgrip for near maximal acute increase on coronary flow in patients with coronary artery disease. *Am J Cardiol* 1981;48:1077.

49. Chan SY, Brunken RC, Czernin J, et al. Comparison of maximal myocardial blood flow during adenosine infusion with that of intravenous dipyridamole in normal men. *J Am Coll Cardiol* 1992;20(4):979–985.

50. Hoffman JI. Determinants and prediction of transmural myocardial perfusion. *Circulation* 1978;58(3):381–391.

51. Becker LC. Conditions for vasodilator-induced coronary steal in experimental myocardial ischemia. *Circulation* 1978;57(6):1103–1110.

52. Forman R, Kirk ES, Downey JM, et al. Nitroglycerin and heterogeneity of myocardial blood flow and ventricular contractile force. *J Clin Invest* 1973;52(4):905–911.

53. Flameng W, Schaper W, Lewi P. Multiple experimental coronary occlusion without infarction. *Am Heart J* 1973;85:767.

54. Flameng W, WΦusten B, Schaper W. On the distribution of myocardial blood flow II. Effects of arterial stenosis and vasodilation. *Basic Res Cardiol* 1974;69(4):435–446.

55. Flameng W, Wusten B, Winkler B, et al. Influence of perfusion pressure and heart rate on local myocardial flow in the collateralized heart with chronic coronary occlusion. *Am Heart J* 1983;89:51.

56. Patterson RE, Kirk ES. Coronary steal mechanisms in dogs with one-vessel occlusion and other arteries normal. *Circulation* 1983;67(5):1009–1015.

57. Hays JT, Mahmarian JJ, Cochran AJ, et al. Dobutamine thallium-201 tomography for evaluating patients with suspected coronary artery disease unable to undergo exercise or pharmacologic stress testing. *J Am Coll Cardiol* 1993;21(7):1583–1590.

58. Krivokapich J, Huang SC, Schelbert HR. Assessment of the effects of dobutamine on myocardial blood flow and oxidative metabolism in normal human subjects using nitrogen-13 ammonia and carbon-11 acetate. *Am J Cardiol* 1993;71(15):1351–1356.

59. Ranhosky A, Kempthorne-Rawson J. The safety of intravenous dipyridamole thallium myocardial perfusion imaging. Intravenous Dipyridamole Thallium Imaging Study Group. *Circulation* 1990;81(4):1205–1209.

60. Lette J, Tatum JL, Fraser S, et al. Safety of dipyridamole testing in 73,806 patients: the Multicenter Dipyridamole Safety Study. *J Nucl Cardiol* 1995;2(1):3–17.

61. Belardinelli L, Linden J, Berne RM. The cardiac effects of adenosine. *Prog Cardiovasc Dis* 1989;32(1):73–97.

62. Rosen J, Stenberg R, Lopez J, et al. Coronary dilation with intravenous dipyridamole and adenosine: a comparative study. *Circulation* 1990;82:III-731(abst).

63. Abreu A, Mahmarian JJ, Nishimura S, et al. Tolerance and safety of pharmacologic coronary vasodilation with adenosine in association with thallium-201 scintigraphy in patients with suspected coronary artery disease. *J Am Coll Cardiol* 1991;18(3):730–735.

64. Cerqueira MD, Verani MS, Schwaiger M, et al. Safety profile of adenosine stress perfusion imaging: results from the Adenoscan Multicenter Trial Registry (see comments). *J Am Coll Cardiol* 1994;23(2):384–389.

65. Lenaers A, Block P, Thiel EV, et al. Segmental analysis of Ti-201 stress myocardial scintigraphy. *J Nucl Med* 1977;18(6):509–516.

66. Massie BM, Botvinick EH, Brundage BH. Correlation of thallium-201 scintigrams with coronary anatomy: factors affecting region by region sensitivity. *Am J Cardiol* 1979;44(4):616–622.

67. Dash H, Massie BM, Botvinick EH, et al. The noninvasive identification of left main and three-vessel coronary artery disease by myocardial stress perfusion scintigraphy and treadmill exercise electrocardiography. *Circulation* 1979;60(2):276–284.

68. McKillop JH, Murray RG, Turner JG, et al. Can the extent of coronary artery disease be predicted from thallium-201 myocardial images? *J Nucl Med* 1979;20(7):714–719.

69. Rigo P, Bailey IK, Griffith LS, et al. Value and limitations of segmental analysis of stress thallium myocardial imaging for localization of coronary artery disease. *Circulation* 1980;61(5):973–981.

70. Ritchie JL, Trobaugh GB, Hamilton GW, et al. Myocardial imaging with thallium-201 at rest and during exercise. Comparison with coronary arteriography and resting and stress electrocardiography. *Circulation* 1977;56(1):66–71.

71. Bailey IK, Griffith LS, Rouleau J, et al. Thallium-201 myocardial perfusion imaging at rest and during exercise. Comparative sensitivity to electrocardiography in coronary artery disease. *Circulation* 1977;55(1):79–87.

72. Rosenblatt A, Lowenstein JM, Kerth W, et al. Post-exercise thallium-201 myocardial scanning: a clinical appraisal. *Am Heart J* 1977;94(4):463–470.

73. Botvinick EH, Taradash MR, Shames DM, et al. Thallium-201 myocardial perfusion scintigraphy for the clinical clarification of normal, abnormal and equivocal electrocardiographic stress tests. *Am J Cardiol* 1978;41(1):43–51.

74. Verani MS, Marcus ML, Razzak MA, et al. Sensitivity and specificity of thallium-201 perfusion scintigrams under exercise in the diagnosis of coronary artery disease. *J Nucl Med* 1978;19(7):773–782.

75. Ritchie JL, Zaret BL, Strauss HW, et al. Myocardial imaging with thallium-201:a multicenter study in patients with angina pectoris or acute myocardial infarction. *Am J Cardiol* 1978;42(3):345–350.

76. Turner DA, Battle WE, Deshmukh H, et al. The predictive value of myocardial perfusion scintigraphy after stress in patients without previous myocardial infarction. *J Nucl Med* 1978;19(3):249–255.

77. Blood DK, McCarthy DM, Sciacca RR, et al. Comparison of

single-dose and double-dose thallium-201 myocardial perfusion scintigraphy for the detection of coronary artery disease and prior myocardial infarction. *Circulation* 1978;58(5):777–788.

78. Carrillo AP, Marks DS, Pickard SD, et al. Correlation of exercise 201thallium myocardial scan with coronary arteriograms and the maximal exercise test. *Chest* 1978;73(3):321–326.

79. Hamilton GW, Trobaugh GB, Ritchie JL, et al. Myocardial imaging with 201thallium: an analysis of clinical usefulness based on Bayes' theorem. *Semin Nucl Med* 1978;8(4):358–364.

80. McCarthy DM, Blood DK, Sciacca RR, et al. Single dose myocardial perfusion imaging with thallium-201: application in patients with nondiagnostic electrocardiographic stress tests. *Am J Cardiol* 1979;43(5):899–906.

81. Caralis DG, Bailey I, Kennedy HL, et al. Thallium-201 myocardial imaging in evaluation of asymptomatic individuals with ischaemic ST segment depression on exercise electrocardiogram. *Br Heart J* 1979;42(5):562–567.

82. Silber S, Fleck E, Klein U, et al. [The value of the thallium-201 scintigram as compared with the exercise electrocardiogram in patients with coronary artery disease but no myocardial infarction (author's translation)]. *Herz* 1979;4(4):359–369.

83. Jengo JA, Freeman R, Brizendine M, et al. Detection of coronary artery disease: comparison of exercise stress radionuclide angiocardiography and thallium stress perfusion scanning. *Am J Cardiol* 1980;45(3):535–541.

84. Caldwell JH, Hamilton GW, Sorensen SG, et al. The detection of coronary artery disease with radionuclide techniques: a comparison of rest-exercise thallium imaging and ejection fraction response. *Circulation* 1980;61(3):610–619.

85. Boucher CA, Zir LM, Beller GA, et al. Increased lung uptake of thallium-201 during exercise myocardial imaging: clinical, hemodynamic and angiographic implications in patients with coronary artery disease. *Am J Cardiol* 1980;46(2):189–196.

86. Iskandrian AS, Mintz GS, Croll MN, et al. Exercise thallium-201 myocardial scintigraphy: advantages and limitations. *Cardiology* 1980;65(3):136–152.

87. Iskandrian AS, Segal BL, Haaz W, et al. Effects of coronary artery narrowing, collaterals, and left ventricular function on the pattern of myocardial perfusion. *Cathet Cardiovasc Diagn* 1980;6(2):159–172.

88. Schicha H, Rentrop P, Facorro L, et al. [Results of quantitative myocardial scintigraphy with thallium-201 at rest and after maximum exercise—critical analysis of predictive value and clinical application (author's translation)]. *Z Kardiol* 1980; 69(1):31–42.

89. Elkayam U, Weinstein M, Berman D, et al. Stress thallium-201 myocardial scintigraphy and exercise technetium ventriculography in the detection and location of chronic coronary artery disease: comparison of sensitivity and specificity of these noninvasive tests alone and in combination. *Am Heart J* 1981; 101(5):657–666.

90. Uhl GS, Kay TN, Hickman JR, Jr. Computer-enhanced thallium scintigrams in asymptomatic men with abnormal exercise tests. *Am J Cardiol* 1981;48(6):1037–1043.

91. Guiney TE, Pohost GM, McKusick KA, et al. Differentiation of false- from true-positive ECG responses to exercise stress by thallium 201 perfusion imaging. *Chest* 1981;80(1):4–10.

92. Melin JA, Piret LJ, Vanbutsele RJ, et al. Diagnostic value of exercise electrocardiography and thallium myocardial scintigraphy in patients without previous myocardial infarction: a Bayesian approach. *Circulation* 1981;63(5):1019–1024.

93. Patterson RE, Horowitz SF, Eng C, et al. Can exercise electrocardiography and thallium-201 myocardial imaging exclude the diagnosis of coronary artery disease? Bayesian analysis of the clinical limits of exclusion and indications for coronary angiography. *Am J Cardiol* 1982;49(5):1127–1135.

94. Faris JV, Burt RW, Graham MC, et al. Thallium-201 myocardial scintigraphy: improved sensitivity, specificity and predictive accuracy by application of a statistical image analysis algorithm. *Am J Cardiol* 1982;49(4):733–742.

95. Kambara H, Kawashita K, Yoshida A, et al. Identification of patients with coronary artery disease using a scoring system of coronary risk factors, electrocardiography and myocardial perfusion imaging. *Jpn Circ J* 1982;46(3):235–244.

96. Brown KA, Boucher CA, Okada RD, et al. Prognostic value of exercise thallium-201 imaging in patients presenting for evaluation of chest pain. *J Am Coll Cardiol* 1983;1(4):994–1001.

97. Cinotti L, Meignan M, Usdin JP, et al. Diagnostic value of image processing in myocardial scintigraphy. *J Nucl Med* 1983; 24(9):768–774.

98. O'Keefe JC, Edwards AC, Wiseman J, et al. Comparison of exercise electrocardiography, thallium-201 myocardial imaging and exercise gated blood pool scan in patients with suspected coronary artery disease. *Aust NZ J Med* 1983;13(1): 45–50.

99. Chairman B, Brevers G, Dupras G, et al. Fluoroscopy when the exercise ECG is strongly positive. *Am Heart J* 1984;108:260.

100. Osbakken MD, Okada RD, Boucher CA, et al. Comparison of exercise perfusion and ventricular function imaging: an analysis of factors affecting the diagnostic accuracy of each technique. *J Am Coll Cardiol* 1984;3(2 pt 1):272–283.

101. Hung J, Chaitman BR, Lam J, et al. Noninvasive diagnostic test choices for the evaluation of coronary artery disease in women: a multivariate comparison of cardiac fluoroscopy, exercise electrocardiography and exercise thallium myocardial perfusion scintigraphy. *J Am Coll Cardiol* 1984;4(1):8–16.

102. Burke JF, Morganroth J, Soffer J, et al. The cardiokymography exercise test compared to the thallium-201 perfusion exercise test in the diagnosis of coronary artery disease. *Am Heart J* 1984;107(4):718–725.

103. Melin JA, Wijns W, Vanbutsele RJ, et al. Alternative diagnostic strategies for coronary artery disease in women: demonstration of the usefulness and efficiency of probability analysis. *Circulation* 1985;71(3):535–542.

104. Canhasi B, Dae M, Botvinick E, et al. Interaction of "supplementary" scintigraphic indicators of ischemia and stress electrocardiography in the diagnosis of multivessel coronary disease. *J Am Coll Cardiol* 1985;6(3):581–588.

105. Del Rio-Meraza A, Vilapando-Gutierrez J, Nava-Lopez G, et al. Correlation between exercise electrocardiographic test, myocardial perfusion test with Tl-201, and contrast coronary arteriography in patients with ischemic heart disease. *Arch Invest Med* 1985;16:175.

106. Hung J, Chaitman BR, Lam J, et al. A logistic regression analysis of multiple noninvasive tests for the prediction of the presence and extent of coronary artery disease in men. *Am Heart J* 1985;110(2):460–469.

107. Rothendler JA, Okada RD, Wilson RA, et al. Effect of a delay in commencing imaging on the ability to detect transient thallium defects. *J Nucl Med* 1985;26(8):880–883.

108. Weiner DA. Accuracy of cardiokymography during exercise testing: results of a multicenter study. *J Am Coll Cardiol* 1985; 6(3):502–509.

109. Amor M, Verdaguer M, Karcher G, et al. [Exertion isotope tests in coronary insufficiency. Comparison with isotopic ventriculography and myocardial scintigraphy]. *Arch Mal Coeur* 1985; 78(1):55–64.

110. Detrano R, Janosi A, Lyons KP, et al. Factors affecting sensitivity and specificity of a diagnostic test: the exercise thallium scintigram. *Am J Med* 1988;84(4):699–710.

111. Okada RD, Boucher CA, Kirshenbaum HK, et al. Improved diagnostic accuracy of thallium-201 stress test using multiple

observers and criteria derived from interobserver analysis of variance. *Am J Cardiol* 1980;46(4):619–624.

112. Atwood JE, Jensen D, Froelicher V, et al. Agreement in human interpretation of analog thallium myocardial perfusion images. *Circulation* 1981;64(3):601–609.

113. Albro PC, Gould KL, Westcott RJ, et al. Noninvasive assessment of coronary stenoses by myocardial imaging during pharmacologic coronary vasodilatation. III. Clinical trial. *Am J Cardiol* 1978;42(5):751–760.

114. Bodenheimer MB, Banka VS, Fooshee CM, et al. Extent and severity of coronary heart disease. Determinations by thallous chloride Tl 201 myocardial perfusion scanning and comparison with stress electrocardiography. *Arch Intern Med* 1979;139(6):630–634.

115. Dunn RF, Kelly DT, Bailey IK, et al. Serial exercise thallium myocardial perfusion scanning and exercise electrocardiography in the diagnosis of coronary artery disease. *Aust NZ J Med* 1979;9(5):547–553.

116. Kaul S, Boucher CA, Newell JB, et al. Determination of the quantitative thallium imaging variables that optimize detection of coronary artery disease. *J Am Coll Cardiol* 1986;7(3):527–537.

117. Goris ML, Gordon E, Kim D. A stochastic interpretation of thallium myocardial perfusion scintigraphy. *Invest Radiol* 1985;20(3):253–259.

118. Van Train KF, Berman DS, Garcia EV, et al. Quantitative analysis of stress thallium-201 myocardial scintigrams: a multicenter trial validation utilizing standard normal limits. *J Nucl Med* 1986;27(1):17–25.

119. Rozanski A, Diamond GA, Berman D, et al. The declining specificity of exercise radionuclide ventriculography. *N Engl J Med* 1983;309(9):518–522.

120. Tamaki N, Yonekura Y, Mukai T, et al. Stress thallium-201 transaxial emission computed tomography: quantitative versus qualitative analysis for evaluation of coronary artery disease. *J Am Coll Cardiol* 1984;4(6):1213–1221.

121. Fintel DJ, Links JM, Brinker JA, et al. Improved diagnostic performance of exercise thallium-201 single photon emission computed tomography over planar imaging in the diagnosis of coronary artery disease: a receiver operating characteristic analysis. *J Am Coll Cardiol* 1989;13(3):600–612.

122. Van Train KF, Maddahi J, Berman DS, et al. Quantitative analysis of tomographic stress thallium-201 myocardial scintigrams: a multicenter trial. *J Nucl Med* 1990;31(7):1168–1179.

123. Leppo J, Boucher CA, Okada RD, et al. Serial thallium-201 myocardial imaging after dipyridamole infusion: diagnostic utility in detecting coronary stenoses and relationship to regional wall motion. *Circulation* 1982;66(3):649–657.

124. Taillefer R, Lette J, Phaneuf DC, et al. Thallium-201 myocardial imaging during pharmacologic coronary vasodilation: comparison of oral and intravenous administration of dipyridamole. *J Am Coll Cardiol* 1986;8(1):76–83.

125. Ruddy TD, Dighero HR, Newell JB, et al. Quantitative analysis of dipyridamole-thallium images for the detection of coronary artery disease. *J Am Coll Cardiol* 1987;10(1):142–149.

126. Timmis AD, Lutkin JE, Fenney LJ, et al. Comparison of dipyridamole and treadmill exercise for enhancing thallium-201 perfusion defects in patients with coronary artery disease. *Eur Heart J* 1980;1(4):275–280.

127. Narita M, Kurihara T, Usami M. Noninvasive detection of coronary artery disease by myocardial imaging with thallium-201—the significance of pharmacologic interventions. *Jpn Circ J* 1981;45(1):127–140.

128. Machecourt J, Denis B, Wolf JE, et al.(Respective sensitivity and specificity of 201 Tl myocardial scintigraphy during effort, after injection of dipyridamole and at rest. Comparison in 70 patients who had undergone coronary radiography). *Arch Mal Coeur* 1981;74(2):147–156.

129. Wilde P, Walker P, Watt I, et al. Thallium myocardial imaging: recent experience using a coronary vasodilator. *Clin Radiol* 1982;33(1):43–50.

130. Ando J, Yasuda H, Kobayashi T, et al. Conditions for "coronary steal" caused by coronary vasodilator in man. *Jpn Heart J* 1982;23(1):79–95.

131. Francisco DA, Collins SM, Go RT, et al. Tomographic thallium-201 myocardial perfusion scintigrams after maximal coronary artery vasodilation with intravenous dipyridamole. Comparison of qualitative and quantitative approaches. *Circulation* 1982;66(2):370–379.

132. Harris D, Taylor D, Condon B, et al. Myocardial imaging with dipyridamole: comparison of the sensitivity and specificity of $^{201}$Tl versus MUGA. *Eur J Nucl Med* 1982;7(1):1–5.

133. Sochor H, Pachinger O, Ogris E, et al. Radionuclide imaging after coronary vasodilation: myocardial scintigraphy with thallium-201 and radionuclide angiography after administration of dipyridamole. *Eur Heart J* 1984;5(6):500–509.

134. Demangeat JL, Wolff F. [Redistribution of 201 Tl after myocardial scintigraphy with dipyridamole: value in the detection of coronary stenosis and ventricular kinetic anomalies]. *Arch Mal Coeur* 1985;78(13):1902–1911.

135. Laarman GJ, Verzijlbergen JF, Ascoop CA. Ischemic ST-segment changes after dipyridamole infusion. *Int J Cardiol* 1987;14(3):384–386.

136. Lam JY, Chaitman BR, Glaenzer M, et al. Safety and diagnostic accuracy of dipyridamole-thallium imaging in the elderly. *J Am Coll Cardiol* 1988;11(3):585–589.

137. Schmoliner R, Dudczak R, Kronik G, et al. Thallium-201 imaging after dipyridamole in patients with coronary multivessel disease. *Cardiology* 1983;70(3):145–151.

138. Okada RD, Lim YL, Rothendler J, et al. Split dose thallium-201 dipyridamole imaging: a new technique for obtaining thallium images before and immediately after an intervention. *J Am Coll Cardiol* 1983;1(5):1302–1310.

139. Walker PR, James MA, Wilde RP, et al. Dipyridamole combined with exercise for thallium-201 myocardial imaging. *Br Heart J* 1986;55(4):321–329.

140. Diamond GA, Forrester JS. Analysis of probability as an aid in the clinical diagnosis of coronary-artery disease. *N Engl J Med* 1979;300(24):1350–1358.

141. Uhl GS, Kay TN, Hickman JR Jr, et al. Detection of coronary artery disease in asymptomatic aircrew members with thallium-201 scintigraphy. *Aviat Space Environ Med* 1980;51(11):1250–1255.

142. Diamond GA, Forrester JS, Hirsch M, et al. Application of conditional probability analysis to the clinical diagnosis of coronary artery disease. *J Clin Invest* 1980;65(5):1210–1221.

143. Dans PE, Weiner JP, Melin JA, et al. Conditional probability in the diagnosis of coronary artery disease: a future tool for eliminating unnecessary testing. *South Med J* 1983;76(9):1118–1121.

144. Christopher T, Konstantinow G, Jones R. Incremental value of clinical assessment supine exercise electrocardiography and biplane exercise radionuclide ventriculography in the prediction of coronary artery disease in men with chest pain. *Am J Cardiol* 1983;52:927.

145. Currie PJ, Kelly MJ, Harper RW, et al. Incremental value of clinical assessment, supine exercise electrocardiography and biplane exercise radionuclide ventriculography in the prediction of coronary artery disease in men with chest pain. *Am J Cardiol* 1983;52(8):927–935.

146. McLaughlin PR, Martin RP, Doherty P, et al. Reproducibility of thallium-201 myocardial imaging. *Circulation* 1977;55(3):497–503.

147. Rehn T, Griffith LS, Achuff SC, et al. Exercise thallium-201 myocardial imaging in left main coronary artery disease: sensitive but not specific. *Am J Cardiol* 1981;48(2):217–223.

148. Maddahi J. Myocardial perfusion imaging for the detection and evaluation of coronary artery disease. In: Skorton DJ, Schelbert HR, Wolf GL, et al., eds. *Marcus cardiac imaging:* a companion to Braunwald's heart disease. Philadelphia: WB Saunders, 1996: 971–996.

149. Brown KA, Rowen M. Prognostic value of a normal exercise myocardial perfusion imaging study in patients with angiographically significant coronary artery disease. *Am J Cardiol* 1993;71(10):865–867.

150. Maddahi J, Abdulla A, Garcia EV, et al. Noninvasive identification of left main and triple vessel coronary artery disease: improved accuracy using quantitative analysis of regional myocardial stress distribution and washout of thallium-201. *J Am Coll Cardiol* 1986;7(1):53–60.

151. Patterson RE, Horowitz SF, Eng C, et al. Can noninvasive exercise test criteria identify patients with left main or 3-vessel coronary disease after a first myocardial infarction. *Am J Cardiol* 1983;51(3):361–372.

152. Abdulla A, Maddahi J, Garcia E, et al. Slow regional clearance of myocardial thallium-201 in the absence of perfusion defect: contribution to detection of individual coronary artery stenoses and mechanism for occurrence. *Circulation* 1985;71(1):72–79.

153. Bateman TM, Maddahi J, Gray RJ, et al. Diffuse slow washout of myocardial thallium-201: a new scintigraphic indicator of extensive coronary artery disease. *J Am Coll Cardiol* 1984; 4(1):55–64.

154. Ladenheim ML, Pollock BH, Rozanski A, et al. Extent and severity of myocardial hypoperfusion as predictors of prognosis in patients with suspected coronary artery disease. *J Am Coll Cardiol* 1986;7(3):464–471.

155. Gibson RS, Watson DD, Carabello BA, et al. Clinical implications of increased lung uptake of thallium-201 during exercise scintigraphy 2 weeks after myocardial infarction. *Am J Cardiol* 1982;49(7):1586–1593.

156. Bingham JB, McKusick KA, Strauss HW, et al. Influence of coronary artery disease on pulmonary uptake of thallium-201. *Am J Cardiol* 1980;46(5):821–826.

157. Kushner FG, Okada RD, Kirshenbaum HD, et al. Lung thallium-201 uptake after stress testing in patients with coronary artery disease. *Circulation* 1981;63(2):341–347.

158. Levy R, Rozanski A, Berman DS, et al. Analysis of the degree of pulmonary thallium washout after exercise in patients with coronary artery disease. *J Am Coll Cardiol* 1983;2(4):719–728.

159. Weiss AT, Berman DS, Lew AS, et al. Transient ischemic dilation of the left ventricle on stress thallium-201 scintigraphy: a marker of severe and extensive coronary artery disease. *J Am Coll Cardiol* 1987;9(4):752–759.

160. Stolzenberg J. Dilatation of left ventricular cavity on stress thallium scan as an indicator of ischemic disease. *Clin Nucl Med* 1980;5(7):289–291.

161. Chouraqui P, Rodrigues EA, Berman DS, et al. Significance of dipyridamole-induced transient dilation of the left ventricle during thallium-201 scintigraphy in suspected coronary artery disease. *Am J Cardiol* 1990;66(7):689–694.

162. Kaul S, Finkelstein DM, Homma S, et al. Superiority of quantitative exercise thallium-201 variables in determining long-term prognosis in ambulatory patients with chest pain: a comparison cardiac catheterization. *J Am Coll Cardiol* 1988;12(1): 25–34.

163. Kaul S, Lilly DR, Gascho JA, et al. Prognostic utility of the exercise thallium-201 test in ambulatory patients with chest pain: comparison with cardiac catheterization. *Circulation* 1988;77(4):745–758.

164. Pollock SG, Abbott RD, Boucher CA, et al. Independent and incremental prognostic value of tests performed in hierarchical order to evaluate patients with suspected coronary artery disease. Validation of models based on these tests. *Circulation* 1992;85(1):237–248.

165. Epstein SE, Palmeri ST, Patterson RE. Current concepts: evaluation of patients after acute myocardial infarction: indications for cardiac catheterization and surgical intervention. *N Engl J Med* 1982;307(24):1487–1492.

166. Gibson RS, Watson DD, Craddock GB, et al. Prediction of cardiac events after uncomplicated myocardial infarction: a prospective study comparing predischarge exercise thallium-201 scintigraphy and coronary angiography. *Circulation* 1983;68(2): 321–336.

167. Gimple LW, Beller GA. Assessing prognosis after acute myocardial infarction in the thrombolytic era. *J Nucl Cardiol* 1994;1(2 pt 1):198–209.

168. Haber HL, Beller GA, Watson DD, et al. Exercise thallium-201 scintigraphy after thrombolytic therapy with or without angioplasty for acute myocardial infarction. *Am J Cardiol* 1993; 71(15):1257–1261.

169. Gibson RS, Beller GA, Gheorghiade M, et al. The prevalence and clinical significance of residual myocardial ischemia 2 weeks after uncomplicated non-Q wave infarction: a prospective natural history study. *Circulation* 1986;73(6):1186–1198.

170. Brown KA, Weiss RM, Clements JP, et al. Usefulness of residual ischemic myocardium within prior infarct zone for identifying patients at high risk late after acute myocardial infarction. *Am J Cardiol* 1987;60(1):15–19.

171. Wilson WW, Gibson RS, Nygaard TW, et al. Acute myocardial infarction associated with single vessel coronary artery disease: an analysis of clinical outcome and the prognostic importance of vessel patency and residual ischemic myocardium. *J Am Coll Cardiol* 1988;11(2):223–234.

172. Leppo JA, O'Brien J, Rothendler JA, et al. Dipyridamole-thallium-201 scintigraphy in the prediction of future cardiac events after acute myocardial infarction. *N Engl J Med* 1984;310(16): 1014–1018.

173. Younis LT, Byers S, Shaw L, et al. Prognostic value of intravenous dipyridamole thallium scintigraphy after an acute myocardial ischemic event. *Am J Cardiol* 1989;64(3):161–166.

174. Gimple LW, Hutter AM Jr, Guiney TE, et al. Prognostic utility of predischarge dipyridamole-thallium imaging compared to predischarge submaximal exercise electrocardiography and maximal exercise thallium imaging after uncomplicated acute myocardial infarction. *Am J Cardiol* 1989;64(19):1243–1248.

175. Brown KA, O'Meara J, Chambers CE, et al. Ability of dipyridamole-thallium-201 imaging one to four days after acute myocardial infarction to predict in-hospital and late recurrent myocardial ischemic events. *Am J Cardiol* 1990;65(3):160–167.

176. Mahmarian J, Cochran A, Marks G, et al. Models for predicting long-term outcome after acute myocardial infarction by quantitative adenosine tomography. *J Nucl Med* 1993;34:54.

177. Hertzer NR, Beven EG, Young JR, et al. Coronary artery disease in peripheral vascular patients. A classification of 1000 coronary angiograms and results of surgical management. *Ann Surg* 1984;199(2):223–233.

178. Mangano D, Browner W, Hollenberg M, et al. Association of perioperative myocardial ischemia with cardiac morbidity and mortality in men undergoing noncardiac surgery. The Study of Preoperative Ischemia Research Group. *N Engl J Med* 1990; 323:389.

179. Boucher CA, Brewster DC, Darling RC, et al. Determination of cardiac risk by dipyridamole-thallium imaging before peripheral vascular surgery. *N Engl J Med* 1985;312(7):389–394.

180. Brown KA, Rowen M. Extent of jeopardized viable

myocardium determined by myocardial perfusion imaging best predicts perioperative cardiac events in patients undergoing noncardiac surgery. *J Am Coll Cardiol* 1993;21(2):325–330.

181. Levinson JR, Boucher CA, Coley CM, et al. Usefulness of semi-quantitative analysis of dipyridamole-thallium-201 redistribution for improving risk stratification before vascular surgery. *Am J Cardiol* 1990;66(4):406–410.

182. Lette J, Waters D, Bernier H, et al. Preoperative and long-term cardiac risk assessment. Predictive value of 23 clinical descriptors, 7 multivariate scoring systems, and quantitative dipyridamole imaging in 360 patients. *Ann Surg* 1992;216(2):192–204.

183. Coley CM, Field TS, Abraham SA, et al. Usefulness of dipyridamole-thallium scanning for preoperative evaluation of cardiac risk for nonvascular surgery. *Am J Cardiol* 1992;69(16):1280–1285.

184. Hendel RC, Whitfield SS, Villegas BJ, et al. Prediction of late cardiac events by dipyridamole thallium imaging in patients undergoing elective vascular surgery. *Am J Cardiol* 1992;70(15):1243–1249.

185. Camp AD, Garvin PJ, Hoff J, et al. Prognostic value of intravenous dipyridamole thallium imaging in patients with diabetes mellitus considered for renal transplantation. *Am J Cardiol* 1990;65(22):1459–1463.

186. Lane SE, Lewis SM, Pippin JJ, et al. Predictive value of quantitative dipyridamole-thallium scintigraphy in assessing cardiovascular risk after vascular surgery in diabetes mellitus. *Am J Cardiol* 1989;64(19):1275–1279.

187. Eagle KA, Singer DE, Brewster DC, et al. Dipyridamole-thallium scanning in patients undergoing vascular surgery. Optimizing preoperative evaluation of cardiac risk. *JAMA* 1987;257(16):2185–2189.

188. Sachs RN, Tellier P, Larmignat P, et al. Assessment by dipyridamole-thallium-201 myocardial scintigraphy of coronary risk before peripheral vascular surgery. *Surgery* 1988;103(5):584–587.

189. Eagle KA, Coley CM, Newell JB, et al. Combining clinical and thallium data optimizes preoperative assessment of cardiac risk before major vascular surgery. *Ann Intern Med* 1989;110(11):859–866.

# ASSESSMENT OF MYOCARDIAL PERFUSION AND VIABILITY WITH TECHNETIUM-99M PERFUSION AGENTS

## DANIEL S. BERMAN
## SEAN W. HAYES
## GUIDO GERMANO

The previous edition of this book documented the many advantages of single photon emission computed tomography (SPECT) over planar imaging in the assessment of myocardial perfusion. In comparison to planar imaging, myocardial perfusion SPECT increases contrast resolution and leads to improved localization of coronary artery disease (CAD) (1). It is estimated that in 1997 over 90% of myocardial perfusion scintigraphy in the United States was performed using SPECT. At the present time, approximately 30% of these procedures are performed with thallium 201 ($^{201}$Tl) alone, 30% with technetium 99m ($^{99m}$Tc) sestamibi alone, 20% with rest $^{201}$Tl/stress $^{99m}$Tc-sestamibi in a dual-isotope protocol, and 20% using $^{99m}$Tc-tetrofosmin, either alone or in combination with $^{201}$Tl.

The high count rate associated with $^{99m}$Tc perfusion agents make them particularly well suited to combined assessment of perfusion and function. With the recent widespread availability of powerful computer systems as well as multidetector cameras, gated myocardial perfusion SPECT has now become common, allowing for the routine simultaneous clinical assessment of regional myocardial perfusion at rest and peak stress, as well as the evaluation of rest and poststress left ventricular volumes, ejection fractions, and regional ventricular function. Thus, the technique of gated myocardial perfusion SPECT using $^{99m}$Tc perfusion agents provides a powerful clinical tool for evaluating a wide variety of clinical questions arising in the assessment of patients with known or suspected CAD.

**D. S. Berman:** Department of Medicine, University of California–Los Angeles School of Medicine; Nuclear Cardiology, Cedars-Sinai Medical Center, Los Angeles, California 90048.

**S. W. Hayes:** Nuclear Cardiology, Cedars-Sinai Medical Center, Los Angeles, California 90048.

**Guido Germano:** Department of Radiological Sciences, University of California–Los Angeles School of Medicine; Department of Medicine, Cedars-Sinai Medical Center, Los Angeles, California 90048.

## $^{99m}$TC MYOCARDIAL PERFUSION AGENTS

### $^{99m}$Tc-Sestamibi

$^{99m}$Tc is produced from a molybdenum-99m generator, has a half-life of 6 hours, and emits monoenergetic gamma rays at 140 keV. The whole-body radiation dose is estimated to be 16 mrad/mCi, in contrast to the higher radiation dose associated with $^{201}$Tl, 240 mrad/mCi. Due to this more favorable radiation dosimetry, much larger doses of $^{99m}$Tc myocardial perfusion imaging agents are used than with $^{201}$Tl (25–30 mCi versus 2–4 mCi).

The strengths and weaknesses of $^{99m}$Tc-sestamibi compared to $^{201}$Tl for myocardial perfusion imaging are understood by comparing their relative physiologic characteristics. $^{99m}$Tc-sestamibi belongs to a class of compounds called isonitriles and is a complex organic compound that behaves physiologically as a monovalent cation. Following its extraction from the blood, $^{99m}$Tc-sestamibi is bound by mitochondria so that there is minimal $^{99m}$Tc-sestamibi myocardial washout over time (2,3). As with $^{201}$Tl, the initial uptake of $^{99m}$Tc-sestamibi is a function of myocardial perfusion to viable tissue. There is a linear relationship between intravenously injected dose per gram of myocardium and myocardial blood flow, from the very low range up to approximately 2 to 2.5 mL/min/g (4). These latter levels are those characteristically associated with maximal treadmill exercise (5). At very high levels of flow, such as those achieved with vasodilator stress (in excess of 3 mL/min/g), a plateau in uptake occurs; this is characteristic of all myocardial perfusion tracers, with the exception of oxygen-15 water. This is because the extraction fraction is reduced at very high flow rates. Since pharmacologic stress testing with adenosine or dipyridamole frequently results in flow rates in the range of 4 mL/min/g (6), on a theoretical basis one would expect that either $^{201}$Tl or $^{99m}$Tc-sestamibi imaging would have difficulties in distinguishing myocardial regions in which the flow increased to 3 mL/min/g from regions in which flow increased to 4 mL/min/g. In other words, both tracers may be limited in detecting coronary lesions with mild hemodynamic significance, as might be expected of lesions causing 50% to 70% luminal diameter narrowing of the coronary artery. [201]Tl has a higher myocardial uptake (as measured by the percent injected dose/gram of myocardium) throughout the range of flow, secondary to a higher extraction fraction than [99m]Tc-sestamibi (approximately 85% compared to 65%) (7,8). [99m]Tc-tetrofosmin has a lower uptake than that of [99m]Tc-sestamibi throughout the medium to higher flow ranges, due to an even lower extraction fraction (approximately 50%) (9,10).

Since [201]Tl is a potassium analog, it redistributes over time. [99m]Tc-sestamibi, on the other hand, demonstrates minimal change in distribution over time. Although reduction in defect contrast over time can occur with [99m]Tc-sestamibi (11,12), for practical clinical purposes this phenomenon is considered of minimal significance, and [99m]Tc-sestamibi imaging is thought to be nearly as accurate when performed up to 2 hours after as when performed 10 to 15 minutes after a stress injection. The higher injected amounts of [99m]Tc-sestamibi, combined with adequate myocardial extraction and prolonged retention in the myocardium, result in better counting statistics with [99m]Tc-sestamibi than with [201]Tl in SPECT imaging. Additionally, owing to the slow washout of [99m]Tc-sestamibi, the effect of more prolonged imaging times associated with SPECT as compared to planar imaging become less important from a clinical standpoint than with [201]Tl. As with [99m]Tc-sestamibi, there is very little change in the myocardial distribution of [99m]Tc-tetrofosmin over time (9).

On theoretical grounds, [201]Tl could be more effective in defining mild coronary stenosis and may be associated with a "deeper" defect contrast (more count reduction compared to normal) than [99m]Tc-sestamibi, while [99m]Tc-sestamibi may show greater defect contrast on stress studies than [99m]Tc-tetrofosmin (13). On the other hand, from a practical standpoint, [99m]Tc-sestamibi and [99m]Tc-tetrofosmin provide greater flexibility than [201]Tl, since they do not require that imaging be accomplished soon after the stress injection for maximal sensitivity. With [201]Tl, imaging must be performed very close to the stress testing, and if soft tissue attenuation or patient motion compromise a study, the benefit of repeating the acquisition is questionable. With [99m]Tc-sestamibi or -tetrofosmin, in contrast, stress testing and tracer injection could take place at a location remote from the imaging laboratory, and image acquisition can simply be repeated when patient motion, soft tissue attenuation, or other artifact, are considered to be responsible for the production of a perfusion defect.

The benefit of being able to repeat images is illustrated in Fig.10.1, which shows stress [99m]Tc-sestamibi acquisition performed with the patient in the supine and prone position. Although the supine images show an apparent perfu-

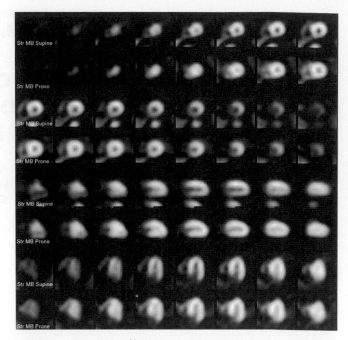

**FIGURE. 10.1.** Stress [99m]Tc-sestamibi (Str MB) single emission photon computed tomography (SPECT) images in the supine and prone positions in a 78-year-old patient with a low likelihood of coronary artery disease (CAD). Prone images are normal, demonstrating that the apparent inferior wall perfusion defect on the supine image is secondary to soft tissue attention. Normal wall motion was noted on gated SPECT.

sion defect, the prone images are normal, demonstrating that the inferior wall defect observed in the supine position was simply secondary to soft tissue attenuation. Our laboratory and others have previously shown that prone imaging is associated with less patient motion and less inferior wall attenuation than supine imaging (14–16). The combination of supine and prone images is also helpful in identifying breast attenuation and attenuation by excessive lateral chest wall fat, due to the shift in position of the attenuating structures that occurs in the prone position. However, since the prone position frequently causes an artifactual anteroseptal defect secondary to increased sternal attenuation in this position, prone imaging is used as an adjunct to, not a replacement for, supine imaging.

## [99m]Tc-Tetrofosmin

The Food and Drug Administration (FDA) recently approved the [99m]Tc myocardial perfusion imaging agent [99m]Tc-tetrofosmin, which is extracted by the myocardium and accumulated in mitochondria in a manner similar to that observed with [99m]Tc-sestamibi. As noted above, the extraction fraction of this agent, however, is slightly lower than that of [99m]Tc-sestamibi. In the canine model, the compound has been shown to have a linear relationship to flow from levels of 2 mL/min/g to near zero, but a marked plateau appears to occur in the relationship between flow rate and uptake above 2 mL/min/g (17). There is less hepatic uptake with this tracer than with [99m]Tc-sestamibi, resulting in more favorable heart/liver ratios early following resting injection (18,19). Despite this difference, optimal imaging following rest injection is at 1 hour after injection. The various acquisition protocols recommended for [99m]Tc-tetrofosmin are the same as those for [99m]Tc-sestamibi.

## Acquisition Protocols for [99m]Tc-Sestamibi and [99m]Tc-Tetrofosmin

Due to the absence of clinically significant redistribution, separate rest and stress injections are standard with either [99m]Tc-sestamibi or [99m]Tc-tetrofosmin SPECT (20,21). A variety of protocols can be used with these agents, including 2-day stress/rest, same-day rest/stress, same-day stress/rest, and dual-isotope. From the standpoint of defect contrast and optimal image quality, the 2-day stress/rest protocol is ideal (Fig. 10.2). With the 2-day stress/rest protocol, both the stress and the rest study are obtained following the injection of high doses of [99m]Tc-sestamibi or [99m]Tc-tetrofosmin, allowing the acquisition of high-quality, high-count images for the accurate assessment of perfusion and function. The principal drawback of this protocol is its requirement for two imaging days, resulting in a delay in the delivery of final information to be used in patient management. The same-day low-dose rest/high-dose stress protocol (22) (Fig. 10.2), perhaps the most commonly employed [99m]Tc-sestamibi or tetrofosmin protocol, has the disadvantage of causing a reduction in stress defect contrast, as approximately 15% of the radioactivity observed at the time of stress imaging comes from the preexisting resting myocardial distribution. The same-day low-dose stress/high-

dose rest sequence (23,24) (Fig. 10.2), on the other hand, has the advantage of requiring image acquisition times essentially identical to those used for [201]Tl imaging, making it easy for a laboratory to alternate between stress/redistribution [201]Tl and stress/rest [99m]Tc-sestamibi or [99m]Tc-tetrofosmin protocols. The principal drawback of this approach is that less than ideal count rates are associated with the most important stress image set, and it is difficult to accurately assess defect reversibility (25). With respect to the assessment of myocardial viability, all stress/rest or rest/stress [99m]Tc-sestamibi or [99m]Tc-tetrofosmin imaging protocols have theoretical limitations in separating severely hibernating myocardium from infarction. These constraints do not apply to [201]Tl, because of its redistribution properties (26,27). Viability assessment with [99m]Tc-sestamibi or [99m]Tc-tetrofosmin may be improved by the administration of nitroglycerin prior to the rest injection study (28).

Given the limitations of standard [99m]Tc agent protocols, our group has developed a rest [201]Tl/stress [99m]Tc sestamibi dual-isotope SPECT approach that has been in place in our institution since 1990 (29), essentially unmodified with the exception of the addition of gated SPECT. Dual-isotope imaging takes advantage of the Anger camera's ability to collect data in different energy windows. The two fundamental types of dual-isotope protocols are referred to as "simultaneous" or "separate" dual-isotope SPECT (Fig. 10.3).

Simultaneous dual-isotope imaging would have many theoretical advantages, compared with conventional stress and rest protocols (27,30). It would halve camera acquisition time and substantially abbreviate the overall study duration for the patient. Furthermore, inherent registration of the stress and rest image sets would reduce the frequency of unrecognized artifacts associated with separate stress and rest image acquisitions. This protocol, however, rests on unproven assumptions, the most important being that the effects of radioisotope crosstalk between the two energy

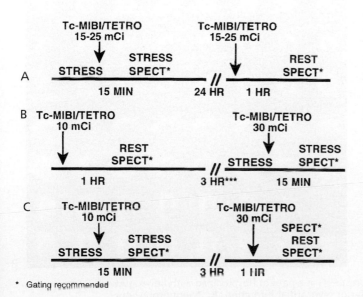

\* Gating recommended

**FIGURE 10.2.** Two-day **(A)**, same-day rest-stress **(B)**, and same-day stress-rest **(C)** [99m]Tc-sestamibi protocols.

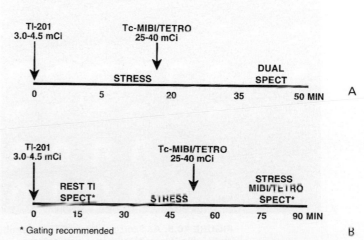

\* Gating recommended

**FIGURE 10.3.** Simultaneous **(A)** and separate acquisition **(B)** dual-isotope rest [201]Tl/stress [99m]Tc-sestamibi SPECT protocols.

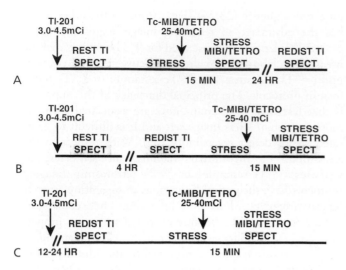

A

B

C

**FIGURE 10.4.** Common protocols for combining redistribution [201]Tl imaging with rest [201]Tl/stress [99m]Tc-sestamibi or tetrofosmin SPECT. **A:** Twenty-four-hour imaging after standard dual-isotope acquisition. **B:** Four-hour redistribution imaging prior to stress. **C:** injection the night before with redistribution [201]Tl SPECT as first acquisition sequence.

acquisition windows is insignificant, or can be accounted for. Kiat et al. (30) demonstrated in a report of patient studies that the downscatter of [99m]Tc-sestamibi or [99m]Tc-tetrofosmin into the lower energy [201]Tl acquisition window causes substantial (approximately 20%) reduction in [201]Tl defect contrast, leading to an overestimation of defect

reversibility. Interesting preliminary data regarding downscatter correction methods has been reported by Kamphuis et al. (31), as well as other groups (32). Until an approach to downscatter correction is validated clinically, however, we do not recommend general use of the simultaneous dual-isotope protocol.

Because of the negligible (2.9%) contribution of [201]Tl into the [99m]Tc energy acquisition window (30) and the fact that the [201]Tl image data set is acquired before [99m]Tc administration, the separate acquisition approach using rest [201]Tl/stress [99m]Tc-sestamibi or -tetrofosmin provides an alternative that does not require correction for cross-contamination between the two radioisotopes. The sensitivity and specificity of this protocol using [99m]Tc-sestamibi have been shown to be approximately 90% each (29). We believe that, for purposes of detecting CAD, all of the sestamibi protocols are likely to be very similar, with possible minimal reduction in sensitivity in the same-day rest/stress protocol due to the resting activity background. Of note, with this protocol, if defects are present on the rest [201]Tl study, redistribution [201]Tl SPECT can be performed before or 24 hours after the [99m]Tc-sestamibi injection (Figs. 10.4, 10.5, and 10.6). The separate acquisition dual-isotope protocol has also been used with rest [201]Tl and [99m]Tc-tetrofosmin.

An additional advantage of the [99m]Tc myocardial perfusion imaging agents is the ease with which ventricular function can be assessed at the time of myocardial perfusion SPECT. Gated SPECT has become routine in the performance of myocardial perfusion SPECT, particularly with

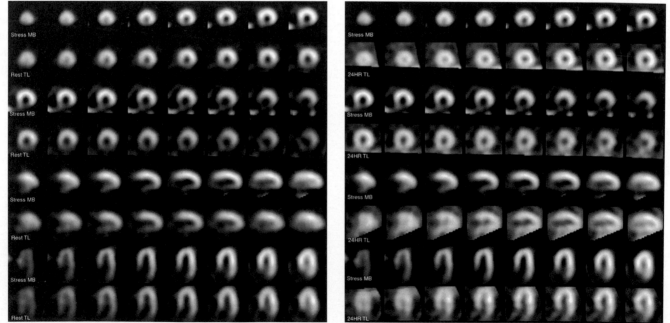

A

B

**FIGURE 10.5. A:** Exercise stress [99m]Tc-sestamibi/rest [201]Tl in a patient hospitalized with new-onset chest pain. Stress/rest images suggested an inferior myocardial infarction. **B:** Twenty-four-hour [201]Tl imaging demonstrates marked reversibility in the inferior wall. Angiography revealed a subtotal stenosis in the middle right coronary artery.

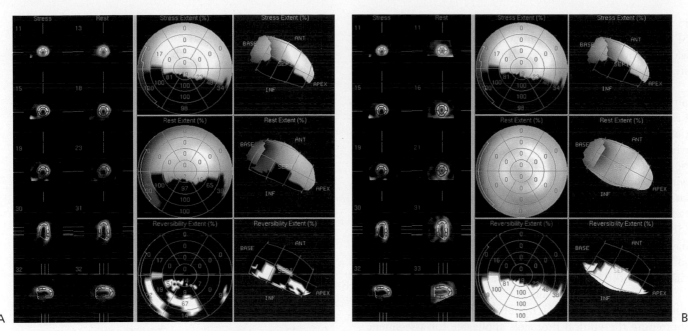

**FIGURE 10.6.** Quantitative perfusion SPECT (QPS) of the patient in Fig. 10.5 showing a large predominantly nonreversible inferior wall defect on stress/rest imaging **(A)**, but normal perfusion on 24-hour imaging **(B)**, demonstrating substantial resting ischemia.

the ⁹⁹ᵐTc agents sestamibi and tetrofosmin. With this approach, the poststress and even the resting phases of the examination can be acquired with electrocardiogram (ECG) gating, allowing the assessment of regional wall motion, left ventricular ejection fraction, and ventricular volumes, in addition to the assessment of regional myocardial perfusion. With the ⁹⁹ᵐTc myocardial perfusion imaging agents, the additional ability to perform first-pass radionuclide angiography at rest or at peak exercise is present. However, the technique of first-pass radionuclide ventriculography as an adjunct to myocardial perfusion SPECT has not become widely utilized, due to the expense of the additional equipment needed and the added complexity of routine use of first-pass exercise radionuclide ventriculography in busy laboratories. Our current protocol for rest ²⁰¹Tl/⁹⁹ᵐTc-sestamibi myocardial perfusion SPECT, which includes gating both at rest and poststress and the routine acquisition of both supine and prone poststress studies, is shown in Fig. 10.7.

## Other ⁹⁹ᵐTc Myocardial Perfusion Agents

⁹⁹ᵐTc-teboroxime belongs to another class of ⁹⁹ᵐTc myocardial perfusion agents, which are neutral lipophilic complexes of boronic acid called BATO (boronic acid adduct of technetium oxime) compounds. Unlike ⁹⁹ᵐTc-sestamibi and ⁹⁹ᵐTc-tetrofosmin, which have lower extraction fractions than ²⁰¹Tl, ⁹⁹ᵐTc-teboroxine appears to have a higher extraction fraction than ²⁰¹Tl. Additionally, it appears that the high extraction fraction with this agent plateaus at a higher flow rate than the other agents (33,34).

These highly desirable extraction characteristics of teboroxime are counterbalanced by the fact that teboroxime washes out very rapidly from the myocardium (35). Although the myocardium can be visualized with this tracer for approximately 20 minutes after injection, the kinetic properties of ⁹⁹ᵐTc-teboroxime require that initial imaging be completed within the first few minutes after tracer injection in order to reflect blood flow distribution at the time of injection. Single detector SPECT imaging and gated SPECT imaging are essentially not feasible with this agent; however, with multiple detector systems, rapid SPECT imaging is feasible. Data from our laboratory demonstrated that a rapid back-

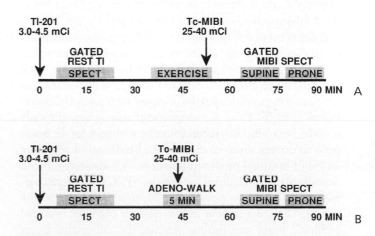

**FIGURE 10.7.** Current Cedars-Sinai Medical Center protocol demonstrating combined supine and prone, separate acquisition dual-isotope gated SPECT acquisition, with exercise **(A)** and pharmacolgic stress **(B)**.

to-back adenosine stress/rest $^{99m}$Tc myocardial perfusion SPECT protocol using a triple detector camera could be accomplished in approximately a half-hour and demonstrated high sensitivity and specificity for CAD (36).

$^{99m}$Tc-NOET (*N*-ethoxy, *N*-ethyl dithiocarbamato nitrido technetium) is a neutral lipophilic myocardial perfusion imaging agent (37) with an excellent extraction fraction across a wide range of flow. Extraction fraction of 85% with this tracer has been observed under hyperemic conditions (38). There appears to be redistribution over time with this tracer, related in part to the absence of intracellular binding and in part to higher circulating blood levels of radioactivity with this tracer compared to $^{99m}$Tc-sestamibi (38). It has been suggested that $^{99m}$Tc-NOEt overall may have kinetic properties and imaging properties very similar to $^{201}$Tl, with the advantage of the higher photon flux associated with the higher injected dose that is possible with a $^{99m}$Tc agent. The redistribution $^{99m}$Tc-NOEt appears to be almost complete after 90 minutes of reflow, potentially shortening the clinical protocols applicable for assessment of myocardial viability with this tracer. A disadvantage compared to $^{99m}$Tc-sestamibi or -tetrofosmin, however, is the relatively rapid redistribution of this tracer, like that of $^{201}$Tl, which makes the agent less forgiving in terms of the ability to repeat imaging should questions arise after the initial acquisition.

$^{99m}$Tc-furifosmin appears to be very similar to $^{99m}$Tc-tetrofosmin (39). Its extraction fraction is lower than that of $^{99m}$Tc-sestamibi. Neither $^{99m}$Tc-NOEt nor $^{99m}$Tc-furifosmin has been approved for clinical use in the United States at this time.

## Patient Preparation for Exercise/Pharmacologic Stress

Most of the above discussion dealt with exercise stress protocols. For all of the radiopharmaceuticals discussed above, pharmacologic stress approaches can also be applied. One of the fundamental advantages of myocardial perfusion SPECT over stress echocardiography is the ability to obtain diagnostic studies in virtually all patients. To this end, appropriate patient preparation is necessary. To derive optimal diagnostic and prognostic information from a study, it is important that a maximal hyperemic state be achieved with myocardial perfusion SPECT. Thus, we recommend that, when clinically feasible, beta-blocking medications be withheld for 48 hours prior to exercise stress to increase the likelihood of achieving ≥85% of maximal predicted heart rate. We also recommend that all patients scheduled for exercise SPECT not ingest caffeine-containing compounds for 24 hours prior to exercise testing. Thus, if a patient fails to achieve ≥85% of maximal predicted heart rate during exercise, the radioactive tracer would not be injected. Rather, pharmacologic stress with adenosine or dipyridamole would be immediately substituted, allowing for diagnostic test results. The sensitivity and specificity and risk stratification information of pharmacologic stress myocardial perfusion SPECT are essentially the same as those observed with exercise stress with all of the available tracers.

## GATED MYOCARDIAL PERFUSION SPECT: INTERPRETATION

A systematic approach to the interpretation and reporting of myocardial perfusion SPECT is essential to the optimal utilization of this modality (40). Since the assessment of perfusion and function are intimately related, this section addresses the interpretation and reporting of the combination of perfusion and function in gated myocardial perfusion SPECT. As with myocardial perfusion SPECT in general, careful attention to all aspects of camera/computer system quality control (verification of camera peaking, detector(s) uniformity, alignment, center of rotation, and closeness to the patient) is essential to ensure the adequacy of gated myocardial perfusion SPECT studies (41).

## Initial Patient Information

Due to the subjective nature of a scan interpretation, it is generally recommended that all scans first be interpreted without knowledge of the patient's clinical state. It is important, however, to know the patient's height, weight, gender, and, if female, bra size, in order to best recognize possible soft tissue artifacts. If the study is an exercise study, the exercise heart rate achieved and the exercise duration should be known.

## Inspection of the Raw Projection Data

One of the most important steps in SPECT interpretation is the review of the raw data, consisting of the projection images prior to filtering and reconstruction. The most useful method for such review is the endless loop "cinematic" display of the rotating projection images. This review ensures that the images were acquired over the appropriate acquisition arc, generally right anterior oblique (RAO) 45 degrees to left posterior oblique (LPO) 45 degrees, and that the heart was within the field of view throughout the entire acquisition. These images also provide useful information regarding count statistics.

### Patient Motion

Careful attention should be paid to patient motion in the vertical (craniocaudal) and lateral (horizontal) direction, since either can be associated with an artifactual defect that may go undetected by simple inspection of the tomographic slices. Moderate motion is frequently associated with artifactual defects (42). Inspection of the rotating projection images can be used to detect patient motion as well as "upward creep" of the heart (43). The latter phenomenon is related to the increased depth of respiration that occurs very early postexercise, which is associated with an average lower position of the diaphragm (and consequently of the heart) in the chest, compared to the normal ventilatory state. This causes the heart to gradually move cephalad during the early portion of SPECT acquisition, resulting in a form of motion artifact in reconstruction. By delaying acquisition until 10 to 15 minutes after exercise stress, this "upward creep" artifact is avoided. When $^{99m}$Tc-sestamibi or -tetrofosmin are employed, scans in which motion is observed can be repeated, preferably in the prone position, without concern for loss of clinical information, whereas a repeat $^{201}$Tl stress SPECT study might, because of the rapid washout of $^{201}$Tl, result in lower contrast of a defect (16). Alternatively, when a validated motion correction algorithm becomes available, this algorithm could be applied to the already obtained data set. Figure 10.8A illustrates an apparent perfusion defect in typical SPECT images reconstructed from projection images, corresponding to moderate motion on visual inspection. Figure 10.8B represents the reconstructed SPECT images from this patient's study using a motion correction algorithm; the reconstructed images demonstrate no perfusion defect.

## Attenuation Artifacts

Inspection of the rotating projection images provides a convenient method for detecting sources of attenuation artifacts.

In female patients, for example, the degree of breast attenuation can be estimated with reasonable accuracy by an experienced observer looking at the projection data. Special attention should be paid, when comparing different data sets side by side, to determine whether the position of the attenuating structure changed between acquisitions. Although most artifactual attenuation perfusion defects are nonreversible on inspection of the tomographic slices, breast attenuation artifacts may appear to be reversible if the breast moved between acquisitions. Other sources of attenuation artifacts observed with the help of the rotating image display include the arms, diaphragm, subdiaphragmatic structures, and general obesity. Many of the attenuation artifacts can be eliminated by repeating the acquisition in the prone position (16), as noted above. An example of supine/prone imaging's ability to clarify diaphragmatic attenuation is shown in Fig. 10.1.

## Extracardiac Uptake

The raw projection data should also be examined for evidence of extracardiac radioactivity uptake, perhaps the most important example of this occurring with occult cancer. An example of a patient with an undiagnosed lung cancer detected by the rotating projection images of a myocardial perfusion SPECT study is shown in Fig. 10.9B, with the tomographic images shown in Fig. 10.9A. Lung cancer, lymphoma, and breast cancer are the most common kinds of cancers detected through this approach.

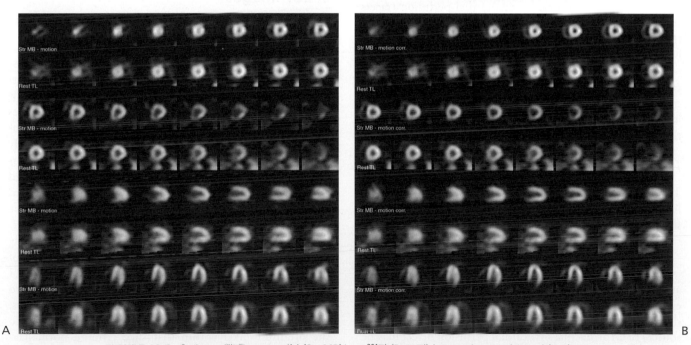

**FIGURE 10.8. A:** Stress $^{99m}$Tc-sestamibi (Str MB)/rest $^{201}$Tl (Rest Tl) images in a patient with a low likelihood of CAD. An apparent reversible inferior perfusion defect is present. Patient motion was noted during acquisition. **B:** Stress $^{99m}$Tc-sestamibi/rest $^{201}$Tl myocardial perfusion SPECT images after motion correction eliminated the inferior artifact, allowing the study to be correctly interpreted as normal.

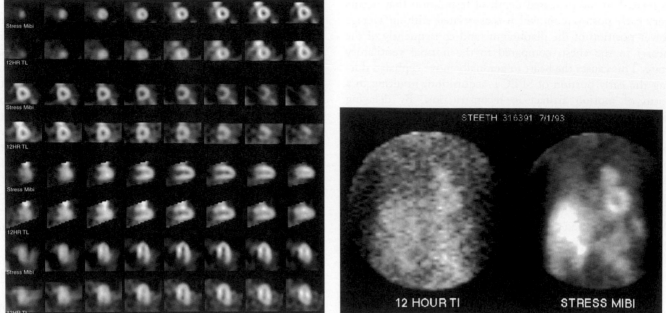

**FIGURE 10.9. A:** Stress [99m]Tc-sestamibi/12-hour redistribution [201]Tl SPECT acquisitions in a patient with a malignant thymoma. Careful inspection of the extracardiac area reveals the increased uptake in the tumor. **B:** Selected anterior view projections from the raw data of the SPECT acquisition. (From Berman D, Germano G. Myocardial perfusion single photon approaches. In: Pohost G, O'Rourke R, et al., eds. *Imaging in cardiovascular disease.* Philadelphia: Lippincott Williams & Wilkins, 2000, in press.)

### Lung Uptake

The degree of lung uptake of myocardial perfusion tracers should be noted from visual inspection of the raw projection images. Quantitative lung/heart ratios for [201]Tl have been shown to have an upper limit of normal of 0.54 (44–46), while preliminary data for [99m]Tc-sestamibi suggests an upper limit of 0.44 (47). In general, there is a strong linear correlation relationship between the degree of lung uptake and the pulmonary capillary wedge pressure at the time of injection (48,49).

### Hepatic/Gastrointestinal Uptake

The degree of myocardial perfusion tracer uptake in the liver and the gastrointestinal tract adjacent to the heart should be noted. If excessive, consideration should be given to repeating image acquisition after a delay of 1 hour, if [99m]Tc-sestamibi or -tetrofosmin is used. The increased uptake in structures adjacent to the heart can be a source of artifacts on the reconstructed tomograms. In particular, either artifactual decrease in the severity of true perfusion defects may occur (due to scatter from the adjacent "hot" source) or an artifactual myocardial perfusion defect may be created by the mathematics of the reconstruction process (cancellation of counts in regions immediately adjacent to "hot" objects) (50).

### Assessment of Myocardial Perfusion from SPECT Images

#### Display

A uniform approach to SPECT image display is recommended, based on the reorientation of images (slices) relative to the axis of orientation of the heart in the chest (51). The reoriented slices are termed the short-axis, vertical long-axis, and horizontal long-axis images. Images from different acquisitions (e.g., stress/rest, rest/redistribution, stress/redistribution) should be appropriately aligned and displayed simultaneously in interleaved fashion. As for image normalization, there are two widely used approaches. Each series (short-axis, vertical long-axis, and horizontal long-axis images) can be normalized to the pixel with the highest count in the entire series (series normalization). This approach provides the most intuitively accurate assessment of the presence, extent, and severity of perfusion defects, although it presents the drawbacks of lack of ideal display for each individual slice, sensitivity to focal hot spots, and insensitivity to basal perfusion defects. Alternatively, each tomographic slice can be normalized to the brightest pixel within that slice ("frame normalization"). This approach provides ideal display of each individual slice and is less sensitive to the problem of basal attenuation.

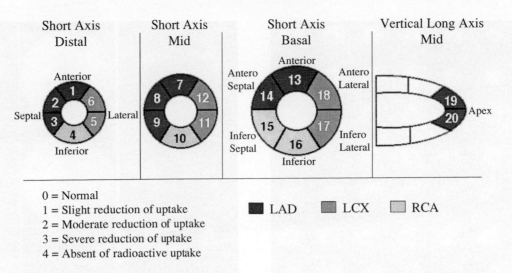

0 = Normal
1 = Slight reduction of uptake
2 = Moderate reduction of uptake
3 = Severe reduction of uptake
4 = Absent of radioactive uptake

■ LAD   ■ LCX   □ RCA

**FIGURE 10.10.** Diaphragmatic representation of the segmental division of the SPECT slices and assignment of individual segments to individual coronary arteries using the 20-segment model. LAD, left anterior descending coronary artery; LCX, left circumflex coronary artery; RCA, right coronary artery. (From Berman D, Germano G. An approach to the interpretation and reporting of gated myocardial perfusion SPECT. In: Germano G, Berman D, eds. *Clinical gated cardiac SPECT.* Armonk, NY: Futura, 1999:147–182, with permission.)

## Twenty-Segment Visual Analysis

The use of a semiquantitative scoring system in which each of 20 segments is scored according to a five-point scheme provides an approach to interpretation that is more systematic and reproducible than simple qualitative evaluation. The 20-segment scoring system we advocate is based on three short-axis slices—distal (apical), middle, and basal—to represent the entire left ventricle, with the apex represented by two segments visualized in a midvertical long-axis image. Each of the 20 segments has a distinct name and number, as indicated in Fig. 10.10. Since the anteroapical and inferoapical segments are visualized in the midventricular vertical long-axis image, the distal short-axis slice is chosen as one that is a few slices into the left ventricle. i.e., not the first slice to contain the ventricular cavity. Each segment is scored as follows: 0 = normal; 1 = slight reduction of uptake (equivocal); 2 = moderate reduction of uptake (usually implies a significant abnormality); 3 = severe reduction of uptake; 4 = absence of radioactive uptake (52). Perfusion defects with scores of 3 or 4 can be reported as consistent with a critical (≥90%) coronary stenosis (53,54).

## Summed Scores

In addition to the segmental visual scores, the 20-segment five-point scoring system lends itself to the derivation of summed scores, which can be considered global indices of perfusion (55). The summed stress score (SSS) is defined as the sum of the stress scores for the 20 segments. The summed rest score (SRS) is defined as the sum of the rest scores or redistribution scores, and the summed differences score (SDS), measuring the degree of reversibility, is defined

as the difference between the summed stress score and the summed rest score. These summed scores are to perfusion what the ejection fraction index is to ventricular function. Based on our previous prognostic work (56,57), summed stress scores <4 are considered normal or nearly normal, summed stress scores of 4 to 8 are considered mildly abnormal, summed stress scores of 9 to 13 moderately abnormal, and summed stress scores >13 severely abnormal. An example of a patient with a moderately abnormal scan (summed stress score of 9) is illustrated in Figs. 10.11 and 10.12.

## Assigning Perfusion Defects to Specific Coronary Artery Territories

As illustrated in Fig. 10.10, the 20 myocardial segments can be ascribed to individual coronary territories (29,58). Specifically, the inferior and basal septal segments are ascribed to the posterior descending coronary artery (Figs. 10.11 and 10.12), the lateral segments to the left circumflex coronary artery (Figs. 10.13 and 10.14), and the middle and distal septal as well as all anterior slices to the left anterior descending coronary artery (Figs. 10.15 and 10.16). Although isolated apical abnormalities are usually associated with left anterior descending artery disease, the apex can also be supplied by the left circumflex or right coronary arteries. If only anterior wall segments are abnormal, sparing the apex and the septum, the abnormalities are usually considered to represent disease of the diagonal branch of the left anterior descending coronary artery (Figs. 10.17 and 10.18).

The coronary assignment is altered for regions at the border between specific vessels territories, depending on the pat-

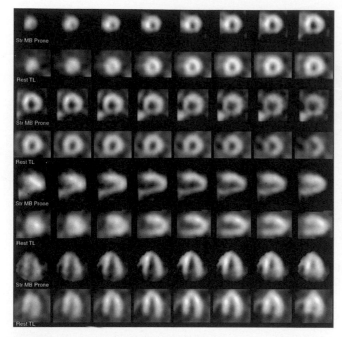

**FIGURE 10.11.** Stress $^{99m}$Tc-sestamibi/rest $^{201}$Tl myocardial perfusion SPECT in a 76-year-old patient with a history of coronary artery bypass surgery 21 years ago, now with typical angina. The study demonstrates a summed stress score of 9 with scores of 3 in the three inferior segments (right coronary artery territory).

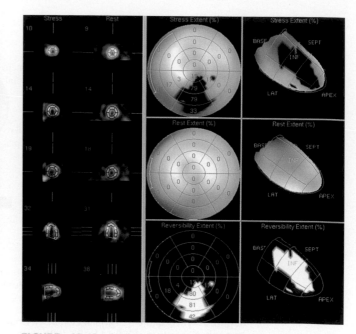

**FIGURE 10.12.** Quantitative perfusion SPECT (QPS) of the patient in Fig. 10.11, indicating the presence of a moderate-size perfusion defect in the distribution of the proximal right coronary artery.

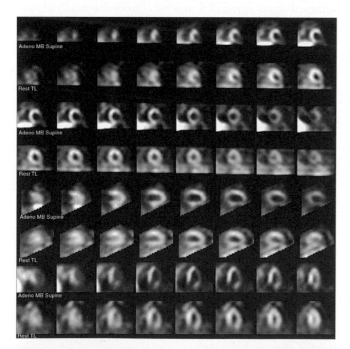

**FIGURE 10.13.** Adenosine $^{99m}$Tc-sestamibi/rest $^{201}$Tl myocardial perfusion SPECT in a 42-year-old patient 3 weeks after a non–Q-wave myocardial infarction. A severe defect is seen throughout the lateral wall (left circumflex coronary artery territory). The summed stress score was 20 and summed rest score was 10, suggesting a myocardial infarction with significant periinfarction ischemia. Immediate catheterization revealed a proximal subtotal stenosis from a high-rising marginal.

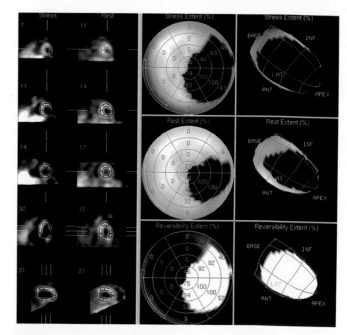

**FIGURE 10.14.** Quantitative perfusion SPECT (QPS) of the patient in Fig. 10.13, demonstrating a large perfusion defect in the distribution of the left circumflex coronary artery.

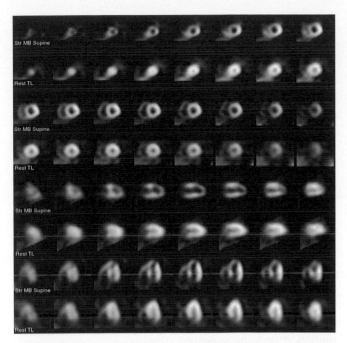

**FIGURE 10.15.** Exercise $^{99m}$Tc-sestamibi/rest $^{201}$Tl myocardial perfusion SPECT in a 75-year-old patient with typical angina. The summed stress score is 24. A severe and extensive reversible perfusion defect is seen throughout the left anterior descending coronary artery territory. There is additional evidence of transient ischemic dilation of the left ventricle. Angiography revealed a 95% stenosis of the left anterior descending coronary artery after the first septal perforator and a 90% stenosis in the first diagonal branch.

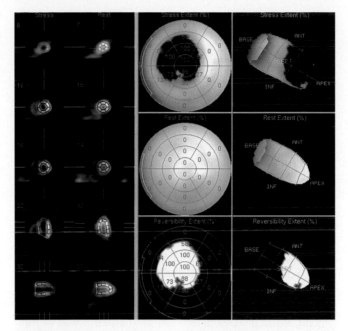

**FIGURE 10.16.** Quantitative perfusion SPECT (QPS) of the patient in Fig. 10.15, demonstrating the presence of a large perfusion defect in the distribution of the proximal left anterior descending coronary artery.

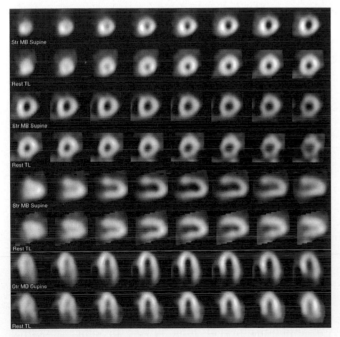

**FIGURE 10.17.** Exercise stress (ST) $^{99m}$Tc-sestamibi/rest $^{201}$Tl myocardial perfusion SPECT in a 60-year-old man with atypical angina. A small reversible defect is seen in the diagonal territory, with scores of 2 in the three anterior segments but no abnormality in the apex. (Adapted from Berman D, Germano G. Myocardial perfusion single photon approaches. In: Pohost G, Berman DS, O'Rourke R, et al., eds. *Imaging in cardiovascular disease.* Philadelphia: Lippincott Williams & Wilkins, 2000, in press.)

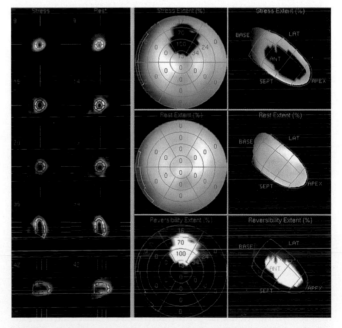

**FIGURE 10.18.** Quantitative perfusion SPECT (QPS) of the patient in Fig. 10.17, demonstrating the presence of a small perfusion defect in the distribution of the diagonal branch of the left anterior descending coronary artery.

tern of perfusion defect abnormality in the adjacent segments. When defects cross the usual coronary territories, judgment is required to determine whether to report multivessel disease as being likely. At times, a dominant perfusion defect in a specific vascular territory will "tail" into a contiguous territory generally assigned to another vessel. In these circumstances, the defect would generally be attributed to the vessel associated with the dominant defect. This pertains most commonly to the inferoseptal and inferolateral walls, but also applies to the anterolateral wall. Regarding the septum, if an inferoseptal defect is present (excluding the basal inferoseptal segment, which is generally a right coronary artery territory), the septal abnormalities would be assigned to the left anterior descending or right coronary artery, depending on which of these vessels had a perfusion defect. Similarly, if an inferolateral or anterolateral defect, but not both, were present in patients with adjacent defects in either the anterior or inferior wall, the lateral wall defect would be assigned to the vessel attributed to the neighboring defect. In general, isolated septal defects (without anterior wall or inferior wall involvement) are rare; isolated lateral wall defects (in the absence of anterior wall or inferior wall defects) would be attributed to the left circumflex coronary artery (58). These are general associations, which may vary in an individual patient based on variations in coronary anatomy.

In determining the overall interpretation (from definitely normal to definitely abnormal), the degree to which an apparent perfusion defect corresponds to a known coronary vascular territory is taken into account. Perfusion defects that fail to correspond to a standard vascular territory are more likely to be artifacts than those corresponding to typical vascular distributions.

## Attenuation Corrected Images

Several camera manufacturers provide hardware and software implementation of attenuation correction protocols (59,60). In general, these attenuation corrections are imperfect, reducing but not eliminating apparent perfusion defects due to soft tissue attenuation in normal patients. In addition, at times, true perfusion defects might be obscured or eliminated by application of these approaches. Because of these limitations, it is currently recommended that attenuation corrected tomographic data sets be visualized simultaneously with noncorrected data sets.

## Automated Quantitative Perfusion Analysis

It is recommended that semiquantitative visual analysis and quantitative analysis be assessed simultaneously. A variety of quantitative approaches have been developed, most of which compute myocardial counts in the various myocardial segments and display these counts using a two-dimensional or three-dimensional polar map (22,61). Most commonly, abnormalities are then defined by comparison of a patient's polar map to the polar maps derived from gender-matched normal patients. Due to the objective and automated nature of the analyses, quantitative assessments are more reproducible than visual assessments and are particularly useful in assessing interval change when patients are evaluated serially. Examples of quantitative analyses, employing quantitative perfusion SPECT (a system developed at Cedars-Sinai Medical Center), are illustrated in Figs. 10.12, 10.14, 10.16, and 10.18. For relatively inexperienced readers, quantitative analysis is helpful in teaching the regional variation associated with myocardial perfusion SPECT and improving interpretive skills. For experienced readers, quantitation serves as a second expert observer, frequently causing a more careful inspection of a regional abnormality that might have been overlooked. Despite the advantages of quantitative analysis, visual analysis is still an integral part of myocardial perfusion SPECT interpretation, since the quantitative analyses have not yet been refined to detect a variety of artifactual patterns easily recognized by visual inspection (e.g., breast attenuation, motion artifact, noncoronary patterns).

## Assessment of Myocardial Viability

The presence of myocardial viability is implied with the myocardial perfusion tracers if the degree of uptake at rest, redistribution, or following nitrate-augmented rest injection is normal or nearly normal. If a region has severely reduced or no uptake of radioactivity in these settings, it is considered to be nonviable. Areas with moderate reduction of counts in these conditions (score 2 at redistribution or nitrate-augmented rest) are usually partially viable, and patients in this group have a variable response in terms of postoperative improvement. Although some have suggested that a single cutoff point (chosen as a percentage of maximal counts in the myocardium) is predictive of viability in a region in question (62,63), we would prefer the use of the number of standard deviations below normal, since the latter would take into account the rather marked normal reduction in counts that occurs in the inferior wall of non–attenuation-corrected myocardial perfusion SPECT images.

## Nonperfusion Abnormalities

In addition to perfusion defects, several nonperfusion abnormalities should be observed and, when present, described. They include size of the left ventricle, transient ischemic dilation (TID) of the left ventricle (64,65), right ventricle myocardial uptake pattern, and right ventricular size. Abnormalities of lung uptake or other abnormal extracardiac activity should be noted (Figure 10.9).

TID is considered present when the left ventricular cavity appears to be significantly larger in the poststress images than in the resting images. The degree of enlargement needed depends on the imaging protocol used. For example, with dual-isotope protocols, the greater Compton scatter associated with [201]Tl causes the myocardial walls to appear intrinsically thicker (and the cavity smaller) in [201]Tl rest images compared to poststress [99m]Tc-sestamibi images (65). Therefore, a greater degree of transient enlargement must be evident for a dual-isotope study to be considered to demonstrate TID. We have found that the upper limits of normal for the TID ratio in dual-isotope imaging is 1.22. Patients who have TID are likely to have severe and extensive CAD (>90% stenosis of the proximal left anterior descending coronary artery, or of multiple vessels) (65). It should be noted that the term *transient ischemic dilation* is imprecise. What is referred to as TID may actually be an apparent cavity dilation secondary to diffuse subendocardial ischemia (obscuring the endocardial border). This phenomenon is likely to explain why TID may be seen for several hours following stress, when true cavity dilation is probably no longer present. TID has similar clinical implications whether it is observed on exercise or pharmacologic stress studies (66). An example of a patient illustrating TID of the left ventricle is shown in Fig. 10.15.

### Final Interpretation of Myocardial Perfusion

We recommend that the interpreter form an overall interpretation of the myocardial perfusion scan prior to incorporation of the clinical information. To minimize the use of an equivocal category, we advocate using a five-point scoring system (normal, probably normal, equivocal, probably abnormal, abnormal), based predominantly on the segmental score, but also on other considerations including the degree to which the scan abnormality conforms to a known vascular coronary territory, the presence of TID or lung uptake, and the heart rate achieved (on exercise studies). This overall interpretation is subjective, but guidelines are provided by the factors listed in Table 10.1.

### Assessment of Ventricular Function from Gated SPECT Images

As with the assessment of myocardial perfusion, a systematic approach to the assessment of ventricular function from the gated SPECT portion of the study is recommended. The use of a systematic approach greatly reduces the chances of misinterpretation.

### Quality Control

As with myocardial perfusion, assessment of adequacy of the technical quality of the data is an integral part of the interpretation of gated SPECT. Inspection of the rotating "summed" projection images is frequently a source of information regarding inadequacy of the data. Observation of "flashing" usually indicates that a gating error has occurred, resulting in the acquisition of a widely different number of cardiac cycles at the different angles along the acquisition arc. Inadequacy of the gating process can also be detected by inspection of the time-volume curve. This curve is derived from quantitative gated SPECT algorithms (67), and provides an assessment of the left ventricular cavity site at the various phases of the cardiac cycle. Figure 10.19 illustrates an example of quantitative gated SPECT results, including the time-volume curve. Note that the frame with the largest volume is the first frame, corresponding to end-diastole, and that the overall curve has a characteristic U-shape. When the time activity curve is clearly inappropri-

**TABLE 10.1. OVERALL INTERPRETATION OF MYOCARDIAL PERFUSION SPECT: VISUAL CRITERIA FOR ABNORMALITY (EXERCISE OR PHARMACOLOGIC TESTING)**

| | |
|---|---|
| Normal | All segments = 0 |
| Probably normal | Few segments = 1 (stress-rest = 1-1) |
| Equivocal | Multiple reversible 1 (stress-rest = 1-0) 1 segment = 2 |
| Probably abnormal | 2 segments = 2 |
| Definitely abnormal | ≥3 segments = 2 ≥1 segments ≥3 |

Weighing toward abnormal if defects are reversible, conform to a standard coronary territory, or are associated with transient ischemic dilation or lung uptake.
From Berman D, Germano G. Myocardial perfusion single photon approaches. In: Pohost G, Berman DS, O'Rourke R, et al., eds. *Imaging in cardiovascular disease*. Philadelphia: Lippincott Williams & Wilkins, 2000, in press.

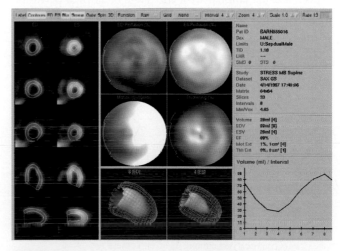

**FIGURE 10.19.** Quantitative gated SPECT (QGS) analysis of the patient in Figs. 10.11 and 10.12. The left ventricular ejection fraction is normal at 69%. There is quantitative evidence of normal left ventricular wall motion with a summed wall motion score (SMS) of 0 and a summed wall thickening score (STS) of 0.

ately timed, the gated SPECT data is generally considered nondiagnostic. The rotating summed projection images should also be evaluated for count statistics; at times, the count density in the overall summed images may be adequate for the interpretation of perfusion SPECT data, but is inadequate for the assessment of wall motion and wall thickening from the individual gated frames.

## Display

We recommend a five-slice display in which three representative short-axis slices (apical, midventricular, and basal), as well as one vertical long-axis and one horizontal long-axis midventricular tomogram, are displayed. The five-slice display is viewed in a cine format, alternating between the contours-on and the contours-off mode of the quantitative algorithm. When appropriate software is available, this alternation is a quality control measure to verify that the endocardial and epicardial surfaces determined by the algorithm were appropriate for computation of left ventricular ejection fraction and left ventricular volumes, and also provides assistance in the accurate scoring of regional function.

## Twenty-Segment Wall Motion Analysis

We recommend that the same 20 segments utilized for perfusion assessment be used for the visual assessment of regional ventricular function. A diagrammatic representation of the five slices chosen for analysis and the six-point motion scoring system is illustrated in Fig. 10.20. As noted, the assignment of the segmental regional wall motion scores is based on what is normal for a given region. This approach assumes that observers are familiar with the range of motion that is normal for a given segment, just as they would be expected to be familiar with the range of normal perfusion in a given segment. Wall motion analysis is performed by

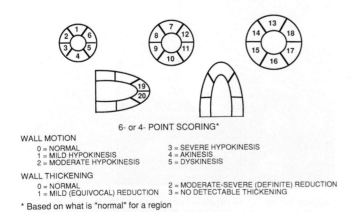

6- or 4- POINT SCORING*

WALL MOTION

| | |
|---|---|
| 0 = NORMAL | 3 = SEVERE HYPOKINESIS |
| 1 = MILD HYPOKINESIS | 4 = AKINESIS |
| 2 = MODERATE HYPOKINESIS | 5 = DYSKINESIS |

WALL THICKENING

| | |
|---|---|
| 0 = NORMAL | 2 = MODERATE-SEVERE (DEFINITE) REDUCTION |
| 1 = MILD (EQUIVOCAL) REDUCTION | 3 = NO DETECTABLE THICKENING |

\* Based on what is "normal" for a region

**FIGURE 10.20.** Diaphragmatic representation of the 20-segment model utilized for analysis of wall motion and wall thickening from gated myocardial perfusion SPECT.

visualizing the endocardial edge of the left ventricle, a process that is aided by the alternation between contours-on and contours-off. As a general rule, most experts recommend the use of a gray scale for the interpretation of regional wall motion.

## Twenty-Segment Wall Thickening Analysis

Visual assessment of wall thickening takes advantage of the direct relationship between the increase in the apparent brightness of a wall during the cardiac cycle [partial volume effect (68)] and the actual increase in its thickness. For purposes of wall thickening evaluation, many investigators recommend the use of a ten-step color scale as opposed to a gray scale. The degree of all thickening is similarly scored with a four-point system (0 = normal to 3 = absent thickening). In general, for a given short-axis slice, there is greater uniformity of absolute thickening than there is of wall motion, due to the greater effect of translational motion of the heart's long axis during systole on perceived regional wall motion than on thickening.

## Discordance Between Wall Motion and Wall Thickening

In general, abnormalities of regional wall motion and wall thickening accompany each other. We have thus found it most convenient to score function in a combined fashion for the 20 segments, only making note of whether wall motion and wall thickening are found to be discordant. The most common cause of discordance between wall motion and wall thickening is found in patients who have undergone bypass surgery; in these cases, abnormal wall motion with preserved thickening of the interventricular septum is an expected normal variant. Similar discordance, between wall motion and wall thickening also occur with a left bundle branch block or ventricular paced rhythm, where preserved thickening with abnormal motion of the interventricular septum is also a common variant. At the edges of a large infarct, normal thickening with minimal or absent motion may be observed in the periinfarction zone, with reduced motion being due to the adjacent infarct. The presence of thickening is considered to be indicative of viable myocardium; conversely, normal wall motion of an abnormally perfused segment that does not thicken could be associated with passive inward motion of a nonviable myocardial region (tethering), due to hypercontractility of adjacent noninfarcted segments.

## Combined Rest/Poststress Regional Function Analysis

When available, the rest and poststress gated images should be compared to identify the development of new wall motion abnormality. Wall motion abnormalities that occur on poststress images but are not seen on resting images imply the presence of ventricular stunning, and are highly specific for the presence of CAD (69,70). If resting gated SPECT studies are not available, a note should still be made of discrete regional wall motion or wall thickening abnormalities, since these can often be indicators of the presence of a severe coronary stenosis (>90% diameter narrowing). This finding might be missed by perfusion defect assessment alone, particularly in patients with a greater degree of ischemia in a region other than that demonstrating the wall motion abnormality (70).

## Quantitative Wall Motion/Wall Thickening Assessment

Ideally, quantitative methods for comparing the degree of wall motion and wall thickening of each segment of the left ventricle to the lower limit of normal would be available, and would augment the visual analysis of ventricular function from gated SPECT data. Algorithms for the automatic quantitative measurement of absolute endocardial motion and relative myocardial thickening between end-diastole and end-systole have been developed and validated at our laboratory (71), and the determination of segment-specific normal limits is currently under way.

## Left Ventricular Volume

It has recently been demonstrated that quantitative assessments of absolute left ventricular cavity volumes correlate well with echocardiography (72–76), thermal dilution catheterization methods (77,78), and magnetic resonance imaging (79). We have also found the absolute measurements of left ventricular volume to be perfectly reproducible (repeated assessment in a given data set) (80) and highly repeatable (repeated data acquisition) (81,82). If a validated method for measuring left ventricular volumes is available on a particular camera-computer system, it is recommended that this measurement be reported as a standard component of gated SPECT analysis. Volume measurements are helpful in prognostication (83), as well as in guiding the use of angiotensin-converting enzyme (ACE) inhibitors (84). Absolute left ventricle volumes tend to be underestimated in patients with very small hearts (partial volume effect).

## Final Interpretation of Ventricular Function

An overall interpretation of the ventricular function component of the gated SPECT examination is recommended, as discussed above for myocardial perfusion, and can be accomplished using the same scale with five gradations (from definitely normal to definitely abnormal). In general, a study would be considered as showing abnormal function if a severe wall motion abnormality is present. If only a

moderate wall motion abnormality is present, the determination as to whether the ventricular function portion of the study should be considered abnormal depends on the ejection fraction.

## Modification of the Interpretation of Perfusion and Function Based on Clinical Information

Having now analyzed the perfusion and function portions of the gated perfusion SPECT examination without knowledge of the patient's clinical state, the observer should incorporate knowledge of all clinically relevant data, including symptoms, risk factors, the results of treadmill testing, and the results of coronary angiography into the final interpretation. By convention, modification of the nuclear interpretation should not change the initial assessment by more than one category of abnormality, using the five-point scale from normal to abnormal (Table 10.2). For example, if the initial interpretation was equivocal, the study could be considered probably normal in a patient with a low prescan likelihood of CAD. Conversely, the equivocal study could be reported as probably abnormal in a high prescan likelihood setting (e.g., typical angina pectoris with multiple risk factors and an abnormal treadmill test). The modification has the effect of improving the overall concordance of information sent to clinicians (a type of "smoothing" function). It is of critical importance to exercise restraint, so that the maximal shift is one category in the five-point scale. Shifting by a greater extent would be confusing, in that it would no longer provide data representative of the scintigraphic study.

## Integration of Information

Table 10.3 lists the items of information that an ideal nuclear cardiology report would contain in addition to the scintigraphic information. The final comprehensive report should represent a synthesis of nuclear and nonnuclear information. We recommend that several summary statements be included as components of the final report, including the following:

**TABLE 10.2. INTERPRETATION OF MYOCARDIAL PERFUSION SPECT SHOWING THE CONVENTION FOR MODIFICATION BASED ON CLINICAL INFORMATION**

| Modify interpretation based on clinical information | | | | |
|---|---|---|---|---|
| Convention: shift by a maximum of 1 degree | | | | |
| Normal | Probably normal | Equivocal | Probably abnormal | Definitely abnormal |

From Berman D, Germano G. Myocardial perfusion single photon approaches. In: Pohost G, Berman DS, O'Rourke R, et al., eds. *Imaging in cardiovascular disease.* Philadelphia: Lippincott Williams & Wilkins, 2000, in press.

**TABLE 10.3. NONSCINTIGRAPHIC INFORMATION THAT SHOULD BE INCORPORATED INTO THE FINAL REPORT**

Incorporate all clinical information and other test results into the final report
- Risk factors
- Presenting symptoms
- Nonnuclear exercise test results
  - Duration
  - Heart rate and blood pressure response
  - Symptoms
  - ST response
- Coronary angiography
- Other imaging tests

From Berman D, Germano G. Myocardial perfusion single photon approaches. In: Pohost G, Berman DS, O'Rourke R, et al., eds. *Imaging in cardiovascular disease.* Philadelphia: Lippincott Williams & Wilkins, 2000, in press.

1. In patients who are not known to have CAD, the postscan likelihood of angiographically significant CAD should be expressed. This likelihood can be calculated by using commercially available programs such as Cadenza (85), or look-up tables (86,87). Table 10.4 lists the adjectives that we associate with the various postscan likelihoods of angiographically significant CAD.
2. In patients with known disease [postangiography, post–myocardial infarction, post–coronary artery bypass graft (CABG), post–percutaneous transluminal coronary angioplasty (PTCA)] undergoing exercise studies, the postscan likelihood is referred to as the likelihood of exercised-induced ischemia. In patients with known disease undergoing pharmacologic stress, the term *likelihood of jeopardized myocardium* is used. This distinction between exercised-induced ischemia and jeopardized myocardium is used since the large majority of patients demonstrating reversible defects (evidence of jeopardized myocardium) with vasodilator stress (dipyri-

**TABLE 10.4. PERCENTAGES AND ADJECTIVES USED TO DESCRIBE THE LIKELIHOOD OF ANGIOGRAPHICALLY SIGNIFICANT CORONARY ARTERY DISEASE**

| Percent Likelihood of >50% Stenosis | Verbal Description |
|---|---|
| <15 | Low |
| 15–29 | Low intermediate |
| 30–69 | Intermediate |
| 70–84 | High intermediate |
| 85–94 | High |
| 95–98 | Very high |
| ≥99 | Virtually diagnostic |

From Berman D, Germano G. Myocardial perfusion single photon approaches. In: Pohost G, Berman DS, O'Rourke R, et al., eds. *Imaging in cardiovascular disease.* Philadelphia: Lippincott Williams & Wilkins, 2000, in press.

damole/adenosine) develop a perfusion imbalance during stress but have not actually developed ischemia (88).

3. The extent, severity, and location of reversible defects should be reported and related to the likely coronary anatomy.
4. The extent and location of fixed defects (which might be referred to as prior myocardial infarction) should be described. In general, the term *myocardial infarction* should be avoided unless late redistribution imaging confirms nonreversibility.
5. Importantly, the final summation should answer the specific question being asked by the referring physician.
6. Using the combined clinical information and scintigraphic scores, it is also recommended that a statement regarding the patient's risk of subsequent cardiac events be considered for inclusion in the final report. We routinely ascribe an annual expected risk of death based on the summed stress score, with the categories <1% per year considered low, 1% to 3% per year intermediate, and >3% per year high.
7. If myocardial viability is being questioned, specific statements regarding the viability of abnormally contracting segments should be included.

### Integration of Information of Perfusion and Function from Gated SPECT

As noted above, data relative to perfusion and function are usually similar. The classic examples of discordance that occur in the interventricular septum in patients who have undergone bypass surgery or in patients with left bundle branch block are expected, but should still be reported.

Unexpected discordance of data should be accompanied by a specific description of the discordance at the end of the final report. In our experience, the most common occurrences of discordance are in patients with cardiomyopathy. For example, if a patient has a very reduced left ventricular ejection fraction, a large left ventricle, and no perfusion defect (the myocardial perfusion SPECT study is normal, but its gated SPECT component is abnormal) we categorize this type of study as "abnormal, with left ventricular enlargement, but no perfusion defects." We would then add, "The findings of severe left ventricular enlargement and severe depression of left ventricular ejection fraction with no associated perfusion defect are most consistent with a dilated nonischemic cardiomyopathic process." In our laboratory, many patients with a report such as this will not undergo subsequent cardiac catheterization.

A somewhat less common but important additional source of discordance between perfusion and function data occurs in patients with ventricular remodeling following myocardial infarction. These patients will typically have large nonreversible perfusion defects with no reversible perfusion defects, but marked left ventricular enlargement and reduction of left ventricular ejection fraction and regional ventricular function out of proportion to the size of the perfusion defect. In those circumstances, a statement such as this is included in the final summation: "The left ventricular enlargement and marked abnormality of left ventricular function are out of proportion to the size of the perfusion defect. These findings are most compatible with ventricular remodeling." Depending on the clinical situation, we may add, "Less likely, but still possible, the patient may have an ischemic cardiomyopathic process with balanced reduction in flow." To make the latter statement, we would usually like to have further evidence of exercise-induced ischemia or jeopardized myocardium, such as marked chest discomfort, ST-segment depression, or unexpected akinesis/dyskinesis in zones with normal resting motion or normal resting perfusion (70).

In dilated nonischemic cardiomyopathic processes and in ventricular remodeling, the portions of the left ventricle demonstrating normal perfusion but abnormal function are usually hypokinetic. When frank akinesis or dyskinesis is noted in zones that appear to have normal perfusion, the final report is weighted toward the possibility of an ischemic cardiomyopathy with balanced reduction in flow, since stress-induced stunning in an ischemic cardiac myopathy would be more likely to explain this discordance

than ventricular remodeling or a nonischemic cardiomyopathic process.

The overall interpretation of gated myocardial perfusion SPECT remains an art. Following the systematic approach recommended in this section allows this art to be refined, and makes the results more reproducible from observer to observer and from center to center.

## CLINICAL APPLICATIONS

### Detection of Coronary Artery Disease

Tables 10.5 and 10.6 present sensitivities and specificities of myocardial perfusion SPECT for the detection of angiographically significant (greater than 50% stenosis) CAD. It should be noted that published reports have consistently demonstrated that the sensitivity of exercise electrocardiography is significantly lower than that of myocardial perfusion SPECT (89). Despite the above-noted differences in the initial extraction characteristics of these tracers, to date, there have been few clinical reports documenting lower sensitivity of the $^{99m}$Tc tracers compared to $^{201}$Tl for the detection of CAD. With respect to specificity, the main difference between $^{201}$Tl and $^{99m}$Tc-sestamibi or -tetrofosmin

**TABLE 10.5. SENSITIVITY AND SPECIFICITY OF EXERCISE MYOCARDIAL PERFUSION SPECT FOR DETECTING CAD (≥50% STENOSIS)**

| Year | First Author | Reference | Isotope | Previous MI | Sensitivity | % | Specificity | % |
|------|-------------|-----------|---------|-------------|-------------|---|-------------|---|
| 1990 | Kiat | 151 | MIBI | 45% | 45/48 | 94 | 4/5 | 80 |
| 1990 | Mahmarian | 152 | Tl | 43% | 192/221 | 87 | 65/75 | 87 |
| 1990 | Nguyen | 153 | Tl | N/R | 19/25 | 76 | 5/5 | 100 |
| 1990 | Van Train | 154 | Tl | 35% | 291/307 | 95 | 30/64 | 47 |
| 1991 | Coyne | 155 | Tl | N/R | 38/47 | 81 | 39/53 | 74 |
| 1993 | Berman | 29 | MIBI/Tl | 0% | 50/52 | 96 | 9/11 | 82 |
| 1993 | Forster | 156 | MIBI | 0% | 10/12 | 83 | 8/9 | 89 |
| 1993 | Chae | 157 | Tl | 42% | 116/163 | 71 | 52/80 | 65 |
| 1993 | Minoves | 158 | MIBI/Tl | 42% | 27/30 | 90 | 22/24 | 92 |
| 1993 | Van Train | 159 | MIBI | 16% | 30/31 | 97 | 6/9 | 67 |
| 1994 | Sylven | 160 | MIBI | 37% | 41/57 | 72 | 5/10 | 50 |
| 1994 | Van Train | 161 | MIBI | 19% | 91/102 | 89 | 8/22 | 36 |
| 1995 | Palmas | 162 | MIBI | 30% | 60/66 | 91 | 3/4 | 75 |
| 1995 | Rubello | 163 | MIBI | 57% | 100/107 | 93 | 8/13 | 62 |
| 1996 | Hambye | 164 | MIBI | 0% | 75/91 | 82 | 28/37 | 76 |
| 1997 | Yao | 165 | MIBI | 55% | 34/36 | 94 | 14/15 | 93 |
| 1997 | Heiba | 166 | MIBI | 31% | 28/30 | 93 | 2/4 | 50 |
| 1997 | Ho | 167 | Tl | 33% | 29/38 | 76 | 10/13 | 77 |
| 1997 | Taillefer | 168 | MIBI | 17% | 23/32 | 72 | 13/16 | 81 |
| 1997 | Van Eck-Smit | 169 | Tetrofosmin | N/R | 46/53 | 87 | 6/7 | 86 |
| 1998 | Budoff | 170 | MIBI | 0% | 12/16 | 75 | 12/17 | 71 |
| 1998 | Santana-Boado | 171 | MIBI | 0% | 92/101 | 91 | 56/62 | 90 |
| 1998 | Acampa | 172 | MIBI | 47% | 23/25 | 92 | 5/7 | 71 |
| 1998 | Acampa | 172 | Tetrofosmin | 47% | 24/25 | 96 | 6/7 | 86 |
| 1998 | Ho | 173 | Tl | 22% | 19/24 | 79 | 15/20 | 75 |
| Total | | | | | 1,515/1,739 | 87 | 431/589 | 73 |

Based on English-language manuscripts providing data with ≥50% stenosis criterion.
N/R, not reported; MIBI, $^{99m}$Tc-sestamibi; Tl, $^{201}$Tl; MI, myocardial infarction.
From Berman D, Germano G. Myocardial perfusion single photon approaches. In: Pohost G, Berman DS, O'Rourke R, et al., eds. *Imaging in cardiovascular disease*. Philadelphia: Lippincott Williams & Wilkins, 2000, in press.

**TABLE 10.6. SENSITIVITY AND SPECIFICITY OF VASODILATOR STRESS PERFUSION SPECT FOR DETECTING CAD (≥50% STENOSIS)**

| Year | Author | Reference | Drug | Isotope | Previous MI | Sensitivity | % | Specificity | % |
|------|--------|-----------|------|---------|-------------|-------------|---|-------------|---|
| 1990 | Nguyen | 153 | Adenosine | Tl | 37% | 49/53 | 92 | 7/7 | 100 |
| 1990 | Verani | 174 | Adenosine | Tl | N/R | 24/29 | 83 | 15/16 | 94 |
| 1991 | Iskandrian | 175 | Adenosine | Tl | 25% | 121/132 | 92 | 14/16 | 88 |
| 1991 | Coyne | 155 | Adenosine | Tl | N/R | 39/47 | 83 | 40/53 | 75 |
| 1991 | Nishimura | 176 | Adenosine | Tl | 13% | 61/70 | 87 | 28/31 | 90 |
| 1995 | Aksut | 177 | Adenosine | Tl | 24% | 358/398 | 90 | 38/45 | 84 |
| 1995 | Miyagawa | 178 | Adenosine | Tl | 15% | 67/76 | 88 | 35/44 | 80 |
| 1996 | Amanullah | 179 | Adenosine | MIBI | 21% | 87/94 | 93 | 28/36 | 78 |
| 1997 | Watanabe | 180 | Adenosine | Tl | 19% | 40/46 | 87 | 21/24 | 88 |
| 1997 | Watanabe | 180 | Dipyridamole | Tl | 23% | 34/41 | 83 | 21/29 | 72 |
| 1997 | Taillefer | 168 | Dipyridamole | MIBI | 11% | 23/32 | 72 | 5/5 | 100 |
| 1997 | He | 181 | Dipyridamole | Tetrofosmin | 52% | 41/48 | 85 | 6/11 | 55 |
| 1997 | Amanullah | 182 | Adenosine | MIBI | 0% | 159/171 | 93 | 37/51 | 73 |
| 1997 | Cuocolo | 183 | Adenosine | Tetrofosmin | 23% | 22/25 | 88 | 1/1 | 100 |
| 1998 | Takeishi | 184 | Adenosine | Tetrofosmin | 17% | 39/44 | 89 | 17/21 | 81 |
| Total | | | | | | 1,164/1,306 | 89 | 313/390 | 80 |

Based on English-language manuscripts providing data with ≥50% stenosis criterion.
N/R, not reported; MIBI, $^{99m}$Tc-sestamibi; Tl, $^{201}$Tl; MI, myocardial infarction.
From Berman D, Germano G. Myocardial perfusion single photon approaches. In: Pohost G, Berman DS, O'Rourke R, et al., eds. *Imaging in cardiovascular disease.* Philadelphia: Lippincott Williams & Wilkins, 2000, in press.

SPECT is considered to be the slightly to moderately reduced susceptibility to artifact due to lower attenuation of $^{99m}$Tc, greater use of gated SPECT with the $^{99m}$Tc perfusion agents, and most importantly, the ability to repeat the SPECT acquisition with these agents when either attenuation or motion artifacts are suspected.

In estimating the true sensitivity and specificity of noninvasive testing, referral or workup bias needs to be taken into account (21,90). In cardiology, this workup bias has been shown to be very powerful. Once a noninvasive test is accepted as being clinically effective, its results strongly influence the performance of subsequent coronary angiography. Referral bias results in an overestimation of test sensitivity, and an underestimation of test specificity. In the extreme case, where the noninvasive test result becomes the gatekeeper to the performance of angiography, its observed sensitivity and specificity will become 100% and 0%, respectively.

Due to the profound impact of the referral bias on specificity, we developed the concept of the normalcy rate and applied it in multiple different clinical studies. First applied in 1981 (91) and named in 1986 (92), the normalcy rate refers to patients with a low likelihood of CAD, based on sequential bayesian analysis of age, sex, symptom classification, and the results of noninvasive stress testing (other than the test in question). We have used the term *normalcy rate* to describe the frequency of normal test results in these patients with a low likelihood of CAD, to differentiate it from specificity, which as noted above refers to the frequency of normal test results in patients with normal coronary angiograms. Low likelihood patients are chosen since they are closer in age and risk factors to patients with CAD undergoing testing than are normal volunteers. (In fact, low likelihood patients are part of a population of patients with suspected CAD prior to their referral.) The normalcy rate has been reported to be in the 80% to 90% range with $^{201}$Tl testing, generally greater than 90% with $^{99m}$Tc-sestamibi SPECT, and would be expected to be similar to the latter for $^{99m}$Tc-tetrofosmin SPECT. As noted above, the better normalcy rate and likely better specificity of the $^{99m}$Tc agents is most probably secondary to the ability to repeat imaging in case of suspected artifactual abnormality. The reported normalcy rate for myocardial perfusion SPECT is illustrated in Table 10.7.

Simple detection of CAD remains one of the most common indications for performing myocardial perfusion SPECT. It is particularly important in certain patients with high-risk occupations, as well as in younger patients in whom the definitive diagnosis of CAD, with its lifelong implications for therapy, may be important, regardless of the likelihood of cardiac events over a 1- to 3-year period. The basis for the diagnostic application of nuclear testing lies in the concept of sequential bayesian analysis of disease probability. This analysis requires knowledge of the pretest likelihood of disease, as well as of the sensitivity and specificity of the test. The pretest likelihood of disease or prevalence of disease varies according to age, sex, symptoms, and risk factors, and can be directly derived from the work of Diamond and Forrester (93), as well as other databases.

Our clinical algorithm for the purpose of simple detection of CAD is illustrated in Fig. 10.21 (94). Patients with a low probability (<0.15) of having angiographically significant (>50% stenosis) CAD can be identified, even before the standard exercise tolerance test (ETT) is performed. Several approaches may be used, including the validated

**TABLE 10.7. NORMALCY RATE OF STRESS SPECT IN PATIENTS WITH A LOW LIKELIHOOD OF CAD**

| Year | Author | Reference | Stress | Isotope | Normalcy Rate | % | Subjects |
|------|--------|-----------|--------|---------|---------------|---|----------|
| 1989 | Maddahi | 185 | Exercise | Tl | 24/28 | 86 | Low likelihood (<5%) of CAD |
| 1989 | Iskandrian | 186 | Exercise | Tl | 123/131 | 94 | Low likelihood (<5%) of CAD |
| 1990 | Kiat | 151 | Exercise | MIBI | 7/8 | 88 | Low likelihood (<5%) of CAD |
| 1990 | Van Train | 154 | Exercise | Tl | 62/76 | 82 | Low likelihood (<5%) of CAD |
| 1992 | Kiat | 16 | Exercise | Tl | 49/55 | 89 | Low likelihood (<5%) of CAD |
| 1993 | Berman | 29 | Exercise | Tl/MIBI | 102/107 | 95 | Low likelihood (<5%) of CAD |
| 1994 | Heo | 187 | Exercise or adenosine | Tl/MIBI | 33/34 | 97 | Low pretest probability (<5%) of CAD |
| 1994 | Van Train | 161 | Exercise | MIBI | 30/37 | 81 | Low likelihood (<5%) of CAD |
| 1995 | Zaret | 188 | Exercise | Tetrofosmin | 56/58 | 97 | Low likelihood (<3%) of CAD |
| 1995 | Kiat | 189 | Arbutamine | Tl | 52/58 | 90 | Low likelihood (<5%) of CAD |
| 1996 | Hendel | 190 | Exercise | Furifosmin | 39/39 | 100 | Low likelihood (<5%) of CAD |
| 1996 | Amanullah | 179 | Adenosine | MIBI | 66/71 | 93 | Low likelihood (<10%) of CAD |
| 1997 | Heo | 191 | Exercise | MIBI | 58/61 | 95 | Low pretest probability (<5%) of CAD |
| Total | | | | | 701/763 | 92 | |

Based on English-language manuscripts.
CAD, coronary artery disease; MIBI, $^{99m}$Tc-sestamibi; Tl, $^{201}$Tl; Tetrofosmin, $^{99m}$Tc-tetrofosmin; Furifosmin, $^{99m}$Tc-furifosmin.
From Berman D, Germano G. Myocardial perfusion single photon approaches. In: Pohost G, Berman DS, O'Rourke R, et al., eds. *Imaging in cardiovascular disease.* Philadelphia: Lippincott Williams & Wilkins, 2000, in press.

CADENZA computer algorithm (85)—a method that determines CAD likelihood based on age, sex, symptom classification, and conventional cardiac risk factors (resting systolic blood pressure, smoking history, glucose intolerance, resting ECG ST-segment abnormalities). Patients with a low pre-ETT likelihood of CAD do not require further diagnostic testing, although continued medical follow-up or a watchful-waiting approach is recommended. Patients with a low-intermediate pre-ETT likelihood of CAD (0.15 to 0.50) should undergo standard ETT as the next diagnostic step. Those who continue to have an intermediate likelihood of CAD after ETT (or those with an indeterminate ETT) and those whose pre-ETT likelihood of CAD was in the 0.50 to 0.85 range (in these patients even a negative ETT would not result in a low likelihood of CAD) will benefit from exercise nuclear testing. Patients

with a high pre-ETT likelihood of CAD (>0.85) are generally considered to have an established diagnosis of CAD, and would not need nuclear stress testing for diagnostic purposes. As described below, nuclear stress testing may be very effective in risk stratification of such patients.

## Risk Stratification/Patient Management

The most rapidly growing area of application of myocardial perfusion SPECT is risk stratification based on increased acceptance of a new paradigm in patient management. A risk-based approach to patients with suspected CAD appears better suited to the modern environment of cost containment and dramatic improvements in medical therapy than the approach focusing on simple diagnosis, in which the patient with disease undergoes coronary angiography and then frequently is revascularized. With the risk-based approach, the focus is not on predicting who has CAD, but on identifying and separating patients at risk for cardiac death, patients at risk for nonfatal myocardial infarction, and patients at low risk for either event. The advantage of this prognostic end point in noninvasive testing is that it defines who has disease and is at risk for an adverse event, thus needing to be treated.

The basic concept in the use of nuclear tests for risk stratification is that they are best applied to patients with an intermediate risk of a subsequent cardiac event, analogous to the optimal diagnostic application of nuclear testing of patients with an intermediate likelihood of having CAD. For prognostic testing, patients known to be at high risk or low risk would not be appropriate patients for cost-effective risk stratification, since they are already risk stratified. For

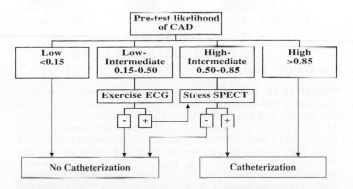

**FIGURE 10.21.** Role of myocardial perfusion SPECT in detection of CAD. (From Germano G, Berman D, eds. *Clinical gated cardiac SPECT.* Armonk, NY: Futura, 1999, with permission.)

purposes of risk assessment, it has been proposed that low risk is defined as a less than 1% cardiac mortality rate per year, high risk as a greater than 3% cardiac mortality rate per year, and intermediate risk as a 1% to 3% cardiac mortality rate per year (94–94a). Since the mortality risk for patients undergoing either coronary artery bypass grafting or angioplasty is greater than 1% per year (95), mildly symptomatic patients with a less than 1% mortality rate would not be candidates for revascularization to improve survival and would be appropriately classified by this rate as at a low risk of death.

The basis for the power of nuclear testing for risk stratification is found in the fact that the major determinants of prognosis in CAD can be assessed by measurements of stress-induced perfusion or function. These measurements include the amount of infarcted myocardium, the amount of jeopardized myocardium (supplied by vessels with hemodynamically significant stenosis), and the degree of jeopardy (tightness of the individual coronary stenosis). An additional important factor in prognostic assessment is the stability (or instability) of the CAD process. This last consideration may help interpret what appears to be a paradox: nuclear tests, which, in general, are expected to be positive only in the presence of hemodynamically significant stenosis, are associated with a very low risk of either cardiac death or nonfatal myocardial infarction when normal; in contrast, it has been observed that most myocardial infarctions occur in regions with premyocardial infarction lesions causing less than 50% stenosis (96,97). It has been postulated that this paradox may be explained by the different response to stress of mild stenoses associated with stable and unstable plaque. For example, it has been shown that unstable plaque is associated with abnormal endothelial function, resulting in a vasoconstrictive response to acetylcholine stimulation, whereas stable mild coronary lesions respond with vasodilation to acetylcholine (98). It is possible that factors released during exercise or vasodilator stress may be similar to acetylcholine in terms of stimulation of a differential endothelial response in stable and unstable plaque. Thus, beyond the ability to define anatomic stenosis, nuclear tests (by virtue of their physiologic assessments) would be able to discern abnormalities of endothelial function associated with high risk, even in the absence of significant stenosis.

## Suspected Chronic Coronary Artery Disease

Ladenheim et al. (99), from our group, have previously documented that the extent and severity of ischemia, as reflected by nuclear variables, are independent prognostic markers and that, for prognostic purposes, exercise myocardial perfusion SPECT provides incremental information over clinical and exercise variables (113).

The most remarkable aspect of this work was that the greatest incremental information for prognosis was pro-

vided not in the patients with intermediate likelihood of disease, but in those with a high likelihood of coronary disease (when this method is not useful for detection of CAD). Exercise 201Tl SPECT was subsequently shown by Iskandrian et al. (100) to provide significant information over clinical information alone or clinical plus exercise information. Furthermore, these authors demonstrated that, once the SPECT information was known, there was no further incremental prognostic information provided by catheterization data (100).

After converting to the use of stress sestamibi imaging as part of the dual-isotope protocol, we felt it important to investigate whether the previous prognostic experience using 201Tl was also applicable to 99mTc-sestamibi imaging. In a study of 1,702 patients, of whom 1,131 had normal scan results, we demonstrated that a normal 99mTc-sestamibi scan is associated with a very low (0.2%) likelihood of cardiac death or myocardial infarction over a 20-month period (Fig. 10.22) (55). Concordant with the results of Ladenheim et al. (99), this study also documented that the greatest separation in event rates between the patients with normal and abnormal test results occurred in patients with a high pretest likelihood of CAD, supporting the use of prognostic testing in this large patient subset.

On the basis of this prognostic data, we devised an optimized nuclear strategy for the assessment of prognosis (Fig. 10.23) (55). With this approach, it is recommended that patients with a low pretest likelihood of CAD not be tested, since their risk was observed to be low (0.8% likelihood of death or myocardial infarction over a 20-month follow-up). The remaining patients would be divided on the basis of

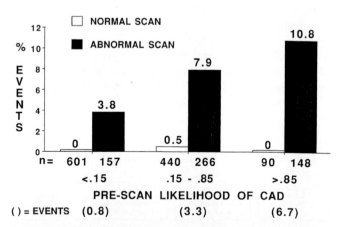

**FIGURE 10.22.** Rate of cardiac events [cardiac death or nonfatal myocardial infarction (MI)] throughout the follow-up period (≥20 ± 5 months) as a function of SPECT results and pre-scan likelihood of CAD (<0.15 = low likelihood; 0.15–0.85 = intermediate likelihood; >0.85 = high likelihood). *Solid bars* = abnormal scan results; *open bars* = normal scan results. (Adapted from Berman DS, Hachamovitch R, Kiat H, et al. Incremental value of prognostic testing in patients with known or suspected ischemic heart disease: a basis for optimal utilization of exercise technetium-99m sestamibi myocardial perfusion single-photon emission computed tomography. *J Am Coll Cardiol* 1995;26:639–647, with permission.)

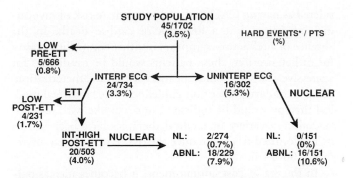

**FIGURE 10.23.** Optimized nuclear strategy for prognostic purposes. Low pre-ETT, low pre-exercise tolerance test likelihood of CAD; interp ECG, interpretable ECG for exercise purposes; uninterp ECG, uninterpretable ECG for exercise purposes; low post-ETT, low postexercise tolerance test likelihood of CAD (<15%); INT-high post-ETT, intermediate to high post-ETT likelihood of CAD ≥15%); NL, normal; ABNL, abnormal. *Cardiac death or nonfatal MI. (Adapted from Berman DS, Hachamovitch R, Kiat H, et al. Incremental value of prognostic testing in patients with known or suspected ischemic heart disease: a basis for optimal utilization of exercise technetium-99m sestamibi myocardial perfusion single-photon emission computed tomography. *J Am Coll Cardiol* 1995;26:639–647, with permission.)

their resting electrocardiogram. If the electrocardiogram could not be interpreted for purposes of stress testing (e.g., left bundle branch block, left ventricular hypertrophy, digoxin, Wolff-Parkinson-White syndrome), direct nuclear testing was highly effective in prognostic stratification. While the overall 20-month event rate in this patient group was 5%, the 50% of the patients who had normal scans enjoyed a 0% event rate over 20 months; the remaining 50% had abnormal scans, which were associated with an 11% event rate over the same period.

In patients with an interpretable exercise ECG response, the overall event rate was lower but still in the intermediate category (3.3% over the 20-month follow-up period). In patients with a low likelihood of CAD following exercise testing, the event rate was also low (1.7% over 20 months), suggesting these patients did not need further nuclear testing. In patients with an intermediate to high postexercise ECG likelihood of CAD, the overall event rate was 4%, and this group was then stratified on a nearly 50-50 basis into patients with a normal scan, in whom the event rate was low (0.7%), and patients with abnormal scans, in whom the event rates were high (7.9%).

In a subsequent publication involving an expanded patient population, our group examined the differences in the prognostic value of $^{99m}$Tc-sestamibi perfusion SPECT in women versus men (101). The combination of clinical, exercise, and nuclear variables yielded incremental prognostic information both in women and men. Of interest, nuclear information added substantially more information in women than in men. Furthermore, the study showed that women were risk stratified more efficiently than men, suggesting the potential for a more cost-efficient strategy in

women using myocardial perfusion SPECT. In that study, the same optimized strategy found to be valid in the overall population worked effectively in women and in men.

Thus, a large number of studies comprising tens of thousands of patients have now clearly documented the effectiveness of nuclear testing for prognostic stratification. What has also been documented is that this risk stratification has an effect on patient outcome. We and others thought that documentation of the postnuclear testing catheterization rate, which governs the rate of revascularization, could be considered an indication of the effect of testing on patient outcome.

After initially describing a low catheterization rate in patients with normal scans (55), we evaluated a population of 2,203 patients with no known CAD (patients with primary myocardial infarction, catheterization, bypass surgery, or angioplasty were excluded) (56). The follow-up was of 18 ± 7 months' duration. In this population, nuclear scanning added dramatically to the prediction of subsequent hard cardiac events. By multivariate analysis, the nuclear result was clearly the overwhelmingly dominant factor determining the subsequent referral to catheterization. Of great clinical importance, the study demonstrated that myocardial perfusion SPECT was most effective in risk stratification and governing management in patients with intermediate clinical risk. In this regard, the data were analyzed as a function of the Duke treadmill score, a composite clinical variable of documented prognostic importance (102). In all patient groups, the subsequent catheterization rates more closely paralleled the nuclear score results than the Duke treadmill score results. However, patients with a low Duke treadmill score had a hard event rate of less than 1%, perhaps not needing nuclear testing. Those with a high Duke treadmill score (representing less than 5% of the population) overall had a high event rate of 7.7% over the 18-month follow-up, and could have been directly catheterized. The majority of the patients in the study, however, fell into the category of an intermediate Duke treadmill score with an intermediate event rate of 2.5%. Within this category, those patients with a normal scan had a very low event rate and were infrequently catheterized, those with moderately abnormal scans had intermediate event rates and an intermediate rate of catheterization, and those with moderately to severely abnormal scans had higher event rates with higher rates of catheterization. Thus, the nuclear tests were able to stratify patients who could not be differentiated according to risk by Duke treadmill score alone. Similar relationships between event rates and catheterization rates were documented in men and women (103). Similar strong relationships between the results of myocardial perfusion SPECT and subsequent catheterization rates have been reported by Bateman et al. (104) and Nallamothu et al. (105).

An important further application of nuclear data derives from observations from multiple randomized trials involving patients with stable angina. To date, no randomized trial has shown that either CABG or PTCA reduces the risk of myocardial infarction in patients with angina. Multiple trials have demonstrated, however, that revascularization can reduce the risk of cardiac death in selected high-risk subsets. Since the annual mortality rate of patients undergoing revascularization is at least 1% (95), it would appear logical that patients who could be predicted to have a rate of cardiac death of less than 1% per year would not warrant revascularization for purposes of improving survival. To determine whether nuclear testing could be utilized to this end, Hachamovitch et al. (57) analyzed 5,183 patients undergoing stress perfusion SPECT testing in our laboratories. Approximately one-third of these patients underwent adenosine stress and two-thirds exercise stress. The follow-up duration was 646 ± 226 days, and 158 nonfatal myocardial infarctions and 119 cardiac deaths were observed in this group. An important result from this study is illustrated in Fig. 10.24, which separately analyzes the nonfatal myocardial infarction and cardiac death rates as a function of the summed stress perfusion scores. Patients with normal scans had relatively low risk for cardiac events, and patients with moderately and severely abnormal scans were at intermediate risk for both cardiac death and myocardial infarction. Importantly, however, patients with mildly abnormal summed stress scores were at intermediate risk for myocardial infarction (2.7% risk of myocardial infarction per year of follow-up), but were at low risk for subsequent mortality (0.8% cardiac death rate per year of follow-up).

Based on the results of this study, patients with a mildly normal scan (summed stress score = 4 to 8) could be con-

sidered as having CAD and an intermediate risk of myocardial infarction, but a low risk of cardiac death. In the absence of a refractory symptom or other compelling reason for catheterization, these patients would be candidates for aggressive risk factor modification without catheterization, using secondary prevention guidelines. Thus maximal medical therapy would be indicated since, unlike with revascularization, a variety of medical therapies have been shown by randomized trials to reduce the risk of myocardial infarction (106–113).

In the era of cost containment, it becomes increasingly important to determine whether noninvasive test results can be cost-effective. To this end, Shaw et al. (114) have evaluated a patient population of 11,372 consecutive stable angina patients, gathered in a large multicenter trial comprising many laboratories around the United States, including our own. In a matched cohort study comparing direct catheterization to myocardial perfusion SPECT with selective catheterization in patients with chronic stable angina, for all levels of pretest clinical risk, there was a substantial reduction (31–50%) in costs using the myocardial perfusion SPECT plus selective catheterization approach. This cost reduction was seen in both the diagnostic (early) and follow-up (late) costs, which included costs of revascularization (Fig. 10.25). The rates of subsequent nonfatal myocardial infarction and cardiac death were virtually iden-

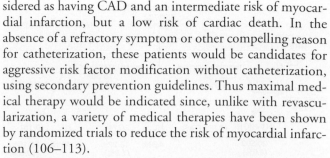

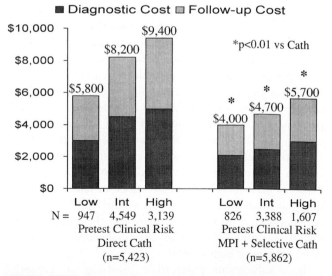

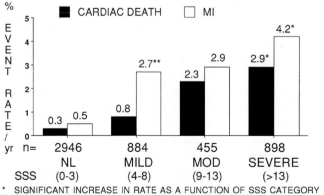

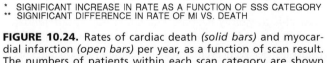

**FIGURE 10.24.** Rates of cardiac death *(solid bars)* and myocardial infarction *(open bars)* per year, as a function of scan result. The numbers of patients within each scan category are shown underneath each pair of columns. *Statistically significant increase as a function of scan result. **Statistically significant increase in rate of myocardial infarction versus cardiac death with scan category. NL, normal; MILD, mildly abnormal; MOD, moderately abnormal; SEVERE, severely abnormal. (From Hachamovitch R, Berman DS, Shaw LJ, et al. Incremental prognostic value of myocardial perfusion single photon emission computed tomography for the prediction of cardiac death: differential stratification for risk of cardiac death and myocardial infarction. *Circulation* 1998;97:535–543, with permission.)

**FIGURE 10.25.** Comparative cost between screening strategies employing direct catheterization (Cath) and myocardial perfusion imaging (MPI) with selective Cath. Low, Int, and High represent low-, intermediate-, and high-risk subsets of the patients with stable angina. Shown are the initial diagnostic costs *(solid bars)* and follow-up costs including costs of revascularization *(gray bars)*. A 30% to 41% reduction in costs was noted in each category. (Adapted from Shaw LJ, Hachamovitch R, Berman DS, et al. The economic consequences of available diagnostic and prognostic strategies for the evaluation of stable angina patients: an observational assessment of the value of precatheterization ischemia. *J Am Coll Cardiol* 1999;33:661–669, with permission.)

tical, when comparing the direct catheterization and myocardial perfusion imaging with selective catheterization approaches in all patient risk subsets. What was significantly different was the rate of revascularization, which was reduced by nearly 50% in the myocardial perfusion imaging with selective catheterization cohort (Fig. 10.26).

Assessing patients by noninvasive testing at one particular point in time does not imply that no follow-up testing is necessary. There can be progression of coronary disease over time, particularly in the absence of aggressive medical therapy. In that regard, our group has preliminarily evaluated the "warranty period" for a normal scan. It appears that for patients who are appropriately referred to testing in the first place (patients with intermediate to high likelihood of CAD), a normal scan result is associated with a very low risk for approximately 2 years. After that the risk rises, suggesting that repeat testing after 2 years should be considered in most patients for prognostic purposes (115).

The foregoing information provides compelling evidence that myocardial perfusion SPECT is effective in the prognostic stratification of patients. It would appear, however, that current data on risk stratification by myocardial perfusion SPECT may actually underestimate the strength of this modality. In all the studies quoted above, patients referred for early revascularization following nuclear testing were excluded from consideration in the prognostic studies. While there is a reason for this exclusion, namely that the event rate may have been altered by the revascularization procedure, the exclusion means that the published data do not reflect the prognostic information data derived from scans performed in the highest risk patient subset. A similar effect occurs to the extent that physicians and patients alter therapy and modify risk factors on the basis of the scan information, thereby likely reducing the event rate that might be observed for a given abnormal scan pattern in a natural history study.

Additionally, recent technical advances in the field of myocardial perfusion SPECT have typically not been included in the prognostic assessments. For example, the impact of quantitative analysis on prognosis has not been studied in any detail, although it has been reported to be equal to semiquantitative analysis, potentially improving the ability to generalize the findings to less experienced laboratories (116). Furthermore, the potent information contained in the ejection fraction assessed from gated SPECT is likely to enhance the prognostic content of myocardial perfusion SPECT (117). A similar gain may occur through consideration of poststress wall motion abnormalities on gated SPECT (70). In addition to the ejection fraction, other important information that can be derived from nuclear studies has not been included in the prognostic assessment, including TID of the left ventricle (64,65), pulmonary uptake of radioactivity as determined by the measurement of lung/heart ratios of radioactivity (47,118), and absolute left ventricular volumes.

## 99mTc-Sestamibi and 99mTc-Tetrofosmin SPECT in Assessing Myocardial Viability

Due to the similarity in the resting myocardial uptake of 99mTc-sestamibi and 99mTc-tetrofosmin, the following comments regarding myocardial viability are likely to apply equally to both agents. In the setting of chronic CAD, nuclear cardiology studies are commonly used to assess viability in patients with abnormal ventricular function. The clinical setting in which this assessment most commonly arises is the evaluation of patients with poor ventricular function, when the likelihood of improvement after revascularization is being considered. This information can be useful in determining the appropriateness of medical management, revascularization, or cardiac transplantation.

In general, the resting distribution of 99mTc-sestamibi provides an effective assessment of myocardial viability, since both perfusion and viability are necessary for the uptake of this tracer. However, since the redistribution of 99mTc-sestamibi in the setting of myocardial ischemia appears to be incomplete, one might expect that 201Tl rest-redistribution imaging might be able to identify patients with reversible resting hypoperfusion (hibernating myocardium), who would appear to have fixed defects by rest 99mTc-sestamibi studies (119). It would also be expected that rest/redistribution myocardial perfusion scintigraphy would be a more accurate approach than 99mTc-sestamibi imaging for detection of viability in

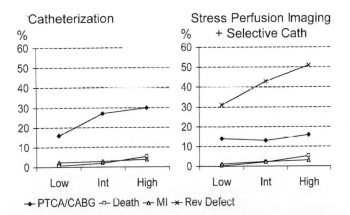

**FIGURE 10.26.** Subsequent event rates in the patient populations in Fig. 10.25. The rates of myocardial infarction (MI) and cardiac death were identical between the populations. What was different was an approximate 50% reduction in revascularization rate in the group approached with myocardial perfusion imaging and selective catheterization. Abbreviations as in Fig. 10.25. Death, cardiac death; REV defect, reversible defect. (Adapted from Shaw LJ, Hachamovitch R, Berman DS, et al. The economic consequences of available diagnostic and prognostic strategies for the evaluation of stable angina patients: an observational assessment of the value of precatheterization ischemia. *J Am Coll Cardiol* 1999;33:661–669, with permission.)

patients with severe hibernation (severe reduction in resting blood flood, downregulation of ventricular function, but preservation of the ability to improve ventricular function with restoration of blood flow) (120,121). Resting myocardial perfusion scintigraphy with $^{99m}$Tc-sestamibi, particularly if augmented by preinjection administration of nitroglycerin (122,123), may nevertheless be as effective as redistribution $^{201}$Tl scintigraphy in assessing myocardial viability (26).

Several studies have documented the ability of $^{201}$Tl and $^{99m}$Tc-sestamibi myocardial perfusion scintigraphy to predict the post-revascularization improvement in abnormal wall motion areas of the myocardium (26,28,62,63,124–128). The relationship between the extent of myocardial viability by $^{201}$Tl scintigraphy and clinical outcome after surgery in ischemic cardiomyopathy has also been investigated (124). Finally, rest/redistribution $^{201}$Tl SPECT has been demonstrated to be of prognostic value in medically treated patients with CAD and left ventricular dysfunction (129). The possibility of further enhancing the viability information of reinjection $^{201}$Tl through the administration of nitroglycerin has been described (130,131). In many of the studies assessing viability, a single cutoff point for myocardial counts in the region in question compared to the maximal observed value is employed, e.g., 50% or 60% of the maximal counts (62,63). Of note, however, is the fact that the inferior wall in non–attenuation-corrected SPECT studies has far fewer counts than the other myocardial regions. This observation would suggest that the ability to predict viability for myocardial perfusion SPECT would be enhanced by approaches that take into account the number of standard deviations below normal in a given region, rather than a single percentage of maximal count uptake.

## Myocardial Viability Protocols

A considerable literature has compared stress-redistribution $^{201}$Tl studies and stress-rest 2-day $^{99m}$Tc-sestamibi studies in patients with chronic coronary syndromes. By visual analyses in two reports comparing stress-rest 2-day $^{99m}$Tc-sestamibi and stress-redistribution $^{201}$Tl SPECT, the extent of exact segmental agreement for normal, reversible, and nonreversible segments was 92% (1,398/1,520 segments) (1,132). Importantly, evidence of nonreversible defects by $^{99m}$Tc-sestamibi was seen in only 1% of patients who had reversible defects by $^{201}$Tl imaging. These comparisons, however, were made only with standard stress-redistribution $^{201}$Tl imaging protocols. A later study (133), using stress-redistribution-reinjection $^{201}$Tl imaging, showed only a 79% agreement, with the 21% of discordant segments largely being irreversible defects by rest $^{99m}$Tc-sestamibi, and showed evidence of viability by both reinjection $^{201}$Tl and $^{18}$F-deoxyglucose (FDG) PET studies. Since the redistribution of $^{99m}$Tc-sestamibi is slower than that of $^{201}$Tl (11), and since the half-life of $^{99m}$Tc is significantly less than

that of $^{201}$Tl, one would expect that redistribution $^{201}$Tl imaging, possibly including late redistribution imaging, would be more effective than $^{99m}$Tc-sestamibi SPECT for assessing hibernating myocardium.

An approach that might minimize this possible difference between the two tracers in the hibernating myocardium would be to utilize nitroglycerin prior to the rest injection of $^{99m}$Tc-sestamibi or $^{99m}$Tc-tetrofosmin. It has been suggested that administration of nitroglycerin prior to the rest injection of $^{201}$Tl (131,134), $^{99m}$Tc-sestamibi (122,123,127,135–137), or $^{99m}$Tc-tetrofosmin (138,139) may improve the detection of viability in hibernating myocardium. The potent effects of nitroglycerin, particularly hypotension, should not be ignored as potential sources of adverse reactions.

In addition, it has recently been shown that low-dose dobutamine $^{99m}$Tc-sestamibi SPECT provides better accuracy for predicting functional recovery than rest SPECT (140). Thus an optimal viability SPECT protocol now consists of rest-redistribution $^{201}$Tl followed by nitroglycerin augmented, low-dose dobutamine $^{99m}$Tc-sestamibi gated SPECT. Our protocol consists of nitroglycerin 0.4 to 0.8 mg sublingually, followed 5 minutes later by the rest injection of $^{99m}$Tc-sestamibi. One hour later a $^{99m}$Tc-sestamibi gated SPECT is acquired, followed immediately with another $^{99m}$Tc-sestamibi gated SPECT acquisition simultaneous with the infusion of low-dose dobutamine (5 mcg/kg/min). Therefore, we can compare wall motion during dobutamine infusion to resting wall motion for improvement and presumed viability.

Another study compared myocardial viability as determined by FDG PET with that determined by rest $^{99m}$Tc-sestamibi SPECT. Of the 418 segments with 51% to 70% of peak $^{99m}$Tc-sestamibi uptake, 55% exhibited evidence of complete viability by positron emission tomography (PET) (141). Of the 238 segments with 31% to 50% of peak uptake, 21% exhibited evidence of viability. In contrast, complete viability was found by PET in only 9% of the defects with ≤30% of peak $^{99m}$Tc-sestamibi uptake. Thus, the accuracy of assessing viability by $^{99m}$Tc-sestamibi may be improved by taking into account the defect severity. This finding has been previously observed with $^{201}$Tl as well (142). Nonetheless, the ability to distinguish subendocardial infarction from hibernating myocardium would not be expected to be possible on the basis of perfusion-defect severity alone.

The dual-isotope approach, by allowing the assessment of $^{201}$Tl redistribution, would allow this distinction. We have demonstrated that incorporation of 24-hour rest-redistribution $^{201}$Tl scintigraphy into the dual-isotope protocol provides detection of an additional 8% to 15% of reversible segments that would go undetected by rest-stress scintigraphy alone (143,143a). As noted above, the injection of tracer on the night before the stress study can eliminate the need for 24-hour studies with this dual-isotope protocol. For inpatients with uncomplicated acute myocardial infarction, this may provide one of the most time-efficient protocols available. In these patients, if postinfarction imaging is safe on a given day, such as day 3, dual-isotope protocols with $^{99m}$Tc-sestamibi in the day-3 stress phase could be completed more rapidly than standard-stress $^{201}$Tl protocols, since the 24-hour post-$^{201}$Tl injection redistribution study, when necessary, is accomplished on day 3 rather than on day 4, thereby potentially decreasing the hospitalization of these patients by 1 day.

## Myocardial Viability Assessment

Table 10.8 illustrates our concept of the relationship between several different myocardial states associated with chronic CAD and the patterns that might be observed in abnormally contracting segments on myocardial perfusion scintigraphy with $^{99m}$Tc-sestamibi or $^{99m}$Tc-tetrofosmin. In the setting of a transmural myocardial infarction, the resting $^{99m}$Tc-sestamibi or $^{99m}$Tc-tetrofosmin uptake (related to resting blood flow) is severely reduced. No reversibility would be expected with either the rest or the stress protocol, and the likelihood of improvement following the revascularization is low. In the setting of a non–Q-wave myocardial infarction, there would be a mild to moderate reduction in resting uptake (depending on the thickness of the infarct), no stress reversibility, and a low likelihood of improvement following revascularization.

In the presence of myocardial hibernation, resting blood flow would be expected to be mildly to even severely reduced, with corresponding reductions in resting $^{201}$Tl or $^{99m}$Tc-perfusion agent uptake (120,121). With $^{201}$Tl, the equilibrium uptake of radioactivity would be expected to be normal, or potentially slightly reduced if true equilibrium was not achieved, or if prolonged hibernation had resulted in cellular degeneration (121). Thus, these patients would demonstrate resting reversibility. For the $^{99m}$Tc agents, this phenomenon can be enhanced by nitroglycerin administration prior to the rest injection of the tracer (122,123). If patients with hibernation are subject to stress, an even greater degree of reduction in flow would be expected, caus-

ing a greater degree of defect reversibility in most cases. The likelihood of improvement with revascularization is great in these patients.

Stunning occurs in the setting of a prolonged episode of severe ischemia (144), with subsequent restoration of flow. It is usually associated with acute CAD, and is most often seen in the setting of aborted myocardial infarction, either by thrombolytic therapy, direct revascularization, or spontaneous thrombolysis. Stunning can also occur in the chronic coronary disease setting, such as following prolonged exercise in patients with high-grade coronary lesions (69,70). In these circumstances, resting myocardial perfusion scintigraphy is generally normal, or minimally reduced, reflecting the return of normal or nearly normal perfusion. However, patients with exercise-induced stunning would be expected to demonstrate marked perfusion defects on the stress study (70). In these patients, the likelihood of improvement in exercise flow and function, as well as postexercise function following revascularization would be high.

It should be noted that the form of stunning observed in conjunction with stress is not generally associated with an abnormality of true resting ventricular function but is discovered as a consequence of measuring ventricular function using stress testing (69,70). For this type of stunning abnormality to improve, revascularization is usually necessary; in contrast, improvement in ventricular function occurs spontaneously over time with the stunning associated with an aborted acute coronary syndrome.

A great deal of attention has been placed on the remodeled left ventricle, usually as a consequence of extensive prior myocardial infarction (145,146). In this circumstance, ventricular function can become diffusely abnormal, even in areas remote from the infarct zone. The area of abnormal contraction associated with remodeling in these patients would be expected to have normal $^{99m}$Tc-sestamibi or $^{99m}$Tc-tetrofosmin uptake, no evidence of reversibility on either stress or rest imaging, and little likelihood of improvement following revascularization. Patients with remodeled left ventricles may have very profoundly reduced

**TABLE 10.8. $^{99m}$TC-SESTAMIBI OR TETROFOSMIN UPTAKE PATTERNS OF HYPOCONTRACTILE MYOCARDIAL SEGMENTS ACCORDING TO THEIR VIABILITY STATUS**

| Viability Status | Rest | Nitrate-Augmented Rest | Stress/Rest Reversibility | Likelihood of Improvement with Revascularization |
|---|---|---|---|---|
| Q wave MI | ↓↓↓ | ↓↓↓ | — | — |
| Non-Q wave MI | ↓ to ↓↓ | ↓ to ↓↓ | — | — |
| Hibernation | ↓ to ↓↓↓↓ | →↓ | ++ | +++ |
| Stunning | → | → | ++ | +++[a] |
| Remodeled | → | → | → | → |
| Nonischemic CM with incidental CAD | → | → | → | → |

CM, cardiomyopathy; MI, myocardial infarction.
[a]Stunning after thrombolysis or direct percutaneous transluminal coronary angioplasty improves spontaneously, whereas the phenomenon of postexercise stunning improves with revascularization.

ventricular function. Given the differential response to revascularization of the remodeled left ventricle and the hibernating left ventricle, the ability of nuclear scanning to differentiate between them becomes important.

Patients with nonischemic cardiomyopathy and concomitant chronic CAD may represent an important patient subset. These patients are frequently discovered by having left ventricular failure, often followed by coronary angiography in which significant (although usually not severe) CAD might be found. Alternatively, there may be historical or electrocardiographic evidence of a small prior myocardial infarction. When CAD is not the principal cause of ventricular dysfunction, the areas of abnormal function will usually have normal or slightly reduced perfusion tracer at rest or stress, and no evidence of reversibility by stress or rest imaging, and will not be expected to improve following revascularization.

It would be highly important to be able to differentiate among the conditions described above, for the purpose of patient management. In that respect, the following general considerations apply when myocardial perfusion scintigraphy is used to help guide patient management decisions: In patients with moderately to severely abnormal left ventricular function, the left ventricle is often enlarged, and there will be a considerable amount of attenuation of $^{201}$Tl, or, to a somewhat lesser extent, $^{99m}$Tc-sestamibi radioactivity. The interpreting physician must take the potential of attenuation into account when interpreting images in this circumstance. Soft tissue attenuation probably explains the frequency with which mild to moderate defects are noted in patients with nonischemic cardiomyopathy and congestive heart failure.

When reversibility of defects is noted on stress/rest studies, the likelihood of post-revascularization improvement of regions with abnormal ventricular function is high. Improvement would also be expected in patients with very severe angiographic CAD (virtually certain to cause severe flow restriction with stress) if normal, mildly reduced, or even moderately reduced tracer uptake is noted on rest scintigraphy, since it could be predicted that such patients would show clear reversibility if stress redistribution imaging were feasible. This inference is commonly made in patients with known coronary anatomy, unstable angina and reluctance to perform stress imaging.

The above circumstances usually lead to straightforward interpretation. Greater difficulty is encountered when there is normal segmental uptake of myocardial perfusion tracers at rest and stress in the setting of severely abnormal ventricular function. The likelihood of improvement in these segments can range from minimal to great, depending on the findings in the rest of the left ventricle. In general, if the patient has reversibility noted in multiple segments, even segments in which reversibility is not noted might improve following revascularization, if a diffuse ischemic cardiomyopathy is present. In these patients, the perfusion tracer content of the most normal region is actually reduced but this fact is not evident (due to the relative perfusion nature of myocardial perfusion SPECT). When the overall degree of reversibility is minimal but a definite perfusion defect is present, the normal tracer content associated with an abnormal contraction pattern is most likely secondary to ventricular remodeling. In these patients, revascularization would not be expected to result in an improvement in ventricular function, although aggressive medical management (e.g., vigorous ACE inhibitor therapy) might improve ventricular size and the patient's symptomatology.

If severely abnormal function is associated with no clear-cut perfusion defects or only very small perfusion defects, it is likely that the patient has a diffuse nonischemic cardiomyopathic process, and if CAD is present, it is most likely incidental. Such patients would not be expected to improve with revascularization therapy.

Another study category that can be difficult to interpret is patients who have a true moderate reduction in radiopharmaceutical uptake at stress and rest imaging. The most common circumstance in which this is observed is in subendocardial infarction that occurred in a region with only a mild coronary lesion secondary to a transient thrombosis or in a region in which successful coronary revascularization was achieved. With $^{201}$Tl imaging, this type of patient may also demonstrate the pattern of reverse redistribution with rest (147,148) or stress imaging (149). The rest or even stress distribution of radioactivity appears normal, due to the failure of autoregulation (148) and the increased blood flow per gram of viable myocardium at rest or stress. The redistribution image, however, is likely to be more reflective of the extent of myocardial viability in these patients. Regions with either moderate nonreversible defect or reverse redistribution would not be expected to improve following revascularization.

Due to the redistribution characteristics of $^{201}$Tl, this agent provides potentially additional information regarding myocardial viability over that provided by the more pure perfusion tracers. In contrast to the $^{99m}$Tc-sestamibi or -tetrofosmin, redistribution imaging has been demonstrated to improve the assessment of myocardial viability in hibernating myocardium. In this regard, late redistribution imaging with $^{201}$Tl (generally considered to be that occurring after 12 hours) may provide additional information over standard 4-hour redistribution imaging. As noted above, however, nitrate-augmented $^{99m}$Tc myocardial perfusion imaging agents may provide similar information to that provided by $^{201}$Tl redistribution imaging for assessment of viability in hibernation.

## ACKNOWLEDGMENTS

The authors gratefully acknowledge the assistance of Jim Gerlach and Xingping (Connie) Kang, M.D., in the preparation of this manuscript, as well as the expert editorial assistance provided by Suzanne Ridgway.

# REFERENCES

1. Kiat H, Maddahi J, Roy LT, et al. Comparison of technetium 99m methoxy isobutyl isonitrile and thallium 201 for evaluation of coronary artery disease by planar and tomographic methods. *Am Heart J* 1989;117:1–11.

2. Li Q-S, Frank TL, Franceschi D, et al. Technetium-99m methoxyisobutyl isonitrile (RP30) for quantification of myocardial ischemia and reperfusion in dogs. *J Nucl Med* 1988;29: 1539–1548.

3. Sinusas AJ, Bergin JD, Edwards NC, et al. Redistribution of $^{99m}$Tc-sestamibi and $^{201}$Tl in the presence of a severe coronary artery stenosis. *Circulation* 1994;89:2332.

4. Nielsen AP, Morris KG, Murdock R, et al. Linear relationship between the distribution of thallium-201 and blood flow in ischemic and nonischemic myocardium during exercise. *Circulation* 1980;61:797–801.

5. Krivokapich J, Smith GT, Huang SC, et al. 13N ammonia myocardial imaging at rest and with exercise in normal volunteers. Quantification of absolute myocardial perfusion with dynamic positron emission tomography. *Circulation* 1989;80:1328–1337.

6. Chan SY, Brunken RC, Czernin J, et al. Comparison of maximal myocardial blood flow during adenosine infusion with that of intravenous dipyridamole in normal men. *J Am Coll Cardiol* 1992;20:979–985.

7. Leppo JA, Meerdink DJ. Comparison of the myocardial uptake of a technetium-labeled isonitrile analogue and thallium. *Circ Res* 1989;65:632–639.

8. Hurwitz GA, Blais M, Powe JE, et al. Stress/injection protocols for myocardial scintigraphy with 99Tcm-sestamibi compared with $^{201}$Tl: implications of early post-stress kinetics. *Nucl Med Commun* 1996;17:400–409.

9. Takahashi N, Reinhardt CP, Marcel R, et al. Myocardial uptake of $^{99m}$Tc-tetrofosmin, sestamibi, and $^{201}$Tl in a model of acute coronary reperfusion. *Circulation* 1996;94:2605–2613.

10. Arbab AS, Koizumi K, Toyama K, et al. Technetium-99m-tetrofosmin, technetium-99m-MIBI and thallium-201 uptake in rat myocardial cells. *J Nucl Med* 1998;39:266–271.

11. Taillefer R, Primeau M, Costi P, et al. Technetium-99m-sestamibi myocardial perfusion imaging in detection of coronary artery disease: comparison between initial (1-hour) and delayed (3-hour) postexercise images. *J Nucl Med* 1991;32:1961–1965.

12. Maurea S, Cuocolo A, Soricelli A, et al. Myocardial viability index in chronic coronary artery disease: technetium-99m-methoxy isobutyl isonitrile redistribution. *J Nucl Med* 1995;36:1953–1960.

13. Soman P, Taillefer R, DePuey E, et al. Improved detection of reversible ischemia by Tc-99m sestamibi compared to Tc-99m tetrofosmin SPECT imaging in mild to moderate coronary artery disease. *J Nucl Cardiol* 1999;6:S35(abst).

14. Esquerré JP, Coca FJ, Martinez SJ, et al. Prone decubitus: a solution to inferior wall attenuation in thallium-201 myocardial tomography. *J Nucl Med* 1989;30:398–401.

15. Segall GM, Davis MJ. Prone versus supine thallium myocardial SPECT: a method to decrease artifactual inferior wall defects. *J Nucl Med* 1989;30:548–555.

16. Kiat H, Van Train KF, Friedman JD, et al. Quantitative stress-redistribution thallium-201 SPECT using prone imaging: methodologic development and validation. *J Nucl Med* 1992; 33:1509–1515.

17. Sinusas AJ, Shi Q, Salzberg MT, et al. Technetium-99m-tetrofosmin to assess myocardial blood flow: experimental validation in an intact canine model of ischemia. *J Nucl Med* 1994;35: 664–671.

18. Jain D, Wackers FJ, Mattera J, et al. Biokinetics of technetium-99m-tetrofosmin: myocardial perfusion imaging agent: implications for a one-day imaging protocol. *J Nucl Med* 1993;34: 1254–1259.

19. Wackers FJ, Berman DS, Maddahi J, et al. Technetium-99m hexakis 2-methoxyisobutyl isonitrile: human biodistribution, dosimetry, safety, and preliminary comparison to thallium-201 for myocardial perfusion imaging. *J Nucl Med* 1989;30:301–311.

20. Berman DS, Kiat H, Maddahi J. The new $^{99m}$Tc myocardial perfusion imaging agents: $^{99m}$Tc-sestamibi and $^{99m}$Tc-teboroxime. *Circulation* 1991;84:17–21.

21. Berman D, Kiat H, Germano G, et al. 99m Tc-sestamibi SPECT. In: DePuey EG, Berman DS, Garcia EV, eds. *Cardiac SPECT imaging*. New York: Raven Press, 1995:121–146.

22. Van Train KF, Areeda J, Garcia EV, et al. Quantitative same-day rest-stress technetium-99m-sestamibi SPECT: definition and validation of stress normal limits and criteria for abnormality. *J Nucl Med* 1993;34:1494–1502.

23. Buell U, Dupont F, Uebis R, et al. 99Tcm-methoxy-isobutyl-isonitrile SPECT to evaluate a perfusion index from regional myocardial uptake after exercise and at rest. Results of a four hour protocol in patients with coronary heart disease and in controls. *Nucl Med Commun* 1990;11:77–94.

24. Heo J, Kegel J, Iskandrian AS, et al. Comparison of same-day protocols using technetium-99m-sestamibi myocardial imaging. *J Nucl Med* 1992;33:186–191.

25. Taillefer R, Gagnon A, Laflamme L, et al. Same day injections of Tc-99m methoxy isobutyl isonitrile (hexamibi) for myocardial tomographic imaging: comparison between rest-stress and stress-rest injection sequences. *Eur J Nucl Med* 1989;15.113–117.

26. Marzullo P, Parodi O, Reisenhofer B, et al. Value of rest thallium-201/technetium-99m sestamibi scans and dobutamine echocardiography for detecting myocardial viability. *Am J Cardiol* 1993;71:166–172.

27. Berman DS, Kiat HS, Van Train KF, et al. Myocardial perfusion imaging with technetium-99m-sestamibi: comparative analysis of available imaging protocols. *J Nucl Med* 1994;35:681–688.

28. Sciagra R, Bisi G, Santoro GM, et al. Comparison of baseline-nitrate technetium-99m sestamibi with rest-redistribution thallium-201 tomography in detecting viable hibernating myocardium and predicting postrevascularization recovery. *J Am Coll Cardiol* 1997;30:384–391.

29. Berman DS, Kiat H, Friedman JD, et al. Separate acquisition rest thallium-201/stress technetium-99m sestamibi dual-isotope myocardial perfusion single-photon emission computed tomography: a clinical validation study. *J Am Coll Cardiol* 1993;22: 1455–1464.

30. Kiat H, Germano G, Friedman J, et al. Comparative feasibility of separate or simultaneous rest thallium-201/stress technetium-99m-sestamibi dual-isotope myocardial perfusion SPECT. *J Nucl Med* 1994;35:542–548.

31. Kamphuis C, Beekman FJ, van Rijk PP, et al. Dual matrix ordered subsets reconstruction for accelerated 3D scatter compensation in single-photon emission tomography. *Eur J Nucl Med* 1998;25:8–18.

32. Cullom S, Liu L, White M. Compensation of attenuation map errors from Tc-99m-sestamibi downscatter with simultaneous Gd-153 transmission scanning. *J Nucl Med* 1996;37:215P(abst).

33. Meerdink DJ, Leppo JA. Experimental properties of technetium-99m agents: myocardial transport of perfusion imaging agents. *Am J Cardiol* 1990;66:9E–15E.

34. Leppo JA, Meerdink DJ. Comparative myocardial extraction of two technetium-labeled BATO derivatives (SQ30217, SQ30214) and thallium. *J Nucl Med* 1990;31:67–74.

35. Chua T, Kiat H, Germano G, et al. Technetium-99m teboroxime regional myocardial washout in subjects with and without coronary artery disease. *Am J Cardiol* 1993;72:728–734.

36. Chua T, Kiat H, Germano G, et al. Rapid back to back adenosine stress/rest technetium-99m teboroxime myocardial perfusion SPECT using a triple-detector camera. *J Nucl Med* 1993; 34:1485–1493.

37. Pasqualini R, Duatti A, Bellande E, et al. Bis(dithiocarbamato) nitrido technetium-99m radiopharmaceuticals: a class of neutral myocardial imaging agents. *J Nucl Med* 1994;35:334.

38. Ghezzi C, Fagret D, Arvieux CC, et al. Myocardial kinetics of TcN-NOEt: a neutral lipophilic complex tracer of regional myocardial blood flow. *J Nucl Med* 1995;36:1069–1077.

39. Gerson MC, Lukes J, Deutsch E, et al. Comparison of technetium 99m Q12 and thallium 201 for detection of angiographically documented coronary artery disease in humans. *J Nucl Cardiol* 1994;1:499–508.

40. Berman D, Germano G. An approach to the interpretation and reporting of gated myocardial perfusion SPECT. In: Germano G, Berman D, eds. *Clinical gated cardiac SPECT.* Armonk, NY: Futura, 1999:147–182.

41. DePuey EG. Artifacts clarified by and caused by gated myocardial perfusion SPECT. In: Germano G, Berman DS, eds. *Clinical gated cardiac SPECT.* Armonk, NY: Futura, 1999;183–237.

42. Prigent FM, Hyun M, Berman DS, et al. Effect of motion on thallium-201 SPECT studies: a simulation and clinical study. *J Nucl Med* 1993;34:1845–1850.

43. Friedman J, Van Train K, Maddahi J, et al. "Upward creep" of the heart: a frequent source of false-positive reversible defects during thallium-201 stress-redistribution SPECT. *J Nucl Med* 1989;30:1718–1722.

44. Aksut SV, Mallavarapu C, Russell J, et al. Implications of increased lung thallium uptake during exercise single photon emission computed tomography imaging. *Am Heart J* 1995; 130:367–373.

45. Jain D, Thompson B, Wackers FJ, et al. Relevance of increased lung thallium uptake on stress imaging in patients with unstable angina and non-Q wave myocardial infarction: results of the Thrombolysis in Myocardial Infarction (TIMI)-IIIB Study. *J Am Coll Cardiol* 1997;30:421–429.

46. Vaccarino RA, Johnson LL, Antunes ML, et al. Thallium-201 lung uptake and peak treadmill exercise first-pass ejection fraction. *Am Heart J* 1995;129:320–329.

47. Bacher-Stier C, Sharir T, Kavanagh P, et al. Post-exercising uptake of TC-99m sestamibi determined by a new automatic technique: validation and application in detection of severe and extensive coronary artery disease and reduced left ventricular function. *J Nucl Med* 2000;41:1190–1197.

48. Liu P, Kiess M, Okada RD, et al. Increased thallium lung uptake after exercise in isolated left anterior descending coronary artery disease. *Am J Cardiol* 1985;55:1469–1473.

49. Martinez EE, Horowitz SF, Castello HJ, et al. Lung and myocardial thallium-201 kinetics in resting patients with congestive heart failure: correlation with pulmonary capillary wedge pressure. *Am Heart J* 1992;123:427–432.

50. Germano G, Chua T, Kiat H, et al. A quantitative phantom analysis of artifacts due to hepatic activity in technetium-99m myocardial perfusion SPECT studies. *J Nucl Med* 1994;35: 356–359.

51. The Cardiovascular Imaging Committee, American College of Cardiology; The Committee on Advanced Cardiac Imaging and Technology, Council on Clinical Cardiology, American Heart Association; and Board of Directors, Cardiovascular Council, Society of Nuclear Medicine. Standardization of cardiac tomographic imaging. *J Am Coll Cardiol* 1992;20:255–256.

52. Berman DS, Kiat H, Van Train K, et al. Technetium 99m sestamibi in the assessment of chronic coronary artery disease. *Semin Nucl Med* 1991;21:190–212.

53. Reisman S, Berman D, Maddahi J, et al. The severe stress thallium defect: an indicator of critical coronary stenosis. *Am Heart J* 1985;110:128–134.

54. Matzer L, Kiat H, Van Train K, et al. Quantitative severity of stress thallium-201 myocardial perfusion single-photon emission computed tomography defects in one-vessel coronary artery disease. *Am J Cardiol* 1993;72:273–279.

55. Berman DS, Hachamovitch R, Kiat H, et al. Incremental value of prognostic testing in patients with known or suspected ischemic heart disease: a basis for optimal utilization of exercise technetium-99m sestamibi myocardial perfusion single-photon emission computed tomography. *J Am Coll Cardiol* 1995;26: 639–647.

56. Hachamovitch R, Berman DS, Kiat H, et al. Exercise myocardial perfusion SPECT in patients without known coronary artery disease: incremental prognostic value and use in risk stratification. *Circulation* 1996;93:905–914.

57. Hachamovitch R, Berman DS, Shaw LJ, et al. Incremental prognostic value of myocardial perfusion single photon emission computed tomography for the prediction of cardiac death: differential stratification for risk of cardiac death and myocardial infarction. *Circulation* 1998;97:535–543.

58. Matzer L, Kiat H, Friedman JD, et al. A new approach to the assessment of tomographic thallium-201 scintigraphy in patients with left bundle branch block. *J Am Coll Cardiol* 1991; 17:1309–1317.

59. Ficaro EP, Fessler JA, Shreve PD, et al. Simultaneous transmission/emission myocardial perfusion tomography. Diagnostic accuracy of attenuation-corrected $^{99m}$Tc-sestamibi single-photon emission computed tomography. *Circulation* 1996;93:463–473.

60. Cullom S, Hendel R, Liu L, et al. Diagnostic accuracy and image quality of a scatter, attenuation and resolution compensation method for Tc-99m cardiac SPECT: preliminary results. *J Nucl Med* 1996;37:81P(abst).

61. Germano G, Kavanagh P, Waechter P, et al. A new automatic approach to myocardial perfusion SPECT quantitation. *J Nucl Med* 1998;39:62P(abst).

62. Bonow R. Assessment of myocardial viability with thallium-201. In: Zaret BL, Beller G, eds. *Nuclear cardiology:* state of the art and future directions, 2nd ed. St. Louis: CV Mosby, 1998: 503–512.

63. Udelson JE, Coleman PS, Metherall J, et al. Predicting recovery of severe regional ventricular dysfunction. Comparison of resting scintigraphy with $^{201}$Tl and $^{99m}$Tc-sestamibi. *Circulation* 1994;89:2552–2561.

64. Weiss AT, Berman DS, Lew AS, et al. Transient ischemic dilation of the left ventricle on stress thallium-201 scintigraphy: a marker of severe and extensive coronary artery disease. *J Am Coll Cardiol* 1987;9:752–759.

65. Mazzanti M, Germano G, Kiat H, et al. Identification of severe and extensive coronary artery disease by automatic measurement of transient ischemic dilation of the left ventricle in dual-isotope myocardial perfusion SPECT. *J Am Coll Cardiol* 1996; 27:1612–1620.

66. Chouraqui P, Rodrigues EA, Berman DS, et al. Significance of dipyridamole-induced transient dilation of the left ventricle during thallium-201 scintigraphy in suspected coronary artery disease. *Am J Cardiol* 1990;66:689–694.

67. Germano G, Kiat H, Kavanagh PB, et al. Automatic quantification of ejection fraction from gated myocardial perfusion SPECT. *J Nucl Med* 1995;36:2138–2147.

68. Smith WH, Kastner RJ, Calnon DA, et al. Quantitative gated single photon emission computed tomography imaging: a counts-based method for display and measurement of regional

and global ventricular systolic function. *J Nucl Cardiol* 1997;4: 451–463.

69. Johnson LL, Verdesca SA, Aude WY, et al. Postischemic stunning can affect left ventricular ejection fraction and regional wall motion on post-stress gated sestamibi tomograms. *J Am Coll Cardiol* 1997;30:1641–1648.

70. Sharir T, Bacher-Stier C, Levin HC, et al. Identification of severe and extensive coronary artery disease by post-exercise regional wall motion abnormalities in Tc technetium-99m sestamibi gated single-photon omission computed tomography. *Am J Cardiol* in press.

71. Germano G, Erel J, Lewin H, et al. Automatic quantitation of regional myocardial wall motion and thickening from gated technetium-99m sestamibi myocardial perfusion single-photon emission computed tomography. *J Am Coll Cardiol* 1997;30: 1360–1367.

72. Zanger D, Bhatnagar A, Hausner E, et al. Automated calculation of ejection fraction from gated Tc-99m sestamibi images-comparison to quantitative echocardiography. *J Nucl Cardiol* 1997;4:S78 (abst).

73. Bateman T, Magalski A, Barnhart C, et al. Global left ventricular function assessment using gated SPECT-201: comparison with echocardiography. *J Am Coll Cardiol* 1998;31:441A(abst).

74. Cwajg E, Cwajg J, He Z, et al. Comparison between gated-SPECT and echocardiography for the analysis of global and regional left ventricular function and volumes. *J Am Coll Cardiol* 1998;31:440A–441A(abst).

75. Mathew D, Zabrodina Y, Mannting F. Volumetric and functional analysis of left ventricle by gated SPECT: a comparison with echocardiographic measurements. *J Am Coll Cardiol* 1998; 31:44A(abst).

76. Akinboboye O, El-Khoury Coffin L, Sciacca R, et al. Accuracy of gated SPECT thallium left ventricular volumes and ejection fractions: comparison with three-dimensional echocardiography. *J Am Coll Cardiol* 1998;31:85A(abst).

77. Germano G, VanDecker W, Mintz R, et al. Validation of left ventricular volumes automatically measured with gated myocardial perfusion SPECT. *J Am Coll Cardiol* 1998;31:43A(abst).

78. Iskandrian A, Germano G, VanDecker W, et al. Validation of left ventricular volume measurements by gated SPECT Tc-99m sestamibi imaging. *J Nucl Cardiol* 1998;5:574–578.

79. He Z, Vick G, Vaduganathan P, et al. Comparison of left ventricular volumes and ejection fraction measured by gated SPECT and by cine magnetic resonance imaging. *J Am Coll Cardiol* 1998;31:44A(abst).

80. Germano G, Berman D. On the accuracy and reproducibility of quantitative gated myocardial perfusion SPECT. *J Nucl Med* 1999;40:810–813.

81. Berman D, Germano G, Lewin H, et al. Comparison of post-stress ejection fraction and relative left ventricular volumes by automatic analysis of gated myocardial perfusion single-photon emission computed tomography acquired in the supine and prone positions. *J Nucl Cardiol* 1998;5:40–47.

82. Germano G, Kavanagh PB, Kavanagh JT, et al. Repeatability of automatic left ventricular cavity volume measurements from myocardial perfusion SPECT. *J Nucl Cardiol* 1998;5: 477–483.

83. White HD, Norris RM, Brown MA, et al. Left ventricular end-systolic volume as the major determinant of survival after recovery from myocardial infarction. *Circulation* 1987;76:44–51.

84. Pfeffer MA, Braunwald E, Moye LA, et al. Effect of captopril on mortality and morbidity in patients with left ventricular dysfunction after myocardial infarction. Results of the survival and ventricular enlargement trial. The SAVE Investigators. *N Engl J Med* 1992;327:669–677.

85. Diamond GA, Staniloff HM, Forrester JS, et al. Computer-assisted diagnosis in the noninvasive evaluation of patients with suspected coronary artery disease. *J Am Coll Cardiol* 1983;1: 444–455.

86. Staniloff HM, Forrester JS, Berman DS, et al. Prediction of death, myocardial infarction, and worsening chest pain using thallium scintigraphy and exercise electrocardiography. *J Nucl Med* 1986;27:1842–1848.

87. Pryor DB, Shaw L, Harrell FE Jr, et al. Estimating the likelihood of severe coronary artery disease. *Am J Med* 1991;90: 553–562.

88. Iskandrian AS, Verani MS, Heo J. Pharmacologic stress testing: mechanism of action, hemodynamic responses, and results in detection of coronary artery disease. *J Nucl Cardiol* 1994;1: 94–111.

89. Fleischmann KE, Hunink MG, Kuntz KM, et al. Exercise echocardiography or exercise SPECT imaging? A meta-analysis of diagnostic test performance. *JAMA* 1998;280:913–920.

90. Rozanski A, Diamond GA, Berman D, et al. The declining specificity of exercise radionuclide ventriculography. *N Engl J Med* 1983;309:518–522.

91. Maddahi J, Garcia EV, Berman DS, et al. Improved noninvasive assessment of coronary artery disease by quantitative analysis of regional stress myocardial distribution and washout of thallium-201. *Circulation* 1981;64:924–935.

92. Van Train KF, Berman DS, Garcia EV, et al. Quantitative analysis of stress thallium-201 myocardial scintigrams: a multicenter trial. *J Nucl Med* 1986;27:17–25.

93. Diamond GA, Forrester JS. Analysis of probability as an aid in the clinical diagnosis of coronary-artery disease. *N Engl J Med* 1979;300:1350–1358.

94. Berman D, Hachamovitch R, Lewin H, et al. Risk stratification in coronary artery disease: implications for stabilization and prevention. *Am J Cardiol* 1997;79:10–16.

94a. Gibbons R, Chatterjee K, Daley J, et al. ACC/AHA/ACP-ASIM guidelines for the management of patients with chronic stable angina. *J Am Coll Cardiol* 1999;33:2092–2197.

95. Comparison of coronary bypass surgery with angioplasty in patients with multivessel disease. The Bypass Angioplasty Revascularization Investigation (BARI) Investigators. *N Engl J Med* 1996;335:217–225.

96. Little WC, Constantinescu M, Applegate RJ, et al. Can coronary angiography predict the site of a subsequent myocardial infarction in patients with mild-to-moderate coronary artery disease? *Circulation* 1988;78:1157–1166.

97. Ambrose JA, Tannenbaum MA, Alexopoulos D, et al. Angiographic progression of coronary artery disease and the development of myocardial infarction. *J Am Coll Cardiol* 1988;12:56–62.

98. Hasdai D, Gibbons RJ, Holmes DR Jr, et al. Coronary endothelial dysfunction in humans is associated with myocardial perfusion defects. *Circulation* 1997;96:3390–3395.

99. Ladenheim ML, Pollock BH, Rozanski A, et al. Extent and severity of myocardial hypoperfusion as predictors of prognosis in patients with suspected coronary artery disease. *J Am Coll Cardiol* 1986;7:464–471.

100. Iskandrian AS, Chae SC, Heo J, et al. Independent and incremental prognostic value of exercise single-photon emission computed tomographic (SPECT) thallium imaging in coronary artery disease. *J Am Coll Cardiol* 1993;22:665–670.

101. Hachamovitch R, Berman DS, Kiat H, et al. Effective risk stratification using exercise myocardial perfusion SPECT in women: gender-related differences in prognostic nuclear testing. *J Am Coll Cardiol* 1996;28:34–44.

102. Mark DB, Hlatky MA, Harrell FE Jr, et al. Exercise treadmill score for predicting prognosis in coronary artery disease. *Ann Intern Med* 1987;106:793–800.

103. Hachamovitch R, Berman DS, Kiat H, et al. Gender-related

differences in clinical management after exercise nuclear testing. *J Am Coll Cardiol* 1995;26:1457–1464.

104. Bateman TM, O'Keefe JH Jr, Dong VM, et al. Coronary angiographic rates after stress single-photon emission computed tomographic scintigraphy. *J Nucl Cardiol* 1995;2:217–223.

105. Nallamothu N, Pancholy SB, Lee KR, et al. Impact on exercise single-photon emission computed tomographic thallium imaging on patient management and outcome. *J Nucl Cardiol* 1995;2:334–338.

106. Randomised trial of cholesterol lowering in 4444 patients with coronary heart disease: the Scandinavian Simvastatin Survival Study (4S). *Lancet* 1994;344:1383–1389.

107. Shepherd J, Cobbe SM, Ford I, et al. Prevention of coronary heart disease with pravastatin in men with hypercholesterolemia. West of Scotland Coronary Prevention Study Group. *N Engl J Med* 1995;333:1301–1307.

108. Pfeffer MA, Sacks FM, MoyΘ LA, et al. Cholesterol and Recurrent Events: a secondary prevention trial for normolipidemic patients. CARE Investigators. *Am J Cardiol* 1995;76:98C–106C.

109. Pasternak RC, Brown LE, Stone PH, et al. Effect of combination therapy with lipid-reducing drugs in patients with coronary heart disease and "normal" cholesterol levels. A randomized, placebo-controlled trial. Harvard Atherosclerosis Reversibility Project (HARP) Study Group. *Ann Intern Med* 1996;125:529–540.

110. Borzak S, Cannon CP, Kraft PL, et al. Effects of prior aspirin and anti-ischemic therapy on outcome of patients with unstable angina. TIMI 7 Investigators. Thrombin Inhibition in Myocardial Ischemia. *Am J Cardiol* 1998;81:678–681.

111. Kober L, Torp-Pedersen C, Carlsen JE, et al. A clinical trial of the angiotensin-converting-enzyme inhibitor trandolapril in patients with left ventricular dysfunction after myocardial infarction. Trandolapril Cardiac Evaluation (TRACE) Study Group. *N Engl J Med* 1995;333:1670–1676.

112. Haim M, Shotan A, Boyko V, et al. Effect of beta-blocker therapy in patients with coronary artery disease in New York Heart Association classes II and III. The Bezafibrate Infarction Prevention (BIP) Study Group. *Am J Cardiol* 1998;81:1455–1460.

113. Ornish D, Brown SE, Scherwitz LW, et al. Can lifestyle changes reverse coronary heart disease? The Lifestyle Heart Trial. *Lancet* 1990;336:129–133.

114. Shaw LJ, Hachamovitch R, Berman DS, et al. The economic consequences of available diagnostic and prognostic strategies for the evaluation of stable angina patients: an observational assessment of the value of precatheterization ischemia. *J Am Coll Cardiol* 1999;33:661–669.

115. Hachamovitch R, Berman D, Kiat H, et al. What is the warranty period for a normal scan? Temporal changes in risk in patients with normal exercise sestamibi SPECT. *Circulation* 1995;92:I-130(abst).

116. Berman DS, Kang X, Van Train KF, et al. Comparative prognostic value of automatic quantitative analysis versus semiquantitative visual analysis of exercise myocardial perfusion single-photon emission computed tomography. *J Am Coll Cardiol* 1998;32:1987–1995.

117. Sharir T, Germano G, Kavanagh PB, et al. Incremental prognostic value of post-stress left ventricular rejection traction and volume by gated myocardial perfusion single photon emission computed tomography. *Circulation* 1999;100:1035–1042.

118. Morise AP. An incremental evaluation of the diagnostic value of thallium single-photon emission computed tomographic imaging and lung/heart ratio concerning both the presence and extent of coronary artery disease. *J Nucl Cardiol* 1995;2:238–245.

119. Marcassa C, Galli M, Cuocolo A, et al. Rest-redistribution thallium-201 and rest technetium-99m-sestamibi SPECT in patients with stable coronary artery disease and ventricular dysfunction. *J Nucl Med* 1997;38:419–424.

120. Tubau JF, Rahimtoola SH. Hibernating myocardium: a historical perspective. *Cardiovasc Drugs Ther* 1992;6:267–271.

121. Elsässer A, Schlepper M, Klövekorn WP, et al. Hibernating myocardium: an incomplete adaptation to ischemia. *Circulation* 1997;96:2920–2931.

122. Galli M, Marcassa C, Imparato A, et al. Effects of nitroglycerin by technetium-99m sestamibi tomoscintigraphy on resting regional myocardial hypoperfusion in stable patients with healed myocardial infarction. *Am J Cardiol* 1994;74:843–848.

123. Maurea S, Cuocolo A, Soricelli A, et al. Enhanced detection of viable myocardium by technetium-99m-MIBI imaging after nitrate administration in chronic coronary artery disease. *J Nucl Med* 1995;36:1945–1952.

124. Pagley PR, Beller GA, Watson DD, et al. Improved outcome after coronary bypass surgery in patients with ischemic cardiomyopathy and residual myocardial viability. *Circulation* 1997;96:793–800.

125. Berger BC, Watson DD, Burwell LR, et al. Redistribution of thallium at rest in patients with stable and unstable angina and the effect of coronary artery bypass surgery. *Circulation* 1979;60:1114–1125.

126. Iskandrian AS, Hakki AH, Kane SA, et al. Rest and redistribution thallium-201 myocardial scintigraphy to predict improvement in left ventricular function after coronary arterial bypass grafting. *Am J Cardiol* 1983;51:1312–1316.

127. Bisi G, Sciagrà R, Santoro GM, et al. Rest technetium-99m sestamibi tomography in combination with short-term administration of nitrates: feasibility and reliability for prediction of postrevascularization outcome of asynergic territories. *J Am Coll Cardiol* 1994;24:1282–1289.

128. Dakik HA, Howell JF, Lawrie GM, et al. Assessment of myocardial viability with $^{99m}$Tc-sestamibi tomography before coronary bypass graft surgery: correlation with histopathology and postoperative improvement in cardiac function. *Circulation* 1997;96:2892–2898.

129. Gioia G, Milan E, Giubbini R, et al. Prognostic value of tomographic rest-redistribution thallium 201 imaging in medically treated patients with coronary artery disease and left ventricular dysfunction. *J Nucl Cardiol* 1996;3:150–156.

130. Basu S, Senior R, Raval U, et al. Superiority of nitrate-enhanced $^{201}$Tl over conventional redistribution $^{201}$Tl imaging for prognostic evaluation after myocardial infarction and thrombolysis. *Circulation* 1997;96:2932–2937.

131. He ZX, Medrano R, Hays JT, et al. Nitroglycerin-augmented $^{201}$Tl reinjection enhances detection of reversible myocardial hypoperfusion. A randomized, double-blind, parallel, placebo-controlled trial. *Circulation* 1997;95:1799–1805.

132. Kahn JK, McGhie I, Akers MS, et al. Quantitative rotational tomography with $^{201}$Tl and $^{99m}$Tc 2-methoxy-isobutyl-isonitrile. A direct comparison in normal individuals and patients with coronary artery disease. *Circulation* 1989;79:1282–1293.

133. Dilsizian V, Perrone-Filardi P, Arrighi JA, et al. Concordance and discordance between stress-redistribution-reinjection and rest-redistribution thallium imaging for assessing viable myocardium. Comparison with metabolic activity by positron emission tomography. *Circulation* 1993;88:941–952.

134. Antonopoulos A, Georgiou E, Kyriakidis M, et al. Early postexercise thallium-201 reinjection after sublingual nitroglycerin augmentation: effects on detection of myocardial ischemia and/or viability. *Clin Cardiol* 1998;21:419–426.

135. Bisi G, Sciagrà R, Santoro GM, et al. Technetium-99m-sestamibi imaging with nitrate infusion to detect viable hibernating myocardium and predict postrevascularization recovery. *J Nucl Med* 1995;36:1994–2000.

136. Greco C, Ciavolella M, Tanzilli G, et al. Preoperative identification of viable myocardium: effectiveness of nitroglycerine-

induced changes in myocardial sestamibi uptake. *Cardiovasc Surg* 1998;6:149–155.

137. Baszko A, Blaszyk K, Cieslinski A, et al. 99Tcm-sestamibi tomoscintigraphy at rest and after nitrate administration in predicting wall motion recovery after revascularization. *Nucl Med Commun* 1998;19:1141–1148.

138. Flotats A, Carrio I, Estorch M, et al. Nitrate administration to enhance the detection of myocardial viability by technetium-99m tetrofosmin single-photon emission tomography. *Eur J Nucl Med* 1997;24:767–773.

139. Peix A, Lopez A, Ponce F, et al. Enhanced detection of reversible myocardial hypoperfusion by technetium 99m-tetrofosmin imaging and first-pass radionuclide angiography after nitroglycerin administration. *J Nucl Cardiol* 1998;5:469–476.

140. Leoncini M, Marcucci G, Silvestri M, et al. Prediction of functional recovery after revascularization: comparison of low-dose dobutamine Tc-99m sestamibi spect with rest spect and dobutamine echocardiography. *J Nucl Cardiol* 1999;6:S51(abst).

141. Altehoefer C, vom Dahl J, Biedermann M, et al. Significance of defect severity in technetium-99m-MIBI SPECT at rest to assess myocardial viability: comparison with fluorine-18-FDG PET. *J Nucl Med* 1994;35:569–574.

142. Bonow RO, Dilsizian V, Cuocolo A, et al. Identification of viable myocardium in patients with chronic coronary artery disease and left ventricular dysfunction. Comparison of thallium scintigraphy with reinjection and PET imaging with 18F-fluorodeoxyglucose. *Circulation* 1991;83:26–37.

143. Kiat H, Biasio Y, Wong F, et al. Frequency of reversible resting hypoperfusion in patients undergoing rest Tl-201/stress Tc-sestamibi separate acquisition dual isotope myocardial perfusion SPECT. *J Am Coll Cardiol* 1993;21:222A(abst).

143a. Sharir T, Berman DS, Lewin HC, et al. Incremental prognostic value of rest-redistribution Tl-201 single photon emission computed tomography. *Circulation* 1999;100:1964–1970.

144. Braunwald E, Kloner RA. The stunned myocardium: prolonged, postischemic ventricular dysfunction. *Circulation* 1982; 66:1146–1149.

145. Rumberger JA. Ventricular dilatation and remodeling after myocardial infarction. *Mayo Clin Proc* 1994;69:664–674.

146. Gaudron P, Eilles C, Kugler I, et al. Progressive left ventricular dysfunction and remodeling after myocardial infarction. Potential mechanisms and early predictors. *Circulation* 1993;87:755–763.

147. Maddahi J, Berman DS. Reverse redistribution of thallium-201. *J Nucl Med* 1995;36:1019–1021.

148. Weiss AT, Maddahi J, Lew AS, et al. Reverse redistribution of thallium-201: a sign of nontransmural myocardial infarction with patency of the infarct-related coronary artery. *J Am Coll Cardiol* 1986;7:61–67.

149. Hecht HS, Hopkins JM, Rose JG, et al. Reverse redistribution: worsening of thallium-201 myocardial images from exercise to redistribution. *Radiology* 1981;140:177–181.

150. Berman D, Germano G. Myocardial perfusion single photon approaches. In: Pohost G, O'Rourke R, Shah P, et al., eds. *Imaging in cardiovascular disease*. Philadelphia: Lippincott Williams & Wilkins, 2000.

151. Kiat H, Van Train KF, Maddahi J, et al. Development and prospective application of quantitative 2-day stress-rest Tc-99m methoxy isobutyl isonitrile SPECT for the diagnosis of coronary artery disease. *Am Heart J* 1990;120:1255–1266.

152. Mahmarian JJ, Boyce TM, Goldbert RK, et al. Quantitative exercise thallium-201 single photon emission computed tomography for the enhanced diagnosis of ischemic heart disease. *J Am Coll Cardiol* 1990;15:318–329.

153. Nguyen T, Heo J, Ogilby JD, et al. Single photon emission computed tomography with thallium-201 during adenosine induced coronary hyperemia: correlation with coronary arteri-

154. Van Train KF, Maddahi J, Berman DS, et al. Quantitative analysis of tomographic stress thallium-201 myocardial scintigrams: a multicenter trial. *J Nucl Med* 1990;31:1168–1179.

155. Coyne E, Belvedere D, Vande Streek PR, et al. Thallium-201 scintigraphy after intravenous infusion of adenosine compared with exercise thallium testing in the diagnosis of coronary artery disease. *J Am Coll Cardiol* 1991;17:1289–1294.

156. Forster T, McNeill AJ, Salustri A, et al. Simultaneous dobutamine stress echocardiography and technetium-99m isonitrile single-photon emission computed tomography in patients with suspected coronary artery disease. *J Am Coll Cardiol* 1993;21: 1591–1596.

157. Chae SC, Heo J, Iskandrian A, et al. Identification of extensive coronary artery disease in women by exercise single-photon emission computed tomography (SPECT) thallium imaging. *J Am Coll Cardiol* 1993;21:1305–1311.

158. Minoves M, Garcia A, Magrina J, et al. Evaluation of myocardial perfusion defects by means of "bull's eye" images. *Clin Cardiol* 1993;16:16–22.

159. Van Train KF, Areeda J, Garcia EV, et al. Quantitative same-day rest-stress technetium-99m-sestamibi SPECT: definition and validation of stress normal limits and criteria for abnormality. *J Nucl Med* 1993;34:1494–1502.

160. Sylven C, Hagerman I, Ylen M, et al. Variance ECG detection of coronary artery disease—a comparison with exercise stress test and myocardial scintigraphy. *Clin Cardiol* 1994;17:132–140.

161. Van Train KF, Garcia EV, Maddahi J, et al. Multicenter trial validation for quantitative analysis of same-day rest-stress technetium-99m-sestamibi myocardial tomograms. *J Nucl Med* 1994;35:609–618.

162. Palmas W, Friedman JD, Diamond GA, et al. Incremental value of simultaneous assessment of myocardial function and perfusion with technetium-99m sestamibi for prediction of extent of coronary artery disease. *J Am Coll Cardiol* 1995;25:1024–1031.

163. Rubello D, Zanco P, Candelpergher G, et al. Usefulness of 99m-Tc-MIBI stress myocardial SPECT bull's eye quantification in coronary artery disease. *Q J Nucl Med* 1995;39:111–115.

164. Hambye AS, Vervaet A, Lieber S, et al. Diagnostic value and incremental contribution of bicycle exercise, first-pass radionuclide angiography, and ⁹⁹ᵐTc-labeled sestamibi single-photon emission computed tomography in the identification of coronary artery disease in patients without infarction. *J Nucl Cardiol* 1996;3:464–474.

165. Yao Z, Liu XJ, Shi R, et al. A comparison of 99m Tc-MIBI myocardial SPET with electron beam computed tomography in the assessment of coronary artery disease. *Eur J Nucl Med* 1997;24.

166. Heiba SI, Hayat NJ, Salman HS, et al. Technetium-99m-MIBI myocardial SPECT: supine versus right lateral imaging and comparison with coronary arteriography. *J Nucl Med* 1997;38:1510–1514.

167. Ho YL, Wu CC, Huang PJ, et al. Dobutamine stress echocardiography compared with exercise thallium-201 single-photon emission computed tomography in detecting coronary artery disease—effect of exercise level on accuracy. *Cardiology* 1997; 88:379–385.

168. Taillefer R, DePuey EG, Udelson JE, et al. Comparative diagnostic accuracy of Tl-201 and Tc-99m sestamibi SPECT imaging (perfusion and ECG-gated SPECT) in detecting coronary artery disease in women. *J Am Coll Cardiol* 1997;29:69–77.

169. Van Eck-Smit BLF, Poots S, Zwinderman AH, et al. Myocardial SPET imaging with 99Tc m-tetrofosmin in clinical practice: comparison of a 1 day and a 2 day imaging protocol. *Nucl Med Commun* 1997;18:24–30.

170. Budoff MJ, Gillespie R, Georgiou D, et al. Comparison of exercise electron beam computed tomography and sestamibi in the evaluation of coronary artery disease. *Am J Cardiol* 1998;81: 682–687.

171. Santana-Boado C, Candell-Riera J, Castell-Conesa J, et al. Diagnostic accuracy of technetium-99m-MIBI myocardial SPECT in women and men. *J Nucl Med* 1998;39:751–755.

172. Acampa W, Cuocolo A, Sullo P, et al. Direct comparison of technetium 99m-sestamibi and technetium 99m-tetrofosmin cardiac single photon emission computed tomography in patients with coronary artery disease. *J Nucl Cardiol* 1998;5: 265–274.

173. Ho Y, Wu C, Huang P, et al. Assessment of coronary artery disease in women by dobutamine stress echocardiography: comparison with stress thallium-201 single-photon emission computed tomography and exercise electrocardiography. *Am Heart J* 1998;135:655–662.

174. Verani MS, Mahmarian JJ, Hixson JB, et al. Diagnosis of coronary artery disease by controlled coronary vasodilation with adenosine and thallium-201 scintigraphy in patients unable to exercise. *Circulation* 1990;82:80–87.

175. Iskandrian AS, Heo J, Nguyen T, et al. Assessment of coronary artery disease using single-photon emission computed tomography with thallium-201 during adenosine-induced coronary hyperemia. *Am J Cardiol* 1991;67:1190–1194.

176. Nishimura S, Mahmarian JJ, Boyce TM, et al. Quantitative thallium-201 single-photon emission computed tomography during maximal pharmacologic coronary vasodilation with adenosine for assessing coronary artery disease. *J Am Coll Cardiol* 1991;18:736–745.

177. Aksut SV, Pancholy S, Cassel D, et al. Results of adenosine single photon emission computed tomography thallium-201 imaging in hemodynamic nonresponders. *Am Heart J* 1995;30:67–70.

178. Miyagawa M, Kumano S, Sekiya M, et al. Thallium-201 myocardial tomography with intravenous infusion of adenosine triphosphate in diagnosis of coronary artery disease. *J Am Coll Cardiol* 1995;26:1196–1201.

179. Amanullah AM, Kiat H, Friedman JD, et al. Adenosine technetium-99m sestamibi myocardial perfusion SPECT in women: diagnostic efficacy in detection of coronary artery disease. *J Am Coll Cardiol* 1996;27:803–809.

180. Watanabe K, Sekiya M, Ikeda S, et al. Comparison of adenosine triphosphate and dipyridamole in diagnosis by thallium-201 myocardial scintigraphy. *J Nucl Med* 1997;38:577–581.

181. He ZX, Iskandrian AS, Gupta NC, et al. Assessing coronary artery disease with dipyridamole technetium-99m-tetrofosmin SPECT: a multicenter trial. *J Nucl Med* 1997;38:44–48.

182. Amanullah AM, Berman DS, Kiat H, et al. Usefulness of hemodynamic changes during adenosine infusion in predicting the diagnostic accuracy of adenosine technetium-99m sestamibi single-photon emission computed tomography (SPECT). *Am J Cardiol* 1997;79:1319–1322.

183. Cuocolo A, Sullo P, Pace L, et al. Adenosine coronary vasodilation in coronary artery disease: technetium-99m tetrofosmin myocardial tomography versus echocardiography. *J Nucl Med* 1997;38:1089–1094.

184. Takeishi Y, Takahashi N, Fujiwara S, et al. Myocardial tomography with technetium-99m-tetrofosmin during intravenous infusion of adenosine triphosphate. *J Nucl Med* 1998;39:582–586.

185. Maddahi J, Van Train K, Prigent F, et al. Quantitative single photon emission computed thallium-201 tomography for detection and localization of coronary artery disease: optimization and prospective validation of a new technique. *J Am Coll Cardiol* 1989;14:1689–1699.

186. Iskandrian AS, Heo J, Kong B, et al. Effect of exercise level on the ability of thallium-201 tomographic imaging in detecting coronary artery disease: analysis of 461 patients. *J Am Coll Cardiol* 1989;14:1477–1486.

187. Heo J, Wolmer I, Kegel J, et al. Sequential dual-isotope SPECT imaging with thallium-201 and technetium-99m-sestamibi. *J Nucl Med* 1994;35:549–553.

188. Zaret BL, Rigo P, Wackers FJT, et al. Myocardial perfusion imaging with [99m]Tc tetrofosmin. *Circulation* 1995;91:313–319.

189. Kiat H, Iskandrian AS, Villegas BJ, et al. Arbutamine stress thallium-201 single-photon emission computed tomography using a computerized closed-loop delivery system. *J Am Coll Cardiol* 1995;26:1159–1167.

190. Hendel RC, Verani MS, Miller DD, et al. Diagnostic utility of tomographic myocardial perfusion imaging with technetium 99m furifosmin (Q12) compared with thallium 201: results of a phase III multicenter trial. *J Nucl Cardiol* 1996;3:291–300.

191. Heo J, Powers J, Iskandrian AE. Exercise-rest same-day SPECT sestamibi imaging to detect coronary artery disease. *J Nucl Med* 1997;38:200–203.

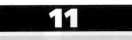
# CLINICAL APPLICATION OF GATED MYOCARDIAL PERFUSION SPECT

**E. GORDON DEPUEY**
**GARY HELLER**
**RAYMOND TAILLEFER**

Gated myocardial perfusion single photon emission computed tomography (SPECT) now provides the ability to assess both myocardial perfusion and ventricular function with scintigraphic imaging. There are a variety of unique and clinically relevant applications of gated SPECT myocardial perfusion imaging. Some have been well validated and are now part of routine clinical practice. Others have been described more recently and await widespread utilization. These, as well as other potential applications of gated perfusion SPECT, are described in this chapter.

## PATIENTS WITH NORMAL PERFUSION SCANS

A normal perfusion study carries a very low risk of future cardiac events including nonfatal myocardial infarction (MI) and cardiac death (1–3). As a screening tool, myocardial perfusion imaging can be extremely useful not only in the diagnosis but also in the prognosis of patients with known or suspected coronary artery disease (CAD). The additions of gated SPECT imaging may provide additional information on ventricular function to further risk-stratify patients presenting for myocardial perfusion imaging. This may be particularly helpful and cost-efficient in patients with no known CAD and no evidence of cardiac valvular disease in establishing the patient's cardiac status. Thus, a patient undergoing screening for evidence of coronary disease with normal perfusion and function may not require further cardiac evaluation (Fig. 11.1).

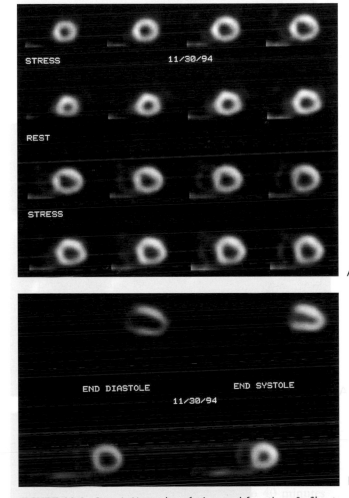

**FIGURE 11.1.** Case 1: Normal perfusion and function. **A:** Short-axis stress and rest tomograms demonstrate normal myocardial perfusion. **B:** Vertical long-axis *(top)* and the short-axis *(bottom)* end-diastolic and end-systolic tomograms demonstrate normal left ventricular wall motion and wall thickening.

E. G. DePuey: Department of Radiology, Columbia University College of Physicians and Surgeons; Division of Nuclear Medicine, Department of Radiology, St. Luke's–Roosevelt Hospital, New York, New York 10025.

G. Heller: Division of Cardiology, Department of Medicine, University of Connecticut School of Medicine, Hartford, Connecticut 06102.

R. Taillefer: Department of Nuclear Medicine, University of Montreal; Department of Nuclear Medicine, Center Hospital of the University of Montreal, H2W 1T8 Montreal, Canada.

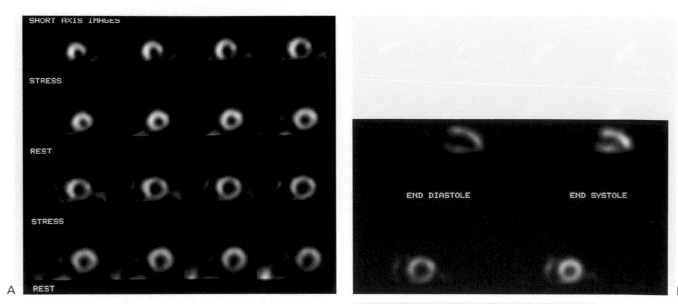

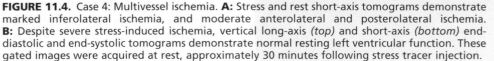

**FIGURE 11.4.** Case 4: Multivessel ischemia. **A:** Stress and rest short-axis tomograms demonstrate marked inferolateral ischemia, and moderate anterolateral and posterolateral ischemia. **B:** Despite severe stress-induced ischemia, vertical long-axis *(top)* and short-axis *(bottom)* end-diastolic and end-systolic tomograms demonstrate normal resting left ventricular function. These gated images were acquired at rest, approximately 30 minutes following stress tracer injection.

in the stress planar projection images, and severe and extensive ischemia (15–17) (Fig. 11.5).

To reconcile the question of whether gated stress perfusion SPECT in a patient with stress-induced ischemia accurately reflects true resting function, two tactics can be employed:

1. Gate the resting perfusion scan. This is a relatively simple matter if a separate-day stress/rest imaging protocol is used. However, if a single-day rest/stress protocol is used, the resting nongated acquisition will have already been completed, and the stress dose will have been administered.

2. Perform a repeat, delayed acquisition of the gated stress SPECT study. By several hours following the termination of stress, poststress stunning, present at 30 to 40 minutes poststress, should be resolved in essentially all patients.

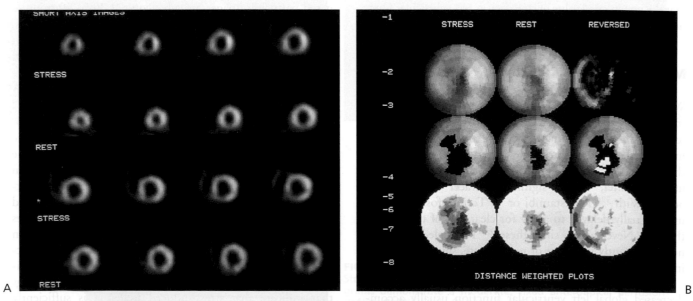

**FIGURE 11.5.** Case 5: Poststress stunning. Stress and rest short-axis tomograms **(A)** and quantitative polar plots **(B)** demonstrate moderate anteroseptal, apical, and inferoapical ischemia with a question of slight inferoapical scarring.

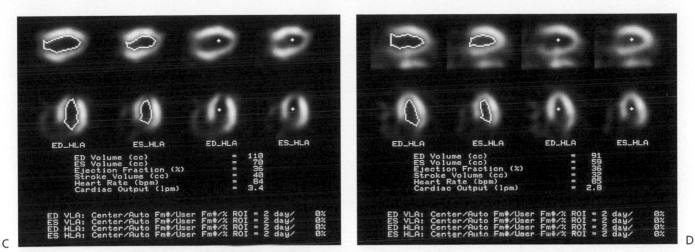

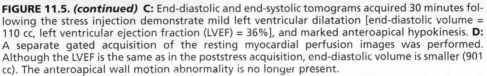

C

D

**FIGURE 11.5. *(continued)* C:** End-diastolic and end-systolic tomograms acquired 30 minutes following the stress injection demonstrate mild left ventricular dilatation [end-diastolic volume = 110 cc, left ventricular ejection fraction (LVEF) = 36%], and marked anteroapical hypokinesis. **D:** A separate gated acquisition of the resting myocardial perfusion images was performed. Although the LVEF is the same as in the poststress acquisition, end-diastolic volume is smaller (90 cc). The anteroapical wall motion abnormality is no longer present.

## ACUTE CORONARY SYNDROMES

Patients in the cardiac care unit (CCU) and the emergency department (ED) with symptoms suggestive of myocardial ischemia and with normal or nondiagnostic electrocardiograms are difficult to assess. The problem is enormous since over 5 million patients with such symptoms present to EDs annually, and over half of them are hospitalized at a cost of $12 billion. The current ED triage process is very inefficient because only a small percentage of the patients who are hospitalized actually have acute MI or unstable angina. Conversely, 5% to 10% of patients with chest pain who are discharged from the ED have unrecognized MI, with an annual mortality of 6% to 8%; others have unstable angina and require subsequent hospitalization (18–23). In addition, many hospitalized patients are also diagnostic dilemmas in regard to cardiac origins of their symptoms (24).

Myocardial perfusion imaging has been proposed as a way to expedite patient care in the CCU (25,26) and to improve triage decisions in the ED (27–32). Acute rest myocardial perfusion imaging may distinguish patients with myocardial ischemia in need of early interventions from low-risk patients not requiring hospitalization. Abnormal acute rest images are highly sensitive in identifying MI in patients injected with radiopharmaceutical during or shortly after an episode of chest pain. This procedure also successfully identifies patients with unstable angina at risk for in-hospital and short-term cardiac events.

Gated SPECT imaging may provide extremely useful information in this setting. However, few data are currently available to confirm this in a formalized evaluation. It should also be recognized that acute myocardial perfusion

imaging involves one image only; therefore, distinction between ischemia and attenuation artifact is extremely difficult. For example, a patient with anterior ischemia may be injected during symptoms but imaged 1 hour later when symptoms were resolved. If gated SPECT imaging were normal, one could not distinguish between attenuation artifact and resolved ischemia as a cause of a perfusion defect. Conversely, if wall motion assessment were abnormal, this information would be quite useful since the likelihood that the perfusion defect represents resting ischemia or scar would be greatly increased (Fig. 11.6).

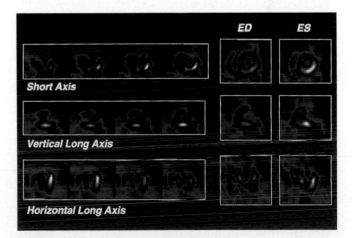

**FIGURE 11.6.** Case 6: Acute chest pain. Perfusion single photon emission computed tomography (SPECT) was performed following sestamibi injection at rest in the emergency department, in this 54-year-old diabetic woman with chest pain and a nondiagnostic electrocardiogram (ECG). An extensive anterior/apical perfusion defect with hypokinesis and markedly decreased wall thickening are supportive of a diagnosis of acute MI.

## CARDIOMYOPATHY

Patients with left ventricular systolic dysfunction need to be categorized as having either ischemic or nonischemic cardiomyopathy because treatment and prognosis differ between the two conditions. Clinical trials indicate that bisoprolol, calcium channel blockers, amiodarone, and digoxin may benefit patients with nonischemic cardiomyopathy but are either ineffective or much less effective in patients with ischemic cardiomyopathy. On the other hand, patients with coronary disease benefit from aggressive risk factor modification. In particular, those with ischemic cardiomyopathy benefit from revascularization of residual viable myocardium (33–44). Although coronary angiography can distinguish between ischemic and nonischemic cardiomyopathy, a noninvasive diagnostic method would be preferable. Previous studies, however, indicate that noninvasive tests cannot reliably classify patients with cardiomyopathy. Myocardial perfusion imaging with [201]Tl or nitrogen-13 ammonia positron emission tomography (PET), and ventricular wall motion assessment with either RNV or echocardiography reveal group differences between ischemic and nonischemic patients; however, considerable overlap has been reported between the groups, limiting the usefulness of these techniques for the classification of individual patients (45–61).

Recent advances in nuclear cardiology offer the potential to overcome the limitations of older methods. Imaging with [99m]Tc agents is less prone to attenuation and scatter artifacts, and produces higher quality images than [201]Tl (62). SPECT improves the sensitivity for perfusion defect localization, and thus the determination of the severity of coronary disease (63). Most importantly, electrocardiogram (ECG)-gated SPECT techniques allow simultaneous evaluation of both myocardial perfusion and ventricular function (64).

Gated SPECT imaging may provide extremely useful information in the evaluation of etiologies of cardiomyopathy. Previous studies with perfusion only, usually with planar imaging, have not successfully stratified ischemic from nonischemic patients. Conversely, evaluation of ventricular function alone also has serious shortcomings in this evaluation. The combination of assessment of ventricular perfusion and function may provide information that is useful and may offset the shortcomings of either modality alone (65–68). Two cases are provided to illustrate this concept (Figs. 11.7 and 11.8).

## ARTIFACTS

Potential artifacts in myocardial perfusion SPECT images can be divided into four general categories:

- artifacts related to SPECT system quality control (69),
- patient motion,
- variation in radiotracer biodistribution (70),
- soft tissue attenuation artifacts.

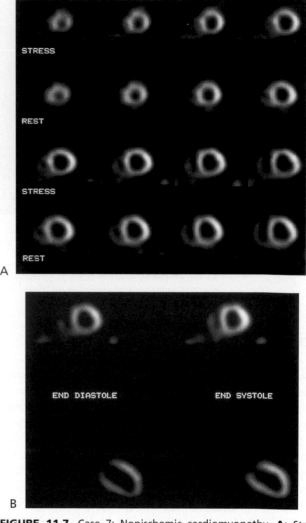

**FIGURE 11.7.** Case 7: Nonischemic cardiomyopathy. **A:** Stress and arrest short-axis tomograms demonstrate left ventricular dilatation, but normal perfusion throughout the left ventricular myocardium. **B:** Short-axis *(top)* and vertical long-axis *(bottom)* end-diastolic and end-systolic tomograms demonstrate diffuse left ventricular hypokinesis.

It is well recognized that nonhomogeneous attenuation from various tissues within the thorax can affect the specificity of SPECT myocardial perfusion imagining (71) (see Chapter 12). Most physicians rely on visual interpretation and quantitative analysis for study interpretation. They learn to integrate in their final data analysis the effects on the perfusion patterns of the presence of different physical factors such as variable spatial resolution of collimated SPECT systems and nonhomogeneous attenuation. Soft tissue attenuation can create significant artifacts. If an observer chooses to interpret studies with a high sensitivity, these artifacts will reduce the specificity or the normalcy rate. On the other hand, if one prefers to interpret

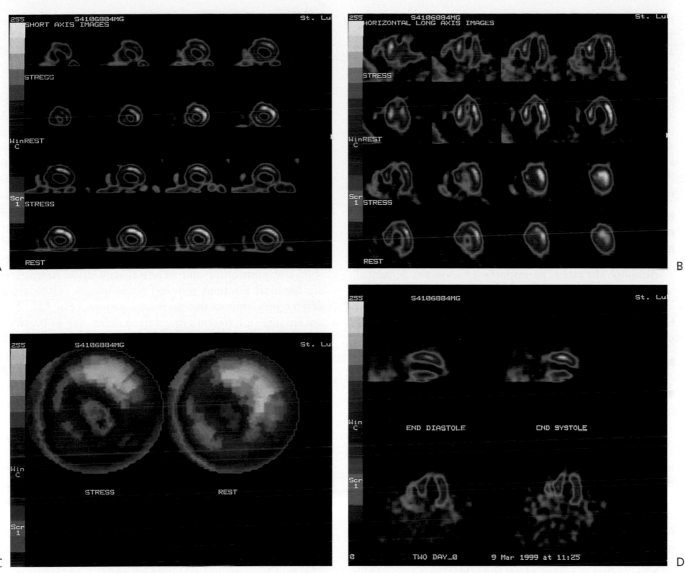

**FIGURE 11.8.** Case 8: Ischemic cardiomyopathy. Stress and rest short-axis **(A)** and vertical long-axis **(B)** tomograms and polar plots **(C)** demonstrate an extensive, reversible inferolateral perfusion defect and a partially reversible apical and anteroseptal defect. These findings are consistent with ischemia and scar in a multivessel distribution. **D:** Vertical long axis *(top)* and horizontal long-axis *(bottom)* end-diastolic and end-systolic tomograms demonstrate decreased to absent thickening of the inferior wall and apex and the diffuse left ventricular hypokinesis. LVEF = 30%.

the images with higher specificity, a high threshold for determining abnormality will be required to avoid interpreting these attenuation artifacts as true myocardial perfusion defects, thereby reducing the sensitivity of the procedure.

Gated perfusion SPECT imaging has been shown to be particularly useful for recognizing and characterizing soft tissue attenuation artifacts and increasing the overall diagnostic certainty of image interpretation in the presence of such artifacts. Several reports have shown significant improvements in test specificity when gated-SPECT images are used for interpretation (72–74).

Depending on the energy level of the photons and the distance they have to travel between their origin and the surface of the gamma camera, the photons may lose their energy and never be detected. This attenuation of photons, if not uniform, will result in substantial artifactual image distortion and ultimately will affect the final diagnosis.

The most frequent sources of significant soft tissue attenuation artifacts in myocardial perfusion imaging are the breast, diaphragm, and lateral chest wall fat. Apical thinning, although not considered as a real attenuation artifact, is also included in this general category of artifacts. The literature has classically divided the soft tissue attenuation artifacts into two general categories: breast attenuation artifact in women and diaphragmatic attenuation artifact in men. It is important, however, to recognize that these artifacts are not gender specific. For example, a fixed inferior wall defect created by diaphragmatic attenuation, although more frequent in men, can also be seen in women, especially in obese patients or in patients with an accentuated abdominal protuberance. Breast attenuation can also be seen in men with gynecomastia. Photon attenuation by the breast depends on three equally important variables:

- the size of the breast,
- its position,
- the density of the breast tissue.

Although the size is an important factor, the density of the breast is also critical. A small but dense breast may cause a more marked attenuation artifact than a large pendulous breast. Furthermore, different positions of the breast will more often create different locations of artifacts:

- Small but dense breast will usually create anterior wall defects.
- Large pendulous breasts will often create lateral wall defects.

Initial reports suggested that artifacts created by breast attenuation lead to only fixed myocardial perfusion defects. It is now recognized that this observation is not always true. If no special care is taken to ensure that images are obtained in identical positions and under identical conditions, large and pendulous breasts, for example, may shift between the rest and the stress studies, thereby creating a falsely reversible defect, a second defect, or a pattern of reverse redistribution. Therefore, optimal imaging conditions must be obtained in order to decrease the likelihood of image distortion from artifacts.

Fortunately, there are different methods or technical procedures that can help the interpreter to distinguish an artifact from a real myocardial perfusion defect. Information about the patient's body habitus is very useful, such as weight and height, chest circumference, bra cup size, position and density of the breast, presence of chest wall fat, abdominal protuberance, and ascites. Careful evaluation of unprocessed analog rotating planar images from the SPECT acquisition, or of the cine display, and the use of markers to define breast contours are helpful. Furthermore, new attenuation and scatter correction methods hold promise in providing another way to decrease the effects of soft tissue attenuation artifacts on the final images. However, all these techniques are not always successful in making the distinction between a soft tissue attenuation artifact and a real perfusion defect.

Initially, it was thought that the introduction of $^{99m}$Tc-labeled myocardial perfusion-imaging agents would solve the problem of attenuation artifacts. Despite the higher energy level of $^{99m}$Tc photons compared to those of $^{201}$Tl, tissue attenuation with $^{99m}$Tc is decreased by a factor of only approximately 15% (69). Although there is less scattered activity with $^{99m}$Tc photons, soft tissue attenuation artifacts are still seen with $^{99m}$Tc-labeled perfusion-imaging agents but to a lesser degree than that of $^{201}$Tl. A major advantage of $^{99m}$Tc-labeled perfusion-imaging agents is their associated high-count density, which allows image acquisition with ECG gating, thereby providing an analysis of regional wall motion and thickening. Attenuation artifacts can be more easily recognized with this technique.

Soft tissue attenuation artifacts and/or normal variants such as diaphragmatic or breast attenuation, and apical thinning often appear as fixed myocardial perfusion defects if patient positioning and technical acquisition parameters are identical for both rest and stress images. These fixed defects may mimic the perfusion pattern of a MI. The uncertainty in differentiating a fixed defect due to previous MI from one due to soft tissue attenuation artifact will result in false-positive studies and will decrease the specificity of myocardial perfusion imaging in detection of CAD. However, with the use of gated SPECT and analysis of wall motion and thickening, it is now possible to determine the cause of a fixed myocardial perfusion defect. If a fixed perfusion defect shows normal or relatively preserved wall motion and wall thickening, it is likely that the defect is secondary to a soft tissue attenuation artifact. In the presence of decreased wall motion and wall thickening, a previous MI is more likely to be the cause of the defect (Figs. 11.9 and 11.10).

Using this rationale, DePuey and Rozanski (72) evaluated 551 consecutive patients referred for the evaluation of CAD (72). Gated $^{99m}$Tc-sestamibi SPECT studies were obtained in all patients. Isolated fixed myocardial perfusion defects were identified in 180 patients (33%). Results from gated SPECT studies were correlated with clinical evidence of MI (based on history and/or ECG Q-waves). Abnormal function was seen in 98 (96%) of 102 patients with fixed defects and clinically documented MI. In 77% of patients with no clinical evidence of MI, function was normal. In the remaining 23% of patients with no clinical evidence of MI, there was decreased function in the defect area, possibly indicating a silent MI. The percentage of patients with unexplained fixed defects (no clinical evidence of MI) decreased from 14% to 3% when patients with fixed defects and normal function were reclassified as normal. They concluded that gated SPECT $^{99m}$Tc-sestamibi imaging could improve the characterization of fixed defects and potentially improve test specificity.

In another study, Smanio et al. (73) showed that the number of borderline interpretations was reduced from 89 to 29 with the addition of gating. In a group of 137 patients with a <10% pretest likelihood of CAD, the addition of

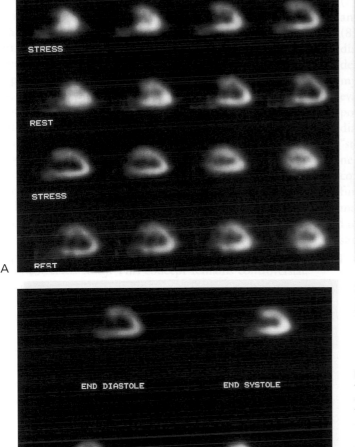

A

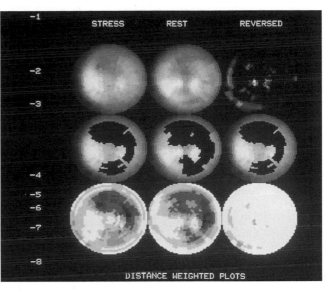

B

C

**FIGURE 11.9.** Case 9: Breast attenuation. Short-axis **(A)** and vertical long-axis **(B)** stress and rest tomograms demonstrate a moderate, fixed perfusion defect in the anterior and lateral walls of the left ventricle. Quantitative polar plots **(C)** accentuate this apparent abnormality. **C.** Vertical long-axis *(top)* and short-axis *(bottom)* end-diastolic and end-systolic images demonstrate entirely normal left ventricular wall motion and wall thickening, including that of the anterior and lateral walls. This finding would strongly favor an attenuation artifact rather than scar as a cause of the apparent fixed perfusion defects.

gated images to the interpretation added significantly to those designated as normal, 74% versus 93% ($p$ <.0001), due to a reduction in borderline normal and abnormal readings. In 49 patients with a previous infarction, the addition of gated images increased the abnormal scan interpretations from 78% to 92%.

In addition, Taillefer et al. (/4) prospectively compared $^{99m}$Tc-sestamibi perfusion SPECT studies with and without gating in 115 female patients (85 patients scheduled for coronary angiography and 30 normal volunteers with a likelihood of CAD <5%) in order to compare their respective sensitivity and specificity. Three blinded observers interpreted all images. SPECT studies were read without and then with ECG gating. When the 34 patients with normal coronary angiography were added to the group of 30

normal volunteers, the specificity for coronary lesions >70% was 84.4% for SPECT perfusion study and 92.2% for gated SPECT imaging. The authors concluded from this study, performed in a patient population having proven CAD, that the diagnostic specificity of $^{99m}$Tc-sestamibi SPECT perfusion imaging could be enhanced by the use of ECG gating.

Thus, assessment of wall motion and wall thickening on gated perfusion SPECT studies can be an important adjunct to the static perfusion study information in cases where the etiology of a fixed myocardial perfusion defect is unknown or of uncertain origin. By differentiating a fixed defect due to a previous MI from one due to soft tissue attenuation artifact, the gated SPECT study improves the specificity of the myocardial perfusion study.

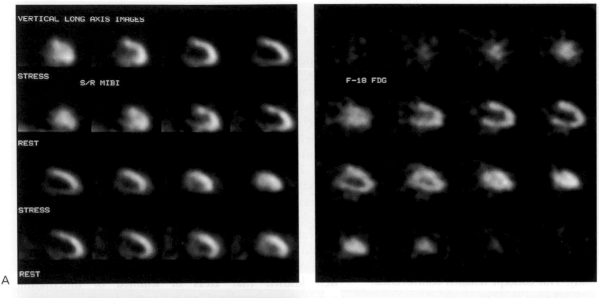

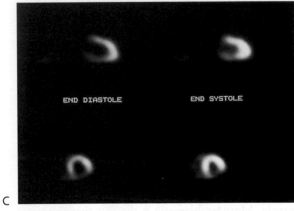

**FIGURE 11.11.** Case 11: Myocardial viability. **A:** Stress and rest $^{99m}$Tc-sestamibi vertical long-axis perfusion tomograms demonstrate a marked fixed inferior wall defect. **B:** 18-F-fluorodeoxyglucose SPECT vertical long-axis tomograms demonstrate normal tracer concentration throughout the inferior wall. This finding is consistent with viability of the inferior myocardium. **C:** Vertical long-axis *(top)* and short-axis *(bottom)* end-diastolic and end-systolic $^{99m}$Tc-sestamibi tomograms demonstrate relatively normal inferior wall motion. Inferior wall thickening is present, but decreased.

## VALUE OF GATING BOTH END-SYSTOLIC AND END-DIASTOLIC IMAGES

The high count density of myocardial perfusion studies using $^{99m}$Tc labeled radiopharmaceuticals allows for acquisition of gated planar or SPECT images synchronized to the patient's ECG. Different qualitative and quantitative assessments can be obtained from a gated SPECT study, such as the evaluation of global and regional myocardial wall motion, systolic wall thickening, and calculation of the left ventricular ejection fraction. Another potential advantage of ECG gating of myocardial perfusion studies is the ability to extract and analyze the end-diastolic images of the complete cardiac cycle. Theoretically, end-diastolic image frames could provide better image resolution by reducing the blurring effect of cardiac motion on the perfusion study. This could improve the sensitivity for detection of myocardial perfusion defects, especially in patients with small and/or hyperdynamic hearts (Fig. 11.12).

At present, there are few data available showing the diagnostic value of the end-diastolic image obtained from both rest and stress studies. Mannting and Morgan-Mannting (95) compared ungated SPECT image and diastolic frames obtained from gated SPECT study in 83 subjects (63 patients and 20 normal volunteers) using a 1-day $^{99m}$Tc-sestamibi injection protocol. They demonstrated that the right ventricle appeared more distinct and with higher contrast in end-diastolic images than in summed (nongated) studies. The left ventricular cavity was also larger, leading to more coronal slices through the ventricular cavity. In end-diastolic frames, myocardial walls are captured in a phase with minimal movement, thereby providing a sharper image. The increase in ventricular cavity size, resulting from exclusion of the systolic obliteration of the cavity in end-diastolic images, improves evaluation of myocardial perfusion, especially in the apical third of the myocardium. This is particularly obvious in patients with small, hyperdynamic hearts and/or thick left ventricle walls. In a subgroup of 50

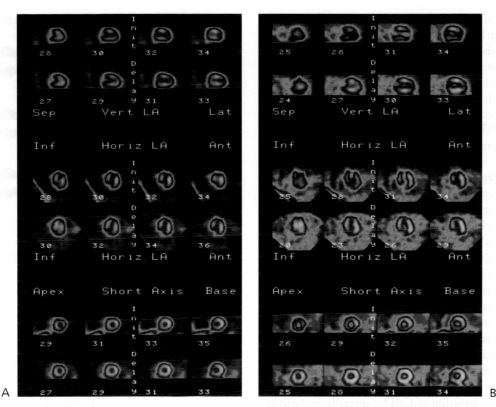

**FIGURE 11.12.** Case 12: Stress and rest end-diastolic gated tomograms. Baseline end-diastolic and end-systolic vertical long-axis tomograms demonstrate apical akinesis. With low-dose dobutamine infusion, there is potentiation of apical wall motion, consistent with myocardial viability. With high-dose dobutamine infusion, apical wall motion further deteriorates, consistent with stress-induced ischemia.

patients in the same study, the authors showed that the quantitative assessment of the extent and the degree of myocardial perfusion abnormalities in rest and stress studies highly correlated in nongated and end-diastolic studies. The severity of small and moderate-sized defects showed a high degree of agreement in nongated and end-diastolic studies, whereas in patients with subtle perfusion abnormalities, the results from diastolic imaging agreed best with clinical data. Unfortunately, there was no correlation in this study with coronary angiography and no data regarding the sensitivity and the specificity of end-diastolic imaging in detection of CAD.

In a prospective study, using ECG gating of both rest and stress studies, 53 female patients were studied to compare the diagnostic accuracy of end-diastolic images to that of the summed images with $^{99m}$Tc-sestamibi SPECT studies (96). All these patients had coronary angiography. A 2-day protocol was used. Sixteen frames per cardiac cycle were acquired using a dual-head gamma camera for both rest and stress studies. Three end-diastolic frames were used to form end-diastolic images, and all 16 frames were summed to obtain a standard myocardial perfusion study. Both the summed and

end-diastolic images were interpreted by three blinded observers during two distinct sessions. The sensitivity for coronary artery detected was 73.7% (28/38) and 84.2% (32/38), respectively, for summed images and end-diastolic images. Three out of four patients with coronary stenoses not detect by summed images but seen with end-diastolic images were considered to have relatively small hearts. The specificity was 86.7% (13/15) and 80.0% (12/15) for summed images and end-diastolic images, respectively. Of a total of 901 myocardial segments, 106 ischemic defects were detected by summed images and 173 by end-diastolic images ($p$ = .001). The segmental agreement between the two techniques was 88.6%. This study, as well as the study from Mannting and Morgan-Mannting (95), confirmed that end-diastolic images can detect more ischemic defects, especially in patients with small hearts. Although there was no statistically significant difference in the specificity between the two types of images, the specificity of end-diastolic imaging potentially may be lower in patients with a dilated left ventricle or in studies with relatively low count densities.

Gated SPECT imaging could be useful in two different ways in the detection of CAD, especially in women

would be enormous radiopharmaceutical, instrumentation, and personnel cost savings. Patient throughput and laboratory efficiency would be dramatically increased. These savings would result in decreased charges for myocardial perfusion SPECT, rendering the technique much more attractive to health care providers and more competitive compared to other modalities such as stress echocardiography.

## INTERPRETING GATED PERFUSION SPECT

Gated SPECT imaging data should be interpreted in conjunction with all acquired data.

Evaluate the unprocessed data for:

- quality of the study,
- presence of patient motion,
- other contributors to artifact such as breast, diaphragm, liver, gut,
- extrinsic information, such as activity in the breast or thorax suggestive of a mitotic process.

Evaluate the processed static tomographic data in the form of cardiac slices (horizontal long, vertical long, and short axis) at rest and stress for:

- extent and severity of ischemic and infarcted myocardium,
- quantitative data in conjunction with the reader's observations.

Evaluate processed gated SPECT data:

- in conjunction with data from the perfusion slices,
- to observe ventricular function in areas of perfusion abnormalities, including infarction and potential attenuation artifacts,
- to evaluate ventricular function including regional and global wall motion abnormalities, as well as visually estimated left ventricular ejection fraction,
- to confirm information using quantitative gated SPECT programs,
- to observe right ventricular function.

## REFERENCES

1. Brown KA. Prognostic value of myocardial perfusion imaging: state of the art and new developments. *J Nucl Cardiol* 1996;3:516–525.
2. Heller GV, Brown KA. Prognosis of acute and chronic coronary artery disease by myocardial perfusion imaging. *Cardiol Clin* 1994;12:271–287.
3. Iskander S, Iskandrian A. Risk assessment using single-photon emission computed tomographic technetium-99m sestamibi imaging. *J Am Coll Cardiol* 1998;32:57–62.
4. Gibson RS, Watson DD, Craddock GB, et al. Prediction of cardiac events after uncomplicated myocardial infarction: a prospective study comparing predischarge exercise thallium-201 scintigraphy and coronary angiography. *Circulation* 1983;68:321–336.
5. Hung J, Goris ML, Nash E, et al. Comparative value of maximal treadmill testing, exercise thallium myocardial perfusion scintigraphy and exercise radionuclide ventriculography for distinguishing high- and low-risk patients soon after acute myocardial infarction. *Am J Cardiol* 1984;53:1221–1227.
6. Leppo JA, O'Brien J, Rothendler JA, et al. Dipyridamole-thallium-201 scintigraphy in the prediction of future cardiac events after acute myocardial infarction. *N Engl J Med* 1984;310:1014–1018.
7. Smeets JP, Rigo P, Legrand V, et al. Prognostic value of thallium-201 stress myocardial scintigraphy with exercise ECG after myocardial infarction. *Cardiology* 1981;68(suppl 2):67–70.
8. DePuey EG, Jones ME, Garcia EV. Evaluation of right ventricular regional perfusion with technetium-99m sestamibi SPECT. *J Nucl Med* 1991;32:1199–1205.
9. Zaret BL, Wackers FJ, Terrin M, et al., and the TIMI investigators. Does left ventricular ejection fraction following thrombolytic therapy have the same prognostic impact described in the prethrombolytic era? Results of the TIMI II trial. *J Am Coll Cardiol* 1991;17:214A.
10. The Multicenter Postinfarction Research Group. Risk stratification and survival after myocardial infarction. *N Engl J Med* 1983;309:331–336.
11. Lee KL, Pryor DB, Pieper KS, et al. Prognostic value of radionuclide angiography in medically treated patients with coronary artery disease: a comparison with clinical and catheterization variables. *Circulation* 1990;82:1705–1717.
12. Palmas W, Friedman JD, Diamond GA, et al. Incremental value of simultaneous assessment of myocardial function and perfusion with technetium-99m sestamibi for predication of extent of coronary artery disease. *J Am Coll Cardiol* 1995;25:1024–1031.
13. Taliercio CP, Clements IP, Zinsmerster AR, et al. Prognostic value and limitations of exercise radionuclide angiography in medically treated coronary artery disease. *Mayo Clin Proc* 1988;63:573–582.
14. Johnson LL, Verdesca SA, Aude WY, et al. Postischemic stunning can affect left ventricular ejection fraction and regional wall motion on post-stress gated sestamibi tomograms. *J Am Coll Cardiol* 1997;30:1641–1648.
15. Stolzenberg J. Dilation of the left ventricular cavity on stress thallium scan as an indicator of ischemic disease. *Clin Nucl Med* 1980;5:289–291.
16. Weiss AT, Berman DS, Lew AS, et al. Transient Ischemic dilation of the left ventricle on stress thallium 201 scintigraphy: a marker of severe and extensive coronary artery disease. *J Am Coll Cardiol* 1987;9:752–759.
17. Chouraqui P, Rodrigues EA, Berman DS, et al. Significance of dipyridamole-induced transient dilation of the left ventricle during thallium-201 scintigraphy in suspected coronary artery disease. *Am J Cardiol* 1990;66:689–694.
18. Schor S, Behar S, Modan B, et al. Disposition of presumed coronary patients from an emergency room. A follow-up study. *JAMA* 1976;236:941–943.
19. Selker HP. Coronary care unit triage decision aids: how do we know when they work? *Am J Med* 1989;87:491–493.
20. McCarthy BD, Beshansky JR, D'Agostino RB, et al. Missed diagnoses of acute myocardial infarction in the emergency department: results from a multicenter study. *Ann Emerg Med* 1993;22:579–582.
21. Weingarten SR, Ermann B, Riedinger MS, et al. Selecting the best triage rule for patients hospitalized with chest pain. *Am J Med* 1989;87:494–500.
22. Lee TH, Rouan GW, Weisberg MC, et al. Clinical characteristics and natural history of patients with acute myocardial infarction sent home from the emergency room. *Am J Cardiol* 1987;60:219–224.
23. Lee TH, Ting HH, Shammash JB, et al. Long-term survival of

emergency department patients with acute chest pain. *Am J Cardiol* 1992;69:145–151.

24. Roberts R, Kleiman NS. Earlier diagnosis and treatment of acute myocardial infarction necessitates the need for a new diagnostic mind-set. *Circulation* 1994;89:872–881.

25. Bilodeau L, Theroux P, Gregoire J, et al. Technetium-99m sestamibi tomography in patients with spontaneous chest pain: correlations with clinical, electrocardiographic and angiographic findings. *J Am Coll Cardiol* 1991;18:1684–1691.

26. Christian TF, Clements IP, Gibbons RJ. Noninvasive identification of myocardium at risk in patients with acute myocardial infarction and nondiagnostic electrocardiograms with technetium-99m sestamibi. *Circulation* 1991;83:1615–1620.

27. Wackers FJTh, Lie KI, Liem KL, et al. Thallium-201 scintigraphy in unstable angina pectoris. *Circulation* 1978;57:738–742.

28. Varetto T, Cantalupi D, Altieri A, et al. Emergency room technetium-99m sestamibi imaging to rule out acute myocardial ischemic events in patients with non-diagnostic electrocardiograms. *J Am Coll Cardiol* 1993;22:1804–1808.

29. Hilton TC, Thompson RC, Williams HJ, et al. Technetium-99m sestamibi myocardial perfusion imaging in the emergency room evaluation of chest pain. *J Am Coll Cardiol* 1994;23:1016–1022.

30. Kontos MC, Jesse RL, Schmidt KL, et al. Value of acute rest sestamibi perfusion imaging for evaluation of patients admitted to the emergency department with chest pain. *J Am Coll Cardiol* 1997;30:976–982.

31. Hilton TC, Fulmer H, Abuan T, et al. Ninety-day follow-up of patients in the emergency department with chest pain who undergo initial single-photon emission computed tomographic perfusion scintigraphy with technetium-99m-labeled sestamibi. *J Nucl Cardiol* 1996;3:308–311.

32. Tatum JL, Jesse RL, Kontos MC, et al. Comprehensive strategy for the evaluation and triage of the chest pain patient. *Ann Emerg Med* 1997;29:116–125.

33. Alderman EL, Fisher LD, Litwin P, et al. Results of coronary artery surgery in patients with poor left ventricular function (CASS). *Circulation* 1983;68:785–795.

34. Gersh BJ, Kronmal RA, Schaff HV, et al. Comparison of coronary artery bypass surgery and medical therapy in patients 65 years of age or older. A nonrandomized study from the Coronary Artery Surgery Study (CASS) registry. *N Engl J Med* 1985;313:217–224.

35. Eleftcriades JA, Tolis G Jr, Levi E, et al. Coronary artery bypass grafting in severe left ventricular dysfunction: excellent survival with improved ejection fraction and functional state. *J Am Coll Cardiol* 1993;22:1411–1417.

36. Scandinavian Simvastatin Survival Study Group. Randomized trial of cholesterol lowering in 4444 patients with coronary heart disease: the Scandinavian Simvastatin Survival Study (4S). *Lancet* 1994;344:1383–1389.

37. CIBIS Investigators and Committee. A randomized trial of β-blockade in heart failure: the Cardiac Insufficiency Bisoprolol Study (CIBIS). *Circulation* 1994;90:1765–1773.

38. Gheorghiade M, Young JB, Uretsky BF, et al. The effects of digoxin withdrawal in patients with stable heart failure due to coronary artery disease compared to primary cardiomyopathy: insights from the PROVED and RADIANCE studies. *Circulation* 1995;92(suppl I):I-142(abst 0672).

39. Singh SN, Fletcher RD, Fisher SG, et al. Amiodarone in patients with congestive heart failure and asymptomatic ventricular arrhythmia. *N Engl J Med* 1995;333:77–82.

40. Singh SN, Fisher SG, Singh BN, et al. Ischemic vs non-ischemic cardiomyopathy: clinical outcome and response to amiodarone. *J Am Coll Cardiol* 1996;27(suppl A):203A(abst 924-67).

41. Figula HR, Gietzen F, Zeymer U, et al. Dilriazem improves cardiac function and exercise capacity in patients with idiopathic

dilated cardiomyopathy. Results from the Diltiazem in Dilated Cardiomyopathy Trial. *Circulation* 1996;94:346–352.

42. O'Connor CM, Puma JA, Gardner LH, et al. A 25-year experience in patients with coronary artery disease (CAD) and chronic heart failure (CHF): outcomes with medical therapy and bypass surgery (CABG). *J Am Coll Cardiol* 1996;27(suppl A):142A(abst 734-6).

43. Packer M, O'Connor CM, Ghali JK, et al. Effect of amlodipine on morbidity and mortality in severe chronic heart failure. *N Engl J Med* 1996;335:1107–1114.

44. Yusuf S, Garg R, Smith T, et al. Which heart failure patients benefit the most from long term digoxin therapy? *Circulation* 1996;94(suppl I):I-23(abst 0131).

45. Saltissi S, Hockings B, Croft DN, et al. Thallium-201 myocardial imaging in patients with dilated and ischaemic cardiomyopathy. *Br Heart J* 1981;46:290–295.

46. Greenberg JM, Murphy JH, Okada RD, et al. Value and limitations of radionuclide angiography in determining the cause of reduced left ventricular ejection fraction: comparison of idiopathic dilated cardiomyopathy and coronary artery disease. *Am J Cardiol* 1985;55:541–544.

47. Wallis DE, O'Connell JB, Henkin RE, et al. Segmental wall motion abnormalities in dilated cardiomyopathy: a common finding and good prognostic sign. *J Am Coll Cardiol* 1984;4:674–679.

48. Shors CM, Kozul VJ, Henderson F. The differential diagnosis of congestive cardiomyopathy and ischemic cardiomyopathy by echocardiography. *Angiology* 1975;26:723–733.

49. Eisenberg JD, Sobel BE, Geltman EM. Differentiation of ischemic from nonischemic cardiomyopathy with positron emission tomography. *Am J Cardiol* 1987;59:1410–1414.

50. Dunn RF, Uren RF, Sadick N, et al. Comparison of thallium-201 scanning in idiopathic dilated cardiomyopathy and severe coronary artery disease. *Circulation* 1982;66:804–810.

51. Eichhorn EJ, Kosinski EJ, Lewis SM, et al. Usefulness of dipyridamole-thallium-201 perfusion scanning for distinguishing ischemic from nonischemic cardiomyopathy. *Am J Cardiol* 1988;62:945–951.

52. Bulkley BH, Hutchins GM, Bailey I, et al. Thallium 201 imaging and gated blood pool scans in patients with ischemic and idiopathic congestive cardiomyopathy: a clinical and pathologic study. *Circulation* 1977;55:753–760.

53. Iskandrian AS, Hakki A-H, Kane S. Resting thallium-201 myocardial perfusion patterns in patients with severe left ventricular dysfunction: differences between patients with primary cardiomyopathy, chronic coronary artery disease, or acute myocardial infarction. *Am Heart J* 1986;111:760–767.

54. Medina R, Panidis IP, Morganroth J, et al. The value of echocardiographic regional wall motion abnormalities in detecting coronary artery disease in patients with or without a dilated left ventricle. *Am Heart J* 1985;109:799–803.

55. Juilliere Y, Marie PY, Danchin N, et al. Radionuclide assessment of regional differences in left ventricular wall motion and myocardial perfusion in idiopathic dilated cardiomyopathy. *Eur Heart J* 1993;14:1163–1169.

56. Chikamori T, Doi YL, Yonezawa Y, et al. Value of dipyridamole thallium-201 imaging in noninvasive differentiation of idiopathic dilated cardiomyopathy from coronary artery disease with left ventricular dysfunction. *Am J Cardiol* 1992;69:650–653.

57. Tauberg SG, Orie JE, Bartlett BE, et al. Usefulness of thallium-201 for distinction of ischemic from idiopathic dilated cardiomyopathy. *Am J Cardiol* 1993;71:674–680.

57a. Wackers FJTh. Comparison of thallium-201 and technetium-99m methoxyisobutyl isonitrile. *Am J Cardiol* 1992;70:30E–34E.

**TABLE 12.1. BODY HABITUS PROFILE**

Patient x-ray date:
Height:
Weight:
Females:
    Chest circumference (inches):
    Bra cup size (A–D):
    Left Mastectomy: No Yes
    Breast prosthesis: No Yes
    Breast Implant: No Yes
    Breast position
        Anterior
        Anterolateral
        Lateral
        Inferolateral

| | | | |
|---|---|---|---|
| Breast density (chest x-ray): - | Low | Moderate | Marked |
| Lateral chest wall fat: | Mild | Moderate | High |
| Abdominal protuberance: | Mild | Moderate | Marked |

    Immediate Images: Bra off, Bra on

    Delayed Images: Bra off, Bra on

    Additional delayed images: Bra off, Bra on

Males
    Chest circumference (inches):
    Gynecomastia: No Yes

| | | | |
|---|---|---|---|
| Pectoral development: | Mild | Moderate | Marked |
| Lateral chest fat: | Mild | Moderate | Marked |
| Abdominal protuberance: | Mild | Moderate | Marked |

Commentos on body habitus:

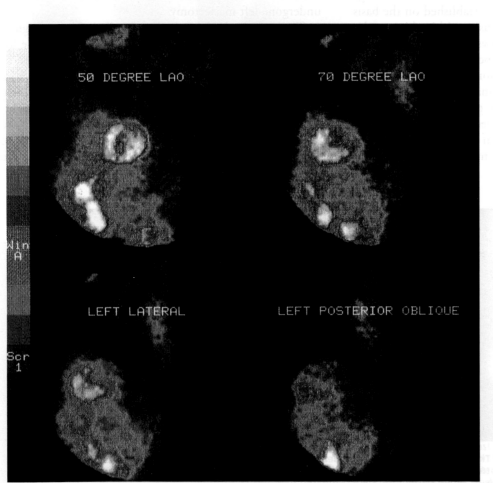

**FIGURE 12.4.** A photopenic, curvilinear, photon-deficient area secondary to breast attenuation, "eclipsing" the superior portion of the left ventricle. The breast "shadow" is noted to extend to regions adjacent to the heart.

imaging palette, the size, thickness, and position of the breasts should be noted. It is important that this notation be made with the patient supine and not upright, since image acquisition is performed with the patient supine.

2. The patient should always be instructed to remove her bra prior to each and every image acquisition. It is useful for the technologist to document that the bra has been removed.

3. A history of mastectomy should be documented, and breast prostheses must be removed, if possible. Any history of breast augmentation should be noted. If a chest x-ray is available, it may be helpful in assessing the density of the implant and its location relative to the left ventricle.

4. Positioning of the patient on the SPECT imaging table should be reproduced as closely as possible for stress and rest images. Since the position of the elevated left arm greatly influences the position of the left breast, the left arm should be positioned identically for each image acquisition. An arm holder is particularly useful to assure reproducible arm positioning.

5. The planar images from which SPECT data are reconstructed should be viewed in a rotating cinematic for-mat. The position of the breast "shadow" should be observed with regard to the portion of the left ventricular myocardium that is eclipsed. Such a shadow is usually noted to extend beyond the heart to overlie the adjacent left hemithorax, and can thereby be differentiated from a true myocardial perfusion defect in these rotating planar images (Fig. 12.4). Moreover, the density of the breast can be estimated from the degree of attenuation of photons emanating from structures within the thorax, including the myocardium and lungs. The constancy (or inconstancy) of the position of the left breast in stress and rest images should be ascertained.

6. In reconstructed SPECT images, an area of markedly decreased photon density may be observed anterior or lateral to the heart in patients with very large or dense breasts (Fig. 12.5). Adjacent to this photopenic defect are frequently observed accentuated streak artifacts due to nonisotropic attenuation (2). The position of the breast is best evaluated from transaxial or horizontal long-axis slices. When such a large area of markedly decreased count density is noted, an attenuation artifact that may mimic a myocardial perfusion defect often

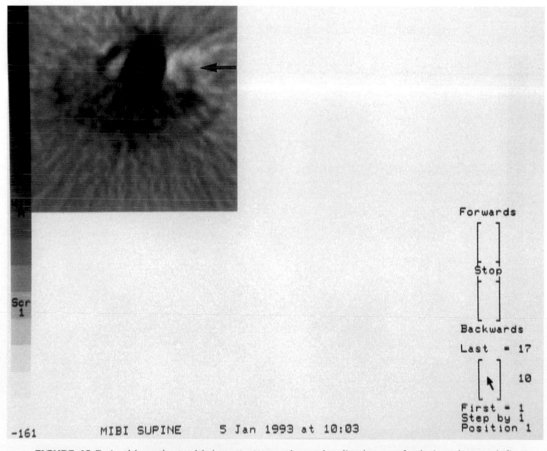

**FIGURE 12.5.** In this patient with breast attenuation, a localized area of relative photon deficiency compared to background activity lies anterolateral and lateral to the left ventricle *(arrow)* in this stress $^{99m}$Tc-sestamibi transaxial slice.

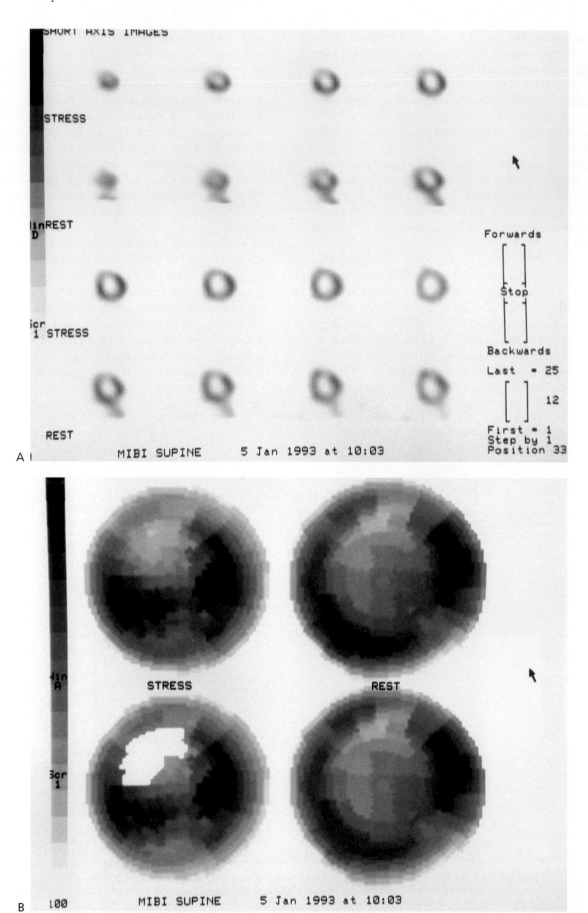

**FIGURE 12.6.** Anterior breast artifact in stress *(left)* and rest *(right)* 99mTc-sestamibi single photon emission computed tomography (SPECT) images. The artifact is fixed in midventricular short-axis slices **(A)** and polar coordinate plots **(B)**.

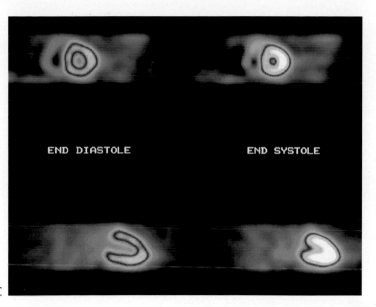

END DIASTOLE          END SYSTOLE

C

**FIGURE 12.6** *(continued).* Gated end-diastolic and end-systolic midventricular short-axis *(top)* and vertical long-axis *(bottom)* slices **(C)** demonstrate normal anterior-wall motion and thickening, thus favoring an attenuation artifact rather than anterior infarction as a cause of the fixed defect.

occurs in the adjacent myocardium. This is especially important since a shifting breast attenuation artifact can mimic reversible perfusion defect (i.e., ischemia) or reverse distribution. Although the planar projection images may be viewed at the computer console in either black and white or color, a linear black and white display may be preferable since lower count density soft tissue activity is better visualized.

7. In the reconstructed SPECT slices and polar coordinate plots, the location of the apparent perfusion defect should be carefully observed with regard to its conformance to a discrete vascular territory. Attenuation artifacts in women with large breasts often involve the anteroseptal, anterior, and contiguous anterolateral walls, often extending to involve the upper half of the lateral wall. Although such a defect could be secondary to disease involving the proximal left anterior descending (LAD) coronary artery, including a very large diagonal branch supplying the lateral wall, or the left anterior descending and proximal branch(es) of the circumflex (first obtuse marginal) artery, such a distribution for a true perfusion defect is unusual, and an artifact should be suspected, particularly if there are no accompanying electrocardiographic (ECG) abnormalities (Fig. 12.6).

Because the attenuation of photons from $^{99m}$Tc by soft tissue is less than for $^{201}$Tl, breast attenuation artifacts are less marked in scans performed with $^{99m}$Tc-labeled myocardial perfusion agents. However, they nonetheless occur, particularly in women with very large or very dense breasts. A unique attribute of $^{99m}$Tc-labeled agents is that they permit performing gated SPECT, owing to the relatively high count density and spatial resolution of the tomographic slices (see Chapter 8). Gated $^{99m}$Tc-sestamibi SPECT is helpful in differentiating breast attenuation artifacts from

scar, since artifacts will demonstrate normal wall motion and wall thickening, whereas infarcts, if they are transmural and sizable, will be hypokinetic with decreased wall thickening (3,4) (Fig. 12.6C). The interpreting physician should also determine if the patient has historical or ECG evidence of anterior myocardial infarction to aid in the differentiation of scar from a breast attenuation artifact. Clinical judgment is important here. Patients with nontransmural myocardial infarctions might show normal wall motion depending on the thickness of the infarct zone.

Attenuation correction for SPECT is now noncommercially available but is still a topic of intense interest and research. The methods for accomplishing it have employed either scatter correction or attenuation correction using a separate transmission image. This approach has been demonstrated to significantly reduce breast attenuation artifacts in phantom and patient studies (6–11).

## Lateral Chest-Wall Fat Attenuation

In obese patients, there may be a considerable accumulation of fat in the lateral chest wall. When such a patient lies supine on the imaging palette, the thickness of soft tissue in the lateral chest wall is further accentuated. Although this tissue thickness may be the same as or greater than that of the breast, chest-wall fat is usually more uniformly distributed. Therefore, the resultant attenuation artifact is usually more diffuse, often involving the entire lateral wall of the left ventricle (Fig. 12.7).

Like breast attenuation artifacts, apparent perfusion defects due to lateral chest-wall fat should be anticipated before the actual inspection of tomographic slices, through awareness of the following points:

1. Height, weight, and chest-wall circumference should be recorded for all patients (Table 12.1). In obese men and

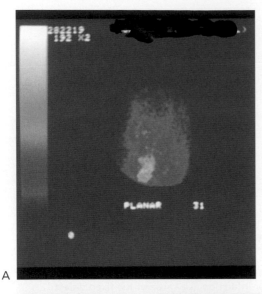

A

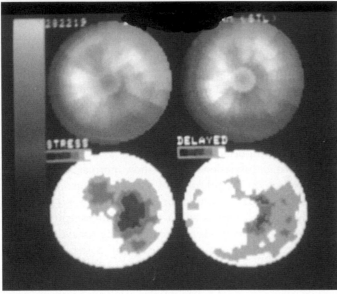

B

**FIGURE 12.7.** **A:** Marked attenuation of the heart in lateral and left posterior oblique planar images used for SPECT reconstruction is frequently observed in obese patients, with photon attenuation due to lateral chest-wall fat. **B:** Lateral chest-wall photon attenuation produced a fixed lateral wall artifact in these stress *(left)* and delayed *(right)* [201]Tl polar maps. The artifact is highlighted in quantitative plots *(bottom row)*. (From *J Nucl Med,* with permission.)

women, lateral chest-wall attenuation artifacts occur frequently, and in general their severity is directly proportional to the chest circumference.

2. The patient should be observed lying supine on the imaging palette, and the degree of lateral chest-wall fat should be estimated as mild, moderate, or marked.

3. In the planar images displayed in rotating cinematic format, the left ventricle will exhibit a markedly decreased count density in lateral and left posterior oblique (LPO) views in patients with excessive lateral chest-wall fat. Although patients with true lateral chest-wall perfusion defects in the distribution of the circumflex coronary artery may exhibit similar findings in the rotating planar images, a perfusion abnormality in the lateral wall is sometimes more often identifiable in the LAO view in

these patients, since lateral chest-wall fat usually lies more posterior when the patient lies supine.

4. As for breast attenuation artifacts, gated [99m]Tc-sestamibi SPECT is useful in differentiating lateral chest-wall attenuation artifacts from true perfusion defects. Normal lateral wall motion and wall thickening strongly favor the former.

5. It is also likely that algorithms for SPECT attenuation correction will substantially reduce attenuation artifacts secondary to lateral wall fat.

## Diffuse Soft Tissue Attenuation

In some obese patients, soft tissue attenuation may be diffuse and not particularly localized as with breast or diaphragmatic attenuation. Under these circumstances, the entire myocardium may be attenuated. Because attenuation within soft tissue is distance-dependent, the more basal portions of the left ventricular myocardium will be attenuated to the greatest degree. Therefore, in obese patients, an apparent circumferential decrease in trace concentration may be present at the base. The artifact may be most pronounced at the base of the lateral/posterior wall, which is furthest from the detector (Fig. 12.8).

## Diaphragmatic Attenuation

The inferior wall of the left ventricle of both men and women normally exhibits a decreased count density. This is most likely due to the attenuation of photons from the inferior wall of the left ventricle by both the left hemidi-

aphragm and to a lesser degree the overlying right ventricle and right ventricular blood pool. In normal men the anterior-to-inferior count-density ratio with $^{201}$Tl SPECT is 1.2:1 (5). For $^{99m}$Tc, the ratio is approximately 1:1 (1). In women, the ratio is approximately unity with both $^{201}$Tl and $^{99m}$Tc. This has been postulated to be due to the counterbalancing of inferior wall attenuation caused by the left hemidiaphragm in women by breast attenuation. However, it is doubtful whether that alone explains the difference, since the inferior-to-lateral wall ratio is also higher in women.

Left hemidiaphragmatic elevation can result in accentuated attenuation and inferior myocardial perfusion artifacts. Diaphragmatic elevation is common in obese patients. In patients with pleural or pulmonary parenchymal disease, atelectasis and loss of lung volume are frequent, and

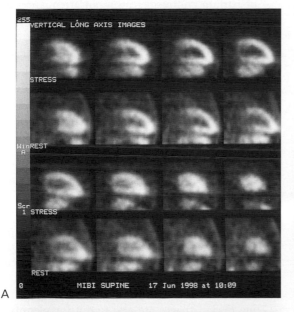

A

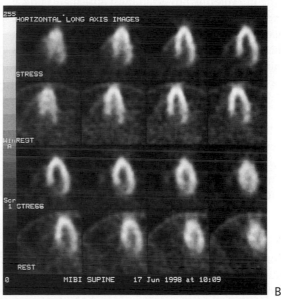

B

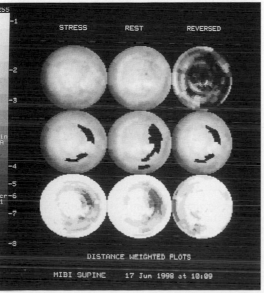

C

**FIGURE 12.8.** Vertical long-axis **(A)** and horizontal long axis **(B)** $^{99m}$Tc-sestamibi stress and rest tomograms obtained in a 320-pound woman with a low clinical likelihood of coronary artery disease. Tracer concentration appears to be decreased at the base of the left ventricle, particularly the base of the lateral wall. Polar plots **(C)** similarly demonstrate an apparent circumferential decrease in activity at the base.

diaphragmatic elevation is often observed. Partial or even complete diaphragmatic paralysis with consequent diaphragmatic elevation may occur following thoracic surgery, including coronary bypass surgery. Gastric dilation will also elevate the left hemidiaphragm. Although restricting the intake of food and liquids during the course of a myocardial perfusion study will considerably decrease the possibility of gastric dilatation, anxious patients may swallow air, particularly during stress, producing such dilation (Fig. 12.9). In patients with left ventricular dilatation, diaphragmatic attenuation may be accentuated. This may be because the dilated heart "sinks" down below the diaphragm, or possibly because the diluted ventricular blood results enhance attenuation of photons from the inferoposterior wall, which must pass through the ventricular cavity to reach the scintillation detector.

Attenuation artifacts due to left hemidiaphragmatic elevation are usually constant (fixed) in stress and rest images. However, the interpreting physician must anticipate clinical circumstances in which the degree of diaphragmatic elevation is inconstant. A change in the position of the left hemidiaphragm may occur, for instance, in a patient who is anxious and swallows air during exercise but expels the air prior to subsequent resting images. This will result in more marked diaphragmatic attenuation in the stress images, mimicking a reversible, ischemic perfusion defect in the inferior wall.

Infrequently, densities below the diaphragm may overlie the left ventricle in planar projections used for SPECT reconstruction and result in attenuation artifacts. In patients with ascites, such as those with liver disease and those undergoing peritoneal dialysis, ascites fluid may accumulate below the left hemidiaphragm, elevating it and resulting in attenuation of photons from the inferior wall of the left ventricle (12). Since ascites fluid may shift in position, attenuation artifacts originating from it are not always fixed. For example, if a patient performs upright exercise, the ascites fluid may shift to the pelvis, resulting in less marked attenuation than in resting images obtained after the patient has lain supine for several hours (Fig. 12.10). A patient imaged under these circumstances would show a pattern of apparent reverse redistribution.

Patients with chest pain often undergo a battery of diagnostic tests, which may include an upper gastrointestinal (GI) series with barium contrast. Occasionally, a loop of bowel containing barium may be superimposed on a portion of the left ventricle in the planar images used for SPECT reconstruction. Although very uncommon, such attenuation artifacts may be localized and mimic inferior wall perfusion defects (Fig. 12.11).

To anticipate and recognize attenuation artifacts caused by the left hemidiaphragm and subdiaphragmatic contents and structures, the following factors should be considered before interpreting SPECT images:

1. The degree of abdominal protuberance should be noted as the patient is lying supine (Table 12.1).
2. The hospital chart should be perused or the patient should be questioned about having conditions predisposing to free peritoneal fluid (e.g., liver disease, peritoneal dialysis, etc.).
3. The patient should be questioned about barium contrast studies within the preceding week. If there is a suspicion of barium contrast creating an attenuation artifact, an abdominal x-ray may help to confirm the presence and location of barium in the bowel.
4. The planar images used for SPECT reconstruction should be reviewed in a rotating cinematic format. The position of the left hemidiaphragm is usually readily identified in the left lateral or LPO views as a curvilinear region of tracer concentration representing the diaphragm itself or as a photopenic defect due to the stomach, which lies immediately below the diaphragm. Attenuation of the inferior or inferoposterior wall of the left ventricle is often evident from these views. To better define the position of the left hemidiaphragm and the associated potential for an attenuation artifact, some laboratories have obtained a separate left lateral planar view (preferably obtained with the patient in the right lateral decubitus position) with a higher count density (13). With the patient in this position, maximal separation between the heart and diaphragm is obtained. The rotating planar images are also useful for identifying ascites fluid below the diaphragm and barium in the bowel, both of which result in foci of marked photon deficiency. As explained above for breast attenuation, diaphragmatic attenuation is usually best appreciated by inspection of projection images displayed using a linear black and white scale.
5. Gated $^{99m}$Tc perfusion SPECT is very useful in differentiating diaphragmatic attenuation artifacts from inferior

**FIGURE 12.9.** Left hemidiaphragmatic elevation may be secondary to gastric dilatation. In this patient who swallowed air during exercise, planar projection images **(A)** reveal a photopenic defect below the left hemidiaphragm secondary to gastric dilatation. The defect is more apparent in stress images *(left)*. Tomographic short-axis *(top left)*, vertical long-axis *(top right)*, and horizontal long-axis slices *(bottom left)* demonstrate a localized photopenic defect in the inferior wall secondary to diaphragmatic attenuation **(B)**. A transaxial slice *(bottom right)*, at the level of the inferior wall, demonstrates a photopenic defect *(arrow)* corresponding to the fundus of the stomach.

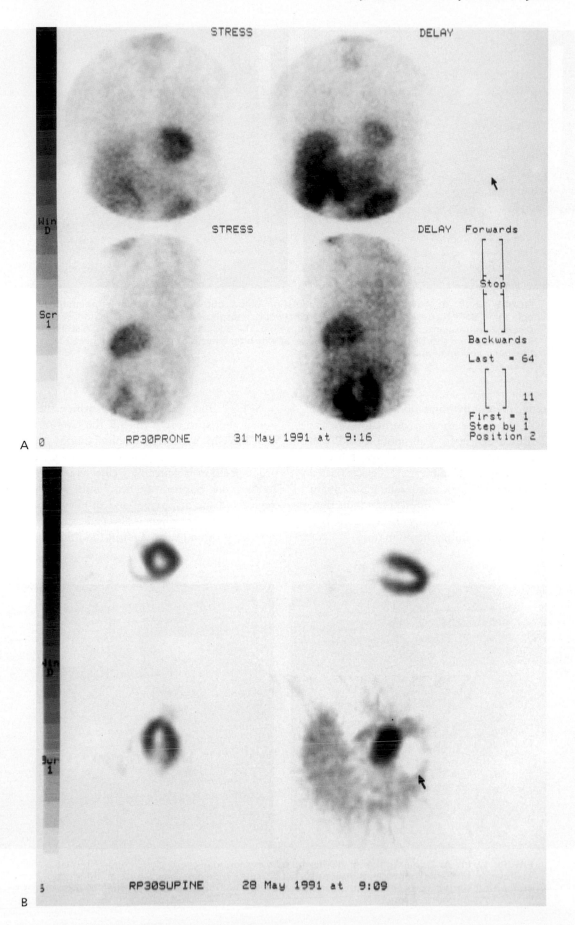

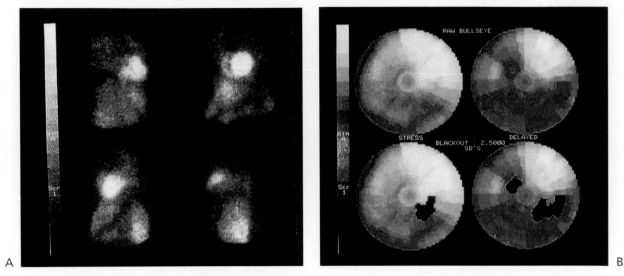

**FIGURE 12.10. A:** Ascites with fluid accumulation below both the right and left hemidi-aphragms. **B:** ²⁰¹Tl stress *(left)* and delayed *(right)* polar maps show an inferolateral artifact secondary to photon attenuation by localized ascites fluid. The artifact is much less marked in stress images obtained shortly after treadmill exercise, at which time much of the ascites gravitated to the lower abdomen and pelvis.

or inferoposterior myocardial infarction. Defects due to attenuation will move and thicken normally, whereas infarcts will exhibit decreased wall motion and wall thickening (Fig. 12.12) (3). As noted above, however, some caution in this regard is appropriate; defects related to small subendocardial myocardial infarctions might move and thicken normally, thus mimicking attenuation, whereas some regions of hibernating myocardium that are viable may not move, simulating infarction.

SPECT image acquisitions in which the patient's position is altered in order to shift the level of the diaphragm and thereby minimize diaphragmatic attenuation have helped to increase diagnostic specificity. Imaging in the prone position is generally well tolerated by patients (14). In the prone position the heart shifts anteriorly to a slight degree and the diaphragm and subdiaphragmatic contents are pushed down. There is also generally less motion of the anterior portion of the chest in the prone position and less

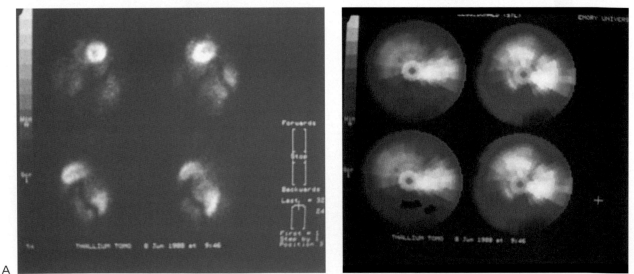

**FIGURE 12.11. A:** Barium in the splenic flexure of the colon may overlie the inferior/inferolateral margin of the left ventricle. **B:** Reconstructed ²⁰¹Tl SPECT images demonstrate an inferolateral artifact secondary to photon attenuation by barium. The artifact is also identified by quantitative analysis *(bottom row)*.

submax
shown
liver ir
immed
is injec
sation.
tracer a
tracer i
tion in
tion, ar
studies
99mTc-
atic, ar
For ph
which
val of a
milk or
hepatic
patient
imagin
ductive
small l
immed
cle. Fo
times r
ance of
As c
tion by
imagin
and sli
prone
abdom
For 201
tracer
occurre
true pe
imagin
washou

upon the inferior wall
to this area, making c
deficient. Therefore,
incorrectly identify de
imposed abdominal vi
The degree of 201T
ate (stress) or delayed
type of study perform
away from the abdom
musculature and myoc
perform adequate exer
age-predicted maximal
and such artifacts seldo
delayed images obtaine
from the heart, and re
and may result in artif
excessive liver uptake n
Similarly, with resting
reinjection protocol us
the liver concentration
cologic stress studies wi
not only in coronary
splanchnic blood flow,
the liver. Unlike exercise
lowed by a progressive
Therefore, in studies v
artifacts due to superin
quent in stress images th
of various imaging states
in the liver is listed in T
cisc, when the liver cor
delayed images, apparer
marked at 4 hours, imita
trast, with pharmacologi
tion of 201Tl is greatest
reversible perfusion abno
201Tl may concentrate
other than the liver, inc
spleen, all of which n
myocardium, particularl
aphragmatic elevation. T
atic in pharmacologic stre

### TABLE 12.2. RELATIVE
### LIVER AS A CAUSE OF
### ARTIFACTS

**Relative 201Tl**
**Concentration**

Exercise (maximal)
Exercise (submaximal)
Pharmacologic stress
Delay, postexercise
Delay, postpharmacologic str

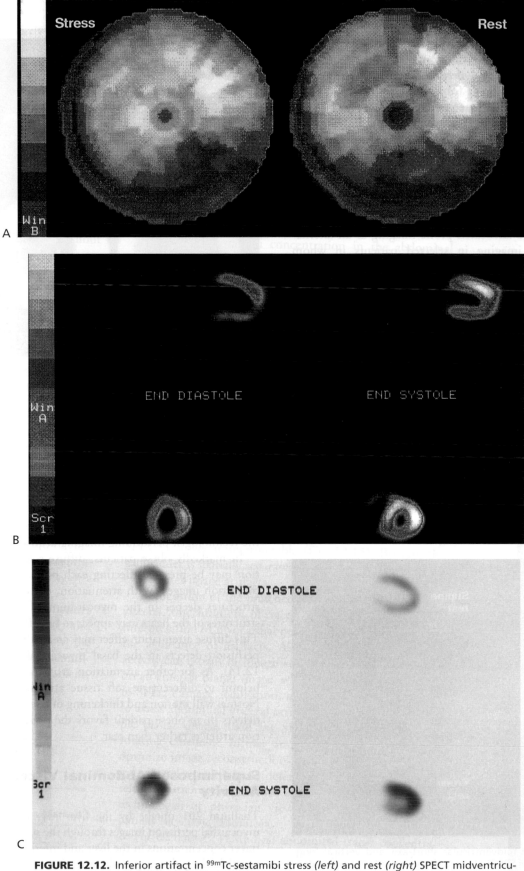

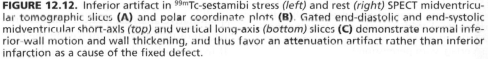

**FIGURE 12.12.** Inferior artifact in 99mTc-sestamibi stress *(left)* and rest *(right)* SPECT midventricular tomographic slices **(A)** and polar coordinate plots **(B)**. Gated end-diastolic and end-systolic midventricular short-axis *(top)* and vertical long-axis *(bottom)* slices **(C)** demonstrate normal inferior-wall motion and wall thickening, and thus favor an attenuation artifact rather than inferior infarction as a cause of the fixed defect.

243

upward creep (
decreases, mini
rior myocardia
supine but tha
represent diaph

Tracer washc
²⁰¹Tl SPECT, n
the prone posit
repeated with t
appreciable trac
the differentiat
reversible ischer
investigators hav
tive to supine
diaphragmatic a
the physician n
prone SPECT r
prone position t
supine position,
metric relationsl
With the more a
wall and septum
increasing the ap
(Fig. 12.13). Bec:
not be compared
purposes of quan
decrease in the
increased sternal

To recognize ar
uation artifacts, it

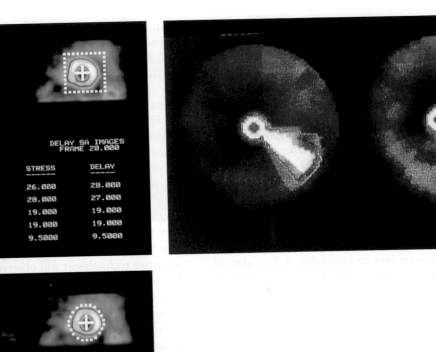

**FIGURE 12.17.** A rectangular box placed around the left ventricle for purposes of polar-map reconstruction may unavoidably include abdominal visceral activity **(A)**. The resultant polar map is normalized to superimposed abdominal visceral activity, with a consequent apparent decrease in count density in the remainder of the left ventricle **(B)**. (From Springer-Verlag, with permission.) In contrast, a circular region conforming closely to the epicardial borders **(C)** excludes abdominal visceral activity and associated artifact.

are the greatest. If a portion of the myocardium is not encompassed, the maximal regional myocardial count density may not be detected in the bull's-eye radius of search, thereby resulting in an artifactually low regional count density in the polar plot. Software is also available to volume-normalize myocardial perfusion images to the region of the myocardium only, thereby effectively eliminating abdominal visceral activity. A deceptively attractive means for eliminating abdominal visceral activity is to place a lead shield or apron over the areas of abdominal uptake. However, since abdominal visceral uptake can closely approximate that in the heart, and since an apron may shift during SPECT image acquisition, there is the potential for attenuating the inferior myocardial wall as well.

## Motion Artifacts

Because of the process of filtered backprojection used for reconstructing SPECT images, cardiac motion relative to the detector can create image misregistration and artifact. Cardiac motion has several sources. As it contracts, the

heart rotates physiologically on its axis. It is unlikely that such motion creates artifacts large enough to be recognized or misconstrued as perfusion abnormalities. By means of ECG gating, frames at end-diastole alone and/or during the isovolumetric phase of contraction, and the period of diastasis, can be selected, thereby potentially minimizing cardiac motion. This technique is applicable to ⁹⁹ᵐTc SPECT but not generally feasible for imaging with ²⁰¹Tl or ⁹⁹ᵐTc-teboroxime because of the lower image count density,

A reversible ²⁰¹Tl SPECT artifact may result from "upward creep" of the heart (18). A patient's rate and depth of respiration increase markedly during dynamic exercise, resulting in more marked diaphragmatic excursion, increased lung volume, and a lower position of the diaphragm. If SPECT image acquisition is begun while the rate and depth of respiration are still increased, the position of the diaphragm and thus of the heart will be low. During the acquisition, as the depth of respiration decreases, the height of the diaphragm will progressively rise, with a gradual upward shift of the heart. Such cardiac motion will not be present in delayed resting images, when the rate of respiration is slower and more regular. Diaphragmatic creep artifacts are common with exercise $^{201}$Tl and $^{99m}$Tc-teboroxime studies, in which exercise SPECT images are acquired immediately after dynamic exercise. A 15-minute delay between exercise and $^{201}$Tl image acquisition helps to allow for the respiratory rate to return to baseline. However, because of the very rapid myocardial washout rate, such a delay is not feasible for $^{99m}$Tc-teboroxime. Diaphragmatic creep artifacts are avoided with pharmacologic stress, which does not significantly increase respiration, and with $^{99m}$Tc-sestamibi or tetrofosmin SPECT, for which there is a delay between exercise and stress image acquisition.

The most common source of motion artifact during SPECT image acquisition is patient movement. Such motion is unpredictable and thus most problematic. Patients may move at any time during the acquisition. The motion may be gradual or abrupt, vertical (axial), horizontal (sideways), or rotational, and may occur once or multiple times. Artifact location, configuration, and severity will depend on all of these factors (19–22). Cooper and colleagues (20) evaluated the effect of patient motion in creating $^{201}$Tl SPECT image artifacts. The visual detectability of artifacts by experienced observers was directly proportional to the magnitude of motion. One-half pixel (3.25 mm) of motion was not visually detectable, one pixel of motion was recognized but judged to be clinically insignificant, and two pixels of motion resulted in artifacts potentially misconstrued as true perfusion defects. By quantitative analysis, two pixels of motion in the axial direction resulted in clinically significant artifacts in 5% of interpretations.

It is likely that cardiac motion subtending distances smaller than the spatial resolution of the camera (11 mm in air for most cameras) will not result in clinically significant artifacts. However, the spatial resolution of the imaging system depends not only on the intrinsic resolution of the camera, but also on the collimator, radioisotope, and image count density. Therefore, since $^{201}$Tl SPECT is usually performed with an all-purpose parallel hole collimator and a relatively low image count density, there may be greater tolerance to patient motion than with $^{99m}$Tc SPECT, for which high-count-density images are obtained with a high-resolution collimator. Moreover, higher resolution filters are used for $^{99m}$Tc SPECT, further accentuating small perfusion defects as well as motion artifacts.

Patient motion is particularly problematic because the location and severity of the resultant artifact depend not only on the magnitude of motion but also on its direction and the location within the 180-degree imaging arc. Cooper and co-workers (20) observed that motion artifacts are more noticeable when axial motion occurs at the midpoint of the 180-degree acquisition. They postulated that this was because the backprojected images were more evenly split between projections of two different distributions of radioactivity, one before and one after movement. These authors also observed that sideways motion results in more marked artifacts when it occurs in the anterior view, when the heart is parallel to the camera, and in the least artifacts in the lateral projection, when the heart is more oblique or perpendicular to the camera.

The most reliable method for detecting the degree, direction, and frequency of cardiac motion is to inspect the rotating planar images at the computer console. An alternate, somewhat less reliable method is to add the individual planar frames to produce a summed image in which the heart forms a horizontal "stripe" as it moves left [45-degree right anterior oblique (RAO) projection] to right (45-degree LPO projection) across the field of view (Fig. 12.18A). Although abrupt downward or upward motion and diaphragmatic creep are reliably detected by this technique, it is difficult to detect sideways motion and "cardiac bounce," or erratic up-and-down motion throughout the acquisition. A third and even less reliable method for detecting cardiac motion is by inspection of the cardiac sinogram. The sinogram can be thought of as a "stack" of planar views in which the $y$ axis has been compressed. In the initial 45-degree RAO projection, the vertically compressed cardiac activity is therefore positioned in the lower left corner of the image. As the heart moves rightward across the field of view, subsequent compressed cardiac images are "stacked" in a sinusoidal configuration (reflecting a one-dimensional projection of an object rotating in a circular or elliptical orbit). Discontinuity of the sinogram indicates patient motion. However, inspection of the sinogram does not make it easily possible to discern the type or direction of motion. Moreover, gradual, continuous motion is usually not apparent on the sinogram.

When cardiac motion occurs, misalignment of data by filtered backprojection often results in telltale artifacts in tomographic slices. The anterior and posterior walls of the left ventricle may appear to be misaligned, with curvilinear tails of activity extending from the myocardium into adjacent background regions (Fig. 12.18B,C).

It is essential that the physician interpreting a cardiac SPECT scan evaluate the study for motion and potential associated artifacts. It is equally or more important for the technologist to assess cardiac motion. If motion is noted during an acquisition, the acquisition may be terminated and restarted. Although this may be impractical for $^{201}$Tl stress studies, reimaging is feasible for delayed $^{201}$Tl studies and with $^{99m}$Tc-sestamibi and $^{99m}$Tc-tetrofosmin. Likewise, if motion is detected using the quality control methods described above, these studies may be reacquired. Therefore, it is important that rotating planar images be viewed before the patient leaves the laboratory, to avoid a repeat visit and reinjection.

Motion artifacts can be avoided or minimized by an alert technologist. The patient should be positioned as comfortably as possible on the imaging table, and should be observed during the entire SPECT acquisition. An arm rest is very helpful for maximizing patient comfort and thus minimizing motion. Nevertheless, patients often cannot hold their arms

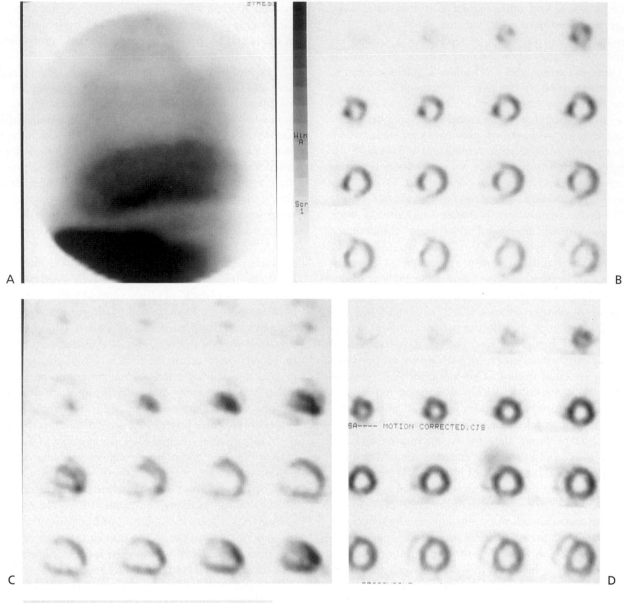

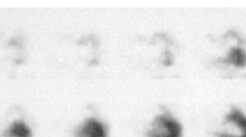

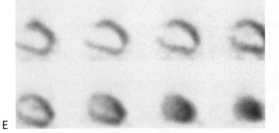

**FIGURE 12.18.** Summed planar images **(A)** in a patient with marked downward motion during 180-degree $^{99m}$Tc-sestamibi SPECT acquisition. Reconstructed short-axis slices **(B)** reveal apparent misalignment of the septal and lateral walls of the left ventricle, contralateral anterior and inferior defects, and "tails" of activity streaming from the defects. Vertical long-axis slices **(C)** have a "double image" pattern. After motion correction, accomplished by shifting individual planar frames upward or downward, short-axis **(D)** and vertical long-axis **(E)** slices demonstrate normal tracer distribution. (From Springer-Verlag, with permission.)

above their heads for the entire acquisition. Since arm movement often results in motion of the torso, the technologist should carefully reposition the patient's arm(s), avoiding any motion of the chest. The technologist should also encourage the patient to maintain a slow, steady rate of respiration. Similarly, coughing should be prevented if possible.

Computer methods to correct cardiac motion are commercially available. Their applicability may be limited if there is considerable concentration of tracer in the liver, which confounds the detection of myocardial borders (23,24). A more reliable method of correcting studies for motion is to manually shift individual image frames, so that the heart remains within a constant, horizontal plane (Fig. 12.18D). Studies can often be salvaged by this means, obviating the need for repeat acquisition, and in some cases, reinjection (Fig. 12.18E).

Automated computer methods for motion detection and correction have been reported. A "cross-correlation" method estimates the distance between successive planar projection images (25). The images are adjusted throughout the acquisition for gradual motion, including the lateral shift between frames, caused by camera rotation. Since abrupt patient motion departs from the expected gradual motion of the heart, both axially and laterally, it can be detected and corrected. A second motion-correction algorithm that has been described—a "diverging squares" method—estimates the coordinates of the center of the heart in each planar projection image (24). By this means the axial and lateral deviation of the center of the heart from its expected position can be determined as a function of camera angle, and deviant planar images can be adjusted accordingly. A third, related method is "two-dimensional fit," whereby a circular ROI is placed about the heart in each planar projection image, and pixels within this region are compared to those in adjacent frames (26). Each of these methods has shown the ability to detect significant patient motion, although axial motion is generally detected more accurately than lateral or rotational patient motion. A different approach to detecting motion has been described using multidetector SPECT and a point source placed on the chest (27). By determining any deviation of the motion of the point source, chest-wall motion can be detected and corrected. However, cardiac motion is not always directly related to chest-wall motion, as is the case for diaphragmatic creep, described above. Nevertheless, despite the development of these methods, to date visual inspection of the rotating planar images remains the most important physician- and technologist-dependent method of quality control in cardiac SPECT.

## Myocardial Hypertrophy

A localized increase in myocardial wall thickness and/or count density may create artifacts because images are normalized to the region of greatest count density for computer and photographic display and also for quantitation.

Since for an object smaller than twice the spatial resolution of the scintigraphic imaging system an increase in size is recognized as an apparent increase in count density, regional myocardial hypertrophy will appear as a localized increase in image count density (28). If the tomographic slice or polar map is normalized to this region of increased count density, regions adjacent to and distant from the "hot spot" will appear to have relatively decreased count densities.

Diffuse myocardial hypertrophy often results from systemic hypertension or the increased volume or pressure overload associated with valvular heart disease. Such hypertrophy results in a generalized increase in uptake of the radiopharmaceuticals used for studying myocardial perfusion. Additionally, a relative increase in septal wall count density is common in hypertensive patients (29). It is not clear whether this relative increase in septal count density is due to some degree of selective septal hypertrophy or to alterations in regional blood flow or metabolism in hypertensive patients. For $^{201}$Tl SPECT in patients with long-standing hypertension, a significant decrease in the lateral-to-septal wall count-density ratio as compared to that in normotensive controls has been reported ($1.02 \pm 0.10$ vs. $1.17 \pm 0.08$, $p \leq .00001$ for exercise images and $1.02 \pm 0.11$ vs. $1.11 \pm 0.08$, $p \leq .00001$ for 3-hour delayed images) (26). Thus, in tomographic slices, raw polar maps, and quantitative plots, the lateral wall often displays a relative decrease in count density, simulating CAD in the territory of the circumflex coronary artery (Fig. 12.19). This defect is usually "fixed" in stress and rest images obtained with either $^{201}$Tl or $^{99m}$Tc-sestamibi, mimicking myocardial infarction. However, occasionally, the septum may appear slightly less intense in resting images, rendering the defect partly reversible and raising a clinical suspicion of ischemia.

The physician interpreting the scan should anticipate this artifact in patients with hypertension or valvular heart disease. Therefore, it is important to obtain appropriate historical information. Similarly, the medical record should be examined for historical or echocardiographic evidence of idiopathic hypertrophic subaortic stenosis (IHSS) or asymmetric septal hypertrophy (ASH), which may produce a similar artifact. Moreover, inspection of the ECG for evidence of left ventricular hypertrophy is worthwhile. However, the standard voltage criteria are relatively insensitive to hypertrophy (30). In gated SPECT studies in hypertensive patients without CAD, areas of relatively decreased count density, usually involving the lateral wall, will move and thicken vigorously.

Localized "hot spots" in the anterolateral and posterolateral wall may arise from a prominence or hypertrophy of the anterior and posterior papillary muscles, respectively. In the case of a prominent posterior papillary muscle, the image will be normalized to the hot spot in the posterior wall, creating a relative decrease in count density

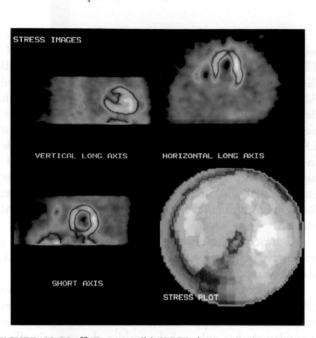

**FIGURE 12.20.** 99mTc-sestamibi SPECT demonstrating a prominent posterior papillary muscle in vertical long-axis, short-axis, and horizontal long-axis slices through the papillary muscle. The polar map demonstrates a localized increase in count density in the midposterior wall.

further from the detector in the left lateral and LPO views. Such alterations in the relationship between the detector and the heart result in an apparent relative increase in septal and anterior count density and a decrease in lateral-wall count density. In contrast, in patients with cardiac levorotation, the lateral wall lies closer to the detector when it is lat-

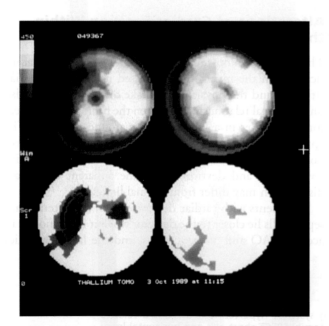

**FIGURE 12.21.** Quantitative exercise *(left)* and delayed *(right)* 201Tl polar maps in a patient with left bundle branch block and angiographically normal coronary arteries demonstrate a reversible septal perfusion defect.

erally positioned, and the septum is more distant from the detector in the RAO and anterior views, resulting in an apparent relative increase in lateral-wall count density and a decrease in septal count density. Therefore, when compared to normal limits, patients with cardiac dextrorotation may demonstrate lateral-wall artifacts, and those with levorotation may exhibit septal artifacts (Fig. 12.22). In general, because the rotational orientation of the heart within the thorax is relatively constant, these artifacts usually appear as fixed defects.

Although such artifacts are uncommon, patients with congenital heart disease or selective dilatation of either the right or left ventricle may demonstrate alterations in cardiac rotation. Similarly, abnormalities in lung volume due to pneumonectomy, atelectasis, or hyperexpansion may alter the position of the heart within the thorax and the SPECT myocardial image pattern. Moreover, chest-wall deformities, such as pectus excavatum, can alter the position of the heart within the thorax. Therefore, the interpreting physician should be aware of factors that may result in cardiac dextrorotation or levorotation in an individual patient. The abnormal orientation of the heart is easily detected by inspection of the rotating images.

Potentially, 360-degree image acquisition could minimize artifacts resulting from cardiac rotation. Likewise, for 180-degree acquisitions, tailoring the rotational arc for each patient so that the best septal LAO view is at the center (90 degrees) of the imaging arc could decrease the possibility of the heart being off-center in the acquisition. However, neither of these techniques has been fully evaluated with regard to the ability to eliminate rotational artifacts.

## TECHNICAL ARTIFACTS

### Errors in Selecting Oblique Cardiac Axes and Subsequent Polar-Map Reconstruction

If the long axis of the left ventricle is defined incorrectly on either the transaxial or midventricular vertical long-axis slice, the geometry of the heart in subsequently reconstructed orthogonal tomographic slices can be distorted. Consequently, the apparent regional count density can be altered in polar maps, resulting in apparent perfusion defects. These may be accentuated by quantitative analyses in which patient data are compared to normal files (Fig. 12.23). In polar map reconstruction, such errors most often occur in basal myocardial regions at the periphery of the bull's-eye plot, due to foreshortening of one of the myocardial walls. Also, the apex, which often demonstrates physiologic thinning and a decreased count density, is displaced from the exact center of the polar plot. The displaced apex may also consequently result in an artifact. When true myocardial perfusion defects are present, particular difficulty may be encountered in correctly position-

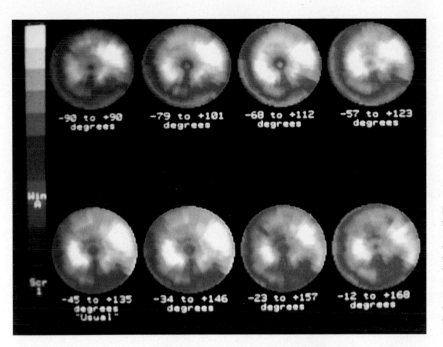

**FIGURE 12.22.** In this 360-degree [201]Tl SPECT study, 180-degree data are reconstructed, varying the start angle to simulate normal cardiac orientation within the thorax *(lower left)*, progressive cardiac levorotation *(upper row,* progressing from *right* to *left)*, and cardiac dextrorotation *(lower row,* progressing from *left* to *right)*. With levorotation there is a relative increase in the lateral-wall count density and a decrease in septal count density. With dextrorotation the converse is present.

ing the ventricular axes. Misregistration of perfusion defects in short-axis slices and polar maps is not infrequently encountered in patients with sizable, severe infarcts (Fig. 12.24).

To avoid such artifacts, the technologist must carefully identify the midpoint of the valve plane and the exact apex

when selecting the ventricular long axes. In cases in which artifacts are questioned, the interpreting physician should review the axes selection. With many commercially available software programs this option is available in the image display/review mode (Fig. 12.25). The axes selected should bisect the apex and the valve plane, and the obliquity of the axes should be identical for stress and rest studies. The interpreting physician should be alerted to the possibility of

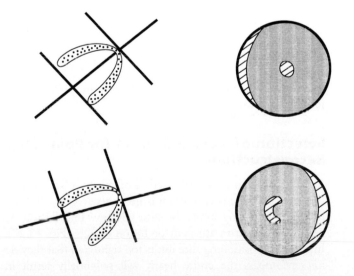

**FIGURE 12.23.** In this normal scan long axis of the left ventricle, correctly selected from the transaxial tomographic midventricular slice, bisects the apex and the valve plane *(top left)*. In the reconstructed polar map *(top right)*, the count density at the base of the septum is decreased due to the membranous septum, and physiologic apical "thinning" results in a decreased count density at the very center of the polar map. When the long axis is selected incorrectly (too oblique) *(bottom left)*, a ventricular wall (in this case the lateral wall) may be foreshortened, and the apical "defect" may be displaced, in this case toward the septum *(lower right)*.

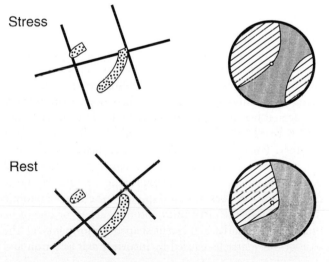

**FIGURE 12.24.** In these transaxial tomograms from a patient with a large anteroapical/anteroseptal myocardial infarction, axes are inconsistent in the stress and rest reconstructions. In the stress image the axis is incorrect and too oblique. The true perfusion defect is displaced septally. The lateral wall is foreshortened, creating an artifactual basal lateral wall defect. In contrast, the axis selected for the rest study is correct. Comparing the resulting stress and rest polar plots, there appears to be ischemia of the basal lateral wall and "reverse distribution" at the apex.

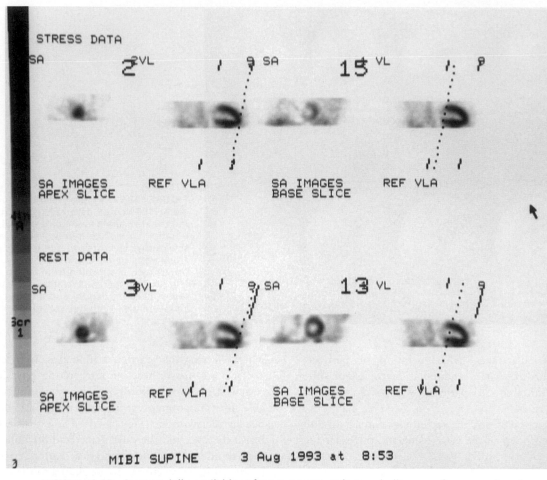

STRESS DATA

SA IMAGES APEX SLICE     REF VLA     SA IMAGES BASE SLICE     REF VLA

REST DATA

SA IMAGES APEX SLICE     REF VLA     SA IMAGES BASE SLICE     REF VLA

MIBI SUPINE     3 Aug 1993 at 8:53

**FIGURE 12.25.** Commercially available software programs (Emory bull's-eye software package) allow for review of the axes selected for tomographic slice and polar-map reconstruction.

incorrect axis selection if the left ventricular cavity appears oblong rather than circular (except for patients with extensive infarct and marked regional dysfunction resulting in cavity deformity) (Fig. 12.26). When polar-map artifacts are created because of incorrect axis selection, the resultant defects frequently do not correspond to a discrete vascular territory. For instance, if the apex is displaced posteriorly, the resultant artifact will be an apparent posteroapical defect. However, such an abnormality would be quite unusual since it does not correspond to the usual anatomic distribution of the circumflex coronary artery or one of its branches. Similarly, a crescent-shaped abnormality at the base of the ventricle, caused by incorrect axis selection and foreshortening of one of the myocardial walls, does not correspond to a usual vascular territory.

## Selection of Apex and Base for Polar Map Reconstruction

Accurate and reproducible selection of the apex and base of the left ventricular myocardium is necessary in stress and rest images. Positioning limits for slice selection that lie too far basally will result in apparent perfusion defects (Fig. 12.27). In contrast, positioning slice limits too tightly, so that they do not encompass the entire heart, will potentially result in underestimation of the size and extent of a defect (Fig. 12.28).

**FIGURE 12.26.** In this normal $^{99m}$Tc-sestamibi SPECT scan, stress short-axis slices (*first* and *third rows*) demonstrate a circular left ventricular cavity. However, in the rest short-axis slices (*second* and *fourth rows*), the cavity appears elliptical, indicative of incorrect selection of the ventricular long axis **(A)**. After reprocessing and correct axis selection, the cavity configuration is the same in stress and rest images **(B)**.

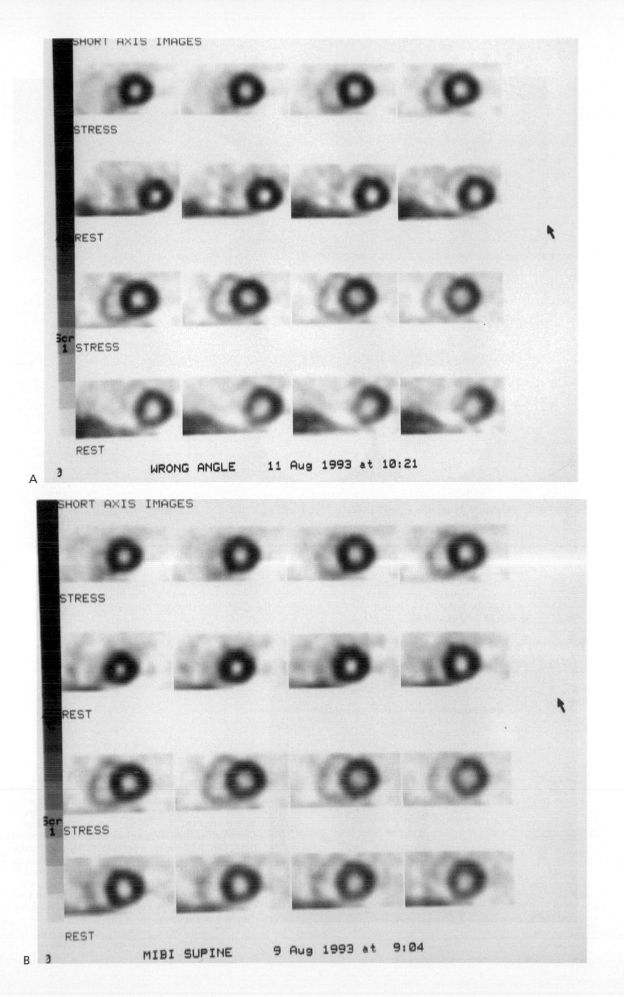

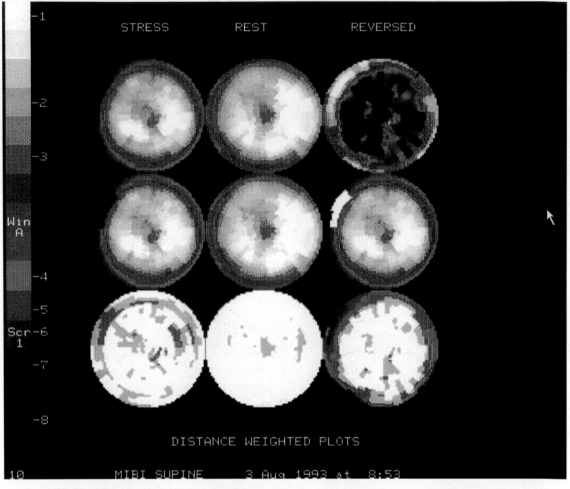

**FIGURE 12.27.** The limits set for selection of the basal myocardial slice in the stress $^{99m}$Tc-sestamibi study were too generous, resulting in a "rim" of apparently hypoperfused myocardium at the base. In the resting images, the basal slice was selected correctly, making the defect appear reversible (ischemic). The circular "rim" of activity in the "difference image" *(upper right)* alerts the reader to this artifact.

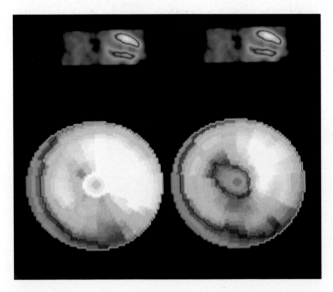

**FIGURE 12.28.** In this patient with a large apical infarct, an apical perfusion defect is present in the stress *(left)* and rest *(right)* vertical long-axis, midventricular $^{99m}$Tc-sestamibi tomographic slices *(upper row)*. The apical limit for slice selection for polar-map reconstruction was too "tight" in the stress study, virtually eliminating the apical perfusion defect from the stress polar map. Slice selection for the rest image was correct, and a large apical defect is apparent in the stress polar map, giving the false impression of "reverse redistribution" in this case.

## Detector Center-of-Rotation and Alignment Errors

If the camera center of rotation (COR) is incorrect, filtered backprojection during SPECT reconstruction will result in image misregistration and apparent misalignment of the myocardial walls. Technically, this is similar to the error created by cardiac motion. However, unlike motion artifacts, those due to COR error are usually more systematic and predictable. The appropriate method for COR analysis is detailed elsewhere in this volume.

The artifacts caused by COR errors are most easily appreciated in transaxial or horizontal long-axis tomographic slices. Errors in the COR in the positive (rightward) direction result in posteroapical defects, whereas errors in the negative (leftward) direction result in anteroapical defects (Fig. 12.29). These defects appear linear, extending through the thickness of the myocardium, and the anterior and posterior walls of the heart appear to be misaligned. The severity of the apparent defect is directly proportional to the magnitude of the COR error.

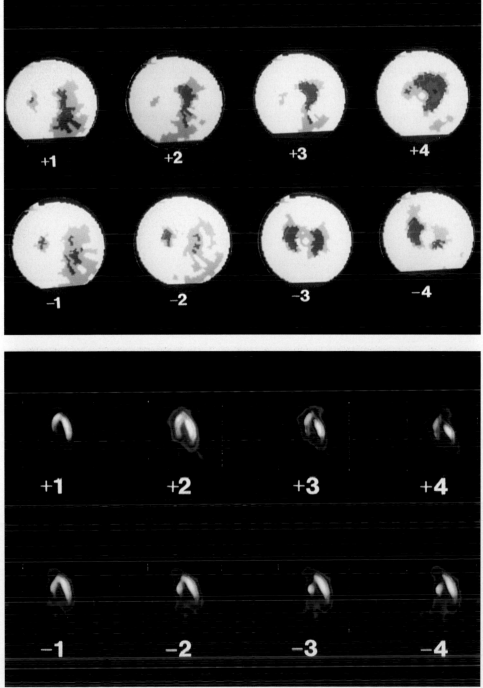

**FIGURE 12.29.** Center of rotation (COR) errors of 1, 2, 3, and 4 pixels in the leftward (negative) and rightward (positive) direction were simulated in the midventricular horizontal long-axis slice of a normal $^{201}$Tl SPECT scan. With COR errors of increasing magnitude, there appears to be progressive misalignment of the septal and lateral walls **(A)**. Anteroapical and posteroapical defects are present with negative and positive COR errors, respectively. Corresponding defects are present in quantitative polar maps **(B)**. (From *J Nucl Med* 1989;30:447, with permission.)

To avoid these artifacts, camera COR checks should be performed according to the camera manufacturer's guidelines. The resultant plots should be inspected regularly by a knowledgeable technologist and physician before the camera is used for patient studies. With the observation of a myocardial defect suspected of representing such an artifact, the COR determination should be repeated immediately. An error similar to that produced by the wrong center of rotation is produced when the detector is not aligned perpendicular to the radius of rotation.

## Flood Field Nonuniformity

Flood field nonuniformity will result in "ring" artifacts in reconstructed SPECT images. These relatively photon-deficient rings may be apparent in tomographic slices, and in severe cases may also appear in polar coordinate maps.

The routine quality-assurance measures required for cameras used in cardiac SPECT are done as described elsewhere in this volume. However, if ring artifacts appear in clinical SPECT images, it may be necessary to reacquire flood-field images in the middle of the day. Identifying the cause of flood-field nonuniformity in SPECT images is sometimes difficult. Malfunction of photomultiplier tubes, computer boards, preamplifiers, and other components critical to the maintenance of flood-field uniformity may not necessarily occur when the camera head orientation is at 0 degrees (parallel to the floor, facing the ceiling) (Fig. 12.30). Malfunction may occur only when the camera head is vertical or facing downward. Therefore, it may be necessary to obtain flood-field images in nonconventional orientations to uncover the source of the problem.

## Arrhythmias and Gating Errors

If arrhythmia is present, or if the heart rate changes during SPECT acquisition, inordinately short or long cardiac cycles will be rejected during eight gated acquisition. If the degree of the regular beat rejection varies during the SPECT acquisition, the number of cardiac cycles acquired for each projection image may vary if each projection image is acquired for the same length of time. Therefore, projec-

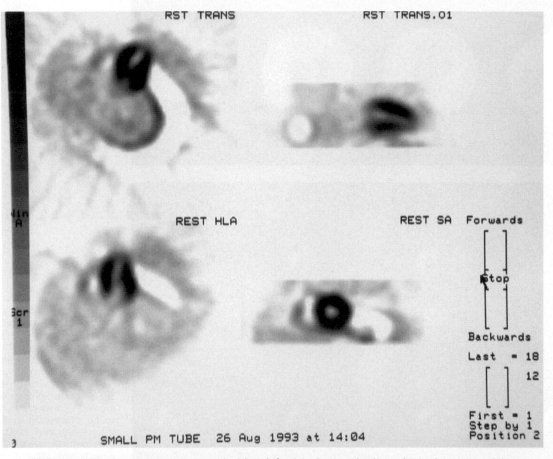

**FIGURE 12.30.** SPECT images acquired with a defective photomultiplier tube in the center of the field of view in a region overlying the heart in the anterior projection image. Concentric "cold" and "hot" ring artifacts are present in the transaxial slice *(upper left).* The rings are seen in various obliquities in the midventricular vertical long-axis *(upper right),* horizontal long-axis *(lower left),* and short-axis *(lower right)* slices.

tion images will vary in count density. When viewed in endless loop cinematic format, the projection images will appear to "flash". Acquisition of a variable number of counts in the projection images may potentially result in errors in filtered backprojection and consequently perfusion artifacts. However, Nichols et al. have reported that only

## TABLE 12.3. GUIDELINES TO INCREASED AWARENESS OF MYOCARDIAL PERFUSION SPECT ARTIFACTS

Clinical history
 Hypertension, valvular heart disease, renal disease
 Increased septal count density; lateral defect
 Breast implants, augmentation
 Anterior fixed defect
 Peritoneal dialysis
 Inferior defect, often less marked in delayed images
 Congenital heart disease, lung disease
 Cardiac rotation, altered septal/lateral count-density ratio
Physical Examination
 Sex, height, weight
 Chest wall, abdominal attenuation
 Chest circumference, bra cup size
 Breast attenuation, anterior defect
 Lateral chest-wall fat
 Fixed lateral defect
 Abdominal protuberance
 Diaphragmatic elevation, inferior defect
 Chest-wall deformity
 Alterations in cardiac rotation
Electrocardiogram
 Left bundle branch block
 Reversible septal defect
 Left ventricular hypertrophy
 Increased septal count density, lateral defect
 Abnormal left ventricular axis
 Alterations in cardiac rotation
 Arrhythmia (marked)
 Variable perfusion defects
Rotating planar images
 Soft-tissue attenuation
 Corresponding fixed defects
 Abdomial viscera overlying heart
 "Hot" inferolateral wall contralateral defect
 Cardiac motion
 Variable artifact
Tomographic slices
 Prominent papillary muscle
 "Hot spot"; contralateral defect
 Ventricular axis selection
 Defects from displaced apex and foreshortened walls
 Slice selection for polar maps
 Apical/basal defects
Camera quality control
 Center of rotation (COR)
 Anteroapical/posteroapical defects
 Flood field nonuniformity
 Concentric "rings"
Image filtering
 Elimination of low frequency data
 Accentuation of trivial variations in count density

with severe arrhythmias associated with atrial fibrillation are clinically significant perfusion artifacts encountered. The effect of gating errors in myocardial perfusion SPECT is detailed further in Chapter 7.

## SUMMARY

The list of technical and clinical circumstances that can result in SPECT image artifacts is considerable (38). To avoid artifacts and to optimize test specificity, both the technologist and interpreting physician must be aware of factors potentially contributing to the creating of artifacts. A summary of these factors and the associated artifacts is presented in Table 12.3.

## REFERENCES

1. Maddahi J, Kiat H, Van Train K, et al. Myocardial perfusion imaging with technetium-99m sestamibi SPECT in the evaluation of coronary artery disease. *Am J Cardiol* 1990;66:55E–62F.
2. Manglos SH, Thomas FD, Gagne GM, et al. Phantom study of breast tissue attenuation in myocardial imaging. *J Nucl Med* 1993;34:992–996.
3. DePuey EG, Rozanski A. Using gated technetium-99m sestamibi SPECT to characterize fixed myocardial defects as infarct or artifact. *J Nucl Med* 1995;36:952–955
4. Smanio PE, Watson DD, Segalla DL, et al. Value of gating of technetium-99m sestamibi single-photon emission computed tomographic imaging. *J Am Coll Cardiol* 1997;29:69–77.
5. DePasquale EE, Nody AC, DePuey EG, et al. Quantitative rotational thallium-201 tomography for identifying and localizing coronary artery disease. *Circulation* 1988;77:316–327.
6. Malko JA, Van Heertum RL, Gullberg GT, et al. SPECT liver imaging using an iterative attenuation correction algorithm and an external flood source. *J Nucl Med* 1986;27:701–705.
7. Bailey DL, Hutton BF, Walter PJ. Improved SPECT using simultaneous emission and transmission tomography. *J Nucl Med* 1987;28:844–851.
8. Galt JR, Cullum SJ, Garcia EV. SPECT quantification: a simplified method of attenuation and scatter correction for cardiac imaging. *J Nucl Med* 1992;33:2232–2237.
9. Manglos SH, Bassano DA, Thomas FD. Cone-beam transmission CT for nonuniform attenuation compensation of SPECT images. *J Nucl Med* 1991;32:1813–1820.
10. Tung C-H, Gullberg GT, Zeng GL, et al. Nonuniform attenuation correction using simultaneous transmission and emission converging tomography. *IEEE Trans Nucl Sci* 1992;39:1134–1143.
11. Manglos SH, Bassano DA, Thomas FD, et al. Imaging of the human torso using cone beam transmission CT implementation on a rotating gamma camera. *J Nucl Med* 1992;33:150–156.
12. Rab ST, Alazraki NP, Guertler-Krawczynska E. Peritoneal fluid causing inferior attenuation on SPECT thallium 201 myocardial imaging in women. *J Nucl Med* 1988;29:1860–1864.
13. Johnstone D, Wackers F, Berger H, et al. Effect of patient positioning on left lateral thallium-201 myocardial images. *J Nucl Med* 1979;20:183–188.
14. Machac J, George T. Effect of 360 SPECT prone imaging on Tl-201 myocardial perfusion studies. *J Nucl Med* 1990;31:812.
15. Kiat H, Van Train KF, Friedman JD, et al. Quantitative stress-redistribution thallium-201 SPECT using prone imaging:

methodologic development and validation. *J Nucl Med* 1992;33:1509–1515.

16. Chua T, Kiat H, Germano G, et al. Rapid back to back adenosine stress/rest technetium-99m teboroxime myocardial perfusion SPECT using a triple-detector camera: development and validation of an optimized clinical protocol. *J Nucl Med* 1993;34(9):1485–1493.

17. Stern S, Greenberg D, Corne R. Effect of exercise supplementation on dipyridamole thallium-201 image quality. *J Nucl Med* 1992;33(suppl):1559.

18. Friedman J, Van Train K, Maddahi J, et al. "Upward creep" of the heart: a frequent source of false-positive reversible defects during thallium-201 stress-redistribution SPECT. *J Nucl Med* 1989;30:1718–1722.

19. Friedman J, Berman DS, Van Train K, et al. Patient motion in thallium-201 myocardial SPECT imaging. An easily identified frequent source of artifactual defect. *Clin Nucl Med* 1988;13:321–324.

20. Cooper JA, Neumann PH, McCandless BK. Effect of patient motion on tomographic myocardial perfusion imaging. *J Nucl Med* 1992;13:1566–1571.

21. Botvinick EH, Yu Yz, O'Connell WJ, et al. A quantitative assessment of patient motion and its effect of myocardial perfusion SPECT Images. *J Nucl Med* 1993;34:303–310.

22. Prigent FM, Hyun M, Berman DS, et al. Effect of motion on thallium-201 SPECT studies: a simulation and clinical study. *J Nucl Med* 1993;34:1845–1850.

23. Eisner RL, Churchwell A, Noever T, et al. Quantitative analysis of the tomographic thallium-201 myocardial bullseye display: critical role of correcting for patient motion. *J Nucl Med* 1988;29:91–97.

24. Geckle WJ, Frank TL, Links JM, et al. Correction for patient and organ movement in SPECT: application to exercise thallium-201 cardiac imaging. *J Nucl Med* 1986;27:899.

25. Eisner RL, Noever T, Nowak D, et al. Use of cross-correlation function to detect patient motion during SPECT imaging. *J Nucl Med* 1987;28:97–101.

26. Cooper JA, Neumann PH, McCandless BK. Detection of patient motion during tomographic myocardial perfusion imaging. *J Nucl Med* 1993;34:1341–1348.

27. Germano G, Chua T, Kavanagh PB, et al. Detection and correction of patient motion in dynamic and static myocardial SPECT using a multi-detector camera. *J Nucl Med* 1993;34:1349–1355.

28. Galt JR, Robbins WL, Eisner RL, et al. Thallium-201 myocardial SPECT quantitation: effect of wall thickness. *J Nucl Med* 1987;27:577.

29. DePuey EG, Guertler-Krawczynska E, Perkins JV, et al. Alterations in myocardial thallium-201 distribution in patients with chronic systemic hypertension undergoing single-photon emission computed tomography. *Am J Cardiol* 1988;62:234–238.

30. Devereux RB, Alonso DR, Lutas EM, et al. Echocardiographic assessment of left ventricular hypertrophy: comparison of necropsy findings. *Am J Cardiol* 1986;57:450–458.

31. DePuey EG, Krawczynska EG, Robbins WL. Thallium-201 SPECT in coronary artery disease patients with left bundle branch block. *J Nucl Med* 1988;29:1479–1485.

32. Burns RJ, Galligan L, Wright LM, et al. Improved specificity of myocardial thallium-201 single-photon emission computed tomography in patients with left bundle branch block by dipyridamole. *Am J Cardiol* 1991;68:504–508.

33. Hirzel HO, Senn M, Nuesch K, et al. Thallium-201 scintigraphy in complete left bundle branch block. *Am J Cardiol* 1984;53:764–769.

34. Matzer LA, Kiat H, Friedman JD, et al. A new approach to the assessment of tomographic thallium-201 scintigraphy in patients with left bundle branch block. *J Am Coll Cardiol* 1991;17:1309–1317.

35. Civelek AC, Gozukara I, Durski K, et al. Detection of left anterior descending coronary artery disease in patients with left bundle branch block. *Am J Cardiol* 1992;70:1565–1570.

36. Rockett JF, Chadwick W, Moinuddin M, et al. Intravenous dipyridamole thallium-201 SPECT imaging in patients with left bundle branch block. *Clin Nucl Med* 1990;6:401–407.

37. Larcos G, Brown ML, Gibbons RJ. Role of dipyridamole thallium-201 imaging in left bundle branch block. *Am J Cardiol* 1991;68:1097–1098.

38. DePuey EG, Garcia EV. Optimal specificity of thallium-201 SPECT through recognition of imaging artifacts. *J Nucl Med* 1989;30:441–449.

# 13

# MYOCARDIAL PERFUSION SCINTIGRAPHY IN CONJUNCTION WITH EXERCISE AND PHARMACOLOGIC STRESS: PROGNOSTIC APPLICATIONS IN THE CLINICAL MANAGEMENT OF PATIENTS WITH CORONARY ARTERY DISEASE

SIU-SUN YAO
ALAN ROZANSKI

Since the introduction of myocardial perfusion imaging into clinical medicine in the late 1970s, this technique has undergone considerable expansion and evolution. Initially, myocardial perfusion imaging was introduced as a noninvasive diagnostic tool in determining the presence or absence of coronary artery disease (CAD). In more recent years, however, the prognostic efficacy of myocardial perfusion imaging has become well established. The ability to distinguish patients at low risk from those at high risk for future cardiac events has become an essential adjunct for clinicians in the management of patients with CAD. This chapter evaluates the prognostic applications of myocardial perfusion single photon emission computed tomography (SPECT), reviews the principles of stress testing as they apply to the prognostic applications of stress myocardial perfusion SPECT, and discusses the clinical applications of myocardial perfusion SPECT.

## CHARACTERIZATIONS OF PATIENT RISK

The assessment of patient prognosis is central to the clinical management of patients with CAD. As illustrated schematically in Fig. 13.1, patients with CAD can be characterized along a continuum of risk for cardiac events. When the risk of cardiac events is low, cardiologists generally employ conservative medical management. Conversely,

S.-S. Yao and A. Rozanski: Division of Cardiology, Columbia University College of Physician's and Surgeons, St. Luke's–Roosevelt Hospital Center, New York, New York 10025.

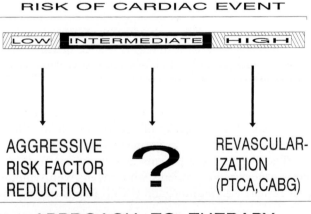

**RISK OF CARDIAC EVENT**

LOW   INTERMEDIATE   HIGH

AGGRESSIVE RISK FACTOR REDUCTION    ?    REVASCULARIZATION (PTCA,CABG)

**APPROACH TO THERAPY**

**FIGURE 13.1.** Schematic diagram of relationship between cardiac risk [for myocardial infarction (MI), cardiac death] and selection of therapy for patients with coronary disease, based on clinical data (the results of clinical history, risk factors, and exercise electrocardiography). When the risk of cardiac events is deemed to be "low" (roughly <2% annualized cardiac event rate), patients are generally treated conservatively and nuclear stress testing is not necessary. Aggressive risk factor modification should be emphasized in these patients, such as the lowering of abnormally elevated serum cholesterol levels. In patients at relatively high risk (arguably above a 6% event rate/year), coronary revascularization may be indicated. In patients at definitely high risk on a clinical basis, radionuclide stress testing is also not necessary. In patients who present with an intermediate risk of cardiac events, however, the choice of therapeutic modalities is often uncertain. As discussed in the text, radionuclide stress testing is particularly useful for placing such patients into appropriate high- and low-risk prognostic subsets, thus clarifying the appropriate therapeutic option in such patients.

**TABLE 13.1. CLINICAL, HEMODYNAMIC, AND EXERCISE VARIABLES THAT CAN CONTRIBUTE TO CARDIAC RISK ASSESSMENT IN CAD PATIENTS**

Hemodynamic and clinical variables
   Age
   Sex
   Prior myocardial infarction
   Chest pain characteristics
   Peak exercise heart rate
   Peak exercise systolic blood pressure
   Exercise duration
   Exercise hypotension
   Exercise induced chest pain
   Dyspnea
Exercise ECG variables
   Magnitude of ST-segment depression
   Slope of ST-segment depression
   Onset of ST-segment depression
   Postexercise duration of ST-segment depression

CAD, coronary artery disease; ECG, electrocardiogram.

when the risk of cardiac events is high, aggressive patient management, such as the performance of coronary bypass surgery or coronary angioplasty, tends to be favored. Between these extremes of risk, however, are a large number of patients who have an intermediate risk of cardiac events, which can be arbitrarily and roughly defined as a likelihood of from 2% to 5% of major cardiac events over the ensuing year. Decision making with regard to such patients is challenging, since the indication for conservative versus aggressive treatment is most uncertain in this group. Thus, the clinician often desires additional prognostic information about such patients to better define the likelihood of cardiac events. It is this group of patients in whom radionuclide stress testing finds its greatest prognostic benefit.

Who then are the patients at intermediate risk? As a gross generalization, patients who present with symptoms and exercise electrocardiogram (ECG) results that are "dis-cordant" fall into the intermediate risk group (1–5). However, characterization of risk on the basis of patient symptoms and exercise ECG results alone is simplistic. Rather, the physician also considers a variety of other clinical data and test parameters in evaluating patient risk, as listed in Table 13.1.

## PRINCIPLES GOVERNING THE PROGNOSTIC APPLICATIONS OF EXERCISE AND PHARMACOLOGIC STRESS MYOCARDIAL PERFUSION SPECT

### The Basis of Risk Assessment: Characterization of the Magnitude of Stress-Induced Ischemia

The prognostic utility of radionuclide stress tests derives from their ability to quantify the magnitude of "jeopardized" myocardium during exercise or during pharmacologic stress testing with dipyridamole or adenosine. Specifically, myocardial perfusion scintigraphy measures two indices of ischemia: ischemic extent and ischemic severity. Ischemic extent indices reflect the area of myocardial mass that becomes ischemic during stress. Ischemic severity indices correlate roughly with the number of stenosed coronary arteries. The number of reversible myocardial perfusion defects seen by SPECT, for example, constitutes a typical variable of ischemic extent. By contrast, ischemic severity indices reflect the magnitude of inducible ischemia within a given myocardial region. This measurement is roughly proportional to the magnitude of stenosis subtending a given myocardial region. For instance, the severity of a perfusion defect reflects the severity of subtending coronary stenoses.

Variables of ischemic extent and severity that can be assessed with stress myocardial perfusion SPECT are shown in Table 13.2. Included in this list are two variables that

**TABLE 13.2. PREDICTORS OF STRESS-INDUCED ISCHEMIA EXTENT AND SEVERITY USING MYOCARDIAL PERFUSION SPECT AND ADJUNCTIVE SCINTIGRAMS**

| Predictor | Ischemia Extent | Ischemia Severity |
|---|---|---|
| Number and/or location of reversible defections | ++++ | |
| Magnitude of defects | | ++++ |
| Delayed redistribution | + | ++++ |
| Lung uptake of isotope[a] | +++ | + |
| Transient LV dilation postexercise[a] | ++++ | ++++ |
| Magnitude of WMA[b] | | ++++ |
| Number/location of WMA[b] | ++++ | |
| Change in LVEF with stress[b] | +++ | ++ |

[a]Best assessed by obtaining a 5-minute and 4-hour anterior planar scintigram before the initiation of SPECT imaging.
[b]Obtained from concomitant rest-exercise first-pass radionuclide ventriculography when employing 99mTC-sestamibi.
LV, left ventricle; WMA, wall-motion abnormality; EF, ejection fraction.

may be assessed by obtaining an early anterior planar scintigram before SPECT imaging: (a) the poststress lung uptake of isotope (6–11) and (b) the transient poststress ischemic dilation of the left ventricle (12). Table 13.2 also includes the information that may be obtained from concomitant rest-exercise first-pass radionuclide ventriculography when technetium 99m ($^{99m}$Tc)-sestamibi is used as the radioisotope for myocardial perfusion imaging. Selected variables of ischemic extent or severity in Table 13.2 are summarized in the following sections.

## Variables Assessed Using Thallium 201 as a Radioisotope

In addition to the extent and severity of defects, three other scintigraphic variables may be assessed using thallium 201 ($^{201}$Tl) for myocardial perfusion imaging:

### Lung Thallium Uptake

In patients without organic heart disease, poststress myocardial perfusion scintigrams generally reveal little or no uptake of $^{201}$Tl within the pulmonary region. In patients with an elevated left ventricular end-diastolic pressure during stress, however, transient uptake of $^{201}$Tl may be noted in the lungs following stress, as indicated in Fig. 13.2. Caution must be applied in interpreting the significance of lung uptake of $^{201}$Tl in the presence of prior infarction, hypertension, valvular heart disease, or underlying cardiomyopathy, since elevated left ventricular end-diastolic pressure of any cause may result in a transient increase in the poststress uptake of lung $^{201}$Tl. Transient $^{201}$Tl uptake in the lungs following stress signifies disease that is functionally and anatomically

more advanced (6–11). The usefulness of this variable resides in its prognostic import. For example, Gill and co-workers (11) evaluated the predictive value of lung $^{201}$Tl uptake in the follow-up of 467 patients referred for planar stress-redistribution myocardial perfusion scintigraphy. A Cox analysis of survival identified increased lung uptake of $^{201}$Tl as the most powerful predictor of cardiac events in a comparison of clinical, hemodynamic, exercise ECG, and exercise $^{201}$Tl variables. The frequency of cardiac events over 5 years among patients with both an abnormal $^{201}$Tl scan and an abnormal increase in pulmonary $^{201}$Tl uptake was markedly higher in the Gill study than in patients with an abnormal $^{201}$Tl scan and normal lung $^{201}$Tl uptake, as shown in Fig. 13.3.

### Transient Left Ventricular Dilation Postexercise

Transient left ventricular dilation following stress may be optimally assessed by obtaining a brief (e.g., 5-minute) planar myocardial image early after stress, before the initiation of SPECT imaging, and comparing it to another planar image obtained during redistribution imaging. Transient left-ventricular dilation following stress is often a short-lived phenomenon, generally resolving well before the completion of SPECT imaging. Thus, the performance of early planar imaging may increase the detection of such transient dilation. Transient poststress ischemic dilation is generally a marker of both extensive and severe CAD, as demonstrated by Weiss et al. (12) (Fig. 13.4). In their study, transient left ventricular dilation following stress had a sensitivity of 60% and a specificity of 95% for detecting the end point of "severe" (i.e., >90%) stenosis in two or more coronary vessels. It is hypothesized that extensive coronary disease is

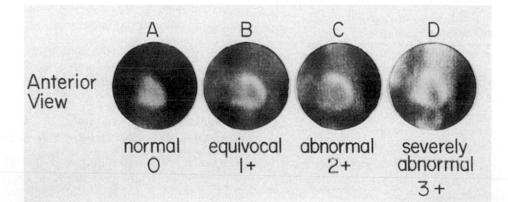

**FIGURE 13.2.** The presence or absence of thallium 201 ($^{201}$Tl) uptake in the lungs is best assessed from anterior-view planar scintigrams. Four grades of increasing lung uptake of $^{201}$Tl poststress are shown in this figure, ranging from 0 (no lung uptake) to 3+ (severe lung uptake, nearly matching the intensity of myocardial uptake). Information about lung uptake can be gathered in conjunction with myocardial perfusion single photon emission computed tomography (SPECT), by obtaining an initial 5-minute anterior-view planar scintigram immediately prior to SPECT imaging. Comparison of immediate poststress and delayed resting planar images also represents the best means to identify transient ischemic dilation of the left ventricle after stress, since such imaging can be performed early thereafter, before transient ischemic dilation disappears. (From Levy R, Rozanski A, Berman DS, et al. Analysis of the degree of pulmonary thallium washout after exercise in patients with coronary artery disease. *J Am Coll Cardiol* 1983;2(4):719–728, with permission.)

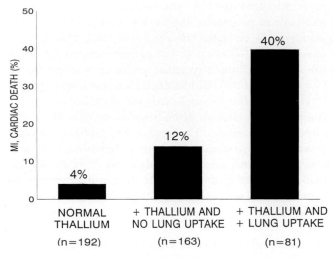

**FIGURE 13.3.** Cardiac event rates (for MI, cardiac death) (vertical axis) were assessed in 467 patients referred for exercise [201]Tl myocardial perfusion scintigraphy (planar technique) and followed for a mean of 4.8 ± 2.5 years. Patients were divided according to three scintigraphic patterns: a normal [201]Tl study *(left bar)*, an abnormal (+) [201]Tl study (fixed or reversible defects) but no evidence of lung uptake of [201]Tl *(middle bar)*, and both an abnormal [201]Tl scan and abnormal lung uptake of [201]Tl immediately after stress *(right bar)*. Note that the patients who had abnormal lung uptake had a markedly increased frequency of cardiac events. (Adapted from Gill JB, Ruddy TD, Newell JB, et al. Prognostic importance of thallium uptake by the lungs during exercise in coronary artery disease. *N Engl J Med* 1987;317(24): 1485–1489.)

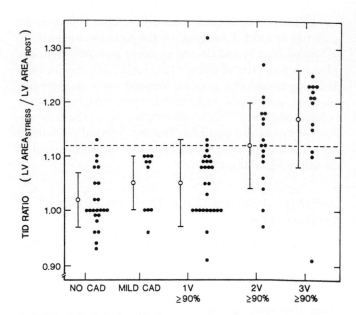

**FIGURE 13.4.** Relationship between the transient ischemic dilation (TID) ratio and the angiographic extent and severity of coronary artery disease (CAD) in five patient groups: (a) no significant angiographic disease; (b) "mild CAD" (all coronary stenoses between 50% and 75%); (c) one major vessel with ≥90% stenosis; (d) two vessels with ≥90% stenoses; and (e) three vessels with ≥90% stenoses. Mean 1 SD values are shown to the left of the individual patient values in each angiographic subgroup. The *horizontal dotted line* indicates the upper normal value for the transient ischemic dilation ratio in this study. Note that virtually all of the abnormal TID ratio values (i.e., those above the *dotted line*) were concentrated among patients who had ≥2 vessels with ≥90% coronary artery stenoses. Hence, the presence of an elevated TID ratio following stress generally signifies the presence of extensive and severe coronary artery stenoses. (From Weiss AT, Berman DS, Lew AS, et al. Transient ischemic dilation of the left ventricle on stress thallium-201 scintigraphy: a marker of severe and extensive coronary artery disease. *J Am Coll Cardiol* 1987; 9(4):752–759, with permission.)

required to cause left ventricular dilation following stress, whereas concomitant severe disease is required to maintain the dilation following exercise, for the duration of the imaging period. Thus, the presence of transient left ventricular dilation following stress should be regarded as an ominous scintigraphic finding, indicative of high-risk CAD. This measurement has also been reported to have similar implications with SPECT acquisition (12a).

### Late Defect Reversibility

Many viable myocardial segments will be associated with "fixed" perfusion defects on conventional 4-hour [201]Tl redistribution imaging. These defects will frequently demonstrate reversibility on 24-hour thallium redistribution imaging (13–15), and an even larger percentage (approximately 30% to 50%) will demonstrate reversibility following the reinjection of [201]Tl at rest (16,17). The rate of regional [201]Tl redistribution is roughly related to the magnitude of stenosis supplying that region: the more severe the underlying stenosis, the slower the rate of reversibility of a defect revealed by [201]Tl (13). Patients with fixed 4-hour defects that reverse at 24 hours are functionally sicker than patients with fixed 4-hour defects that fail to reverse at 24 hours (15), manifesting a significantly greater frequency of ischemic responses to exercise ECG than those with late fixed defects. Thus, the delayed redistribution of [201]Tl is a

marker of ischemic severity, indicating an increased likelihood of a severe subtending stenosis. So far, however, the potential prognostic significance of delayed redistribution of thallium has not been reported.

### Variables Assessed Using [99m]Tc-Sestamibi

The use of [99m]Tc-sestamibi instead of [201]Tl for myocardial perfusion scintigraphy can affect consideration of some of the scintigraphic variables mentioned above. First, since [99m]Tc-sestamibi imaging is frequently delayed for ≥30 minutes after stress, the ability to assess transient ischemic dilation of the left ventricle could be reduced. However, the lung-to-heart uptake ratios with [99m]Tc-sestamibi imaging, similar to the lung uptake of [201]Tl, are positively correlated with left ventricular ejection fraction and predictive of left ventricular dysfunction (18,18a).

Second, the presence of fixed defects at rest with [99m]Tc-sestamibi may sometimes be problematic since fixed defects with $^{99m}$Tc-sestamibi can also occur in zones of viable myocardium, due to resting myocardial hypoperfusion (19). The viability of such fixed defects can be identified by performing a separate rest-redistribution $^{201}$Tl scintigraphy study on another day (19), as illustrated in Fig. 13.5. Some institutions utilize a routine dual-isotope imaging approach in which a stress $^{99m}$Tc-sestamibi image is compared to a redistribution $^{201}$Tl image in all patients (20). The thallium isotope is injected first, at rest, with redistribution imaging performed at an appropriate interval thereafter. This redistribution $^{201}$Tl study replaces the resting $^{99m}$Tc-sestamibi study in all patients. Alternatively, both stress and rest myocardial perfusion SPECT may be performed using $^{99m}$Tc-sestamibi, and delayed thallium redistribution imaging is reserved for the subgroup of patients manifesting fixed defects with $^{99m}$Tc-sestamibi and residual questions regarding the potential presence of viability in these fixed defect zones. It is the standard practice of our laboratory to perform redistribution $^{201}$Tl scintigraphy on a subsequent day, 3 hours after the rest injection of the isotope, if there is an indication to assess the viability of fixed defects seen in a stress-rest $^{99m}$Tc-sestamibi myocardial perfusion study. Common indications for performing a redistribution thallium study following the identification of fixed $^{99m}$Tc-sestamibi defects include the assessment of patients who develop chest pain or ECG evidence of ischemia during stress testing, and patients in whom complete information about myocardial viability is central to patient management (e.g., consideration of whether or not to perform angioplasty for a coronary stenosis that subtends a region manifesting only fixed defects with $^{99m}$Tc-sestamibi).

Third, electrocardiographic gated acquisition of the perfusion myocardium can be performed with $^{99m}$Tc-sestamibi to simultaneously assess myocardial perfusion and resting left ventricular function. $^{99m}$Tc-sestamibi gated SPECT allows visual analysis of left ventricular wall motion and thickening, and left ventricular ejection fraction can be accurately calculated from either automatic or manually generated end-systolic and end-diastolic volumes (112–114). This technique of automatic quantification of ejection fraction from gated myocardial perfusion images has been well validated, when compared with conventional radionuclide measurements of ejection fraction (113). Recently, normal limit values for left ventricular volume and ejection fraction have been derived from patients with a low Bayesian pretest likelihood of CAD (114a,b). Notably, a significant gender discrepancy has been observed, with females manifesting significantly higher resting left ventricular ejection fraction measurements and smaller left ventricular volumes, when compared to males (114a–c).

The combined assessment of myocardial perfusion during exercise, and associated resting wall motion and global left ventricular function at rest can be used together to distinguish between attenuation-related artifacts and myocardial scar in zones manifesting fixed $^{99m}$Tc-sestamibi defects (28). Furthermore, gated $^{99m}$Tc-sestamibi SPECT imaging can aid in the detection of occult left ventricular dysfunction in patients with CAD and without prior myocardial infarction (MI), since resting left ventricular dysfunction in such patients usually signifies multivessel CAD (28a). Reports also suggest that the presence of global and regional left ven-

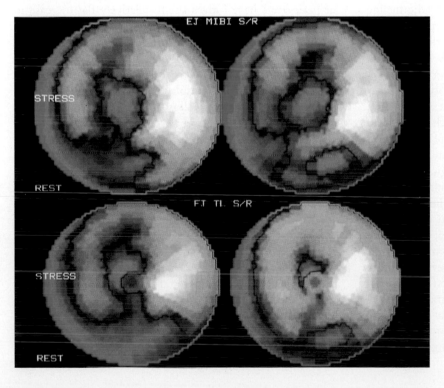

**FIGURE 13.5.** Four polar maps of myocardial perfusion are noted. The top two polar maps represent myocardial perfusion following stress *(top left)* and at rest *(top right)* in a patient undergoing stress-rest $^{99m}$Tc-sestamibi myocardial perfusion SPECT to evaluate the likelihood and magnitude of jeopardized myocardium. There is moderate hypoperfusion in the septum following stress, and severe hypoperfusion in portions of the anterior wall, inferior wall, and apex. No improvement is noted on the resting polar map images. The bottom two graphs represent the polar maps of myocardial $^{201}$Tl uptake following rest $^{201}$Tl injection *(bottom left)* and following redistribution imaging 4 hours later *(bottom right)*. The initial $^{201}$Tl image *(bottom left)* corresponds with the rest $^{99m}$Tc-sestamibi image *(top right)*, but the septal defect reverses on the polar map of $^{201}$Tl redistribution *(bottom right)*. Hence, this patient has resting septal ischemia, which is the cause for the underestimation of jeopardized myocardium following the rest $^{99m}$Tc-sestamibi injection. This potential limitation to $^{99m}$Tc-sestamibi imaging can be overcome by our combined $^{99m}$Tc-sestamibi/$^{201}$Tl imaging protocol for indicated patients, as discussed in the text.

tricular dysfunction in patients with reversible perfusion defects, as measured by $^{99m}$Tc-sestamibi gated SPECT, may represent postischemic stunning (28b). In addition, follow-up studies indicate that the use of gated left ventricular ejection fraction yields incremental prognostic value over myocardial perfusion scintigraphy alone for risk stratification of CAD patients (28c).

Regional and global left ventricular function during rest and exercise can also be measured by using the technique of first-pass radionuclide ventriculography with $^{99m}$Tc-sestamibi. This could be accomplished either with a dedicated first-pass camera system in conjunction with treadmill exercise (21,22), or by employing bicycle exercise in conjunction with either a multicrystal camera, or with a conventional single-crystal camera system that is equipped with an ultrahigh-sensitivity collimator (23). Such studies require that $^{99m}$Tc-sestamibi be injected in bolus fashion at rest and peak stress. Studies indicate that the combined assessment of exercise first-pass left ventricular function and myocardial perfusion enhances the prognostic efficacy of $^{99m}$Tc-sestamibi SPECT imaging (24–27). The use of first-pass exercise radionuclide ventriculography in conjunction with rest/stress myocardial perfusion SPECT, however, has been limited in some locations due to restricted reimbursement for both perfusion and functional stress studies at one time.

### Reporting the Magnitude of Jeopardized Myocardium

Because of its clinical importance, information about the extent and severity of jeopardized myocardium should be incorporated into the routine reporting of radionuclide stress test results. For example, a conventional practice is to divide the short axis of the left ventricle into three regions: apical, midventricular, and basal (Fig. 13.6). In addition, the apex is assessed from the vertical long-axis slices. A semiquantitative score may then be applied to grade visually assessed defects. Our approach is to assess the reduction in regional uptake of isotope in each of the 20 myocardial segments shown in Fig. 13.6 on a five-point scale, as follows: 0 = none, 1 = mild, 2 = moderate, 3 = severe, and 4 = complete reduction in regional uptake. Comparison of the stress and rest scores provides the physician with a quantitative estimation of the degree of reversibility of each myocardial defect. From the location of defects, it can be estimated which coronary vessels are the most likely "culprit" lesions for the induction of myocardial ischemia (32). In addition, whenever 5-minute planar images are obtained before the performance of SPECT imaging, the presence or absence of transient poststress dilation of the left ventricular, or of pulmonary uptake of isotope, should be reported on a routine basis, because of their added value in characterizing the magnitude of stress-induced ischemia.

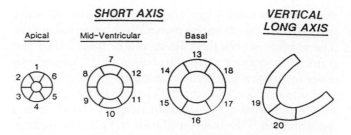

**FIGURE 13.6.** For scoring of defects on myocardial scintigraphy, the short-axis myocardial scintigram is divided into three zones, as indicated. Each short-axis zone is further divided into six myocardial regions, to evaluate the anterior wall (regions 1, 7, 13), anteroseptal wall (regions 2, 8, 14), inferoseptal wall (regions 3, 9, 15), inferior wall (regions 4, 10, 18), inferolateral wall (regions 5, 11, 17), and high lateral wall (regions 6, 12, 18). The apex (regions 19, 20) of the left ventricle is best assessed from the midvertical long-axis views. We use a five-point scale to evaluate the magnitude of diminished $^{201}$Tl or $^{99m}$Tc-sestamibi uptake in each of these 20 myocardial segments on each stress and rest study (see text). (From Palmas W, Bingham SP, Diamond GA, et al. Incremental prognostic value of exercise thallium-201 myocardial SPECT late afer coronary artery bypass surgery. *J Am Coll Cardiol* 1995;25:403–409.

## The Exponential Relationship Between Ischemic Magnitude and the Likelihood of Cardiac Events

The relationship between the magnitude of inducible myocardial ischemia and the likelihood of cardiac events is not linear. Rather, previous investigation has shown that the magnitude of ischemia has an exponential relationship to the occurrence of subsequent cardiac events (33). Accordingly, patients who demonstrate only mild ischemia at peak stress have only a small, relatively flat increase in the likelihood of cardiac events as compared to patients who manifest no scintigraphic evidence of inducible ischemia. By contrast, once ischemia progresses to a moderate magnitude, the likelihood of cardiac events begins to increase sharply. For example, Ladenheim and colleagues (33) performed a 1-year follow-up of 1,689 patients without prior MI who underwent exercise planar $^{201}$Tl myocardial perfusion scintigraphy for diagnostic or prognostic purposes. The frequency of "hard" cardiac events (i.e., MI/cardiac death) and late (>60 days) bypass surgery after testing (a proxy for worsening clinical status) were recorded as cardiac events. Stepwise logistic regression identified three independent predictors of cardiac events in this study: (a) the number of reversible $^{201}$Tl perfusion defects (a measure of ischemic extent), (b) the magnitude of reversible $^{201}$Tl defects (a measure of ischemic severity), and (c) the heart rate achieved during stress. Both ischemic extent and ischemic severity were exponentially related to the cardiac event rate (Fig. 13.7). The interrelationship between these two variables and their further relationship to achieved heart rate in predicting cardiac events is shown on orthogonal axes in Fig. 13.8.

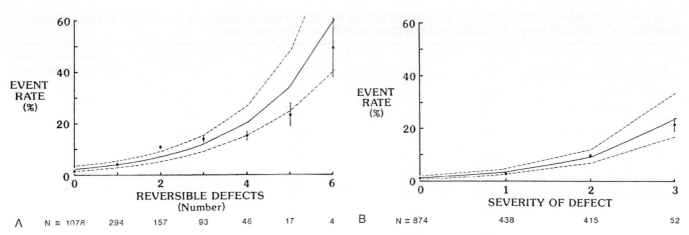

**FIGURE 13.7. A:** Relationship between cardiac event rate (vertical axis) and number of reversible ²⁰¹Tl defects (horizontal axis) in patients with suspected coronary disease who were followed for 1 year. The 15 segments that are normally assessed on a planar thallium scan were condensed into six myocardial regions for this analysis: anterior, septal, inferior, posterolateral, apical, and inferoapical. Thus, the number of reversible defects could range from 0 to 6. The number of reversible defects was exponentially related to the cardiac event rate. **B:** Relationship between cardiac event rate and severity of hypoperfusion. For this analysis, the magnitude of ²⁰¹Tl defects was scored according to a four-point scale: 0 = no defect; 1 = mild defect; 2 = moderate defect; 3 = severe defect. This variable was also exponentially related to the cardiac event rate, but with a lower range of magnitude for this variable compared to that for extent (compare the event-rate range to that for extent of defect in Fig. 13.7A). (From Ladenheim ML, Pollock BH, Rozanski A, et al. Extent and severity of myocardial hypoperfusion as predictors of prognosis in patients with suspected coronary artery disease. *J Am Coll Cardiol* 1986;7(3):464–471, with permission.)

Based on the published prognostic literature, four points may be derived that can serve as general rules of thumb for the utilization of scintigraphic testing in clinical practice:

1. The presence of a normal scintigraphic study at a high level of stress confers a very benign prognosis. For example, in the study by Ladenheim and colleagues (33), the annualized cardiac event rate was 1.3% in patients with a normal scintigraphic study. The same finding has been validated in a series of 16 other studies (Table 13.3) involving over 5,500 patients that evaluated annualized cardiac event rates during the follow-up of patients who had normal findings during the performance of exercise myocardial perfusion scintigraphy for suspected CAD (5,11,34–40,42,42a,51,72,74,172,172a). This benign prognosis appears to persist even in patients with strongly positive exercise electrocardiograms or angiographically significant CAD (42,42a,74,172a).

2. An equivocal scintigraphic study generally also conveys a benign prognosis. For instance, Berman et al. (41) reported on a cohort of patients referred for exercise ⁹⁹ᵐTc-sestamibi SPECT who were followed for a mean period of 20 ± 5 months (41). Among 1,702 patients, no hard events occurred in the 87 patients with an equivocal scan. Similar results were recently reported in a preliminary study of 505 patients by Yao et al. (41a) with a mean follow-up duration of 19 ± 7 months. Equivocal studies were present in 61 (12%) of SPECT studies. They were grouped as either small defects according to semiquantitative visual analysis or due to

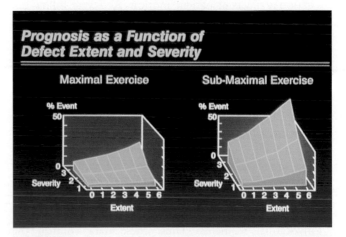

**FIGURE 13.8.** The combined effect of ischemic "extent" (number of reversible defects) (*x* axis) and ischemic severity (magnitude of myocardial hypoperfusion) (*y* axis) on cardiac event rates at 1 year (*z* axis). The patients were divided into 1,414 who were able to exercise to ≥85% of maximal predicted heart rate (*left graph*) and 275 who were unable to achieve 85% of the predicted rate (*right graph*). Note that the event-rate axis for the *right graph* is half that for the *left graph*. In the low heart-rate achievers, the average peak heart rate was only 76% of the maximal predicted heart rate. In both groups, the cardiac event rate rose as a curvilinear function of extent and severity of ischemia. Hence, patients who had both severe and extensive myocardial hypoperfusion with exercise had a cardiac event rate that was an order of magnitude higher than that of patients who had only extensive ischemia without concomitant severe ischemia, or vice versa. The cardiac event rate was at least threefold greater in the low-versus high heart-rate achievers. (From Ladenheim ML, Pollock BH, Rozanski A, et al. Extent and severity of myocardial hypoperfusion as predictors of prognosis in patients with suspected coronary artery disease. *J Am Coll Cardiol* 1986;7(3):464–471, with permission.)

**TABLE 13.3. ANNUALIZED CARDIAC EVENT RATES IN PATIENTS WITH NORMAL EXERCISE MYOCARDIAL PERFUSION SCINTIGRAPHY STUDIES FOLLOWING REFERRAL FOR TESTING**

| Investigators | Year | Stress Isotope | No. of Patients | Mean Follow-Up (Months) | Annualized Cardiac Event Rate (MI/Death) |
|---|---|---|---|---|---|
| Brown et al. (34) | 1983 | $^{201}$Tl | 61 | 44 | 0.8 |
| Pamelia et al. (35) | 1985 | $^{201}$Tl | 345 | 34 | 1.1 |
| Wackers et al. (36) | 1985 | $^{201}$Tl | 95 | 22 | 1.2 |
| Ladenheim et al. (33) | 1986 | $^{201}$Tl | 851 | 12 | 1.3 |
| Staniloff et al. (51) | 1986 | $^{201}$Tl | 374 | 12 | 0.5 |
| Gill et al. (11) | 1987 | $^{201}$Tl | 192 | 58 | 0.8 |
| Heo et al. (37) | 1987 | $^{201}$Tl | 519 | 27 | 0.5 |
| Koss et al. (38) | 1987 | $^{201}$Tl | 309 | 36 | 0.5 |
| Kaul et al. (72) | 1988 | $^{201}$Tl | 39 | 64 | 0.5 |
| Bairey et al. (5) | 1989 | $^{201}$Tl | 144 | 12 | 2.1 |
| Fleg et al. (39) | 1990 | $^{201}$Tl | 352 | 55 | 0.9 |
| Brown et al. (74) | 1993 | $^{201}$Tl | 176 | 24 | 0.9 |
| Schalet et al. (42) | 1993 | $^{201}$Tl | 164 | 34 | 0.0 |
| Fattah et al. (42a) | 1994 | $^{201}$Tl | 97 | 32 | 1.2 |
| Raiker et al. (40) | 1994 | $^{99m}$Tc sestamibi | 208 | 13.5 | 0.5 |
| Hachamovitch et al. (172) | 1995 | $^{99m}$Tc sestamibi | 1,623 | 18.8 | 0.3 |
| Pavin et al. (172a) | 1997 | $^{201}$Tl | 171 | 104.2 | 1.7 |
| Total | | | 5720 | 31.1 | 0.77 |

MI, myocardial infarction; $^{201}$Tl, thallium 201.

technical problems arising from, most commonly, attenuation artifacts or patient motion. At 1 year follow-up, there was only one confirmed cardiac event (MI) that was present in the subgroup with technical problems. Thus, despite the lack of diagnostic certainty with equivocal studies, they are associated with a benign prognosis even in patients with a high likelihood of CAD.

3. Because the extent and severity of myocardial ischemia are independent predictors of cardiac events, they provide incremental information in risk stratification. Thus, as illustrated in Fig. 13.8, when patients have both extensive and severe ischemia, the likelihood of cardiac events is increased by an order of magnitude over that for extensive but nonsevere ischemia, or severe ischemia of discretely localized distribution without inducible ischemia in other myocardial segments. Thus, these data confirm the importance, discussed above, of fully characterizing variables relating to the extent and severity of ischemia when interpreting stress myocardial perfusion SPECT studies.

4. Clinical parameters may powerfully modify the assessment of cardiac risk associated with stress myocardial perfusion defects. For instance, peak heart rate had a strong influence on the likelihood of cardiac events, independent of the defect size on myocardial scintigrams, as demonstrated by Ladenheim et al. (33). When patients are divided into those who did and did not achieve an adequate peak heart rate (i.e., ≥85% of the maximal predicted heart rate), the cardiac event rate for a given magnitude of myocardial ischemia was approximately threefold greater for patients who could not exercise to ≥85% of their maximal predicted heart rate. Such data illustrate the importance of incorporating clinical data into the assessment of cardiac risk when analyzing the results of myocardial perfusion scintigraphy.

## Substitution of Pharmacologic Stress Testing for Risk Stratification

In general, the performance of myocardial perfusion scintigraphy with exercise as opposed to pharmacologic stress is preferable for prognostic purposes. Important prognostic variables associated with exercise ECG testing include exercise capacity (43,44), exercise-inducible chest pain (45) or hypotension (46), and the ECG response to exercise (47–51), particularly the heart rate threshold (43,44,47,48) and postexercise duration of stress-induced ST-segment depression (47,49). These variables cannot be assessed when pharmacologic instead of exercise testing is employed.

However, the performance of myocardial perfusion scintigraphy in conjunction with pharmacologic stress testing, either with dipyridamole (52–55) or with adenosine (56–59), has essentially the same sensitivity and specificity for detecting CAD as does exercise myocardial perfusion scintigraphy. Moreover, studies done with both modalities indicate that the magnitude of ischemic defects induced by exercise is not underestimated by those induced by pharmacologic stress. Further, it appears that a normal scintigraphic study in association with pharmacologic stress is associated with the same low risk of cardiac events as is a normal exercise myocardial perfusion study (60,61). Dipyridamole or adenosine SPECT is commonly employed as the pharmacologic stress agent, given its ease of use. However, myocardial perfusion scintigraphy can also be performed in conjunction with dobutamine or arbutamine

**TABLE 13.4. USE OF RADIONUCLIDE STRESS TESTING IN PATIENT-MANAGEMENT DECISIONS**

Risk assessment in patients with a high likelihood of CAD
Selection of therapy in patients with angiographically documented CAD
   Selection of medical therapy versus revascularization
   Identification of "culprit" lesions prior to coronary angioplasty
   Evaluation of "borderline" coronary artery stenosis
Risk stratification of post-MI patients
   Predischarge exercise testing
   Predischarge pharmacologic stress testing
   Evaluation of patients following thrombolysis
Predischarge evaluation of patients with unstable angina
Risk stratification of the elderly
Risk stratification of patients with congestive heart failure and/or left ventricular dysfunction
Evaluation of patients following treatment modalities for CAD
   Percutaneous coronary intervention
   Coronary artery bypass surgery
   Medical therapy
Risk stratification of patients prior to elective noncardiac surgery

CAD, coronary artery disease; MI, myocardial infarction.

stress, but is generally reserved for patients with asthma or chronic obstructive lung disease (62–66). Despite the theoretical advantages of exercise in assessment prognosis, excellent risk stratification has been reported with adenosine sestamibi SPECT, with results similar to those observed with exercise (62a).

## CLINICAL APPLICATIONS OF STRESS MYOCARDIAL PERFUSION SPECT

Based on its strongly documented prognostic efficacy, myocardial perfusion scintigraphy has emerged as a key guide for major medical decisions involving patients with suspected or known CAD (24,67–70). The most common clinical applications of stress myocardial perfusion scintigraphy in patients with suspected or documented CAD are listed in Table 13.4. Each of these applications is reviewed in the following sections.

### Risk Assessment in Patients with a High Likelihood of Coronary Artery Disease

Patients with a high pretest likelihood of having CAD do not need to undergo radionuclide stress testing for diagnostic purposes (24). However, they are at intermediate risk prognostically for a cardiac event (1–5); this leaves the physician uncertain as to the best management (medical therapy versus coronary revascularization) in many of these patients. However, management decisions can be optimized by assessing both ischemic extent and severity in this patient cohort. For example, Bairey et al. (5) performed on 1-year follow-up of 190 patients who underwent exercise $^{201}$Tl scintigraphy after presenting with typical angina, no history of prior MI (MI), and a negative exercise ECG test. Such patients constitute a typical intermediate-risk group,

with a 1-year cardiac event rate of 6%. The results of follow-up in this patient population are shown in Fig. 13.9. Patients who had an abnormal $^{201}$Tl test had a 1-year overall cardiac event rate of 15%, whereas patients who had normal $^{201}$Tl scintigraphy with adequate stress had a 1-year cardiac event rate of approximately 2%. Among the sub-

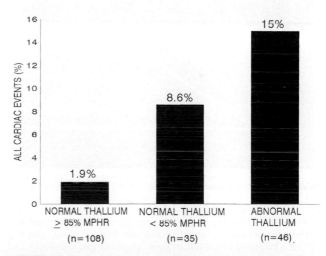

**FIGURE 13.9.** The vertical axis represents the frequency of cardiac events at 1 year (cardiac death, MI, late revascularization) in patients with typical angina and negative exercise electrocardiogram (ECG) tests, according to the results of exercise $^{201}$Tl testing (horizontal axis). A normal $^{201}$Tl study with adequate stress (85% of maximal predicted heart rate) *(left bar)* identified a low-risk subgroup (<2% cardiac event rate). By contrast, an abnormal thallium study *(right bar)* identified a group with a very high subsequent cardiac event rate (15%) within 1 year of testing. Among the patients with a normal $^{201}$Tl study and "inadequate" stress (achieving <85% of maximal predicted heart rate) *(middle bar)*, an intermediate cardiac event rate (8%) was observed. (Adapted from Bairey CN, Rozanski A, Maddahi J, et al. Exercise thallium-201 scintigraphy and prognosis in typical angina pectoris and negative exercise electrocardiography. *Am J Cardiol* 1989;64:282–287.)

group with a normal [201]Tl study but failure to achieve an adequate heart rate, however, the cardiac event was intermediate. These data emphasize the importance, for prognostic and diagnostic purposes, of achieving an adequate level of stress when performing exercise myocardial perfusion scintigraphy. Thus, it is generally recommended that, when a patient undergoing exercise myocardial perfusion scintigraphy cannot achieve an adequate target heart rate, the test is discontinued before injection of the radioisotope, and pharmacologic stress testing is employed instead.

The results of Bairey and colleagues (5) are compatible with bayesian theory. Bayesian analysis predicts that when the pretest likelihood of disease or ischemia is high, tests with a relatively low sensitivity to disease or ischemia will be associated with an accentuated false-negative rate (Fig. 13.10). In such a patient, one would predict that a negative exercise ECG response would not be a reliable predictor of no ischemia, and therefore would also not be a reli-

able predictor of low risk. Increasingly, the literature bears out this relationship.

Other analyses have also demonstrated the prognostic efficacy of stress myocardial perfusion scintigraphy in patients with a high pretest likelihood of having CAD (4,69). Thus, even though radionuclide stress tests are not indicated for diagnostic purposes in patients presenting with a high pretest likelihood of CAD, these tests are very useful in such patients for purposes of risk stratification (i.e., decision making). Figure 13.11 represents a typical case example of the use of stress myocardial perfusion SPECT for prognostic purposes in a patient who already had a high pretest likelihood of CAD.

### Evaluation of Patients with Borderline Coronary Stenosis

It is not uncommon during the performance of coronary angiography to identify borderline coronary stenoses (around 40% to 60%) in the absence of more severe lesions (71). Uncertainty about the significance of these lesions may be augmented by the inherent error associated with visual estimation of the severity of stenosis. Thus, in a patient with a borderline stenosis, the physician may be unsure about whether or not to attribute the patient's symptoms to this lesion. In such patients, the results of stress myocardial perfusion SPECT can be very useful to the physician. The induction of perfusion abnormalities in the distribution of a borderline lesion would indicate that the lesion is hemodynamically significant. The lack of inducible ischemia would indicate that the patient is at low risk for cardiac events, and would allow the physician to assure the patient with respect to symptoms and prognosis, while concomitantly instituting relevant measures for coronary risk-factor reduction so as to retard the progression of lesions.

### Selection of Therapy in Patients with Angiographically Documented Coronary Artery Disease

Even when the results of angiography are known, radionuclide stress tests may provide incremental information for patient risk stratification (72–78). Since radionuclide stress tests provide physiologic measurements, they may be used to test the hemodynamic significance of coronary stenoses, including those of borderline significance. When radionuclide stress testing among patients with angiographically documented CAD yields normal results during adequate stress, the likelihood of subsequent cardiac events is low (42a,74,75). Brown and Rowen (74), for example, reported only two cardiac events during a mean follow-up of 24 months among 75 consecutive patients who manifested a normal exercise myocardial perfusion scintigraphy study in conjunction with angiographic evidence of significant CAD (an annualized cardiac event rate of only 0.7%/year). The first study to demonstrate the complementary nature of

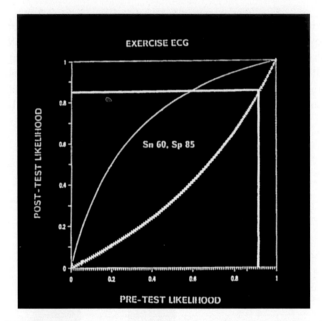

**FIGURE 13.10.** Bayesian curves relating pretest likelihood of CAD (*x* axis) to posttest CAD likelihood (*y* axis) for a positive *(top, thinner curve)* and negative exercise electrocardiogram (ECG) response *(lower, thicker curve)*. This figure is used to illustrate the relationship between a negative exercise ECG response and the posttest likelihood of cardiac disease when the pretest likelihood of disease is high before the performance of exercise ECG. The pretest CAD likelihood is determined from Bayesian analysis of patient age, sex, symptoms, and coronary artery risk factors. The posttest likelihood of disease is determined from Bayes' theorem, which can be applied when test sensitivity, test specificity, and disease prevalence are known. Note that when the pretest likelihood of disease is very high with a negative exercise ECG *(thick vertical line)*, the posttest likelihood of CAD remains high. We demonstrated that these negative exercise ECG responses represent prognostically, two distinct groups of patients: (a) those who are physiologically nonischemic and at low cardiac risk (identified by a negative exercise thallium study), and (b) those who are truly ischemic and at high risk for events. Patients in this latter subgroup are identified by a positive exercise [201]Tl study (see text for details).

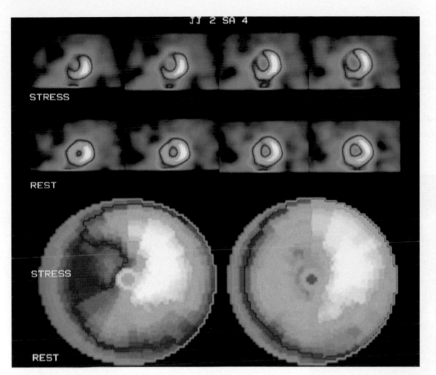

**FIGURE 13.11.** Sequential short-axis slices, using $^{99m}$Tc-sestamibi, following dipyridamole stress *(top row)* and at rest *(second row)*, and the corresponding polar maps following dipyridamole stress *(bottom left)* and at rest *(bottom right)* in a 69-year-old man with a high pretest likelihood of CAD (typical angina, multiple risk factors). Testing was not necessary for diagnostic purposes. Rather, it was performed to determine the need for coronary angiography and subsequent revascularization. Following stress there was a severe anteroseptal wall myocardial perfusion defect, reversing on the rest scintigrams. The polar maps are concordant with the myocardial scintigrams. Subsequent cardiac catheterization revealed a totally occluded lesion in the proximal portion of the left anterior descending coronary artery. There was also a milder lesion in the left circumflex coronary artery. On the basis of these results, the patient was revascularized.

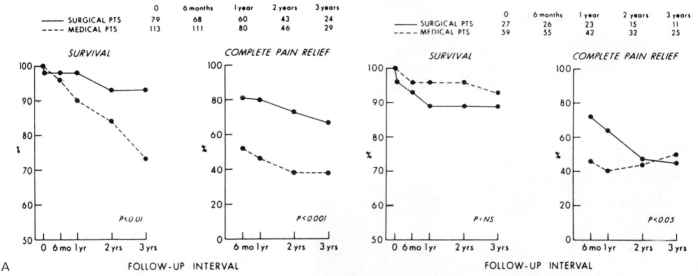

**FIGURE 13.12. A:** Life-table curves comparing patient survival *(left)* and incidence of complete pain relief *(right)* in 192 patients with CAD and ischemic left ventricular dysfunction during rest-exercise first-pass radionuclide ventriculography. Patients are divided into those who underwent coronary bypass surgery *(solid lines)* and those who were treated medically *(dotted lines)*. There was a significant increase in survival and more complete pain relief among patients treated surgically than among those treated medically in this cohort. **B:** Corresponding life-table curves for the 86 patients with coronary disease who had normal rest-exercise radionuclide ventriculography. In the absence of exercise-inducible ischemia, there was no survival benefit in those undergoing coronary bypass surgery. Further, whereas there was initially greater complete pain relief with bypass surgery, this benefit was lost within 2 years. (From Jones RH, Floyd RD, Austin EH, et al. The role of radionuclide angiocardiography in the preoperative prediction of pain relief and prolonged survival following coronary artery bypass grafting. *Ann Surg* 1983;197(6):743–753, with permission.)

anatomic and physiologic data derived from radionuclide imaging for risk assessment was that reported by Jones et al. (76). They found that a nonischemic response during exercise radionuclide ventriculography identified a cohort of patients who did not benefit from coronary bypass surgery, because of an already low risk of cardiac events in medically managed patients who did not have inducible ischemia (Fig. 13.12) (76). Such data have led to the growing recog-

nition that decisions about bypass surgery or coronary angioplasty should not rely solely on the results of coronary angiography among patients with CAD and symptoms of stable angina. Rather, the most informed decisions relating to such patients should incorporate consideration of both anatomic and physiologic factors. Because of the documented low risk of cardiac events among patients with CAD and stable anginal symptoms who demonstrate nor-

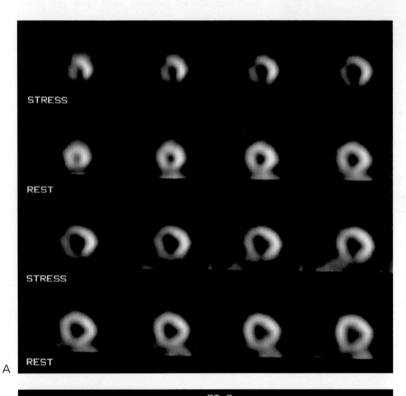

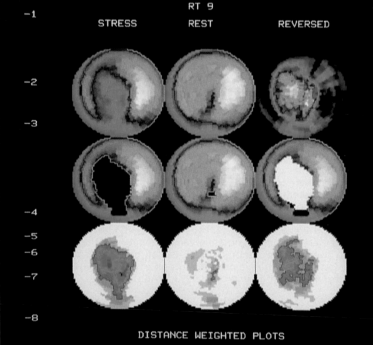

**FIGURE 13.13. A:** Short-axis scintigrams in a 51-year-old man with a history of CAD, documented by coronary angiography 3 days prior to the performance of a myocardial perfusion study. The coronary angiogram revealed complete occlusion of the right coronary artery, complete occlusion of the proximal left anterior descending coronary artery, and a borderline stenosis of the left circumflex coronary artery. The subsequent exercise $^{99m}$Tc-sestamibi study was ordered to assess the physiologic significance of the lesions noted on angiography (the physician wrote that "results of this study will be vital in determining the final recommendation of medical therapy versus coronary bypass surgery.") For this figure and all corresponding figures showing four rows of short-axis slices, the *first* and *third rows* represent poststress images and the *second* and *fourth rows* represent the corresponding short-axis tomograms at rest. The scintigrams begin with representative apical slices *(top left)* and extend to demonstrate basal slices *(bottom right)*. The poststress myocardial scintigram reveals severe and extensive septal and inferior-wall myocardial perfusion defects in this patient, reversing on the rest $^{99m}$Tc-sestamibi scintigrams. These results indicate that the left anterior descending and right coronary artery lesions subtend severely jeopardized myocardium, pointing to the need for myocardial revascularization. The patient therefore underwent coronary bypass surgery. **B:** Corresponding polar maps. This and subsequent figures displaying 3 × 3 polar maps, are grouped by rows and columns. The *left column* of images displays, from *top* to *bottom:* (a) the perfusion map; (b) perfusion map with superimposed blacked-out abnormal territories; and (c) a severity polar map, with the severity of defects depicted by a color code corresponding to the number of standard deviations below normal limits. The *second column* of maps displays the corresponding polar maps at rest. The *third column* of maps shows reversed $^{99m}$Tc-sestamibi distributions, used to indicate zones of defect reversibility. The second map in the *right column* demonstrates zones of reversible defects in white "islands," superimposed on the poststress, blacked-out regions. Perfusion defects are color coded according to a linear scale (not shown), in which the most normal zones are in white and yellow and the most abnormal zones are shaded with an increasing blue to black intensity. Note the marked septal and inferior-wall abnormalities on the poststress polar map *(top row, left column)*, reversing at rest *(top row, middle column)*. This region is blacked out after stress *(middle row, left column)* and identified as reversible on the reversibility map *(middle row, right column)*.

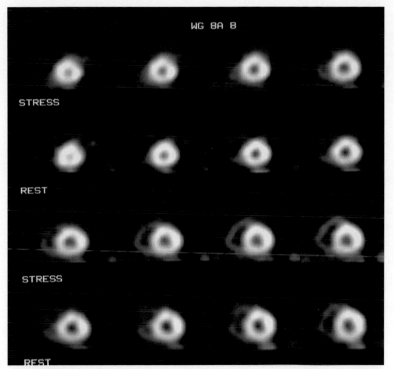

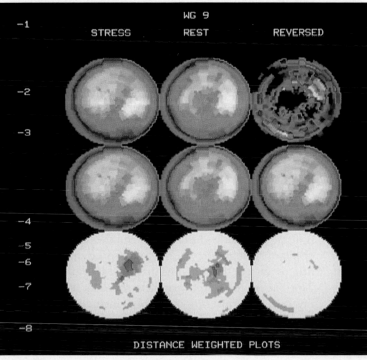

**FIGURE 13.14. A:** Myocardial scintigrams for a 53-year-old man with multiple coronary risk factors and typical angina of recent onset. The patient underwent cardiac catheterization, which revealed an 80% to 90% stenosis of the distal right coronary artery and a 75% stenosis in the middle left anterior descending coronary artery. To assess the physiologic significance of these lesions, an exercise $^{99m}$Tc-sestamibi study was ordered. The patient exercised for 9 minutes to a peak heart rate of 142 beats per minute, and had no chest pain or ST-segment depression. The myocardial scintigrams are normal. Hence, the patient was consigned to conservative medical management. **B:** Corresponding polar maps, indicating normal myocardial perfusion during exercise and at rest.

mal myocardial perfusion scintigraphy during adequate stress testing, it is now generally difficult to justify the performance of coronary angioplasty or coronary bypass surgery in such patients.

Figures 13.13 and 13.14 illustrate examples of the application of stress myocardial perfusion SPECT in guiding clinical decisions in patients with angiographically doc-

umented CAD. Because of its ability to assess the hemodynamic significance of coronary stenosis, stress myocardial perfusion SPECT may also be used to identify the culprit coronary lesions in patients who are candidates for coronary angioplasty and the physiologic significance of borderline coronary stenosis (in the range of 30–60% stenosis).

## Risk Stratification of Post-MI Patients

Patients with an uncomplicated acute MI are generally referred for noninvasive stress testing prior to hospital discharge. The subgroup of post-MI patients who demonstrate extensive or severe ischemia on such testing are subject to immediate catheterization and revascularization because of their documented high risk for cardiac events (79).

### Predischarge Exercise Testing

Whereas exercise ECG may be used in isolation to assess ischemia in post-MI patients, there is a decided advantage to using combined perfusion imaging and ECG monitoring for assessing such risk. Perfusion imaging is innately more sensitive for detecting myocardial ischemia and more accurate in quantifying its magnitude. For example, Gibson et al. (80) compared the prognostic efficacy of exercise ECG, stress-redistribution myocardial perfusion scintigraphy with $^{201}$Tl, and cardiac catheterization, all performed prior to hospital

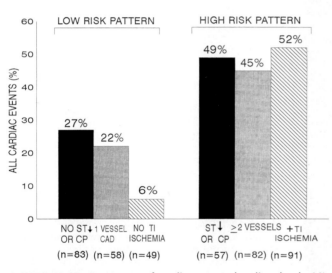

**FIGURE 13.15.** Frequency of cardiac events (cardiac death, MI, development of class III/IV angina) (vertical axis) over a mean follow-up period of 15 ± 2 months for 140 patients undergoing submaximal exercise $^{201}$Tl study and coronary angiography following uncomplicated acute MI. The test results are divided into those associated with low-risk *(left bars)* and high-risk patterns *(right bars)*. A high-risk pattern included ST-segment depression or chest pain with exercise, angiography showing multivessel disease, or a $^{201}$Tl scan showing reversible defects or lung uptake of $^{201}$Tl. Each of these high-risk patterns was associated with a comparable, high frequency of subsequent cardiac events. Markedly different results were noted, however, in the efficacy of these tests for predicting a low risk of events. Thus, whereas a nonischemic $^{201}$Tl study was associated with only a 6% cardiac event rate during the follow-up period, the absence of chest pain or ST-segment depression during ECG, and a cardiac catheterization study manifesting only single-vessel disease were still both associated with a relatively high frequency of subsequent exercise events. (From Gibson RS, Watson DD, Craddock GB, et al. Prediction of cardiac events after uncomplicated myocardial infarction: a prospective study comparing predischarge exercise thallium-201 scintigraphy and coronary angiography. *Circulation* 1983;68(2):321–336, with permission.)

discharge, in 140 patients with an uncomplicated acute MI. The patients were followed for a mean of 15 ± 12 months. The results of the follow-up are shown in Fig. 13.15. Test results that were typical of a high risk were associated with the same frequency of cardiac events, while strikingly different results were noted among these tests for the prediction of a low risk. Both a negative exercise ECG response and the absence of multivessel coronary disease were unreliable predictors of low risk. Only a nonischemic $^{201}$Tl study (i.e., no reversible defects or lung uptake) proved to be an accurate predictor of low risk, as summarized in Fig. 13.15.

Another advantage of myocardial perfusion scintigraphy over exercise ECG is that it may be used to assess the presence and magnitude of residual, jeopardized myocardium within the infarct zone. For instance, the presence of $^{201}$Tl redistribution within infarct zones predicts a significantly increased risk for re-infarction (81). In fact, Wilson and colleagues (82) found the infarct zone was the most important factor in predicting recurrent cardiac events among post-MI patients with single-vessel disease. Similarly, using multivariate analysis, Brown et al. (83) found that redistribution of $^{201}$Tl within the infarct zone was the only significant predictor of subsequent cardiac events in the cohort of post-MI patients. Thus, when post-MI patients undergo stress myocardial perfusion SPECT prior to hospital discharge, the presence and extent of defect reversibility within the infarct zone should be routinely assessed and reported to the referring physician. Also, because of the potential importance of excluding jeopardized myocardium within the infarct zone, a high percentage of patients manifesting fixed defects on stress-redistribution $^{201}$Tl or stress-rest $^{99m}$Tc-sestamibi myocardial perfusion SPECT will be candidates for additional delayed $^{201}$Tl imaging at rest. Figure 13.16 demonstrates the identification of a high-risk patient by stress myocardial perfusion SPECT following MI.

### Predischarge Pharmacologic Stress Testing

A number of studies have established the prognostic efficacy of pharmacologic stress testing in association with myocardial perfusion scintigraphy in post-MI patients (84–89). The pattern of results parallels those noted for exercise myocardial perfusion scintigraphy, including the relatively low risk of cardiac events in patients without evidence of defect reversibility or ischemia, and the increased frequency of cardiac events in patients who manifest evidence of defect reversibility within the initial infarct zone (88).

Pharmacologic stress testing with dipyridamole or adenosine can also be performed safely on days 3 to 5 after hospital admission for acute MI (88,88a). This approach can be used to institute a significant shortening of hospital stay among unstable angina patients, thus reducing health care costs. In an important multicenter study, Brown et al. demonstrated superior risk stratification by very early dipyridamole sestamibi SPECT compared with predischarge low-level exercise SPECT in patients with uncom-

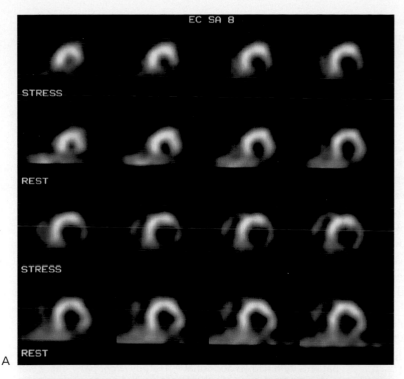

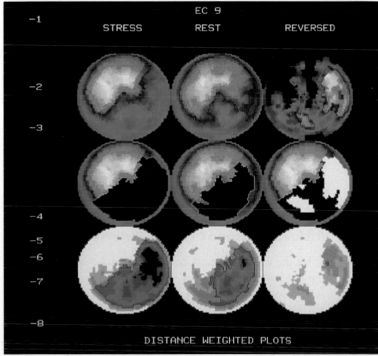

**FIGURE 13.16. A:** Short-axis myocardial scintigrams in a 61-year-old man with a history of recent infarction and recurrent chest pain undergoing an exercise $^{99m}$Tc-sestamibi study. The myocardial scintigrams reveal severe and extensive lateral and inferior-wall defects after exercise. The inferior defect is nonreversible on rest $^{99m}$Tc-sestamibi imaging, but there is extensive reversibility in the adjacent lateral wall. These findings corresponded to the angiographic findings in this patient (totally occluded right coronary artery, high-grade left circumflex lesion, and normal left anterior descending coronary artery). Based on these findings, the patient underwent subsequent coronary bypass surgery. **B:** Corresponding polar maps, indicating the fixed inferior-wall defect, with adjacent reversible lateral-wall defect.

plicated acute myocardiol infarction (82a). Importantly, this risk stratification was as effective with reperfused patients as in patients not receiving reperfusion therapy.

## Evaluation of Patients Following Thrombolysis

The use of thrombolysis has altered the natural history of acute MI, decreasing mortality. The specific assessment of stress myocardial perfusion scintigraphy in postthrom-

bolytic patients has been limited (90–93). Dakik and co-workers (93) have assessed the prognostic efficacy of exercise $^{201}$Tl myocardial perfusion SPECT in a study of 71 patients receiving thrombolytic therapy for acute MI. All of the patients underwent coronary angiography. The mean follow-up period was $26 \pm 18$ months. The ejection fraction and size of $^{201}$Tl perfusion defects were the only significant predictor of future cardiac events by multivariate analysis. The combination of ejection fraction and thallium tomography added significant incremental prognostic information to the clinical data, whereas angiography did not further improve a model that included clinical, ejection fraction, and tomographic variables.

## Assessment of Patients Following Treatment for Unstable Angina

Myocardial perfusion scintigraphy may also be used to assess the likelihood of cardiac events among patients presenting with unstable angina. Several studies have demonstrated that myocardial perfusion imaging can provide accurate differentiation of high- versus low-risk patients following the medical treatment of unstable angina (94–97, 177). For example, Brown et al. (94) performed a follow-up study (for a mean of 39 ± 11 months) in 52 consecutive patients with unstable angina who responded to medical therapy and then underwent exercise [201]Tl myocardial perfusion scintigraphy within 1 week of hospital discharge. Among the 23 patients with reversible [201]Tl defects in their study, the subsequent incidence of cardiac events (MI or death) was 26%, versus an event rate of only 3% in the 29 patients in whom reversible defects were not induced during stress. Stratmann et al. (177) evaluated risk stratification of medically treated patients with unstable angina by exercise myocardial perfusion SPECT with [99m]Tc-sestamibi. The patients were followed for a mean of 12 ± 7 months after SPECT imaging. An abnormal [99m]Tc-sestamibi perfusion study with a reversible perfusion defect was a very strong predictor of cardiac events by multivariate analysis.

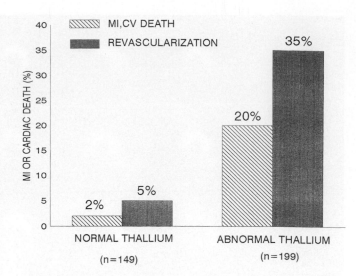

**FIGURE 13.18.** The frequency of subsequent MI and/or cardiac death among 348 elderly patients (mean age = 75 ± 4 years) followed for a mean of 23 ± 15 months after the performance of dipyridamole [201]Tl scintigraphy. Among the 149 patients with a normal [201]Tl study *(left bars)* there was a very low frequency of subsequent cardiac events, and relatively few patients underwent myocardial revascularization. By contrast, among the 199 patients who had an abnormal [201]Tl study *(right bars)*, there was a striking frequency of subsequent cardiac events, occurring in more than one-third of these patients; 20% of these patients underwent myocardial revascularization. (Adapted from Shaw L, Chaitman BR, Hilton TC, et al. Prognostic value of dipyridamole thallium-201 imaging in elderly patients. *J Am Coll Cardiol* 1992; 19(7):1390–1398.)

The risk for a cardiac event was 25% in patients with a reversible perfusion defect as opposed to 2% for those with a normal study. These data suggest that stress myocardial perfusion scintigraphy may be safely used for risk stratification among patients who are medically treated for unstable angina.

## Risk Assessment in the Elderly

With the average life expectancy in the United States having increased to >75 years, risk stratification of the elderly is an increasing reason for stress-test referral. While advanced age is correlated with an increased risk for cardiac disease, prognostic assessment in elderly patients assumes importance because of a somewhat higher threshold for aggressive coronary revascularization. There is established prognostic efficacy for radionuclide stress testing in elderly patients. Iskandrian and colleagues (98) conducted a 2-year follow-up of 449 patients following the performance of exercise [201]Tl myocardial perfusion scintigraphy. The mean age of the patient population was 65 years. As indicated in Fig. 13.17, exercise [201]Tl myocardial perfusion scintigraphy was a very effective method for risk stratification in this geriatric population. Shaw et al. (99) followed 348 elderly patients for a mean of 2 years after pharmacologic stress testing with dipyridamole for

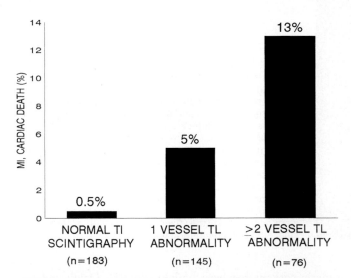

**FIGURE 13.17.** Frequency of MI and/or cardiac death among elderly patients with a mean age of 65 years during a mean follow-up of 2 years after exercise [201]Tl testing according to the results of exercise [201]Tl testing. The cardiac event rate was very low in the patients with a normal exercise [201]Tl study *(left bar)*, intermediate in those with [201]Tl defects localized to one vessel territory *(middle bar)*, and high in those with [201]Tl defects in two or more vascular territories *(right bar)*. (Adapted from Iskandrian AS, Heo J, Decoskey D, et al. Use of exercise thallium-201 imaging for risk stratification of elderly patients with coronary artery disease. *Am J Cardiol* 1988;61:269–272.)

risk stratification. The mean age of the population in their study was 10 years more than that of the patients studied by Iskandrian and colleagues, but the results were very similar. As shown in Fig. 13.18, there was a very low cardiac event rate in patients with a normal $^{201}$Tl dipyridamole study and a very high cardiac event rate among those with an abnormal study. Thus, myocardial perfusion scintigraphy with either exercise or pharmacologic stress is an effective means for risk stratification in the elderly population.

## Assessment of Patients with Congestive Heart Failure and/or Left Ventricular Dysfunction

Since congestive heart failure (CHF) represents an important source of morbidity and mortality among CAD patients, there is a strong emphasis on identifying its treatable components, such as myocardial ischemia. The presence of an ischemic cardiomyopathy may be suspected if there are typical anginal symptoms, a documented prior MI, or pathologic Q waves on the resting ECG. These criteria, however, are often inadequate for differentiating an ischemic from a nonischemic cardiomyopathy in individual patients. Consequently, there has been considerable interest in evaluating imaging techniques for this differentiation.

Because wall-motion imaging must be used with caution for this evaluation (100), investigators have also assessed the role of $^{201}$Tl scintigraphy and positron emission tomography (PET) for this differentiation.

Table 13.5 summarizes ten comparative studies of myocardial perfusion and/or metabolic function in patients with ischemic and idiopathic dilated cardiomyopathy (101–108a). A number of potential imaging criteria were investigated for their usefulness, including the nature of fixed perfusion defects. These studies suggest that large and severe fixed myocardial perfusion defects might serve as a relatively specific marker for ischemic cardiomyopathy. (On a worldwide basis, however, Chagas' disease would also be in the differential diagnosis of large severe fixed defects.) Mild to moderate perfusion defects, by contrast, may be seen in either ischemic or nonischemic cardiomyopathy patients. Another scintigraphic variable, $^{201}$Tl defect reversibility, was not found to be a reliable discriminator of ischemic from nonischemic cardiomyopathy in most of these studies, but these studies preceded the current use of $^{201}$Tl reinjection to assess the reversibility of fixed defects at 4-hour redistribution imaging. In addition, most of the studies in Table 13.5 are based on the planar $^{201}$Tl imaging technique. Thus, further investigation may determine that myocardial perfusion SPECT imaging, and (when necessary) the incorporation of delayed $^{201}$Tl imag-

**TABLE 13.5. COMPARISON OF PERFUSION AND/OR METABOLIC TRACERS FOR COMPARING ISCHEMIC CARDIOMYOPATHY DILATED NONISCHEMIC CARDIOMYOPATHY**

| | | Useful Discriminating Criteria | | | Patient number | | | |
|---|---|---|---|---|---|---|---|---|
| Investigators | Year | Ischemic Cardiomyopathy | Dilated Nonischemic Cardiomyopathy | Imaging Technique | Large Defects | Severe Defects | Redistribution | Lung Uptake |
| Bulkley et al. (101) | 1977 | 13 | 8 | Resting planar $^{201}$Tl | Yes | — | — | — |
| Sallissi et al. (102) | 1981 | 13 | 11 | EX planar $^{201}$Tl | Yes | — | No[a] | — |
| Dunn et al. (103) | 1982 | 15 | 10 | EX planar $^{201}$Tl | No | Yes | No | No |
| Iskandrian et al. (104) | 1986 | 20 | 15 | Resting planar $^{201}$Tl | Yes | Yes | [b] | No |
| Eisenberg et al. (105) | 1987 | 10 | 10 | PET imaging ($^{11}$C-palmitate) | Yes | Yes | — | — |
| Eichhorn et al. (106) | 1988 | 10 | 12 | Dip planar $^{201}$Tl | Yes | — | — | — |
| Mody et al. (107) | 1991 | 11 | 10 | PET imaging ($^{13}$N-ammonia, 18-FDG) | Yes | Yes | [c] | — |
| Chikamori et al. (107a) | 1992 | 77 | 55 | Dip planar $^{201}$Tl | Yes | Yes | Yes | — |
| Taubert et al. (108) | 1993 | 31 | 20 | EX planar $^{201}$Tl | Yes | Yes | No | Yes |
| Danias et al. (108a) | 1998 | 13 | 24 | EX SPECT $^{99m}$Tc | Yes | Yes | Yes | — |

—, not specifically evaluated.
[a]However, reverse redistribution was confined only to patients with ischemic cardiomyopathy.
[b]Redistribution within defects was uncommon, but occurred only in patients with ischemic cardiomyopathy.
[c]"Mismatch" (decreased perfusion, FDG uptake relatively preserved) was more common and extensive with ischemic cardiomyopathy.
EX, FDG, fluorodeoxyglucose; PET, positron emission tomography; $^{99m}$Tc, technetium 99m; $^{201}$Tl, thallium 201.

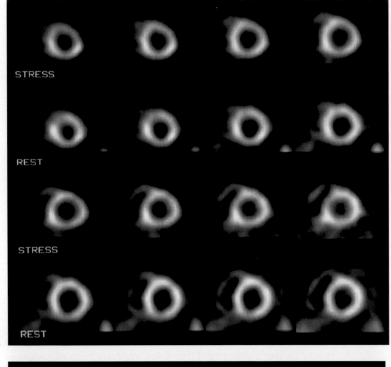

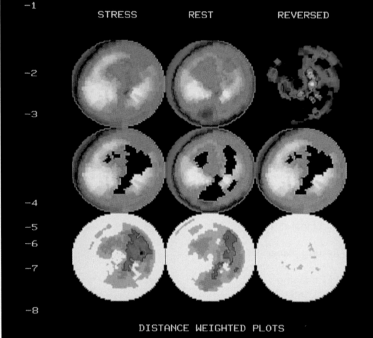

**FIGURE 13.19. A:** Exercise $^{99m}$Tc-sestamibi testing was performed in this 78-year-old woman presenting with a history of congestive heart failure and classic anginal symptoms. The myocardial scintigrams revealed significant left ventricular dilation, but no significant perfusion defects were noted. The gated SPECT images revealed generalized hypokinesis. This combination of scintigraphic findings is characteristic of nonischemic cardiomyopathy. **B:** The corresponding polar maps were normal in this patient with nonischemic cardiomyopathy.

ing after the resting reinjection of $^{201}$Tl, may optimize the ability of this imaging technique to differentiate between ischemic and idiopathic cardiomyopathy (108a,b). In addition, the combined assessment of myocardial perfusion (defect extent, severity, and reversibility) and left ventricular function (regional wall motion abnormalities) with $^{99m}$Tc-sestamibi gated SPECT imaging can further help to distinguish between patients with ischemic cardiomyopathy and patients with nonischemic dilated cardiomyopathy

(108a). Figures 13.19 and 13.20 demonstrate characteristic scintigraphic patterns in patients with nonischemic and ischemic cardiomyopathy, respectively.

Furthermore, $^{201}$Tl scintigraphy can be used for prognostic purposes in patients with ischemic heart disease and left ventricular dysfunction. In such patients, resting wall-motion abnormalities are often assessed for myocardial viability on the presumption that the detection of "hibernating myocardium" identifies patients who are at greater

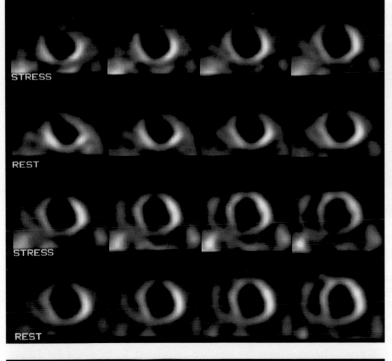

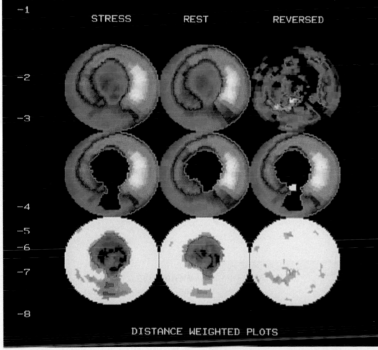

**FIGURE 13.20. A:** A dipyridamole [99m]Tc-sestamibi study was performed in this 76-year-old man with a history of atypical angina, congestive heart failure, and a MI 14 years previously. The left ventricle was markedly enlarged. Following dosing with dipyridamole, there was an extensive and severe anterior-wall defect with septal and inferior-wall hypoperfusion as well. There was no defect reversibility at rest. Such extensive and severe defects are typically seen in patients with ischemic cardiomyopathy but not in those with nonischemic cardiomyopathy. **B:** The corresponding polar maps characterize the extent and severity of the fixed anterior-, septal-, and inferior-wall defects noted above.

risk for subsequent cardiac events. For example, Eitzman and colleagues (109) have provided a prognostic analysis for the detection of hibernating myocardium. For this purpose they used PET in 82 patients with CAD and impaired left ventricular function. Nitrogen-13 ammonia was used to assess myocardial blood flow and 18-fluorodeoxyglucose (FDG) was used to assess myocardial metabolism. Concurrent decreases in blood flow and FDG uptake (matched defects) were used to identify zones of myocardial fibrosis, while decreased blood flow with a relatively increased FDG uptake (mismatch) identified viable, hibernating myocardium. Patients were followed for an average of 1 year. The results of Eitzman and colleagues' analysis are shown in Fig. 13.21. Among the patients with matched defects (i.e., presumably no hibernating myocardium), there was a low 1-year cardiac event rate, regardless of revascularization. Among patients with "mismatch" (i.e., hibernating myocardium), however,

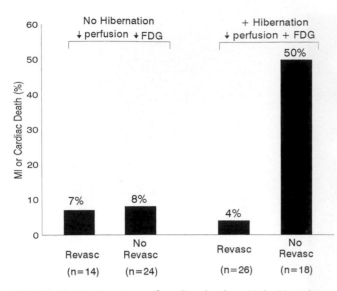

**FIGURE 13.21.** Frequency of cardiac death or MI in 82 patients with CAD followed for an average of 1 year after undergoing positron emission tomography (PET). 13N-ammonia was used to measure myocardial perfusion and 18-fluorodeoxyglucose (FDG) was used to assess metabolic function. The mean resting left ventricular ejection fraction was 34% ± 13%. Corresponding matched defects identified zones with necrosed myocardium *(left two bars)*, whereas defects with "mismatch" (decreased perfusion, but with presence of FDG uptake [+]) defined zones manifesting hibernating myocardium *(right two bars)*. Among the patients without evidence of hibernating myocardium, the cardiac event rate was low, with or without the performance of myocardial revascularization (revasc). Among patients with hibernating myocardium, however, there was a very high cardiac event rate in the absence of myocardial revascularization. Hence, the identification of hibernating myocardium appears to identify a high-risk subgroup among CAD patients with resting left ventricular dysfunction. (Adapted from Eitzman D, Al-Aouar Z, Kanter HL, et al. Clinical outcomes of patients with advanced coronary artery disease after viability studies with positron emission tomography. *J Am Coll Cardiol* 1992;20(3):559–565.)

there was a very high 1-year cardiac event rate if myocardial revascularization was not performed, whereas the cardiac event rate was low if revascularization was performed. Thus, as previously presumed, these data provide objective evidence of the prognostic importance of detecting hibernating myocardium. Other, subsequent reports, also based on PET imaging, appear to confirm these findings (110,111).

Given these observations, the prognostic efficacy of myocardial perfusion SPECT can be determined among patients with significant resting left ventricular dysfunction. Such assessment should incorporate the most optimized means for assessing myocardial viability. As mentioned earlier, this would include the use of a postreinjection study or a rest-redistribution study for evaluating fixed defects on ²⁰¹Tl scintigrams. For ⁹⁹ᵐTc-sestamibi scintigraphy, fixed defects could also be evaluated by performing a separate rest ²⁰¹Tl study (19). Other ancillary data may also aid the assessment of myocardial viability with ⁹⁹ᵐTc, such as the evaluation of wall thickening and segmental wall motion from gated SPECT myocardial perfusion images. In addition, studies indicate that resting left ventricular ejection fraction may be reliably calculated from gated ⁹⁹ᵐTc-sestamibi SPECT images (112–114). Figure 13.22 illustrates a method for determining ejection fraction from a gated ⁹⁹ᵐTc-sestamibi SPECT study in a patient with a history of typical angina and CHF (112).

Thus, the combined assessment of myocardial perfusion defects, segmental wall motion, and resting left ventricular ejection fraction can be made from myocardial perfusion SPECT with ⁹⁹ᵐTc-sestamibi. Current study is ongoing to determine the utility of combined assessment of perfusion and function in the risk assessment of CAD patients with resting left ventricular dysfunction.

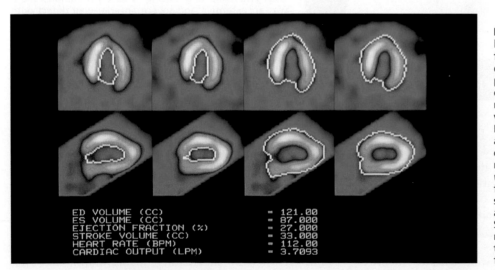

**FIGURE 13.22.** Resting left ventricular ejection fraction was obtained from the gated ⁹⁹ᵐTc-sestamibi myocardial perfusion scintigrams for the patient with nonischemic cardiomyopathy shown in Figure 13.22. Using midventricular horizontal *(top)* and vertical *(bottom)* long-axis slices, from R-wave-triggered end-diastolic *(left)* and end-systolic frames *(right)*, endocardial borders and valve planes were manually determined, as outlined in *white*. The left ventricular ejection fraction was computed by the Simpson's rule method, corrected for the average point-spread function of the SPECT camera. By this method, the resting left ventricular ejection fraction was 27% in this congestive heart failure (CHF) patient.

## Evaluation of Treatment Modalities in Patients with Coronary Artery Disease

### Evaluation of Patients Following Percutaneous Coronary Revascularization

At least two clinical reasons exist for selecting stress myocardial perfusion SPECT over exercise ECG for the routine evaluation of patients who have had percutaneous coronary interventions: (a) the desirability of a highly sensitive test for detecting ischemia over time because of the presence of coronary angioplasty or stent restenosis, and (b) the extent and severity of potential residual ischemia following restenosis may help govern the indication for repeat intervention. Along these lines, stress myocardial perfusion SPECT is well suited for characterizing the extent of residual jeopardized myocardium in patients following coronary intervention, according to the principles discussed earlier in this chapter. In this regard, a number of clinical studies have

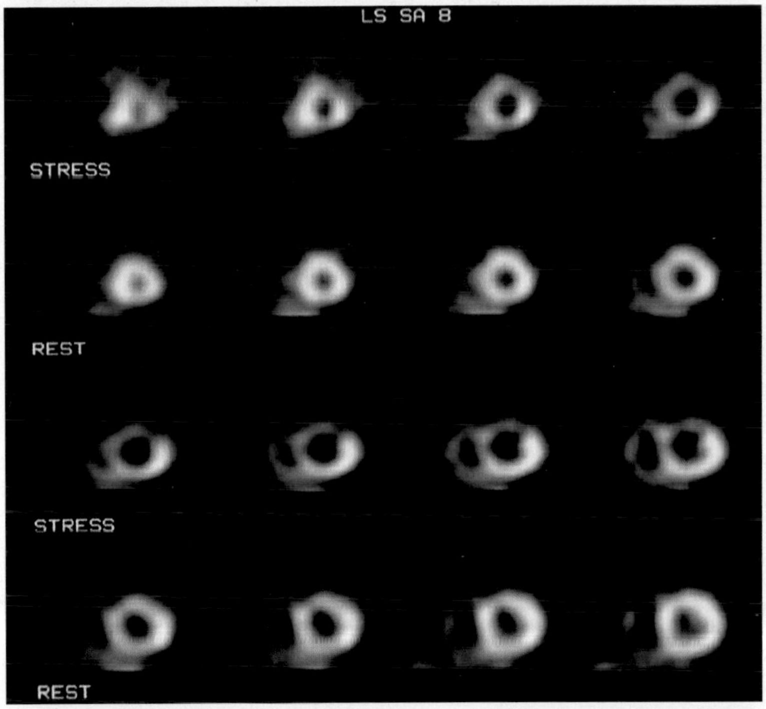

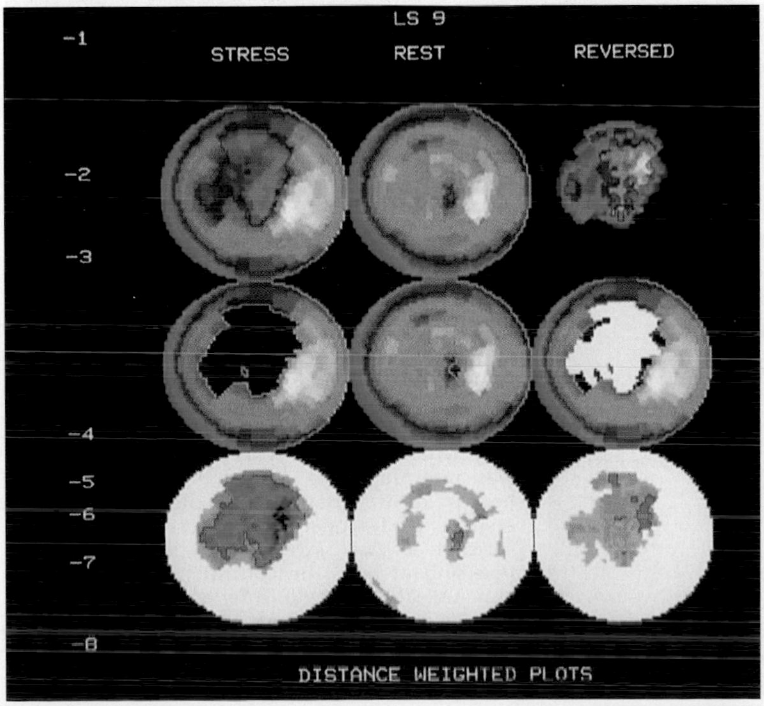

**FIGURE 13.23. A:** Exercise myocardial perfusion scintigraphy was performed in this 60-year-old man who had undergone coronary angioplasty for a lesion of the middle left anterior descending coronary artery 7 weeks previously. The postangioplasty study indicates severe and extensive anterior- and septal-wall defects, reversing at rest. Hence, restenosis is certain, with significant myocardium at jeopardy. **B:** The polar maps indicate corresponding severe hypoperfusion in the anterior and anteroseptal walls and apex after-exercise, reversing at rest.

documented the usefulness of stress myocardial perfusion SPECT for identifying restenosis in patients following coronary angioplasty (115–121). Figure 13.23 illustrates the use of stress myocardial perfusion SPECT to assess the possibility of restenosis, and the associated magnitude of jeopardized myocardium, in a patient with recurrent symptoms following coronary angioplasty.

Manyari and colleagues (122) reported a high frequency of false-positive transient myocardial perfusion defects (i.e., transient defects occurring in conjunction with successfully reperfused arteries) when exercise myocardial perfusion scintigraphy was performed in the first few weeks after the performance of coronary angioplasty. They postulated that transient abnormalities in coronary vasomotor tone, resulting from trauma to the coronary vascular wall in association with the angioplasty procedure, may be the cause of this phenomenon. Accordingly, patients following coronary angioplasty are most commonly initially evaluated by exercise myocardial perfusion SPECT at 4 to 6 weeks after the angioplasty procedure. However, Iskandrian et al. (123) have suggested that myocardial perfusion SPECT may be effectively performed early after angioplasty, in association with pharmacologic stress), without the increased false-positive rate reported by Manyari and associates. Given the potential importance, this issue requires further evaluation.

## Evaluation of Patients Following Coronary Artery Bypass Surgery

A number of studies have demonstrated that stress myocardial perfusion scintigraphy may be used to assess patients following coronary artery bypass graft (CABG) surgery (124–127). Generally, patients who are asymptomatic after recent CABG are not candidates for radionuclide stress testing, since early graft closure in patients following CABG is relatively infrequent. Rather, stress testing in such patients can generally be performed with ECG monitoring alone to determine safety and exercise tolerance for participation in cardiac rehabilitation programs. However, when patients develop typical angina symptoms after recent CABG surgery, radionuclide stress testing may be indicated to evaluate the possibility of postoperative graft closure. Further, at a point late after CABG surgery, the possibility of new atherosclerotic disease within coronary grafts begins to increase considerably. Thus, stress SPECT perfusion imaging is also used in patients who present with new anginal symptoms late after CABG surgery, to exclude or confirm the presence of inducible ischemia and to stratify patients into low-, intermediate-, and high-risk groups for future cardiac events (126a). For example, Palmas and co-workers (127) evaluated the prognostic efficacy of exercise $^{201}$Tl SPECT in 294 postbypass patients who underwent $^{201}$Tl testing ≥5 years after having coronary bypass surgery (127). $^{201}$Tl scintigraphy was assessed for its incremental prognostic value by first forcing the more readily available clinical and nonnuclear exercise data into a multivariate model. Among the nonscintigraphic variables, shortness of breath and peak exercise heart rate were the most important clinical predictors of subsequent MI and cardiac death. Two variables related to $^{201}$Tl imaging, however, were shown to add significant incremental information to the assessment of risk in this population: the $^{201}$Tl summed reversibility

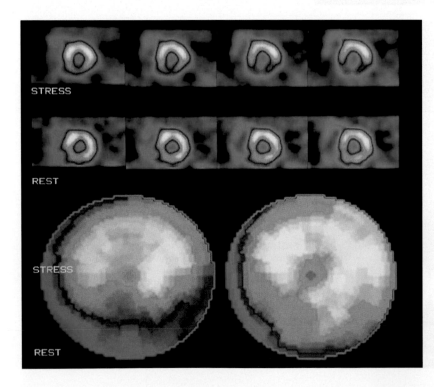

**FIGURE 13.24.** Middle and basal short-axis scintigrams *(top)* with corresponding polar maps *(bottom)* for a 67-year-old man who underwent coronary bypass surgery 11 years previously. The patient was referred for a stress $^{99m}$Tc-sestamibi study because of new chest pain symptoms and a recent episode of syncope. The myocardial scintigrams indicate a basal inferior-wall defect poststress, reversing at rest. The corresponding polar maps also indicate the basal inferior defect poststress. But the overall magnitude of inducible ischemia is not severe. Thus, the patient's physician elected to treat this patient's chest pain syndrome with conservative medical management.

score (a global measure of ischemic index), and abnormal lung uptake of [201]Tl following stress. Thus, as in other patient subgroups, measurement of the magnitude of ischemia by myocardial perfusion scintigraphy represents an important prognostic index in the late postbypass patient. Palmas and colleagues' study also confirms the advantage of combining planar and SPECT imaging wherever possible, since lung uptake in this study was assessed from a routine 5-minute planar image obtained just prior to the initial SPECT acquisition.

Figure 13.24 presents a case in which stress myocardial perfusion SPECT was used to assess anginal symptoms 11 years after coronary bypass surgery.

## Evaluation of Medical Therapy

In clinical practice, radionuclide stress tests are not commonly used to evaluate the efficacy of antiischemic medications after the initiation of medical therapy. Rather, newly treated patients are commonly followed without further stress testing, by evaluating the reduction of anginal symptoms with therapy. However, because of the high frequency of "silent" ischemia during daily activity in ischemic CAD patients (128–131), there is reason to question whether the reduction of angina per se is a satisfactory end point for evaluating the efficacy of antiischemic drug therapy in clinical practice. In addition, in recent years hepatic hydroxymethylglutaryl coenzyme A (HMG-CoA) reductase inhibitor cholesterol lowering agents have become an essential adjuvant in both primary and secondary prevention of CAD. However, the investigative use of radionuclide stress testing for evaluating the antiischemic effects of drug therapy has generally been quite limited (132–138).

## Assessment of Cardiac Risk for Patients Undergoing Elective Noncardiac Surgery

Ischemic heart disease is a major cause of morbidity and mortality among patients undergoing elective noncardiac surgery. For example, as summarized by Mangano and colleagues (139), cardiac deaths account for approximately one-half of all deaths associated with elective noncardiac surgery in the United States each year (140). Nevertheless, most patients with known CAD can safely undergo major noncardiac surgery, since the presence of anatomic coronary disease is not per se a contraindication to elective noncardiac surgery. However, myocardial perfusion SPECT is essential in assessing risk for a cardiac event prior to elective noncardiac surgery.

Stress myocardial perfusion scintigraphy is the most accurate method for preoperative risk stratification among patients with suspected or known CAD. Since most preoperative patients are too sick to exercise, the published clinical experience has centered on the use of pharmacologic

stress testing in these patients. Boucher and co-workers (141) were the first to report on the clinical utility of dipyridamole [201]Tl myocardial perfusion scintigraphy for such preoperative risk assessment. Among the 16 patients in the study who had reversible [201]Tl defects on dipyridamole scintigraphy preoperatively, 8 (50%) had a postoperative event. By contrast, among the 32 patients without a reversible defect, none sustained a postoperative event.

In addition, many investigators have evaluated the preoperative use of myocardial perfusion scintigraphy in association with pharmacologic stress, using either dipyridamole or adenosine (60,141–168). In the majority of these studies, pharmacologic stress testing resulted in an efficacious demarcation of high- from low-risk patients. Subsequently, the use of [99m]Tc-sestamibi (165,166) instead of [201]Tl, and dobutamine rather than dipyridamole or adenosine as the pharmacologic agent (167), have also described an effective identification of high-risk preoperative patients by scintigraphic means. Table 13.6 summarizes data from 15 prognostic studies, included because they satisfied the following criteria: (a) scintigraphic results could be divided into those that were normal, showed fixed defects, or showed reversible defects (with or without associated fixed defects) and (b) the frequency of "hard" perioperative events (i.e., MI and/or cardiac death) was specifically reported. This table shows that approximately 5% of surgical cases are canceled due to an abnormal preoperative dipyridamole study indicating an unacceptable risk of surgery. However, a very low frequency of perioperative cardiac events (1.2%) exists among patients who had a normal myocardial perfusion scintigraphy study. By contrast, the frequency of major perioperative cardiac events (MI or cardiac death) was approximately 15% among patients who manifested reversible myocardial perfusion defects on their preoperative dipyridamole [201]Tl study. Among patients with fixed defects, the cardiac event rate was approximately 5%, an intermediate value, despite most of these studies being performed prior to the routine evaluation of fixed myocardial perfusion defects with a subsequent reinjection [201]Tl study at rest. Approximately 30% to 50% of "fixed" myocardial perfusion defects can be expected to show reversibility after the reinjection of thallium at rest (16,17). Fixed defects of only a small extent and/or low clinical risk are two factors that could potentially explain the intermediate likelihood of cardiac events in association with fixed myocardial perfusion defects.

As mentioned earlier in this chapter, the magnitude of jeopardized myocardium has an exponential relationship to the likelihood of subsequent cardiac events. Given this relationship, it is natural to ask whether patients with mild defects on dipyridamole scintigraphy may safely undergo noncardiac surgery. A study by Lette and associates (60) helps to address this question. They followed 355 operative patients, stratified according to the magnitude of abnormalities on preoperative dipyridamole [201]Tl scintigraphy.

**TABLE 13.6. PERIOPERATIVE CARDIAC EVENT RATES FOLLOWING THE PERFORMANCE OF DIPYRIDAMOLE MYOCARDIAL PERFUSION SCINTIGRAPHY**

| Investigators | Year | No. of patients | Operation Canceled | Dipyridamole [201]Tl results and perioperative events (MI, death) | | |
|---|---|---|---|---|---|---|
| | | | | Normal (Events/No. of Patients) | Fixed Defects (Events/No. of Patients) | Reversible Defects (Events/No. of Patients) |
| Boucher et al. (141) | 1985 | 54 | 6 | 0/20 | 0/12 | 3/16 |
| Leppo et al. (142) | 1987 | 100 | 11 | 1/40 | 0/7 | 14/42 |
| Sachs et al. (160) | 1988 | 46 | — | 0/26 | 0/6 | 2/14 |
| Lane et al. (150) | 1989 | 101 | — | 0/20 | 0/10 | 9/71 |
| Eagle et al. (168) | 1989 | 230 | 30 | 0/51 | 2/67 | 13/82 |
| Stratmann et al. (162) | 1990 | 35 | — | 1/17 | 0/8 | 1/10 |
| Younis et al. (164) | 1990 | 131 | 20 | 0/51 | 2/20 | 6/40 |
| McEnroe et al. (168a) | 1990 | 95 | 8 | 2/46 | 3/15 | 1/26 |
| Mangano et al. (154) | 1991 | 60 | — | 1/20 | 1/18 | 1/22 |
| Lette et al. (152) | 1990 | 66 | 6 | 0/30 | 0/9 | 9/21 |
| Lette et al. (165) | 1992 | 355[a] | — | 2/162 | 0/32 | 28/161 |
| Brown et al. (144) | 1993 | 231 | — | 1/121 | 1/33 | 10/77 |
| Baron et al.[b] (168b) | 1994 | 468 | 11 | 16/203 | 12/94 | 14/160 |
| Bry et al. (168c) | 1994 | 237 | 9 | 0/97 | 5/30 | 12/101 |
| Koutelou et al. (168d) | 1995 | 106 | — | 0/49 | 0/10 | 5/47 |
| Total | | 1,847 | 90/1,847 (4.9%) | 9/750 (1.2%) | 14/277 (5.1%) | 114/730 (15.6%) |

[a]Separate population.
[b]Not included in total.
MI, myocardial infarction.

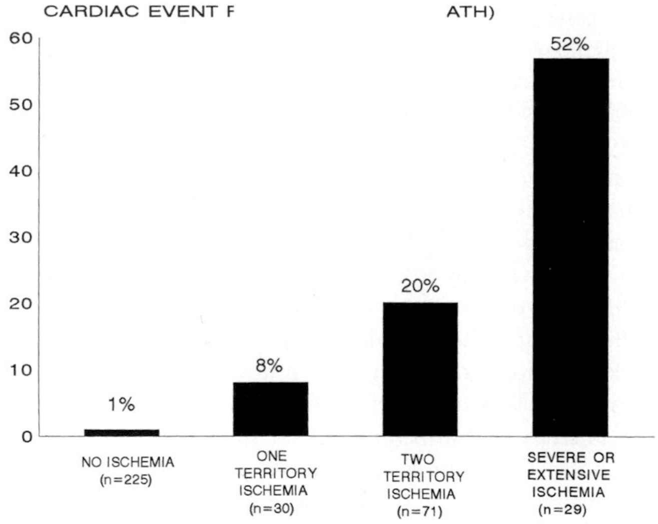

**FIGURE 13.25.** Perioperative rate of MI and/or cardiac death following the performance of major noncoronary surgery (vertical axis) for 355 patients stratified according to the magnitude of reversible defects during preoperative dipyridamole [201]Tl scintigraphy. The cardiac event rate was only 1% in the 225 patients with a normal dipyridamole study, versus 8% in patients with reversible defects localized to one vascular territory. The frequency of perioperative events increased markedly in patients with a greater magnitude of ischemia. These data were noted despite the exclusion of patients who underwent myocardial revascularization because of an abnormal dipyridamole [201]Tl study. (Adapted from Stratmann HG, Younis LT, Wittry MD, et al. Dipyridamole technetium-99m sestamibi myocardial tomography in patients evaluated for elective vascular surgery: prognostic value for perioperative and late cardiac events. *Am Heart J* 1995;131(5):923–929.)

Figure 13.25 illustrates that there was a marked increase in cardiac event rates as the magnitude of [201]Tl abnormality increased. However, among patients with reversible [201]Tl defects within the distribution of only a single vessel, the perioperative cardiac event rate was 8%, an intermediate risk value. This result is somewhat troublesome, since many patients manifesting abnormal studies do so in only one vascular territory. However, it is possible that a low-risk subgroup could readily be identified within this intermediate-risk subgroup by characterizing the extent and severity of defects occurring within single vascular territories. Further study of this possibility appears warranted. Figure 13.26 illustrates a case example in which stress myocardial perfusion SPECT was used to assess perioperative risk in a CAD patient scheduled for elective noncardiac surgery.

A number of the studies described above also compared the prognostic efficacy of myocardial perfusion scintigraphy during pharmacologic stress to other clinical and test variables, using multivariate analyses (142–144,150,151). In each study, the results of myocardial perfusion scintigraphy were found to be the single most important variable in risk stratification. Nevertheless, there still arises the question of how much incremental information pharmacologic stress testing adds when all available clinical information is considered together. To answer this question, Eagle et al. (168) evaluated 200 patients who underwent dipyridamole [201]Tl myocardial perfusion scintigraphy before peripheral vascular surgery. They reviewed the hospital records of these patients for the occurrence of perioperative cardiac events (MI, cardiac death, ischemic pulmonary edema, unstable angina). Five clinical variables were significant univariate predictors of perioperative events: (a) ECG Q-waves, (b) a history of ventricular ectopy requiring therapy, (c) diabetes requiring therapy, (d) advanced age (>70 years), and (e) a history of angina. Figure 13.27 shows the interrelationship between clinical variables, the results of dipyridamole $^{201}$Tl

scintigraphy, and cardiac events. In patients with a very low clinical risk profile (i.e., none of the risk factors cited above) and in those with a high-risk clinical profile (three or more risk factors), the cardiac event rates were correspondingly low and very high, respectively. However, in patients with one or two risk factors, dipyridamole $^{201}$Tl scintigraphy provided a striking differentiation of risk, heralding a 3% versus a 30% rate of perioperative events among the inter-

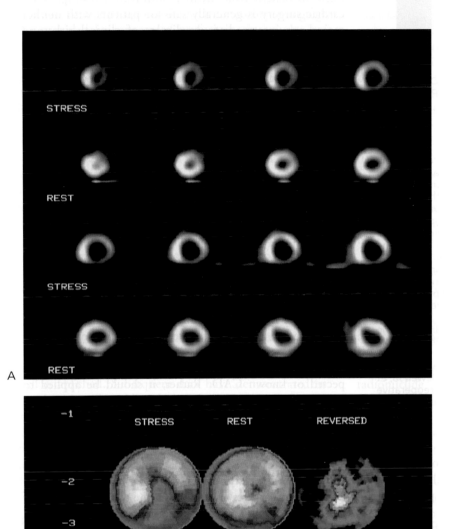

**FIGURE 13.26.** An exercise $^{99m}$Tc-sestamibi study was performed on this 65-year-old man with a history of chronic angina, to clear the patient for the removal of a basal cell carcinoma in the ear. The poststress scintigrams were markedly abnormal with severe lateral- and inferior-wall myocardial perfusion defects extending from the apex to the base of the short-axis slices. The defects were nearly completely reversible at rest. Hence, this patient was identified as being at high preoperative risk and was thus referred for coronary angiography. Angiography demonstrated high-grade lesions within the right coronary and left circumflex arteries, and moderate disease in the proximal left anterior descending artery. Coronary artery bypass surgery was therefore recommended.

myocardial revascularization. The potential effects of this bias on evaluating prognostic efficacy are reviewed elsewhere (185).

Stress myocardial perfusion scintigraphy has become a central guide in decision making with regard to CAD patients. Stress myocardial perfusion SPECT is commonly used either before consideration of coronary revascularization or after its performance, to optimize decision making for CAD patients. Stress myocardial perfusion scintigraphy is also used after myocardial revascularization procedures, to evaluate therapeutic efficacy; following the stabilization of acute ischemic syndromes, to determine subsequent risk; and before the performance of elective noncardiac surgery, to identify the high-risk subset of CAD patients who will require coronary revascularization prior to elective surgery.

Thus, myocardial perfusion scintigraphy has become an important instrument in defining cardiac risk and in identifying patients who are most likely to benefit from additional invasive diagnostic testing and potential coronary revascularization. Myocardial perfusion imaging has demonstrated significant incremental prognostic value when added to clinical and adjuvant testing data. The cost-effective role of myocardial perfusion scintigraphy to serve as a gatekeeper to the cardiac catheterization laboratory will be determined by studies that further establish its impact on clinical outcome and patient management.

# REFERENCES

1. Rozanski A, Berman DS. Silent myocardial ischemia: II. Prognosis and implications for the clinical assessment of patients with coronary artery disease. *Am Heart J* 1987;114(3):627–638.
2. Diamond GA, Staniloff HM, Forrester JS, et al. Computer-assisted diagnosis in the non-invasive evaluation of patients with suspected coronary artery disease. *J Am Coll Cardiol* 1983;1(2):444–455.
3. Rozanski A, Berman D. Uses of stress-redistribution thallium scintigraphy for the diagnosis, prognostic assessment, and management of patients with coronary artery disease. *Cardiovasc Perspect* 1988;3:1–3.
4. Ladenheim ML, Kotler TS, Pollock BH, et al. Incremental prognostic power of clinical history, exercise electrocardiography and myocardial perfusion scintigraphy in suspected coronary artery disease. *Am J Cardiol* 1987;59:270–277.
5. Bairey CN, Rozanski A, Maddahi J, et al. Exercise thallium-201 scintigraphy and prognosis in typical angina pectoris and negative exercise electrocardiography. *Am J Cardiol* 1989;64:282–287.
6. Boucher CA, Zir LM, Beller GA, et al. Increased lung uptake of thallium-201 during exercise myocardial imaging: clinical, hemodynamic and angiographic implications in patients with coronary artery disease. *Am J Cardiol* 1980;46(2):189–196.
7. Bingham JB, McKusick KA, Strauss HW, et al. Influence of coronary artery disease on pulmonary uptake of thallium-201. *Am J Cardiol* 1980;46:821–826.
8. Levy R, Rozanski A, Berman DS, et al. Analysis of the degree of pulmonary thallium washout after exercise in patients with coronary artery disease. *J Am Coll Cardiol* 1983;2(4):719–728.
9. Gibson RS, Watson DD, Carabello BA, et al. Clinical implica-
tions of increased lung uptake of thallium-201 during exercise scintigraphy 2 weeks after myocardial infarction. *Am J Cardiol* 1982;49:1586–1593.
10. Liu P, Kiess M, Okada RD, et al. Increased thallium lung uptake after exercise in isolated left anterior descending coronary artery disease. *Am J Cardiol* 1985;55:1469–1473.
11. Gill JB, Ruddy TD, Newell JB, et al. Prognostic importance of thallium uptake by the lungs during exercise in coronary artery disease. *N Engl J Med* 1987;317(24):1485–1489.
12. Weiss AT, Berman DS, Lew AS, et al. Transient ischemic dilation of the left ventricle on stress thallium-201 scintigraphy: a marker of severe and extensive coronary artery disease. *J Am Coll Cardiol* 1987;9(4):752–759.
12a. Mazzanti M, Germano G, Kiat H, et al. Identification of severe and exclusive coronary artery disease by automatic measurement of transient ischemic dilation of the left ventricle in dual-isotope myocardial perfusion SPECT. *J Am Coll Cardiol* 1996;27:1612–1620.
13. Gutman J, Berman DS, Freeman M, et al. Time to completed redistribution of thallium-201 in exercise myocardial scintigraphy: relationship to the degree of coronary artery stenosis. *Am Heart J* 1983;106(5):989–995.
14. Kiat H, Berman DS, Maddahi J, et al. Late reversibility of tomographic myocardial thallium-201 defects: an accurate marker of myocardial viability. *J Am Coll Cardiol* 1988;12(6):1456–1463.
15. Yang LD, Berman DS, Kiat H, et al. The frequency of late reversibility in SPECT thallium-201 stress redistribution studies. *J Am Coll Cardiol* 1990;15(2):334–340.
16. Dilsizian V, Rocco TP, Freedman NMT, et al. Enhanced detection of ischemic but viable myocardium by the reinjection of thallium after stress-redistribution imaging. *N Engl J Med* 1990;323(3):141–146.
17. Bonow RO, Dilsizian V, Cuocolo A, et al. Identification of viable myocardium in patients with chronic coronary artery disease and left ventricular dysfunction: comparison of thallium scintigraphy with reinjection and PET imaging with 18F-fluorodeoxyglucose. *Circulation* 1991;83(1):26–37.
18. Giubbini R, Campini R, Milan E, et al. Evaluation of technetium-99m-sestamibi lung uptake: correlation with left ventricular function. *J Nucl Med* 1995;36(1):58–63.
18a. Bacher-Stier C, Sharir T, Kavanagh PB, et al. Post-exercise lung uptake of Tc-99m sestamibi determined by a new automatic technique: validation and application in detection of severe and extensive coronary artery disease and reduced left ventricular function. *J Nucl Med* 2000;41:1190–1197.
19. DePuey EG, Rozanski A, Parmett S, et al. The adjunctive value of rest/delayed Tl-201 SPECT to demonstrate reversibility of fixed Tc-99m sestamibi perfusion defects. *J Nucl Med* 1993;34:64–65P(abst).
19a. Mazzanti M, Germano G, Kiat H, et al. Identification of severe and extensive coronary artery disease by automatic measurement of transient ischemic dilation of the left ventricle in dual-isotope myocardial perfusion SPECT. *J Am Coll Cardiol* 1996;27:1612–1620.
20. Sharir T, Berman DS, Lewin HC, et al. Incremental prognostic value of rest-redistribution Tl-201 single-photon emission computed tomography. *Circulation* 1999;100:1964–1970.
21. Jones RH, Borges-Neto S, Potts JM. Simultaneous measurement of myocardial perfusion and ventricular function during exercise from a single injection of technetium-99m sestamibi in coronary artery disease. *Am J Cardiol* 1990;66:68E–71E.
22. Stowers SA, Thompson RC, Williams HJ, et al. Comparison of Tc-99m sestamibi perfusion, regional contraction, and peak left ventricular ejection fraction in the diagnosis of coronary artery disease. *J Nucl Med* 1992;33:847(abst).

23. Nichols K, DePuey EG, Gooneratne N, et al. First pass ventricular ejection fraction using a single crystal nuclear camera. *J Nucl Med* 1994;35(8):1292–1300.

24. Rozanski A, Berman DS. The efficacy of cardiovascular nuclear medicine studies. *Semin Nucl Med* 1987;17(2):104–120.

25. Rozanski A. Applications of exercise radionuclide ventriculography in the clinical management of patients with coronary artery disease. *J Thorac Imaging* 1990;5(3):37–46.

26. Morris DD, Rozanski A, Berman DS, et al. Noninvasive prediction of the angiographic extent of coronary artery disease following myocardial infarction: comparison of clinical, bicycle exercise electrocardiographic, and ventriculographic parameters. *Circulation* 1984;70(2):192–201.

27. Rozanski A, Hestrin L, Resser KT, et al. The magnitude of exercise-induced wall motion abnormality during exercise radionuclide ventriculography: relationship to the severity of coronary artery stenosis. *Dyn Cardiovasc Imaging* 1987;1(1):70–79.

28. DePuey EG, Rozanski A. Using gated technetium-99m sestamibi SPECT to characterize fixed myocardial defects as infarct or artifact. *J Nucl Med* 1995;36(6):952–955.

28a. Yao S, Chandra P, Dorbala S, et al. Assessment of occult left ventricular dysfunction in coronary artery disease patients without prior myocardial infarction by technetium-99m sestamibi myocardial perfusion gated SPECT. *J Nucl Med* 1998;39(5):87P(abst).

28b. Johnson LL, Verdesca SA, Aude WY, et al. Postischemic stunning can affect left ventricular ejection fraction and regional wall motion on post-stress gated sestamibi tomograms. *J Am Coll Cardiol* 1997;30(7):1641–1648.

28c. Sharir T, Germano G, Kavanagh PB, et al. Incremental prognostic value of post-stress left ventricular ejection fraction and volume by gated myocardial perfusion single photon emission computed tomography. *Circulation* 1999;100:1035–1042.

29. Palmas W, Friedman JD, Diamond GA, et al. Incremental value of simultaneous assessment of myocardial function and perfusion with technetium-99m sestamibi for the prediction of coronary artery disease. *J Am Coll Cardiol* 1995;25(5):1024–1031.

30. Palmas W, Denton TA, Berman DS, et al. Enhancement of prognostic ability of thallium-201 myocardial perfusion scintigraphy by addition of left ventricular functional information. *J Am Coll Cardiol* 1993;21:359A(abst).

31. Thompson RC, Stowers SA, Flipse TR, et al. The clinical impact of routine addition of stress first pass radionuclide angiography to Tc-sestamibi perfusion imaging. *Circulation* 1993;88:I-440(abst).

32. Maddahi J, Van Train KF, Prigent F, et al. Quantitative single photon emission computed thallium-201 tomography for detection and localization of coronary artery disease: optimization and prospective validation of a new technique. *J Am Coll Cardiol* 1989;114(7):1689–1699.

33. Ladenheim ML, Pollock BH, Rozanski A, et al. Extent and severity of myocardial hypoperfusion as predictors of prognosis in patients with suspected coronary artery disease. *J Am Coll Cardiol* 1986;7(3):464–471.

34. Brown KA, Boucher CA, Okada RD, et al. Prognostic value of exercise thallium-201 imaging in patients presenting for evaluation of chest pain. *J Am Coll Cardiol* 1983;1(4):994–1001.

35. Pamelia FX, Gibson RS, Watson DD, et al. Prognosis with chest pain and normal thallium-201 exercise scintigrams. *Am J Cardiol* 1985;55:920–926.

36. Wackers FJ, Russo DJ, Russo D, et al. Prognostic significance of normal quantitative planar thallium-201 stress scintigraphy in patients with chest pain. *J Am Coll Cardiol* 1985;6(1):27–30.

37. Heo J, Thompson WO, Iskandrian AS. Prognostic implications of normal exercise thallium images. *Am J Noninvas Cardiol* 1987;1:209–212.

38. Koss JH, Kobren SM, Grunwald AM, et al. Role of exercise thallium-201 myocardial perfusion scintigraphy in predicting prognosis in suspected coronary artery disease. *Am J Cardiol* 1987;59:531–534.

39. Fleg JL, Gerstenblith G, Zonderman AB, et al. Prevalence and prognostic significance of exercise-induced silent myocardial ischemia detected by thallium scintigraphy and electrocardiography in asymptomatic volunteers. *Circulation* 1990;81(2):428–436.

40. Raiker K, Sinusas AJ, Wackers FJT, et al. One-year prognosis of patients with normal planar or single-photon emission computed tomographic technetium 99m-labeled sestamibi exercise imaging. *J Nucl Cardiol* 1994;1(5):449–456.

41. Berman DS, Hachamovitch R, Kiat H, et al. Incremental value of prognostic testing in patients with known or suspected ischemic heart disease: a basis for optimal utilization of exercise technetium-99m sestamibi myocardial perfusion single-photon emission computed tomography. *J Am Coll Cardiol* 1995;26(3):639–647.

41a. Yao S, Chandra P, Dorbala S, et al. Assessment of type, frequency, and prognostic value of equivocal test responses during myocardial perfusion SPECT studies. *Circulation* 1998;98(17):I-653(abst).

42. Schalet BD, Kegel JG, Heo J, et al. Prognostic implications of normal exercise SPECT thallium images in patients with strongly positive exercise electrocardiograms. *Am J Cardiol* 1993;72:1201–1203.

42a. Fattah AA, Kamal AM, Pancholy S, et al. Prognostic implications of normal exercise tomographic thallium images in patients with angiographic evidence of significant coronary artery disease. *Am J Cardiol* 1994;74:769–771.

43. Weiner DA, McCabe CH, Ryan TJ. Prognosis assessment of patients with coronary artery disease by exercise testing. *Am Heart J* 1983;105(5):749–755.

44. McNeer JF, Margolis JR, Lee KL, et al. The role of the exercise test in the evaluation of patients for ischemic heart disease. *Circulation* 1978;57(1):64–70.

45. Ellestad MH, Wan MKC. Predictive implications of stress testing: follow-up of 2,700 subjects after maximum treadmill stress testing. *Circulation* 1975;51:363–369.

46. Hammermeister KE, DeRouen TA, Dodge HT, et al. Prognostic and predictive valve of exertional hypotension in suspected coronary heart disease. *Am J Cardiol* 1983;51:1261–1266.

47. Goldschlager NS, Selzer A, Cohn K. Treadmill stress tests as indicators of presence and severity of coronary artery disease. *Ann Intern Med* 1976;85(3):277–286.

48. Schneider RM, Seaworth JF, Dohrman ML, et al. Anatomic and prognostic implications of an early positive treadmill exercise test. *Am J Cardiol* 1982;50:682–688.

49. Reisman S, Rozanski A, Maddahi J, et al. Prolonged postexercise ST segment depression is an indicator of hemodynamically severe and extensive coronary artery disease (CAD). *J Am Coll Cardiol* 1986;7:163A(abst).

50. Dagenais GR, Rouleau JR, Christen A, et al. Survival of patients with a strongly positive exercise electrogram. *Circulation* 1982;65(3):452–456.

51. Staniloff HM, Forrester JS, Berman DS, et al. Prediction of death, myocardial infarction, and worsening chest pain using thallium scintigraphy and exercise electrocardiography. *J Nucl Med* 1986;27(12):1842–1848.

52. Josephson MA, Brown G, Hecht HS, et al. Noninvasive detection and localization of coronary stenoses in patients: comparison of resting dipyridamole and exercise thallium-201 myocardial perfusion imaging. *Am Heart J* 1982;103(6):1008–1018.

53. Huikuri IIV, Korhonen UR, Airaksinen J, et al. Comparison of

dipyridamole-handgrip test and bicycle exercise test for thallium tomographic imaging. *Am J Cardiol* 1988;61:264–268.

54. Varma SK, Watson DD, Beller GA. Quantitative comparison of thallium-201 scintigraphy after exercise and dipyridamole in coronary artery disease. *Am J Cardiol* 1989;64:871–877.

55. Gimple LW, Hutter AM, Guiney TE, et al. Prognostic utility of predischarge dipyridamole-thallium imaging compared to predischarge submaximal exercise electrocardiography and maximal exercise thallium imaging after uncomplicated acute myocardial infarction. *Am J Cardiol* 1989;64:1243–1248.

56. Nguyen T, Heo J, Ogilby D, et al. Single photon emission computed tomography with thallium-201 during adenosine-induced coronary hyperemia: correlation with coronary arteriography, exercise thallium imaging and two-dimensional echocardiography. *J Am Coll Cardiol* 1990;16(6):1375–1383.

57. Coyne EP, Belvedere DA, Vande Streek PR, et al. Thallium-201 scintigraphy after intravenous infusion of adenosine compared with exercise thallium testing in the diagnosis of coronary artery disease. *J Am Coll Cardiol* 1991;17(6):1289–1294.

58. Nishimura S, Mahmarian JJ, Boyce TM, et al. Equivalence between adenosine and exercise thallium-201 myocardial tomography: a multicenter, prospective, crossover trial. *J Am Coll Cardiol* 1992;20(2):265–275.

59. Gupta NC, Esterbrooks DJ, Hilleman DE, et al. Comparison of adenosine and exercise thallium-201 single-photon emission computed tomography (SPECT) myocardial perfusion imaging. *J Am Coll Cardiol* 1992;19(2):248–257.

60. Lette J, Waters D, Cerino M, et al. Preoperative coronary artery disease risk stratification based on dipyridamole imaging and a simple three-step, three-segment model for patients undergoing noncardiac vascular surgery or major general surgery. *Am J Cardiol* 1992;69:1553–1558.

61. Hendel RC, Layden JJ, Leppo JA. Prognostic value of dipyridamole thallium scintigraphy for evaluation of ischemic heart disease. *J Am Coll Cardiol* 1990;15(1):109–116.

62. Pennell DJ, Underwood SR, Swanton RH, et al. Dobutamine thallium myocardial perfusion tomography. *J Am Coll Cardiol* 1991;18(6):1471–1479.

62a. Hachamovitch R, Berman DS, Kiat H, et al. Incremental prognostic value of adenosine stress myocardial perfusion single-photon emission computed tomography and impact on subsequent management in patients with or suspected of having myocardial ischemia. *Am J Cardiol* 1997;80:426–433.

63. Hays JT, Mahmarian JJ, Cochran AJ, et al. Dobutamine thallium-201 tomography for evaluating patients with suspected coronary artery disease unable to undergo exercise or pharmacologic stress. *J Am Coll Cardiol* 1993;21(7):1583–1590.

64. Kiat H, Iskandrian AS, Villegas BJ, et al. Arbutamine stress thallium-201 single-photon emission computed tomography using a computerized closed-loop delivery system: multicenter trial for evaluation of safety and diagnostic accuracy. *J Am Coll Cardiol* 1995;26(5):1159–1167.

65. Soman P, Khattar R, Senior R, et al. Inotrophic stress with arbutamine is superior to vasodilator stress with dipyridamole for the detection of reversible ischemia with Tc-99m sestamibi single-photon emission computed tomography. *J Nucl Cardiol* 1997;4(5):364–371.

66. Shehata AR, Ahlberg AW, Gillam LD, et al. Direct comparison of arbutamine and dobutamine stress testing with myocardial perfusion imaging and echocardiography in patients with coronary artery disease. *Am J Cardiol* 1997;80:716–720.

67. Iskandrian AS, Hakki AH, Kane-Marsch S. Prognostic implications of exercise thallium-201 scintigraphy in patients with suspected or known coronary artery disease. *Am Heart J* 1985;110 (1):135–143.

68. Beller GA, Gibson RS. Sensitivity, specificity, and prognosis sig-

nificance of noninvasive testing for occult or known coronary disease. *Prog Cardiovasc Dis* 1987;29(4):241–270.

68a. Stratmann HG, Younis LT, Wittry MD, et al. Dipyridamole technetium-99m sestamibi myocardial tomography in patients evaluated for elective vascular surgery: prognostic value for perioperative and late cardiac events. *Am Heart J* 1995;131(5): 923–929.

69. Kotler TS, Diamond GA. Exercise thallium-201 scintigraphy in the diagnosis and prognosis of coronary artery disease. *Ann Intern Med* 1990;113(9):684–702.

70. Brown KA. Prognostic value of thallium-201 myocardial perfusion imaging. A diagnostic tool comes of age. *Circulation* 1991;83(2):363–381.

71. Brown KA, Osbakken M, Boucher CA, et al. Positive exercise thallium-201 test responses in patients with less than 50% maximal coronary stenosis: angiographic and clinical predictors. *Am J Cardiol* 1985;55:54–57.

72. Kaul S, Finkelstein DM, Homma S, et al. Superiority of quantitative exercise thallium-201 variables in determining long-term prognosis in ambulatory patients with chest pain: a comparison with cardiac catheterization. *J Am Coll Cardiol* 1988;12 (1):25–34.

73. Kaul S, Lilly DR, Gascho JA, et al. Prognostic utility of the exercise thallium-201 test in ambulatory patients with chest pain: comparison with cardiac catheterization. *Circulation* 1988;77(4):745–758.

74. Brown KA, Rowen M. Prognostic value of a normal exercise myocardial perfusion imaging study in patients with angiographically significant coronary artery disease. *Am J Cardiol* 1993;71:865–867.

75. Bonow RO, Kent KM, Rosing DR, et al. Exercise-induced ischemia in mildly symptomatic patients with coronary-artery disease and preserved left ventricular function: identification of subgroups at risk of death during medical therapy. *N Engl J Med* 1984;311(21):1339–1345.

76. Jones RH, Floyd RD, Austin EH, et al. The role of radionuclide angiocardiography in the preoperative prediction of pain relief and prolonged survival following coronary artery bypass grafting. *Ann Surg* 1983;197(6):743–753.

77. Pollock SG, Abbott RD, Boucher CA, et al. Independent and incremental prognostic value of tests performed in hierarchical order to evaluate patients with suspected coronary artery disease. *Circulation* 1992;85(1):237–248.

78. Iskandrian AS, Chae SC, Heo J, et al. Independent and incremental prognostic value of exercise single-photon emission computed tomographic (SPECT) thallium imaging in coronary artery disease. *J Am Coll Cardiol* 1993;22(3):665–670.

79. DeBusk RF, Blomqvist G, Kouchoukos NT, et al. Identification and treatment of low-risk patients after acute myocardial infarction and coronary-artery bypass graft surgery. *N Engl J Med* 1986;314(3):161–166.

80. Gibson RS, Watson DD, Craddock GB, et al. Prediction of cardiac events after uncomplicated myocardial infarction: a prospective study comparing predischarge exercise thallium-201 scintigraphy and coronary angiography. *Circulation* 1983;68(2): 321–336.

81. Gibson RS, Beller GA, Gheorghiade M, et al. The prevalence and clinical significance of residual myocardial ischemia 2 weeks after uncomplicated non-Q wave infarction: a prospective natural history study. *Circulation* 1986;73(6):1186–1198.

82. Wilson WW, Gibson RS, Nygaard TW, et al. Acute myocardial infarction associated with single vessel coronary artery disease: an analysis of clinical outcome and the prognostic importance of vessel patency and residual ischemic myocardium. *J Am Coll Cardiol* 1988;11(2):223–234.

83. Brown KA, Weiss RM, Clements JP, et al. Usefulness of resid-

ual ischemic myocardium within prior infarct zone for identifying patients at high risk late after acute myocardial infarction. *Am J Cardiol* 1987;60:15–19.

84. Leppo JA, O'Brien J, Rothendler JA, et al. Dipyridamole-thallium-201 scintigraphy in the prediction of future cardiac events after acute myocardial infarction. *N Engl J Med* 1984;310(16):1014–1018.

85. Gimple LW, Hutter AM, Guiney TE, et al. Prognostic utility of predischarge dipyridamole-thallium imaging compared to predischarge submaximal exercise electrocardiography and maximal exercise thallium imaging after uncomplicated acute myocardial infarction. *Am J Cardiol* 1989;64:1243–1248.

86. Pirelli S, Inglese E, Suppa M, et al. Dipyridamole-thallium 201 scintigraphy in the early post-infarction period. (Safety and accuracy in predicting the extent of coronary disease and future recurrence of angina in patients suffering from their first myocardial infarction). *Eur Heart J* 1989;9:1324–1331.

87. Younis LT, Byers S, Shaw L, et al. Prognostic value of intravenous dipyridamole thallium scintigraphy after an acute myocardial ischemic event. *Am J Cardiol* 1989;64:161–166

88. Brown KA, O'Meara J, Chambers CE, et al. Ability of dipyridamole-thallium-201 imaging one to four days after acute myocardial infarction to predict in-hospital and late recurrent myocardial ischemic events. *Am J Cardiol* 1990;65:160–167.

88a. Mahmarian JJ, Mahmarian AC, Marks GF, et al. Role of adenosine thallium-201 tomography for defining long-term risk in patients after acute myocardial infarction. *J Am Coll Cardiol* 1995;25(6):1333–1340.

89. Mahmarian JJ, Pratt CM, Nishimura S, et al. Quantitative adenosine $^{201}$Tl single-photon emission computed tomography for the early assessment of patients surviving acute myocardial infarction. *Circulation* 1993;87(4):1197–1210.

90. Weiss AT, Maddahi J, Shah PK, et al. Exercise-induced ischemia in the streptokinase-reperfused myocardium: relationship to extent of salvaged myocardium and degree of residual coronary stenosis. *Am Heart J* 1989;118(1):9–16.

91. Tilkemeier PL, Guiney TE, LaRaia PJ, et al. Prognostic value of predischarge low-level exercise thallium testing after thrombolytic treatment of acute myocardial infarction. *Am J Cardiol* 1990;66:1203–1207.

92. Haber HL, Beller GA, Watson DD, et al. Exercise thallium-201 scintigraphy after thrombolytic therapy with or without angioplasty for acute myocardial infarction. *Am J Cardiol* 1993;71:1257–1261.

93. Dakik HA, Mahmarian JJ, Kimball KT, et al. Prognostic value of exercise 201thallium tomography in patients treated with thrombolytic therapy during acute myocardial infarction. *Circulation* 1996;94(11):2735–2742.

94. Brown KA. Prognostic value of thallium-201 myocardial perfusion imaging in patients with unstable angina who respond to medical treatment. *J Am Coll Cardiol* 1991;17(5):1053–1057.

95. Hillert MC, Narahara KA, Smitherman TC, et al. Thallium 201 perfusion imaging after the treatment of unstable angina pectoris-relationship to clinical outcome. *West J Med* 1986;145(3):335–340.

96. Freeman MR, Chisholm RJ, Armstrong PW. Usefulness of exercise electrocardiography and thallium scintigraphy in unstable angina pectoris in predicting the extent and severity of coronary artery disease. *Am J Cardiol* 1988;62:1164–1170.

97. Stratmann HG, Tamesis B, Wittry MD, et al. Dipyridamole sestamibi myocardial tomography: an independent predictor of adverse outcome in unstable angina patients. *Circulation* 1993;88:I-487(abst).

98. Iskandrian AS, Heo J, Decoskey D, et al. Use of exercise thallium-201 imaging for risk stratification of elderly patients with coronary artery disease. *Am J Cardiol* 1988;61:269–272.

99. Shaw L, Chaitman BR, Hilton TC, et al. Prognostic value of dipyridamole thallium-201 imaging in elderly patients. *J Am Coll Cardiol* 1992;19(7):1390–1398.

100. Greenberg JM, Murphy JH, Okada RD, et al. Value and limitations of radionuclide angiography in determining the cause of reduced left ventricular ejection fraction: comparison of idiopathic dilated cardiomyopathy and coronary artery disease. *Am J Cardiol* 1985;55:541–544.

101. Bulkley BH, Hutchins GM, Bailey I, et al. Thallium 201 imaging and gated cardiac blood pool scans in patients with ischemic and idiopathic congestive cardiomyopathy. *Circulation* 1977;55(5):753–760.

102. Saltissi S, Hockings B, Croft DN, et al. Thallium-201 myocardial imaging in patients with dilated and ischaemic cardiomyopathy. *Br Heart J* 1981;46:290–295.

103. Dunn RF, Uren RF, Sadick N, et al. Comparison of thallium-201 scanning in idiopathic dilated cardiomyopathy and severe coronary artery disease. *Circulation* 1982;66(4):804–810.

104. Iskandrian AS, Hakki A-H, Kane S. Resting thallium-201 myocardial perfusion patterns in patients with severe left ventricular dysfunction: Differences between patients with primary cardiomyopathy, chronic coronary artery disease, or acute myocardial infarction. *Am Heart J* 1986;111(4):760–767.

105. Eisenberg JD, Sobel BE, Geltman EM. Differentiation of ischemic from nonischemic cardiomyopathy with positron emission tomography. *Am J Cardiol* 1987;59:1410–1414.

106. Eichhorn EJ, Kosinski EJ, Lewis SM, et al. Usefulness of dipyridamole-thallium-201 perfusion scanning for distinguishing ischemic from nonischemic cardiomyopathy. *Am J Cardiol* 1988;62:945–951.

107. Mody FV, Brunken RC, Stevenson LW, et al. Differentiating cardiomyopathy of coronary artery disease from nonischemic dilated cardiomyopathy utilizing positron emission tomography. *J Am Coll Cardiol* 1991;17(2):373–383.

107a. Chikamori T, Doi YL, Yonezawa Y, et al. Value of dipyridamole thallium-201 imaging in noninvasive differentiation of idiopathic dilated cardiomyopathy from coronary artery disease with left ventricular dysfunction. *Am J Cardiol* 1992;69:650–653.

108. Tauberg SG, Orie JE, Bartlett BE, et al. Usefulness of thallium-201 for distinction of ischemic from idiopathic dilated cardiomyopathy. *Am J Cardiol* 1993;71:674–680.

108a. Danias PG, Ahlberg AW, Clark BA, et al. Combined assessment of myocardial perfusion and left ventricular function with exercise technetium-99m sestamibi gated single-photon emission computed tomography can differentiate between ischemic and nonischemic dilated cardiomyopathy. *Am J Cardiol* 1998;82:1253–1258.

108b. Yao S, Diamond GA, Chandra P, et al. Prospective validation of a quantitative method to differentiate ischemic versus nonischemic cardiomyopathy by Tc-99m sestamibi SPECT. *J Nucl Med* 1999;40(5);125P(abst).

109. Eitzman D, Al-Aouar Z, Kanter HL, et al. Clinical outcomes of patients with advanced coronary artery disease after viability studies with positron emission tomography. *J Am Coll Cardiol* 1992;20(3):559–565.

110. Besozzi MC, Brown MD, Hubner KF, et al. Retrospective post therapy evaluation of cardiac function in 208 coronary artery disease patients evaluated by positron emission tomography. *J Nucl Med* 1992;33:885(abst).

111. Maddahi J, DiCarli M, Davidson M, et al. Prognostic significance of PET assessment of myocardial viability in patients with left ventricular dysfunction. *J Am Coll Cardiol* 1992;19:142A(abst).

112. DePuey EG, Nichols K, Dobrinsky C. Left ventricular ejection fraction assessed from gated technetium-99m-sestamibi SPECT. *J Nucl Med* 1993;34(11):1871–1876.

113. Germano G, Kiat H, Kavanagh, et al. Automatic quantification of ejection fraction from gated myocardial perfusion SPECT. *J Nucl Med* 1995;36(11):2138–2147.

114. Nichols K, DePuey EG, Rozanski A. Automation of gated tomographic left ventricular ejection fraction. *J Nucl Cardiol* 1996;3:475–482.

114a. Nichols K, Rozanski A, Malhotra S, et al. Normal limits of left ventricular function parameters from myocardial perfusion gated SPECT. *J Nucl Med* 1996;37(5):105P(abst).

114b. Kang X, Berman DS, Germano G, et al. Normal parameters of left ventricle volume and ejection fraction measured by gated myocardial perfusion SPECT. *J Am Coll Cardiol* 1999;33(2):409A(abst).

114c. Yao S, Chandra P, Cohen R, et al. Factors influencing resting left ventricular ejection fraction measurements by technetium-99m sestamibi myocardial perfusion gated SPECT. *J Nucl Med* 1998;39(5):45P(abst).

115. Breisblatt WM, Barnes JV, Weiland F, et al. Incomplete revascularization in multivessel percutaneous transluminal coronary angioplasty: the role for stress thallium-201 imaging. *J Am Coll Cardiol* 1988;11(6):1183–1190.

116. DePuey EG. Myocardial perfusion imaging with thallium-201 to evaluate patients before and after percutaneous transluminal coronary angioplasty. *Circulation* 1991;84(3, suppl I):I-59–I-65.

117. Hecht HS, Shaw RE, Chin HL, et al. Silent ischemia after coronary angioplasty: evaluation of restenosis and extent of ischemia in asymptomatic patients by tomographic thallium-201 exercise imaging and comparison with symptomatic patients. *J Am Coll Cardiol* 1991;17(3):670–677.

118. Hirzel HO, Nuesch K, Gruentzig AR, et al. Short- and long-term changes in myocardial perfusion after percutaneous transluminal coronary angioplasty assessed by thallium-201 exercise scintigraphy. *Circulation* 1981;63(5):1001–1007.

119. Miller DD, Liu P, Strauss HW, et al. Prognostic value of computer-quantitated exercise thallium imaging early after percutaneous transluminal coronary angioplasty. *J Am Coll Cardiol* 1987;10(2):275–283.

120. Scholl JM, Chaitman BR, David PR, et al. Exercise electrocardiography and myocardial scintigraphy in the serial evaluation of the results of percutaneous transluminal coronary angioplasty. *Circulation* 1982;66(2):380–390.

121. Wijns W, Serruys PW, Reiber JHC, et al. Early detection of restenosis after successful percutaneous transluminal coronary angioplasty by exercise-redistribution thallium scintigraphy. *Am J Cardiol* 1985;55:357–361.

122. Manyari DE, Knudtson M, Kloiber R, et al. Sequential thallium-201 myocardial perfusion studies after successful percutaneous transluminal coronary artery angioplasty: delayed resolution of exercise-induced scintigraphic abnormalities. *Circulation* 1988;77(1):86–95.

123. Iskandrian AS, Lemlek J, Ogilby JD, et al. Early thallium imaging after percutaneous transluminal coronary angioplasty: tomographic evaluation during adenosine-induced coronary hyperemia. *J Nucl Med* 1992;33(12):2086–2089.

124. Greenberg BH, Hart R, Botvinick EH, et al. Thallium-201 myocardial perfusion scintigraphy to evaluate patients after coronary bypass surgery. *Am J Cardiol* 1978;42:167–176.

125. Ritchie JL, Narahara KA, Trobaugh GB, et al. Thallium-201 myocardial imaging before and after coronary revascularization. *Circulation* 1978;56(5):830–836.

126. Gibson RS, Watson DD, Taylor GJ, et al. Prospective assessment of regional myocardial perfusion before and after coronary revascularization surgery by quantitative thallium-201 scintigraphy. *J Am Coll Cardiol* 1983;1(3):804–815.

126a. Nallamothu N, Johnson JH, Bagheri B, et al. Utility of stress single-photon emission computed tomography (SPECT) perfusion imaging in predicting outcome after coronary artery bypass grafting. *Am J Cardiol* 1997;80:1517–1521.

127. Palmas W, Bingham S, Diamond GA, et al. Incremental prognostic value of exercise thallium-201 myocardial single photon emission computed tomography late after coronary artery bypass surgery. *J Am Coll Cardiol* 1995;25(2):403–409.

128. Stern ST, Tzivoni D. Early detection of silent ischemic heart disease by 24 hour electrocardiographic monitoring of active subjects. *Br Heart J* 1974;36:481–486.

129. Deanfield JE, Maseri A, Selwyn AP, et al. Myocardial ischaemia during daily life in patients with stable angina: its relation to symptoms and heart rate changes. *Lancet* 1983;1:753–758.

130. Rozanski A, Berman DS. Silent myocardial ischemia: I. Pathophysiology, frequency of occurrence, and approaches toward detection. *Am Heart J* 1987;114(3):615–626.

131. Klein J, Rodriguez EA, Berman DS, et al. The prevalence and functional significance of transient ST-segment depression during daily life activity: comparisons of ambulatory ECG with stress redistribution thallium-201 SPECT. *Am Heart J* 1993;125(5):1247–1257.

132. Dehmer GJ, Falkoff M, Lewis SE, et al. Effect of oral propranolol on rest and exercise left ventricular ejection fraction, volumes, and segmental wall motion in patients with angina pectoris. Assessment with equilibrium gated blood pool imaging. *Br Heart J* 1981;45:656–666.

133. Marshall RC, Wisenberg G, Schelbert HR, et al. Effect of oral propranolol on rest, exercise and postexercise left ventricular performance in normal subjects and patients with coronary artery disease. *Circulation* 1981;63(3):572–583.

134. Zacca NM, Verani MS, Chahine RA, et al. Effect of nifedipine on exercise-induced left ventricular dysfunction and myocardial hypoperfusion in stable angina. *Am J Cardiol* 1982;50:689–695.

135. Rainwater J, Steele P, Kirch D, et al. Effect of propranolol on myocardial perfusion images and exercise ejection fraction in men with coronary artery disease. *Circulation* 1982;65(1):77–81.

136. Borer JS, Bacharach SL, Green MV, et al. Effect of nitroglycerin on exercise-induced abnormalities of left ventricular regional function and ejection fraction in coronary artery disease: assessment by radionuclide cineangiography in symptomatic and asymptomatic patients. *Circulation* 1978;57(2):314–320.

137. Cohn PF, Brown EJ, Swinford R, et al. Effect of beta blockade on silent regional left ventricular wall motion abnormalities. *Am J Cardiol* 1986;57:521–526.

138. Bairey CN, Krantz DS, DeQuattro V, et al. Effect of beta-blockade on low heart rate-related ischemia during mental stress. *J Am Coll Cardiol* 1991;17(6):1388–1395.

139. Mangano DT, Browner WS, Hollenberg M, et al. Association of peri-operative myocardial ischemia with cardiac morbidity and mortality in men undergoing noncardiac surgery. *N Engl J Med* 1990;323(26):1781–1788.

140. National Center for Health Statistics Health, United States, 1988. *Advance data for vital and health statistics.* DHHS publication no. PHS 89–1232. Washington, DC: Government Printing Office, 1989:10–17,66,67,100,101.

141. Boucher CA, Brewster DC, Darling RC, et al. Determination of cardiac risk by dipyridamole-thallium imaging before peripheral vascular surgery. *N Engl J Med* 1985;312(7):389–394.

142. Leppo J, Plaja J, Gionet M, et al. Noninvasive evaluation of cardiac risk before elective vascular surgery. *J Am Coll Cardiol* 1987;9(2):269–276.

143. Brown KA, Rimmer J, Haisch C. Noninvasive cardiac risk stratification of diabetic and nondiabetic uremic renal allograft candidates using dipyridamole-thallium-201 imaging and radionuclide ventriculography. *Am J Cardiol* 1989;64:1017–1021.

144. Brown KA, Rowen M. Extent of jeopardized viable

myocardium determined by myocardial perfusion imaging best predicts perioperative cardiac events in patients undergoing noncardiac surgery. *J Am Coll Cardiol* 1993;21(2):325–330.

145. Camp AD, Garvin PJ, Hoff J, et al. Prognostic value of intravenous dipyridamole thallium imaging in patients with diabetes mellitus considered for renal transplantation. *Am J Cardiol* 1990;65:1459–1463.

146. Cambria RP, Brewster DC, Abbott WM, et al. The impact of selective use of dipyridamole-thallium scans and surgical factors on the current morbidity of aortic surgery. *J Vasc Surg* 1992; 15(1):43–51.

147. Cutler BS, Leppo JA. Dipyridamole thallium-201 scintigraphy to detect coronary artery disease before abdominal aortic surgery. *J Vasc Surg* 1987;5(1):91–100.

148. Hendel RC, Whitfield SS, Villegas BJ, et al. Prediction of late cardiac events by dipyridamole thallium imaging in patients undergoing elective vascular surgery. *Am J Cardiol* 1992;70: 1243–1249.

149. Kettunen R, Huikuri HV, Heikkila J, et al. Preoperative diagnosis of coronary artery disease in patients with valvular heart disease using technetium-99m isonitrile tomographic imaging together with high-dose dipyridamole and handgrip exercise. *Am J Cardiol* 1992;69:1442–1445.

150. Lane SE, Lewis SM, Pippin JJ, et al. Predictive value of quantitative dipyridamole-thallium scintigraphy in assessing cardiovascular risk after vascular surgery in diabetes mellitus. *Am J Cardiol* 1989;64:1275–1279.

151. Lette J, Waters D, Lapointe J, et al. Usefulness of the severity and extent of reversible perfusion defects during thallium-dipyridamole imaging for cardiac risk assessment before noncardiac surgery. *Am J Cardiol* 1989;64:276–281.

152. Lette J, Waters D, Lassonde J, et al. Postoperative myocardial infarction and cardiac death. Predictive value of dipyridamole-thallium imaging and five clinical scoring systems based on multifactorial analysis. *Ann Surg* 1990;84–90.

153. Madsen PV, Vissing M, Munck O, et al. A comparison of dipyridamole thallium 201 scintigraphy and clinical examination in the determination of cardiac risk before arterial reconstruction. *Angiology* 1992;43(4):306–311.

154. Mangano DT, London MJ, Tubau JF, et al. Dipyridamole thallium-201 scintigraphy as a preoperative screening test. A reexamination of its predictive potential. *Circulation* 1991;84(2): 493–502.

155. Marwick TH, Underwood DA. Dipyridamole thallium imaging may not be a reliable screening test for coronary artery disease in patients undergoing vascular surgery. *Clin Cardiol* 1990; 13:14–18.

156. McFallas EO, Doliszny KM, Grund F, et al. Angina and persistent exercise thallium defects: independent risk factors in elective vascular surgery. *J Am Coll Cardiol* 1993;21(6):1347–1352.

157. McPhail NV, Ruddy TD, Calvin JE, et al. A comparison of dipyridamole-thallium imaging and exercise testing in the prediction of postoperative cardiac complications in patients requiring arterial reconstruction. *J Vasc Surg* 1989;10(1):51–56.

158. Reifsnyder T, Bandyk DF, Lanza D, et al. Use of stress thallium imaging to stratify cardiac risk in patients undergoing vascular surgery. *J Surg Res* 1992;52(3):147–151.

159. Rose EL, Liu XJ, Henley M, et al. Prognostic value of noninvasive cardiac tests in the assessment of patients with peripheral vascular disease. *Am J Cardiol* 1993;71:40–44.

160. Sachs RN, Tellier P, Larmignat P, et al. Assessment by dipyridamole-thallium-201 myocardial scintigraphy of coronary risk before peripheral vascular surgery. *Surgery* 1988;103(5):584–587.

161. Shaw L, Miller DD, Kong BA, et al. Determination of perioperative cardiac risk by adenosine thallium-201 myocardial imaging. *Am Heart J* 1992;124(4):861–869.

162. Stratmann HG, Mark AL, Williams GA. Thallium-201 perfusion imaging with atrial pacing or dipyridamole stress testing for evaluation of cardiac risk prior to nonvascular surgery. *Clin Cardiol* 1990;13:611–616.

163. Younis LT, Byers S, Shaw L, et al. Prognostic importance of silent myocardial ischemia detected by intravenous dipyridamole thallium myocardial imaging in asymptomatic patients with coronary artery disease. *J Am Coll Cardiol* 1989;14(7): 1635–1641.

164. Younis LT, Aguirre F, Byers S, et al. Perioperative and long-term prognostic value of intravenous dipyridamole thallium scintigraphy in patients with peripheral vascular disease. *Am Heart J* 1990;119(6):1287–1292.

165. Stratmann HG, Younis LT, Wittry MD, et al. Dipyridamole technetium-99m sestamibi myocardial tomography in patients evaluated for elective vascular surgery: prognostic value for perioperative and late cardiac events. *Am Heart J* 1995;131(5): 923–929.

166. Stratmann HG, Younis LT, Wittry MD, et al. Dipyridamole technetium 99m sestamibi myocardial tomography for preoperative cardiac risk stratification before major or minor nonvascular surgery. *Am Heart J* 1996;132(3):536–541.

167. Zellner JL, Elliott BM, Robison JG, et al. Preoperative evaluation of cardiac risk using dobutamine-thallium imaging in vascular surgery. *Ann Vasc Surg* 1990;4(3):238–243.

168. Eagle KA, Coley CM, Newell JB, et al. Combining clinical and thallium data optimizes preoperative assessment of cardiac risk before major vascular surgery. *Ann Intern Med* 1989;110(11): 859–866.

168a. McEnroe CS, O'Donnell TF, Yeager A, et al. Comparison of ejection fraction and Goldman risk factor analysis to dipyridamole-thallium 201 studies in the evaluation of cardiac morbidity after aortic aneurysm surgery. *J Vasc Surg* 1990;11(4):497–504.

168b. Baron JF, Mundler O, Bertrand M, et al. Dipyridamole-thallium Scintigraphy and gated radionuclide angiography to assess cardiac risk before abdominal aortic surgery. *N Engl J Med* 1994;330(10):663–669.

168c. Bry JDL, Belkin M, O'Donnell TF et al. An assessment of the positive predictive value and cost-effectiveness of dipyridamole myocardial scintigraphy in patients undergoing vascular surgery. *J Vasc Surg* 1994;19(1):112–124.

168d. Koutelou MG, Asimacopoulos PJ, Mahmarian JJ, et al. Preoperative risk stratification by adenosine thallium 201 single-photon emission computed tomography in patients undergoing vascular surgery. *J Nucl Cardiol* 1995;2:389–394.

169. Goldman L, Caldera DL, Nussbaum SR, et al. Multifactorial index of cardiac risk in noncardiac surgical procedures. *N Engl J Med* 1977;297(16):845–850.

170. Foster ED, Davis KB, Carpenter JA, et al. Risk of noncardiac operation in patients with defined coronary disease: the coronary artery surgery study (CASS) registry experience. *Ann Thorac Surg* 1986;41(1):42–49.

171. Eagle KA, Brundage BH, Chaitman BR, et al. Guidelines for perioperative cardiovascular evaluation for noncardiac surgery. Report of the American College of Cardiology/American Heart Association task force on practice guidelines (committee on perioperative cardiovascular evaluation for noncardiac surgery). *J Am Coll Cardiol* 1996;27(4):910–948.

172. Hachamovitch R, Berman DS, Kiat H, et al. Exercise myocardial perfusion SPECT in patients without known coronary artery disease. Incremental prognostic value and use in risk stratification. *Circulation* 1996;93(5):905–914.

172a. Pavin D, Delonca J, Siegenthaler M, et al. Long-term (10 years) prognostic value of a normal thallium-201 myocardial exercise scintigraphy in patients with coronary artery disease documented by angiography. *Eur Heart J* 1997;18:69–77.

173. Pancholy SB, Fattah AA, Kamal AM, et al. Independent and incremental prognostic value of exercise thallium single-photon emission computed tomographic imaging in women. *J Nucl Cardiol* 1995;2(2):110–116.

174. Hachamovitch R, Berman DS, Kiat H, et al. Effective risk stratification using exercise myocardial perfusion SPECT in women: gender-related differences in prognostic nuclear testing. *J Am Coll Cardiol* 1996;28(1):34–44.

175. Amanullah AM, Berman DS, Erel J, et al. Incremental prognostic value of adenosine myocardial perfusion single photon emission computed tomography in women with suspected coronary artery disease. *Am J Cardiol* 1998;82:725–730.

176. Mahmarian JJ, Mahmarian AC, Marks CF, et al. Role of adenosine thallium-201 tomography for defining long-term risk in patients after acute myocardial infarction. *J Am Coll Cardiol* 1995;25(6):1333–1340.

177. Stratmann HG, Younis LT, Wittry MD, et al. Exercise technetium-99m myocardial tomography for the risk stratification of men with medically-treated unstable angina pectoris. *Am J Cardiol* 1995;76:236–240.

178. Hachamovitch R, Berman DS, Kiat H, et al. Incremental prognostic value of adenosine stress myocardial perfusion single-photon emission computed tomography and impact on subsequent management in patients with or suspected of having myocardial ischemia. *Am J Cardiol* 1997;80:426–433.

179. Hachamovitch R, Berman DS, Shaw L, et al. Incremental prognostic value of myocardial perfusion single photon emission computed tomography for the prediction of cardiac death. Differential stratification for risk of cardiac death and myocardial infarction. *Circulation* 1998;97:535–543.

180. Steingart RM, Wassertheil-Smoller S, Tobin JN, et al. Nuclear exercise testing and the management of coronary artery disease. *J Nucl Med* 1991;32(5):753–758.

181. Bateman TM, O'Keefe JH , Dong VM, et al. Coronary angiographic rates after stress single-photon emission computed tomographic scintigraphy. *J Nucl Cardiol* 1995;2(3):217–223.

182. Nallamothu N, Pancholy SB, Lee KR, et al. Impact on exercise single-photon emission computed tomographic thallium imaging on patient management and outcome. *J Nucl Cardiol* 1995;2(4):334–33.

183. Hachamovitch R, Berman DS, Kiat H, et al. Gender-related differences in clinical management after exercise nuclear testing. *J Am Coll Cardiol* 1995;26(6):1457–1464.

184. Shaw LJ, Miller DD, Romeis JC, et al. Gender differences in the noninvasive evaluation and management of patients with suspected coronary artery disease. *Ann Intern Med* 1994;120:559–566.

185. Rozanski A. Referral bias and the efficacy of radionuclide stress tests: problems and solutions. *J Nucl Med* 1992;33(12):2074–2079.

# COST-EFFECTIVENESS OF MYOCARDIAL PERFUSION SPECT

## RORY HACHAMOVITCH
## LESLEE J. SHAW

Coronary heart disease (CHD) and its associated entities are responsible for a devastating proportion of all deaths throughout Westernized countries. In the United States, it is the single largest killer of both men and women; every 29 seconds an American will suffer a coronary event, and approximately, once a minute, an American will die from such an event. Coronary disease resulted in 476,124 deaths in the United States in 1996, a number that increases to more than 725,000 (of over 2,000,000 deaths total in the United States) if related syndromes are included (1). Although widespread, the mortality rates associated with this disease have decreased markedly over the years. The age-adjusted mortality rate of myocardial infarctions, for example, has decreased from 226.4 per 100,000 in 1950 to 124.1 per 100,000 in 1987 and that from cerebrovascular events from 88.8 per 100,000 to 30.7 per 100,000 during the same time period (1). Similarly, during the 19-year follow-up of the NHLBI's (National Heart, Lung and Blood Institute) Honolulu Heart program, the age-adjusted annual CHD mortality rate (per 1,000) decreased from 4.7 to 2.9 with an estimated annual decline of 2.7% (1).

In large part, the decline in cardiovascular morbidity and mortality over the past several decades can be attributed to improvements in diagnostic and therapeutic options available for physicians to treat these diseases. A wide range of new pharmacotherapeutic agents are currently available, targeting a number of mechanisms that contribute to the development and progression of coronary artery disease (CAD). Newer technologies, particularly for revascularization, have also been developed. These newer procedures have flourished and are being applied in ever-increasing numbers. Cardiac catheterizations have increased in use from about 300,000 per year in 1979 to more than 1.2 million in 1996 with similar increases in coronary artery bypass surgery procedures (about 100,000 to 600,000 over the same time interval) and percutaneous coronary interventional angioplasty procedures (about 40,000 to 150,000) (1). Although the application of this new technology has impacted on cardiovascular survival, the cost implications of this technology have been enormous (2,3); 170 of US Health Care expenditures.

Health care expenditures, as a percent of the US gross domestic product (a measure of resource consumption), will have increased from 4% almost four decades ago to an estimated 20% by the end of this decade (1). A major factor contributing to the rising cost of health care has been the development and use of new technology (2,3). Rising health care costs have spawned regulatory efforts to control resource consumption. Provider systems such as managed care have instituted mechanisms to decrease extraneous resource use based on the premise that there is a tremendous overuse of health care services (4–10). More recently, at the state level, action had been taken to eliminate reimbursement for components of stress myocardial perfusion imaging examination, such as the pharmacologic stress agent (Michigan, 1998) or the simultaneous performance of peak exercise first-pass imaging (New York, 1998). These resulting economic pressures are forcing a rethinking of the application of a number of medical procedures.

It is this collision of technology and cost that has spurred the growth of research focusing on the evaluation of the processes of health care, attempting to define the effectiveness and quality of care and its associated cost and impact. This approach has spawned numerous labels—among the more popular, outcomes research or health services research. The origins of outcome assessment are deeply rooted in epidemiologic research. The Institute of Medicine defined outcomes assessment as a field of inquiry in which the effects of the organization, financing, and management of health care services on the delivery, quality, cost, access to, and outcomes of such services are examined (11). As the health care environment is rapidly changing with an emphasis on

R. Hachamovitch: Department of Medicine (Division of Cardiology), New York Hospital–Cornell Medical Center, New York, New York 10021.

L. J. Shaw: Emory Center for Outcomes Research, Emory University, Atlanta, Georgia 30322.

containing costs and increasing regulation, outcomes assessment becomes an important mechanism to assess balance and the effects of new initiatives on health care quality. Furthermore, as health care has becoming increasingly complex, outcomes are an important component in understanding the process and efficacy of patient care within medical specialties.

The evaluation of CHD utilizes a number of testing modalities that require evaluation to determine their relative added values within a testing strategy. The future of nuclear cardiology within the framework of economic restraint will depend upon the ability of nuclear imaging to provide tremendous clinical information in a cost effective manner when compared to other diagnostic modalities.

## OUTCOMES RESEARCH: METHODOLOGIC CONSIDERATIONS FOR ECONOMIC ANALYSES

For the purpose of providing a framework within which to understand the current literature regarding the cost-effectiveness of stress myocardial perfusion imaging and its limitations, we will discuss the basis for evaluating effectiveness of testing and understanding clinically relevant risk stratification and review some basic concepts of cost analyses and accounting.

### Regression Modeling Techniques

Development of one or more set(s) of variables may be defined by a statistical model (reviewed in refs. 12–17). An equation that includes multiple variables is called a multivariable model. Conceptually, a multivariable model includes all statistically significant factors related to an outcome assessed simultaneously. This equation can be applied to understand whether confounding is present, to predict outcomes, or to evaluate the drivers of an outcome. Thus, a multivariable model may also be considered an equation in which all of the included factors aim to solve the formula and estimate a given outcome. In most cases, outcome comparisons have not controlled for a uniform set of variables within regression analyses. Thus, differences in outcome may be attributable to a true difference or to unaccounted-for variability in a predictive model. It is the ability of multivariable models to adjust for these differences in underlying patient characteristics that has led to their popularity and wide application. By "leveling the playing field," multivariable models allow comparisons to be made within both observational and randomized data sets that may otherwise not been possible due to multiple sources of confounding.

A major advantage of this type of analysis is that it preserves all of the available statistical power from the entire patient data set. However, a disadvantage of this type of analysis is that the results are less clinically intuitive. Many physicians are also of the opinion that regression methods do not mirror clinical reasoning, a process based on "heuristics"—so-called rules of thumb. This approach can also be applied to economic analyses to determine the predictors of cost or of length of stay, and to determine what patient or physician characteristics are predictors after adjustment for other factors.

## Important Considerations in Regression Analysis

### Type of Multivariable Model to Use

A number of multivariable models are available on most statistical software programs. The most basic models are a linear regression model for end points that are continuous variables (e.g., extent of CAD, patient height, cost of care) and a logistic regression model for end points that are binary (disease versus no disease, normal scan versus abnormal scan). Note that this latter model is usually not used for modeling events. Instead, the modeling of various types of survival is accomplished with models that incorporate data regarding both whether an event occurred (cardiac death, no cardiac death) and when the event occurred (as measured in a unit of time after the index test). This is most commonly done with a Cox proportional hazards model (a model that makes a number of assumptions, including that the risk of two groups being compared are proportional or parallel over time). Other models are also available for multivariable modeling of survival but are less commonly used. The reader is referred to a number of reviews for further information regarding these models (13–15,17a).

### End Points and Outcomes

The end points or outcomes that are studied and analyzed can be generally divided into three types or categories (Table 14.1). Anatomic end points can vary enormously between studies. Often the presence of hemodynamically significant CAD is used as an end point. Variation in definitions based on lesion location (left main versus other arteries; branch disease versus main arteries) or severity (lesions of ≥50% versus ≥70%) is often present. The presence of significant lesions are often an important step for the diagnosis of CAD. However, defining severe and/or extensive CAD may be more important for the use of tests by specialists or in populations with known CAD. Thus, anatomic end points can include varying definitions of severe disease as outlined in Table 14.2.

As can be seen in Table 14.1, a wide range of events can be considered outcomes in a prognosis study. The selection of which end points to incorporate in a study is dependent on a number of considerations including the size of the study and the patients to be enrolled (in studies evaluating

## TABLE 14.1. SPECTRUM OF POTENTIAL END POINTS

Anatomic
    Presence of coronary artery disease (CAD) (≥50% vs. ≥70% threshold)
    Presence of multivessel CAD (≥50% or ≥70% lesions in >1 coronary artery or a ≥50% lesion in
        the left main coronary artery)
    Presence of severe CAD (e.g., two-vessel CAD with proximal left anterior artery lesion,
        three-vessel or left main CAD)
    Presence of three vessel or left main CAD
Prognostic
    Death
    Cardiac death
    Myocardial infarction (MI)
    Stroke
    Catheterization
    Coronary artery bypass surgery or percutaneous transluminal coronary angioplasty
    Hospitalization for
        Unstable angina
        Congestive heart failure (CHF)
        Other cardiac event
    Recurrent angina
Functional
    Exercise tolerance
    Exercise time until occurrence of symptoms
    Anginal status
    Quality of life
    Activity of daily living
    Anginal class

low-risk or smaller populations, an insufficient number of events may occur if cardiac death or myocardial infarction are the sole end points) and the question under consideration (a study focusing on patients with mild CAD or its prevention may wish to focus on ischemia and its related end points and away from cardiac death, congestive heart failure, and strokes as end points). Finally, since trials of therapy usually focus on one of these end points, the evaluation of noninvasive testing toward these events may yield insight into the application of this testing.

### Unconventional Outcomes–The Importance of Functional Variables

Functional end points have been used less frequently in the past, but are becoming the focus of a number of current studies. Particularly with the development of therapeutic options for the prevention of CAD, the use of these "softer" end points may be more useful. Subtle changes in disease status can be evaluated with this approach that may be missed or require too large a population if "harder" end points are used. In addition, these markers allow evaluation of the quality of the patient's life and, by addressing this issue, can help incorporate this consideration into clinical studies.

Quality of life has become an important and essential outcome variable that is considered a significant end point of medical care (16,18,19). The focus of cardiovascular patient care is not cure but rather management of chronic illness including alleviation of symptoms, improvement of functional capabilities, and retardation of disease progression. Historically, quality of life measures in cardiovascular studies focused on reduction of anginal symptoms and return to work. Health-related quality of life is characterized by its application to well-being and satisfaction associated with how an individual's life is affected by disease, accidents, and treatment. Regarding the psychometric approach and evaluation of global aspects of quality of life, four areas

## TABLE 14.2. DEFINITIONS OF ANATOMICALLY SEVERE CORONARY ARTERY DISEASE (CAD)

| Definition | Potentially useful for the evaluation of: |
| --- | --- |
| Three-vessel or left main CAD | Identification of patients who would benefit from CABG |
| Two-vessel CAD with proximal LAD; three-vessel/left main CAD | Identification of patients who would benefit from CABG and PTCA |
| Proximal LAD; otherwise ≥2-vessel CAD | Identification of patients who would benefit from CABG and PTCA |

CABG, coronary artery bypass graft; LAD, left anterior descending; PTCA, percutaneous transluminal coronary angioplasty.

are highly relevant for patients with CHD: physical, functional, emotional, and social.

For the diagnosis of angina, the Rose questionnaire has been frequently used in studies (18), although the Seattle Angina Questionnaire (SAQ) has gained popularity, particularly for serial evaluation of anginal symptoms (20,21). A number of other evaluation instruments have been developed for CAD patients and widely applied such as the Duke Activity Status Index for assessment of functional status (22) and the Minnesota Living with Heart Failure Questionnaire (23).

Quality of life measures may be substituted for more conventional or traditional outcomes. When used as outcomes, they can quantitate patient symptoms, function, or status. Whereas prognosis end points specify how many patients have experienced particular events, functional status measures describe the quality of people's lives. These two outcomes, event status and functional status, provide different but complementary descriptions of treatment outcomes. Consequently, it would be very useful to distill the broad characteristics of quality of life into a single value that can be combined with mortality to describe the overall outcome of treatment.

## INCREMENTAL PROGNOSTIC VALUE: A CONCEPTUAL BASIS

The measurement of the value of noninvasive testing has shifted from a focus on demonstrating the greater value of the results of these tests compared to clinical and historical data, to focusing on the added or incremental value of these tests over that information known about the patient prior to the test. This assessment has become central to the evaluation of the role of nuclear testing (12,17,24). The measurement of incremental prognostic value addresses whether the information provided by testing is unique relative to that already provided by variables that are already known or less expensive to obtain. This can be assessed relative to whether the test results are predictive of patient outcome after known clinical information is considered, if the application of the test result effectively risk stratifies the cohort in question, or if the application of the test as part of a testing strategy will result in a lowering of cost compared to a strategy not using the modality. This latter application of the test is termed the incremental economic value of nuclear testing (i.e., Does the use of myocardial perfusion imaging result in greater cost-benefit or cost-utility when used as part of an overall patient strategy?) as compared to the incremental statistical or clinical value of the test (12). This approach leads to the development of patient strategies that minimize the expense of testing by referring for testing only those patients not at low or very high risk as judged on the basis of previous information.

These analyses are based on a different approach from the one that has often been used in the past. Patient information must now be considered in a hierarchical fashion, beginning with clinical patient characteristics (very inexpensive), followed by exercise electrocardiogram (ECG) testing (inexpensive), and only then considering data from nuclear testing (moderately expensive) and cardiac catheterization (more expensive) (12,16,17,24). The approach to this analysis begins with a model focusing on all relevant clinical, historical, functional status, and comorbidity status information known prior to the nuclear test. A second model may further include the results of exercise treadmill testing (ETT), thus evaluating the added value of variables derived from this test over the baseline clinical information alone. Finally, the variables associated with stress myocardial perfusion imaging can be added. This stepwise approach mimics the order in which clinical information is accumulated by physicians and is equally legitimate for diagnostic, prognostic, economic, and functional outcomes.

This incremental value of a test may be assessed by several statistical tests including the change in model chi-square, the improvement in test accuracy (e.g., sensitivity), the change in the C-index, or receiver operating characteristics (ROC) curves (12–17,24). Incremental value statistics that use multivariable models, controlling for historical or pretest information, are superior to statistical tests that assess only univariable outcome status.

### Economic Analyses

It is important to consider the types of economic analyses available to the investigator and the manner in which cost data should be evaluated. Health economics focuses on the evaluation of cost and its interaction with patient outcomes (e.g., cardiovascular events) and status (e.g., quality of life, functional status) (25). Whereas this approach can take a macroeconomic perspective by focusing on the economic impact of health care policy changes, for purposes of this review, the focus will be microeconomic: What is the cost of testing and associated patient care as it relates to the use of stress myocardial perfusion imaging? Further, how do we optimize the application and utilization of these tests as a part of a strategy of clinical care (12,16,17)?

### Types of Economic Analyses

A number of economic analyses have been defined that compare health care choices on the basis of differences in the impact of treatments relative to their comparative cost (reviewed in refs. 25–27). Ideally, this analytic approach helps define for policymakers the most efficient use of potentially limited societal resources. Four related techniques are most commonly used: cost-effectiveness, cost-savings, benefit, and cost-utility analyses (Table 14.3).

These three approaches are similar in that they express a relationship between the change in a health measure for two

## TABLE 14.3. TYPES OF COST ANALYSES

| Type | Benefit or Outcome | Assumptions | Measure |
|---|---|---|---|
| Cost minimization | Assume equivalent outcomes | No change in outcome or benefit | Lowest net cost |
| Cost benefit | Convert to monetary terms | All outcomes, benefits, and costs translated to monetary terms | Change in cost ($\Delta$cost) |
| Cost effectiveness | Years of life gained; events identified; cases of disease identified | Difference in effectiveness can be defined and measured | $\Delta$Cost/$\Delta$Effectiveness |
| Cost utility | QALY | Able to define and measure different health states | $\Delta$Cost/$\Delta$QALY |

QALY, quality adjusted life years.

strategies versus the difference in cost for the two. For example, patients presenting with suspected CAD may be referred for either noninvasive testing or catheterization. If the costs and outcomes for a strategy using stress myocardial perfusion imaging in patients with suspected CAD needs to be evaluated and compared to those costs and outcomes associated with a conventional approach of referral for catheterization, one of these analytic approaches can be used. In a general sense, each of these approaches compares a benefit or impact of a clinical strategy to the change in cost of care with the strategy. Thus, a generalized formula can be stated for this class of tests:

$$\frac{(\text{Cost}_{\text{New Strategy}}) - (\text{Cost}_{\text{Conventional Strategy}})}{(\text{Impact}_{\text{New Strategy}}) - (\text{Impact}_{\text{Conventional Strategy}})}$$

Although the determination of costs is similar for all three approaches, it is the definition of the impact of the strategy or its benefit that varies (25).

### Cost-Effectiveness Analyses

Cost-effectiveness analyses usually express the impact of a clinical strategy in familiar units of survival—most commonly, life years gained. With respect to the assessment of noninvasive testing, however, it is unclear how to extract life years gained for a diagnostic rather than therapeutic modality. Thus, in the absence of data relating the use of a test to a therapy, alternative end points include the number of events identified (of all patients undergoing testing and having an abnormal result, how many went on to have events) or diagnoses of CAD made.

### Cost-Utility Analyses

An alternative end point to survival is that of patient benefit defined by an estimate of the number of years of life with perfect health. By measuring patient health state preferences (assuming that a patient is willing to forgo additional years of life for enhanced quality of life in those remaining years, how many fewer years of life patient is willing to live if he or she is in perfect health), patient benefit can be measured by translating anticipated survival time to years of life adjusted for their quality. This subgroup of cost-effectiveness analyses relate the cost of achieving quality-adjusted

life years (QALYs) with various clinical strategies, thus determining the lowest cost per QALY.

The use of QALYs is a fundamental concept in expected utility theory, a theory of rational preferences among risky options that can be used to describe and understand patients' decision-making processes. A utility is a description of patients' health status that has an upper bound of "perfect" health and a lower bound that is usually considered to be death. To quantify a utility, numerical values are assigned to health states along a continuum of 0 to 1, where 0 represents death and 1 represents a state completely free of disease. In essence, a utility represents the distillation of all aspects of a patient's quality of life into a single numerical value between 0 and 1. According to expected utility theory, QALY is defined by multiplying a health state utility by the patients' survival. Therefore, the QALY utility model incorporates the trade-off between patient longevity and quality of life by integrating mortality and attitudes toward morbidity into a single measure.

### Cost-Benefit Analyses

In this comparison of strategies, the impact data are converted into economic terms, for example, the dollar value of gaining years of life or functional status versus the cost of obtaining them. Although these analyses are difficult to perform and often controversial, they can be readily compared to other potential societal investments, since all terms are reduced to their monetary equivalent. Thus, the use of stress myocardial perfusion imaging can be compared to the use of seat belts, vaccinations, and other health policy decisions. This approach defined a "most bang for the bucks" type of definition for the comparison of strategies (25).

### Cost Minimization

In addition, another approach that can be used is cost savings analysis. This approach, also known as a cost minimization analysis, addresses the question of which strategy is the most efficient of two or more under evaluation. The assumption is made that the strategies to be compared have similar benefits or outcomes. For example, patients presenting with suspected CAD are referred for either noninvasive testing or catheterization. After correcting for differences in underlying patient characteristics, no differences in survival are found.

The investigators then compare the cost associated with each strategy. Since no difference is present with respect to outcomes, the comparison will reveal which clinical approach, in this example, will yield a greater cost savings with use.

This type of analysis assumes that there is no differences in the effectiveness of testing or in subsequent outcomes between the strategies to be evaluated. Instead, the focus is strictly on the numerator portion of the equation shown above. The analysis is thus reduced to a comparison of the total costs associated with the two strategies. This type of comparison can be applied to strategies at varying time points, e.g., the cost of referring all patients for catheterization after acute myocardial infarction versus referring only those patients with inducible ischemia as assessed at 6 months, 1 year, and 5 years. As in all economic comparisons, caution must be taken not to claim cost superiority for a strategy due to cost shifting. This phenomenon consists of cost savings achieved by delaying or deferring care of patients until a later time point. Hence, short-term cost savings is achieved, but an increase in costs is noted on long-term follow up when the deferred medical care is given. The analyses described above are summarized in Table 14.3.

## Considerations Regarding Cost

Important considerations in constructing or interpreting economic analyses include realistic pricing of the tests compared, inclusion of as many of the associated costs of testing as possible, and appropriate selection of the accuracy of testing. Finally, the importance of the threshold for abnormality takes on particular importance in cost analysis because of its impact on the need for subsequent expensive invasive testing.

### *Cost Versus Charge Data*

In many economic analyses, the economic data considered are based on charges for health care. It is extremely important to remember the difference between charges, reimbursement, and cost. Charges represent the set price of a good or service provided. This monetary amount is an artificial contrivance; in a tight marketplace the charge can be reduced to be more competitive, in economically more liberal settings it can be raised (26,27). Charges should not be considered to be or used as surrogates of cost. The amount actually received for the service performed, the reimbursement, has in recent years tended to be unrelated to the charge. For purposes of analysis, "usual, customary, and reasonable" costs are often considered. But reimbursements tend to be based on set schedules, occasionally negotiated, that are both unaffected by the billed amount and usually lower. Finally, cost is the amount of money required to replace the good or service in question. For example, to determine the true cost of performing a nuclear study, the labor costs, materials used, and cost of the camera and space

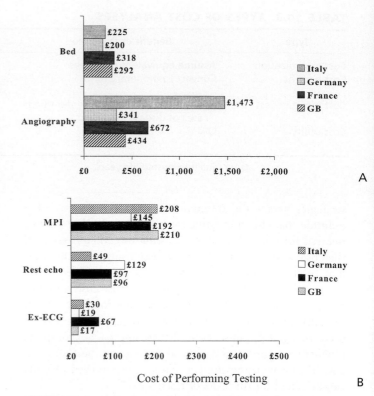

**FIGURE 14.1. A:** Costs of a hospital bed (per day) and angiography in four European countries as determined in the EMPIRE study. Significant intercountry variation is present. Values expressed in pounds sterling. **B:** Costs of stress myocardial perfusion imaging (MPI), resting echocardiography (rest echo), and exercise electrocardiographic treadmill testing (Ex-ECG) in four European countries as determined in the EMPIRE study. Values expressed in pounds sterling. (Data courtesy of Dr. Richard Underwood.)

should all be considered irrespective of the charge or reimbursement of the procedure (16).

In Fig. 14.1, the true costs of various medical expenses are shown for various European countries as determined by the EMPIRE study. Clearly, given the remarkable range of values for the procedures shown, the most cost-efficient strategy will vary not only as a function of test performance, new technology, availability, etc., but as a function of the country studied as well.

### *Direct Versus Indirect Costs*

In performing a cost analysis, it is important to differentiate between direct and indirect costs. Direct costs, in calculating the costs of performing a single photon emission computed tomography (SPECT) study, for example, include the actual costs of the labor and materials used in the performance of the test, while indirect costs include the rent and utilities that may be paid on the space used. In an analysis of a strategy of care, direct costs include the procedures performed on the patient, while indirect costs include the loss of productivity of the patient during the illness.

Indirect costs should not be confused with induced costs. The latter refers to savings or cost due to a procedure that resulted from a strategy examined; for example, if fewer percutaneous transluminal coronary angioplasties are performed because of noninvasive testing used as screening to identify low-risk patients, the costs savings of this strategy are a negative induced cost (26,27).

## Fixed Versus Variable Costs

Fixed costs are said to be those that are present and independent of patient volume and of a single cost over a defined range of patient volume. The latter part of this definition must be present. For example, a laboratory has a single camera and technologist and is capable of performing eight studies a day. The cost of the space and the SPECT camera are considered to be a fixed cost over a range of zero to eight studies done per day. If demand were to increase, additional technologists, space, or cameras may be necessary; the addition of these resources constitutes an increase in the fixed cost, but would also alter the range of patient volume that the laboratory is capable of handling. Variable costs represent additional consumables that may fluctuate during daily use as a function of the number of patients tested (within the predefined range of patients), for example, the amount intravenous tubing and electrocardiographic leads will vary whether no patients or eight patients are tested, while the cost of the SPECT camera, the space used, and the technologist will not (26,27).

## Cost Accounting Techniques

One of two cost accounting approaches are generally used in estimating cost data. The first, a "bottom-up" approach determines the cost of each resource based on actual or estimated costs. The costs of the physician professional component may be estimated using the resource-based relative value scale (RBRVS) methodology. From hospitals with centralized professional billing, all physician services (defined by CPT codes and modifiers) and physician charges over the entire episode of care can be collected. Using the relative value weights from the Medicare Fee Schedule, relative value units (RVUs) may be assigned to each CPT code and the total RVUs summarized. To convert the service RVUs into cost estimates, conversion factors from Medicare, Blue Cross-Blue Shield (BCBS), or the Health Insurance Association of America (HIAA) data are available. Although this approach is time-consuming and expensive, it tends to be more accurate and is preferred by many investigators (26,27).

The alternative approach is a "top-down" approach in which costs are derived from line-item charges appearing on the patient's bill. Cost, in this approach, is defined as the amount on the bill multiplied by a cost-charge ratio unique to the particular hospital or department. For example, in a hospital-wide cost-to-charge ratios approach, the total cost of each hospitalization is calculated as the product of the total billed charges during the hospital episode found in the claims data base and the hospital's overall cost-to-charge ratio available from the Medicare cost report (25,26). This method tends to be the preferred avenue for clinical trials collecting cost data.

## Improved Economic Analysis

Over the last few years, there has been an increased understanding of the cost-efficiency of nuclear imaging, in particular posttest resource use patterns. However, the information currently available is insufficient to determine the cost-effectiveness of all forms of nuclear imaging in a variety of patient cohorts as derived from patient-specific, controlled clinical trials. Furthermore, as nuclear imaging precipitates additional care in at-risk patients, it is important to document both the direct costs of inpatient and outpatient care. The costs associated with outpatient care in particular have not been examined. This is especially the case for medications used and additional noninvasive testing performed. Although usually ignored, the costs associated with lost productivity of patients after events and procedures need to be considered.

## CLINICAL APPLICATION OF OUTCOMES RESEARCH

To understand outcomes research as applied to nuclear cardiology, it is important to understand the concept of risk and its measurement. Risk may be defined as using what is known to forecast future disease and event risk. Risk estimation plays an important role in all steps of patient evaluation and care including testing and therapeutic selection, disease monitoring, and subsequent follow-up.

It is important to describe a priori the levels of risk that are to define the intensity of care to be recommended, particularly that of low risk. What level of risk is sufficiently low that a patient can be referred for no further evaluative testing, and is it acceptable to recommend risk factor modification as the primary therapy? The generally accepted definitions are those first set forth by the Agency for Health Care Policy Research's unstable angina guidelines (28). The definitions of low, intermediate, and high risk are based on a series of patients with stable angina presenting to Duke University for evaluation. Low risk was defined as a risk of less than 1% per year of follow-up. Although originally defined as a risk of cardiac death, in an attempt to achieve a more conservative threshold in light of the lower risk patients referred for noninvasive testing (e.g., less symptomatic patients characteristic of noninvasive testing), a threshold of less than 1% risk of cardiac death or myocardial infarction is usually used (29–31). By achieving this low level of risk, a cohort of patients at low risk for adverse outcomes, and probably low cost of care, can be removed from the screening process and not tested further.

Patients at 2% to 5% event rates per year are defined as intermediate risk, and those with event rates of 5% or more are deemed high risk. Although intervention and aggressive treatment is recommended for the latter, it was originally considered that the former may benefit from intervention, but may not require this intervention immediately. Using these definitions of risk and their implications for recommended care, an evaluative approach to screening can be considered.

## RISK STRATIFICATION

### Measuring Minimum Requirements for Acceptable Risk Stratification

Although statistically significant risk stratification can be achieved by any of a number of modalities, based on the prognostic studies performed to date, certain criteria emerge as minimal standards for clinically acceptable risk stratification by a noninvasive modality.

- A low-risk study should be associated with a very low event rate. As described above, the criteria generally referred to are those listed in the unstable angina guidelines (28) that categorize a mortality rate of <1% as low risk. This is usually extended to a 1% annualized rate of cardiac death or myocardial infarction given the lower risk profile of patients referred for noninvasive testing.
- Not only should the event rate associated with an abnormal test result be statistically significantly greater than that associated with a normal scans, but the relative risk and its confidence interval with an abnormal scan relative to a normal scan should greatly exceed 1. This relative risk defines the effectiveness of the stratification. This takes on greater importance as the cost-effectiveness of noninvasive testing tends to parallel the effectiveness of the stratification achieved. Enhanced stratification results in more patients in the low-risk group (lower cost of care) and

fewer patients in the high-risk group (a higher cost group that will have more resource utilization over time) (24).

For example, in Fig. 14.2, from a study using exercise sestamibi SPECT, among patients with no known CAD prior to testing the effectiveness of stratification is greater in women than men and is greater in older patients than younger patients (24). The threshold for optimal risk stratification is specific to the particular end point of interest (e.g., cardiac death versus nonfatal myocardial infarction and the effectiveness of stratification varies with end points). This finding significantly affects the application of nuclear testing as part of a testing strategy (24,30,32,33).

## ECONOMIC IMPLICATIONS OF CHOOSING THE APPROPRIATE TEST CANDIDATES

Selection of appropriate patients for testing is the first important step in the process of cost-effective risk stratification. Traditional "clinical wisdom" dictated that patients with a low pretest likelihood of CAD needed no further testing; patients with a high likelihood of CAD would not benefit from further noninvasive testing and should be referred for catheterization for definitive diagnosis; and patients with an intermediate likelihood of CAD could be reclassified into either low- or high-likelihood groups (12,24,29,30,32–34) by ETT or nuclear testing. This reasoning is based on bayesian theory, where the posttest probability is a function of the patient's pretest clinical risk. The patient's posttest probability is directly related to pretest probability of disease or event risk such that, when the pretest clinical risk is low, few outcomes may be estimated due to low disease and event prevalence, and the shifting of posttest probabilities is minimal. Using this reasoning, the greatest shift in posttest probabilities of disease lies in patients whose initial pretest clinical risk may be classified as intermediate risk. Using bayesian theory, patients who are asymptomatic or have nonanginal symptoms have a low pretest likelihood of CAD (<10% to 20% likelihood) and are unlikely to be reclassified to high probability irrespective of test results. Similarly, patients with high pretest likelihood of CAD (>80% to 90% likelihood) are unlikely to be reclassified as low risk on the basis of further testing. Importantly, it is patients with intermediate likelihood of CAD (likelihood between 10% and 90% or 20% and 80%) who will most benefit from further testing since, barring equivocal results, they will be reclassified by the test result as having either high or low probability of CAD.

This approach, however, changes when using a risk-based approach. As with a bayesian approach, patients with a low pretest risk (since a risk-based rather than anatomic end point is being considered) are at very low risk and probably do not require additional testing. As above, patients with intermediate risk are appropriately stratified by nuclear testing. However, unlike the scheme described above,

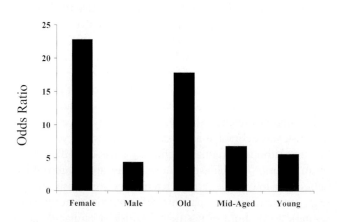

**FIGURE 14.2.** Odds ratios for hard events in abnormal relative to normal scans. All patients are without prior history of coronary artery disease (CAD) at the time of nuclear testing. Old, greater than 70 years; mid-aged, 55 to 70 years; young, less than 55 years.

patients at high risk of adverse outcomes can be stratified into a low-risk group by a normal scan and a higher risk group with an abnormal scan. Thus, the difference in these two approaches is that with a risk-based approach, both intermediate- and high-risk patients can be effectively stratified with respect to risk and need for subsequent care, while in an anatomic approach referral for catheterization would be suggested in the latter group. With respect to implications for cost, the latter approach has significant potential for cost savings since fewer interventions would be required in a strategy that identifies a greater number of patients as not needing further testing rather than immediate referral for catheterization.

## ACHIEVING COST MINIMIZATION VIA A STRATEGY OF RISK STRATIFICATION

The optimal application of testing for the identification of patients at low risk and not in need of further evaluation versus those at need for more aggressive treatment requires a predefined approach or strategy that, by maximizing efficiency, will achieve cost saving. In the context of patient cardiovascular risk evaluation, the results from each step of the clinical screening process must be integrated into an overall assessment of the patient's risk for relevant clinical outcomes. This process describes a stepwise, incremental increase in clinically applicable information, as shown in Fig. 14.3. The evaluative process outlined in this figure can be summarized as applying low cost, prognostically important, clinical and historical data to initially risk stratify a larger population, then applying sequential testing of patients still considered to be at risk, eventually isolating a smaller group of high-risk patients. The order of the individual tests that are used is based on the relative costs of these tests; at each step of testing, the technologic complexity and economic cost of the test increase. How-

ever, as patients at low risk are removed from the process at each step, more expensive testing is limited to fewer patients.

The application of cost analysis to the comparison of clinical strategies with and without nuclear testing is of particular importance. These analyses can distinguish between testing that yields important information while improving cost-effectiveness or cost-utility versus those strategies that add information but result in a strategy that cannot be justified financially.

## CURRENT LITERATURE REGARDING THE COST-EFFECTIVENESS OF NUCLEAR TESTING

### Anatomy-Based Versus Risk-Based Clinical Strategies

The potential differences between bayesian and risk-based approaches to clinical screening strategies are described above. In the latter, noninvasive testing would be indicated in a high likelihood of CAD (or intermediate- to high-risk) cohort if (a) normal scans are still associated with low risk (thus patients could be reclassified as low risk) and (b) a sufficient number of patients would be reclassified as low risk by normal studies, thus not at need for further testing, for the strategy to be cost-effective.

The risk-based approach to this group was confirmed by a report evaluating nuclear testing in 1,944 patients with either high prescan likelihood of CAD or previous myocardial infarction (MI) (35). Those patients with either normal or mildly abnormal SPECT studies were at low risk of cardiac death. In all, 1,189 of these patients, or 61% of the overall cohort, could be reclassified as low risk for cardiac death on the basis of nuclear testing and probably not in need of catheterization unless refractory symptoms occur. In an anatomy-based strategy, however, these patients would have been referred for catheterization and, possibly, revascularization for treatment of their coronary anatomy despite the absence of risk for an adverse outcome. By avoiding referral for catheterization in this population, a significant cost saving could be appreciated.

The economic advantages of an outcomes-based strategy has also been reported. Christian and colleagues (36) demonstrated that myocardial perfusion scintigraphy was cost-ineffective for identifying patients with left main or three-vessel CAD in a population of patients with normal resting ECGs and coronary artery anatomic patterns associated with improved outcomes when treated with coronary artery bypass surgery. However, a similar analysis was performed using a prognostic end point (37). In this analysis of 3,058 patients, the cost of identifying patients at risk of cardiac death or myocardial infarction was $5,179 per event, $3,652 if testing was limited to patients at intermediate to high likelihood of CAD. In comparison (Fig. 14.4), Christian and colleagues report a cost of $20,550 per event for identification of an

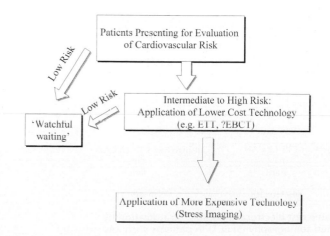

**FIGURE 14.3.** Outline of a hierarchical testing strategy in which technologically complex, higher cost tests are applied following optimal risk stratification with lower cost technology.

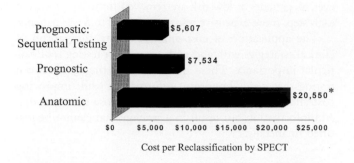

**FIGURE 14.4.** Cost per reclassification of nuclear testing for identification of left main/three vessel CAD (anatomic end point) versus that of intermediate- to high-risk patients tested with nuclear (prognostic end point) or with exercise ECG testing followed by nuclear testing in patients with abnormal exercise ECG tests.

anatomic end point. This comparison demonstrates the greater economic efficiency of a prognostic strategy.

## Cost Implications of Incorporating Stress SPECT in a Testing Strategy

We evaluated the application of stress myocardial perfusion imaging to varying patient subgroups with respect to the ability of the test to risk-stratify patients in a cost-effective manner (29). In this study, those patients with normal resting electrocardiograms, if screened with clinical evaluation alone as a first step, could be risk stratified into low [≤1% per year hard event (HE) rate] and intermediate to high clin-

ical risk groups (based on the pre-ETT likelihood of CAD). Those patients with intermediate to high clinical risk profiles would be candidates for exercise treadmill testing. Those patients within this subgroup with abnormal exercise test responses (intermediate to high post-ETT likelihood of CAD) have an intermediate- to high-risk profile and would be candidates for nuclear testing, while those with a low post-ETT likelihood of CAD would be at low risk and not in need of further testing (hard event rate of 0.93% per year of follow up). We then evaluated the ability of nuclear testing to risk stratify these three patient subgroups—low pre-ETT likelihood of CAD, low post-ETT likelihood of CAD, and those patients with an intermediate to high post-ETT likelihood of CAD. As seen in Fig. 14.5, nuclear testing was able to risk stratify all three patient groups. However, the effectiveness of stratification varied in these groups. In patients with a low pre-ETT likelihood of CAD, 548 patients were tested to identify three patients who had hard events, 231 patients with a low post-ETT likelihood of CAD were tested to identify four patients who had hard events, and 503 patients with an intermediate to high likelihood of CAD were tested to identify 18 who would have hard events. Clearly, the clinical effectiveness of testing increased as the underlying risk of the population increased.

The cost per hard event detected is also shown in Fig. 14.5. As clinical effectiveness increased, cost of testing decreased and the cost-effectiveness increased. Thus, clinical and cost-effectiveness appeared to parallel each other in this patient cohort. A similar pattern was found in those

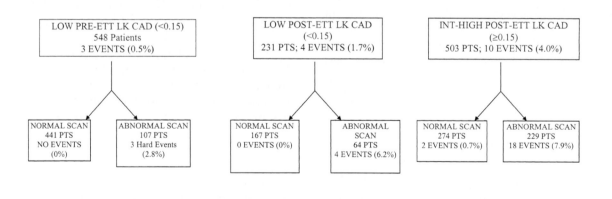

| | Low Pre-ETT Lk CAD | Low Post-ETT Lk CAD | Int-High Post-ETT Lk CAD |
|---|---|---|---|
| Pre-Scan Risk | 0.3% | 1.7% | 4.0% |
| % of all hard events detected by an abnormal scan | 100% | 100% | 90% |
| Cost per HE detected ($/HE) | $253,307 / HE | $93,310 / HE | $59,096 / HE |

**FIGURE 14.5.** Outcomes in patients with interpretable rest electrocardiograms. Stratification by the results of stress single photon emission computed tomography (SPECT) in patients with low pre–exercise treadmill testing (ETT), low post-ETT, and intermediate to high post-ETT likelihood of CAD is shown. The table shows prescan risk (hard event rate before stratification), the percent of all hard events (HE) that occurred that were detected by an abnormal scan, and the cost (per event) of testing. Events, hard events (cardiac death or myocardial infarction); int-high, intermediate to high; lk CAD, likelihood of CAD; pts, patients.

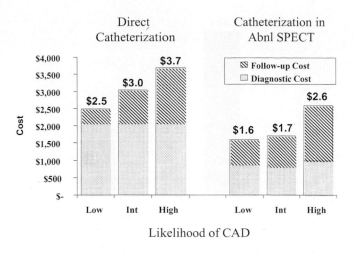

**FIGURE 14.6.** Short-term (diagnostic) and long-term (follow-up) costs of care in patients undergoing initial myocardial perfusion imaging followed by catheterization in patients with abnormal scans versus direct referral for catheterization. Int, intermediate.

patients with abnormal resting ECGs. Further, this study also demonstrated that by adding nuclear testing to a testing algorithm, the overall costs of the testing algorithm decreased. This was achieved by identifying those patients at low risk for adverse outcomes (normal SPECT result) who would not benefit from catheterization despite their clinical risk (likelihood of CAD).

The cost implications of these results were further examined in a multicenter registry of patients presenting with anginal symptoms who were evaluated for the presence of CAD. Comparing 5,826 patients undergoing stress SPECT imaging followed by catheterization in the setting of an abnormal scan to 5,423 patients referred directly for catheterization, Shaw and colleagues (32) found no difference in short- or long-term outcomes in patients for these two clinical approaches after adjusting for clinical risk. A cost-savings of 30% to 41% was found using the strategy of initial SPECT imaging compared to direct referral for catheterization (Fig. 14.6), with variation as a function of clinical risk group examined. These savings were present with respect to both diagnostic costs as well as long-term follow-up costs of care due to a significantly lower rate of normal coronary anatomy at the time of angiography and revascularization rates. Thus, lower overall costs, more efficient use of catheterization, and probable reduction in the rate of unnecessary revascularization were found with the use of SPECT imaging as an initial testing strategy.

## Cost Implications of Shifting the End Point Used

We recently evaluated a population of 5,280 patients who underwent dual-isotope SPECT using either exercise or pharmacologic stress (31). The results of myocardial perfusion SPECT using a dual-isotope approach added incremental value over prescan information for the prediction of both

cardiac death and hard event. The results of this protocol appeared to result in an interesting pattern of risk stratification—increasing rates of both cardiac death and MI occurred with worsening scan results. However, those patients with mildly abnormal scans were found to be at intermediate risk for MI (2.7% per year) although at low risk for cardiac death (0.8% per year), suggesting the possibility that differential risk for MI and cardiac death can be defined by noninvasive testing. Based on these results, patients with mildly abnormal scans would be ideal candidates for medical therapy but would probably not benefit from revascularization unless refractory symptoms were present.

This same study revealed that a clinical strategy limiting referral for catheterization to those patients with moderate and severely abnormal scans, and limiting catheterization in patients with mildly abnormal scans to those with refractory symptoms, would result in a 33.5% cost savings without significant impact on outcomes.

This finding was further evaluated (38). As shown in Fig. 14.7, patients with normal and mildly normal studies had a low risk (<1% per year) of cardiac death, as described above. The mortality rates of patients with moderately to severely abnormal scans are shown as a function of the scan findings, fixed defects without ischemia, mild to moderate amounts of ischemia, and severe ischemia. Patients with fixed defects in the absence of ischemia had the highest mortality rates, while patients with ischemia had similar outcomes irrespective of the amount of ischemia present. This lack of difference in mortality rates as a function of the amount of ischemia present is probably due in part to the rates of referral for revascularization that differ between these groups.

The cost of care per patient is shown by a similar categorization in Fig. 14.8. An interesting pattern of cost of care is seen in this figure. Patients with normal scans had a very low cost of care. Interestingly, patients with mildly abnormal scans had a greater cost of care than patients with moderate

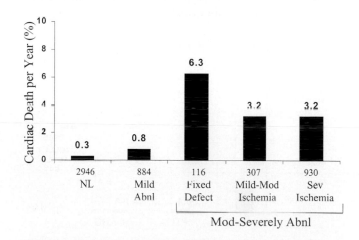

**FIGURE 14.7.** Rates of cardiac death following stress SPECT as a function of normal, mild, and moderate to severely abnormal scan results. The moderate to severely abnormal scan categories are further broken down by the type of defects present—fixed, mild to moderate ischemia, and severe ischemia.

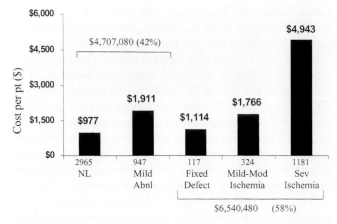

**FIGURE 14.8.** Cost of care per patient (based on Medicare reimbursement) following stress SPECT as a function of normal, mild, and moderate to severely abnormal scan results. The moderate to severely abnormal scan categories are further broken down by the type of defects present—fixed, mild to moderate ischemia, and severe ischemia. As shown, 42% of all costs were derived from patients with normal or mildly abnormal scans, while 58% of costs were due to cost of care in the moderate to severely abnormal scan categories.

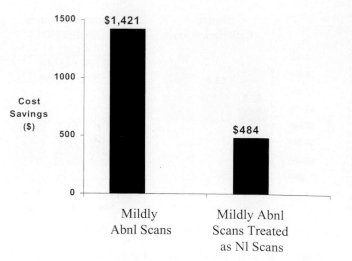

**FIGURE 14.10.** Cost of care per patient (based on Medicare reimbursement) following stress SPECT in patients with mildly abnormal scans *(left)* versus estimated costs in mildly abnormal scans treated as normal scans *(right;* lower rate of referral to interventions).

to severely abnormal scans but no ischemia. Finally, patients with moderate to severely abnormal scans but with mild to moderate or severe amounts of inducible ischemia had the greatest cost of care. Comparing Figs. 14.7 and 14.8, it becomes apparent that the cost of care is driven not by risk, but by physicians' referral patterns that appear to be based on the presence of inducible ischemia. Whether this pattern can be improved upon by focusing on outcomes is the next step.

Focusing first on resource utilization in patients with normal and mildly abnormal scans, we find that despite the low risk of cardiac death in both, the rates of referral for catheterization, percutaneous transluminal coronary angioplasty, and coronary artery bypass surgery were significantly higher in the patients with mildly abnormal scans (Fig. 14.9). Indeed, these rates were higher than in those patients with moderate to severely abnormal scans without ischemia. As

shown in Fig. 14.10, a dramatic cost savings could be attained if patients with mildly abnormal scans would not be referred for catheterization unless refractory symptoms were present. This cost savings would be present in patients with both intermediate and high likelihood of CAD (Fig. 14.11). As shown in Fig. 14.7, the risk in these patients is MI, not cardiac death; thus, aggressive medical management alone would impact their outcomes more than referral for catheterization with an eye to performing revascularization.

As mentioned earlier, those patients with a low likelihood of CAD could probably not be referred for nuclear testing in light of their low risk for adverse outcomes. By

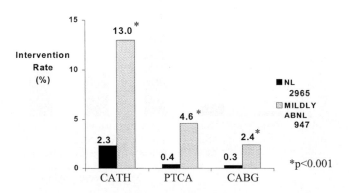

**FIGURE 14.9.** Rates of interventions in patients with normal or mildly abnormal scans. CATH, catheterization; PTCA, percutaneous transluminal coronary angioplasty; CABG, coronary artery bypass surgery.

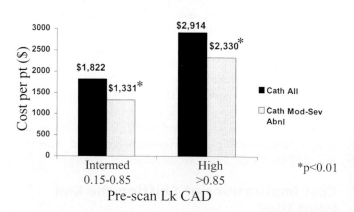

**FIGURE 14.11.** Cost of care per patient (based on Medicare reimbursement) following stress SPECT in patients with intermediate likelihood of CAD *(left)* and high likelihood of CAD *(right),* comparing costs of catheterization in all abnormal studies *(black bars)* versus catheterization only of moderate to severely abnormal scans *(gray bars).*

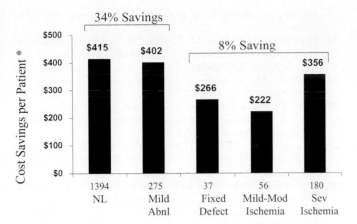

**FIGURE 14.12.** Potential cost savings associated with adoption of a strategy of (1) no referral to SPECT for patients with a low likelihood of CAD, (2) screening of patients with exercise ETT prior to stress SPECT (referral to SPECT only of patients with intermediate to high post-ETT likelihood of CAD), and (3) referral to catheterization only of those patients with moderate to severely abnormal scans.

combining the cost savings described above achieved by not performing catheterization or revascularization in patients with mildly abnormal scans, in addition to not performing nuclear testing and subsequent referrals for catheterization in patients with low likelihood of CAD, the total savings become substantial, as shown in Fig. 14.12. In all, savings of over $400 per patient can be achieved in the cohort with normal and mildly abnormal scans and somewhat lower cost savings in those patients with more abnormal scans. In the former group, about 34% of the costs of care could be avoided with this outcomes-based strategy of care, and 8% cost savings in the latter group.

## EFFECTIVE HEALTH POLICY WITH EVIDENCE-BASED MEDICINE

As health care has become increasing technologically sophisticated, the development of nuclear medicine techniques is a result of the advances that have been accrued in medicine today. Over the past several decades, advances in nuclear medicine have led to the development of higher resolution imaging cameras, new radioisotopes, and computer software developments that have enhanced automation and accuracy of nuclear cardiology techniques. These advances have been achieved with an increase in test cost that exceed the cost of other imaging modalities. Although the increased cost has been accompanied by marked increases in test accuracy, the parallel development of outcomes data is by far the achievement that clearly demarcates the cost-benefit that may be attained with nuclear cardiology. New techniques are needed to justify its regular clinical application.

## How to Live with Cost Containment: A Guide For Clinicians

Having reviewed the basis of economic analyses and a portion of the published data, what can be gleaned by the clinician to apply to daily practice? The limited data we have suggest that cost-effective test use usually is also clinically effective. A number of rules of thumb can be suggested to direct the use of noninvasive testing:

1. Prior to the use of any noninvasive test, the practicing physician should ask whether appropriate patient screening has been performed. Patient clinical risk should be carefully determined; this evaluation should include the results of physical examination, a carefully taken history, a resting ECG, and any other available relevant clinical information.

2. If noninvasive testing is to be performed, a sequential, stepwise approach should be taken. Testing should be applied by use of less expensive tests initially, followed by technologically more advanced (and more expensive) tests in those individuals found to be at intermediate to high risk by the previous step. At each step of testing, those patients found to be at low risk (less than 1% risk of adverse outcomes per year) require no further testing; however, aggressive risk factor modification should not be forgotten in those patients. Thus, at each step of an optimal testing algorithm, the majority of patients will require no further testing, while a minority are sent on to additional tests.

3. At the current time, an exercise ECG should be considered to be the first step in testing for both men and women who have resting ECGs that are not interpretable for an exercise treadmill test. A stress myocardial perfusion scan is probably the next best test if the practitioner has expertise in its use. If not, other stress imaging modalities should be considered.

4. A cardiac catheterization is the final common diagnostic step for all patients. Care should be taken, however, that the referral for catheterization is an appropriate one. As discussed above, not all patients with abnormal scans require this step, and many may have equivalent or superior outcomes with lower cost of care by use of aggressive medical therapy without catheterization.

## REFERENCES

1. American Heart Association. http://www.amhrt.org/.
2. Ginzberg E. *Health services research.* Cambridge, MA: Harvard University Press, 1991.
3. Fuchs U. *The future of health policy.* Cambridge, MA: Harvard University Press, 1993.
4. Brook RH, Kosecoff JB, Park RE, et al. Diagnosis and treatment of coronary disease: comparison of doctors' attitudes in the USA and the UK. *Lancet* 1988;1:750–753.

5. Chassin MR, Kosecoff J, Solomon DH, et al. How coronary angiography is used. Clinical determinants of appropriateness. *JAMA* 1987;258:2543–2547.

6. Mozes B, Shabtai E. The appropriateness of performing coronary angiography in two major teaching hospitals in Israel. *Int J Qual Health Care* 1994;6:245–249.

7. Leape LL, Hilborne LH, Park RE, et al. The appropriateness of use of coronary artery bypass graft surgery in New York State. *JAMA* 1993;269:753–760.

8. Hilborne LH, Leape LL, Bernstein SJ, et al. The appropriateness of use of percutaneous transluminal coronary angioplasty in New York State. *JAMA* 1993;269:761–765.

9. Kahn KL, Kosecoff J, Chassin MR, et al. Measuring the clinical appropriateness of the use of a procedure. Can we do it? *Med Care* 1988;26:415–422.

10. Bernstein SJ, Hilborne LH, Leape LL, et al. The appropriateness of use of coronary angiography in New York State. *JAMA* 1993; 269:766–769.

11. Vibbert S, Reichard, J. *The medical outcomes and guidelines sourcebook.* Washington, DC: Faulkner & Gray, 1992.

12. Hachamovitch R, Berman DS, Morise AP, et al. Statistical, epidemiological and fiscal issues in the evaluation of patients with coronary artery disease. *Q J Nucl Med* 1996;40:35–46.

13. Harrell FE Jr, Lee KL, Califf RM, et al. Regression modelling strategies for improved prognostic prediction. *Stat Med* 1984;3: 143–152.

14. Harrell FE Jr, Lee KL, Matchar DB, et al. Regression models for prognostic prediction: advantages, problems, and suggested solutions. *Cancer Treat Rep* 1985;69:1071–1077.

15. Harrell FE Jr, Lee KL, Mark DB. Multivariable prognostic models: issues in developing models, evaluating assumptions and adequacy, and measuring and reducing errors. *Stat Med* 1996; 15:361–387.

16. Shaw LJ, Eisenstein EL, Hachamovitch R, et al. A primer of biostatistic and economic methods for diagnostic and prognostic modeling in nuclear cardiology: Part II [see comments]. *J Nucl Cardiol* 1997;4:52–60.

17. Shaw LJ, Hachamovitch R, Eisenstein EL, et al. A primer of biostatistic and economic methods for diagnostic and prognostic modeling in nuclear cardiology: Part I. *J Nucl Cardiol* 1996;3: 538–545.

17a. Greenland S. Modeling and variable selection in epidemiologic analysis. *Am J Public Health* 1989;79:340–349.

18. Rose G, Blackburn H. *Cardiovascular survey methods.* Geneva: World Health Organization, 1986.

19. Wenger N, Furberg CD. Cardiovascular Disorders. In: Spilker B, ed. *Quality of life assessments in clinical trials.* New York: Raven Press, 1990:335–345.

20. Spertus JA, Winder JA, Dewhurst TA, et al. Development and evaluation of the Seattle Angina Questionnaire: a new functional status measure for coronary artery disease. *J Am Coll Cardiol* 1995;25:333–341.

21. Spertus JA, Winder JA, Dewhurst TA, et al. Monitoring the quality of life in patients with coronary artery disease. *Am J Cardiol* 1994;74:1240–1244.

22. Nelson CL, Herndon JE, Mark DB, et al. Relation of clinical and angiographic factors to functional capacity as measured by the Duke Activity Status Index. *Am J Cardiol* 1991;68: 973–975.

23. Rector TS, Kubo SH, Cohn JN. Validity of the Minnesota Living with Heart Failure questionnaire as a measure of therapeutic response to enalapril or placebo. *Am J Cardiol* 1993;71: 1106–1107.

24. Hachamovitch R, Shaw LJ, Berman DS. Prognostic assessment in chronic coronary artery disease. In: *American College of Cardiology highlights.* 1997;Summer:4–8.

25. Jacobs P. *The economics of health and medical care,* 4th ed. Gaithersburg, MD: Aspen, 1997.

26. Mark D. Medical economics in cardiovascular medicine. In: Topol E, ed. *Textbook of cardiovascular medicine.* Philadelphia: Lippincott-Raven, 1998:1033–1061.

27. Drummond M, Jefferson TO. Guidelines for authors and peer reviewers of economic submissions to the BMJ. *BMJ* 1996;313: 275–283.

28. Braunwald EMD, Jones RH, Cheitlin MD, et al. *Unstable angina: diagnosis and management.* AHCPR publication number 94-0602. Washington, DC: U.S. Department of Health and Human Services, 1994.

29. Berman DS, Hachamovitch R, Kiat H, et al. Incremental value of prognostic testing in patients with known or suspected ischemic heart disease: a basis for optimal utilization of exercise technetium-99m sestamibi myocardial perfusion single-photon emission computed tomography [published erratum appears in *J Am Coll Cardiol* 1996;27(3):756]. *J Am Coll Cardiol* 1995;26: 639–647.

30. Hachamovitch R, Berman DS, Kiat H, et al. Exercise myocardial perfusion SPECT in patients without known coronary artery disease: incremental prognostic value and use in risk stratification. *Circulation* 1996;93:905–914.

31. Hachamovitch R, Berman DS, Shaw LJ, et al. Incremental prognostic value of myocardial perfusion single photon emission computed tomography for the prediction of cardiac death: differential stratification for risk of cardiac death and myocardial infarction. *Circulation* 1998;97:535–543.

32. Shaw LJ, Hachamovitch R, Berman DS, et al. The economic consequences of available diagnostic and prognostic strategies for the evaluation of stable angina patients: an observational assessment of the value of precatheterization ischemia. Economics of Noninvasive Diagnosis (END) Multicenter Study Group. *J Am Coll Cardiol* 1999;33:661–669.

33. Hachamovitch R, Berman DS, Kiat H, et al. Incremental prognostic value of adenosine stress myocardial perfusion single-photon emission computed tomography and impact on subsequent management in patients with or suspected of having myocardial ischemia. *Am J Cardiol* 1997;80:426–433.

34. Berman DS, Hachamovitch R. Risk assessment in patients with stable coronary artery disease: incremental value of nuclear imaging. *J Nucl Cardiol* 1996;3:S41–49.

35. Hachamovitch R, Kiat H, Amanullah A, et al. Nuclear testing in patients with high pre-scan likelihood of CAD or previous MI: is there benefit from added prognostic value. *J Am Coll Cardiol* 1996;27:100A.

36. Christian TF, Miller TD, Bailey KR, et al. Exercise tomographic thallium-201 imaging in patients with severe coronary artery disease and normal electrocardiograms [see comments]. *Ann Intern Med* 1994;121:825–832.

37. Hachamovitch R, Berman DS, Kiat H, et al. SPECT in patients with normal rest ECG: incremental prognostic value and enhanced risk classification. *J Nucl Med* 1996;37:116.

38. Hachamovitch R, Shaw LJ, Kiat H, et al. Economic implications of a SPECT strategy for the identification of patients at risk of cardiac death. *J Nucl Med* 1996;37:14.

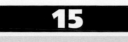

# F-18 FLUORODEOXYGLUCOSE (FDG) SPECT

## FRANS C. VISSER
## JEROEN J. BAX
## MARTIN P. SANDLER

Heart failure is an increasing problem in cardiology, as its increased incidence and prevalence indicate. Despite optimal treatment with, among others, angiotensin-converting enzyme (ACE) inhibitors and beta-blockers, morbidity and mortality remain high. There is increasing awareness that the ventricular function of heart failure patients with left ventricular dysfunction due to coronary artery disease may improve after revascularization if jeopardized but viable tissue is present (1–3).

Currently, numerous Thallium 201 ([201]Tl) redistribution/reinjection and stress/rest Technetium 99m ([99m]Tc)-isonitrile protocols are available and have been validated for the detection of myocardial viability and post-revascularization functional recovery (4–16).

We recently performed a meta-analysis of all the publications in which patients underwent viability studies, were revascularized, and had functional follow-up after revascularization (17). We focused only on the detection of regional improvement of ventricular function because the data on global function (ejection fraction) improvement were too limited. The diagnostic value in terms of sensitivity and specificity of [201]Tl stress-reinjection, [201]Tl rest-redistribution, [99m]Tc-MIBI, and [18]fluorodeoxyglucose ([18]FDG) PET (positron emission tomography) studies was calculated. The pooled analysis (Table 15.1) indicates that of all the different nuclear protocols, the sensitivity to detect improvement of regional ventricular function is high with values ranging from 83% to 90%. In contrast, the specificity to detect absence of functional recovery was low for [201]Tl reinjection (47%) and for [201]Tl rest-redistribution (54%) and highest for FDG PET (73%). This indicates that the best technique to reliably detect viability is FDG imaging. However, PET studies are costly, and the availability of PET centers is too limited to meet the increasing demand of viability studies.

Recent developments in scintigraphic camera technology (18–24) and clinical data from different centers (25–28) have shown that FDG SPECT in combination with cardiac perfusion agents provides an acceptable alternative to PET for the detection of viable tissue.

This chapter discusses the imaging and camera characteristics for FDG SPECT imaging, patient preparation, imaging protocols, and outcome data.

## CAMERAS

### Camera and Collimator Modifications

In recent years, scintillation cameras have been optimized for low-energy imaging below 200 keV. The need for imaging of 511-keV photons made it necessary to apply technology that was developed for low-energy imaging to high-energy imaging applications.

For this purpose, the energy range of the pulse-height analyzer was expanded. Manufacturers have introduced the high-energy mode by reducing the high voltage and recalibrating the pulse-height analyzer. This resulted in some difficulty in imaging at low energies (e.g., 70 keV for [201]Tl) when simultaneous imaging of low and high energies was desired. However, acceptable simultaneous imaging at 140 and 511 keV has been accomplished using this technique (29).

Flood-field uniformity is energy dependent, and low- and medium-energy linearity and sensitivity correction maps are used to produce images of excellent uniformity. Extending the diagnostic range to 511 keV therefore requires linearity and sensitivity correction maps in the high-energy range. This can be done by using the medium-energy maps but is better accomplished by generating new high-energy maps.

F. C. Visser: Department of Cardiology, Free University Hospital, 1081 HV Amsterdam, The Netherlands.

J. J. Bax: Department of Cardiology, University Hospital, Leiden, The Netherlands.

M. P. Sandler: Department of Radiology and Radiological Sciences, Vanderbilt University Medical Center, Nashville, Tennessee.

**TABLE 15.1. DIAGNOSTIC VALUE OF THE DIFFERENT NUCLEAR PROTOCOLS**

| | No. of Patients | Mean LVEF (%) | Range LVEF (%) | Sensitivity (%) | CI Sensitivity (%) | Specificity (%) | CI Specificity (%) | DA % |
|---|---|---|---|---|---|---|---|---|
| FDG PET | 332 | 40 | 32–53 | 88 | 84–91 | 73 | 69–77 | 80 |
| [201]Tl reinjection | 209 | 36 | 31–46 | 86 | 83–89 | 47 | 43–51 | 63 |
| [201]Tl RR | 145 | 35 | 27–39 | 90 | 87–93 | 54 | 49–60 | 74 |
| [99m]Tc MIBI | 207 | 43 | 34–52 | 83 | 78–87 | 69 | 63–74 | 76 |

CI, 95% confidence intervals; DA, diagnostic accuracy; LVEF, left ventricular ejection fraction; [201]Tl RR, [201]Tl rest-redistribution; FDG PET, [18]fluorodeoxyglucose positron emission tomography; MIBI, sestamibi.

Collimator design for high-energy imaging with SPECT is relatively straightforward. For this purpose, septal thickness needs to be increased to absorb the high-energy photons; for adequate sensitivity, the hole diameters must be increased; and to maintain reasonable spatial resolution, the hole length must be increased (29). These modifications typically result in very heavy collimators with low sensitivity and medium resolution as compared to conventional low-energy, high-resolution collimators. Table 15.2 summarizes the range of parameters reported for currently available collimators. It must be noted that the quoted septal penetration values are calculated for a single septum. Septal penetration may actually account for 30% to 50% of detected events in a clinical situation.

Although high-energy collimators weigh in excess of 300 lb (136.4 kg) each, current systems appear to support this additional weight adequately without modifications to the gantries. However, it is important to measure the center of rotation (COR) using the high-energy collimators and routinely to perform COR corrections, if necessary.

Radiation leakage through the detector housing is also of concern, especially in older systems being upgraded to perform 511-keV imaging, and leakage testing should be performed. Manufacturers are now fabricating systems with shielding designed for high-energy imaging.

## Crystal Thickness

Currently available scintillation cameras typically use ³/₈-inch-thick (9.525 mm) NaI(Tl) crystals. However, although these crystals have a photopeak efficiency of approximately 84% at 140 keV, the photopeak efficiency at 511 keV is approximately 13%. Because of the demand for increased efficiencies at 511 keV, manufacturers have increased the crystal options to ¹/₂ (12.7 mm), ⁵/₈ (15.875 mm), and ³/₄ inch (19.05 mm). If high-energy imaging were the only goal, obviously the thicker the crystal the better. However, increasing crystal thickness typically results in degraded intrinsic spatial resolution at lower energies. Recent data indicate that these degradations are not clinically significant because although the intrinsic spatial resolution of 201Tl and [99m]Tc is degraded by 0.5 mm (30), the extrinsic spatial resolution with a low-energy, high-resolution collimator is only degraded by 0.2 mm at 10 cm from the collimator face.

## Dual-Head Cameras

Imaging studies with phantoms and in patients comparing 180- versus 360-degree SPECT image acquisition of the myocardium have shown that superior image resolution is obtained with 180-degree acquisition (23), as is the case for [201]Tl and [99m]Tc imaging protocols. Thus, dual-head cameras with fixed 180-degree geometries have limited advantages over single-head cameras for this application. However, dual-head cameras in a 90-degree geometry (either fixed or variable) provide twice the sensitivity of a single-head camera for 180-degree acquisition. This added sensitivity permits the use of new high-energy collimators with improved spatial resolution (and reduced sensitivity). High-energy collimators are now in use that have the same spatial resolution at 140 keV as the LEHR (low energy, high resolution) colli-

**TABLE 15.2. PARAMETERS OF CURRENTLY AVAILABLE COLLIMATORS**

| Collimator | Weight (lb) | FWHM at 10 cm (mm) | Sensitivity (cpm/μCi) | Septal Penetration (%) | Septal Thickness (mm) | Hole Length (mm) | Hole Diameter (mm) |
|---|---|---|---|---|---|---|---|
| LE | 88 | 7.2 | 160 | 0.2 | 0.2 | 35 | 1.5 |
| HE | 224–475 | 8.2–17.0 | 43–150 | 3.9–7.3 | 1.7–3.4 | 60–104 | 2.5–5.1 |

LE, low-energy; high-resolution collimator; HE, high-energy collimator; FWHM, full width at half maximum.

mators used for low-energy imaging. This added sensitivity also permits the performance of simultaneous, dual-isotope gated SPECT, which makes it possible to evaluate ischemia, metabolism, wall motion, and ejection fraction from a single data acquisition.

## Artifacts

As stated earlier, one of the primary applications of high-energy imaging is the simultaneous acquisition of images of $^{99m}$Tc and $^{18}$F. One concern about the dual-isotope technique is the contribution to the $^{99m}$Tc window from downscatter caused by the presence of $^{18}$F. Phantom measurements performed on a cardiac phantom containing a solution of $^{99m}$Tc and $^{18}$F in a 3.2:1 ratio showed that the downscatter contributed only 5.9% of the total counts in the $^{99m}$Tc window (28). In five patients without coronary artery disease who underwent dual-isotope SPECT, the contribution of $^{18}$F was 3.7% or 6.6% of the total counts in the $^{99m}$Tc window (28). Thus, in patients with normal perfusion and metabolism, the downscatter effect was judged to be insignificant. However, in patients with ischemic heart disease manifested by decreased global perfusion and/or increased metabolism, the possibility exists of errors in the quantification of ischemic regions (29).

It is possible to correct for downscatter of $^{18}$F into the $^{99m}$Tc window as proposed by Yang et al. (31). For this purpose, a third window (scatter window) needs to be added to the dual-isotope protocol, using a 20% window centered on the 170-keV backscatter peak. By assessment of $^{18}$F scatter in the 140-keV $^{99m}$Tc window in combination with the scatter of $^{99m}$Tc in the scatter window, MIBI images can be corrected. However, comparison of the corrected and uncorrected images of 25 patients at the Vanderbilt University Medical Center showed that there was no difference in the diagnostic information content in the corrected versus uncorrected images.

Simultaneous imaging of $^{201}$Tl and $^{18}$F is more complex. The low-energy (70 keV) of $^{201}$Tl and the lower activities commonly used (2–4 mCi) make the downscatter effect more significant, and the energy recalibration used for high-energy imaging often makes it difficult to effectively resolve the $^{201}$Tl photopeak, as previously described.

Attenuation of photons from the inferior wall of the left ventricle by the diaphragm frequently results in an artifact with cardiac SPECT. This is more apparent with low-energy photon emitters such as $^{201}$Tl and $^{99m}$Tc and may result in a misdiagnosis of ischemia. One approach to identifying this problem is to image the patient in the prone position, in addition to the routine supine position, and to compare the two sets of images. Attenuation of the inferior wall may occur in the supine position but will generally be reduced in prone imaging. A second approach is to use an external source to obtain a transmission image that can then be used to perform an attenuation correction of the emission data

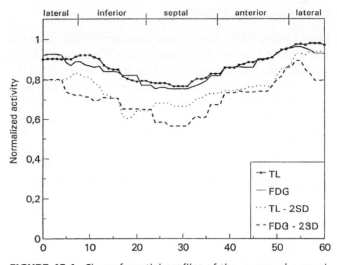

**FIGURE 15.1.** Circumferential profiles of the averaged normalized segmental (*n* = 60) values of the midventricular thallium 201 ($^{201}$Tl) and F-18 fluorodeoxyglucose (FDG) slices. No significant differences in tracer activities were observed. (From reference 32, with permission.)

from $^{99m}$Tc. Several manufacturers are now offering either a fixed or scanning line source (usually gadolinium 153) to perform this correction geometrically. In dual-isotope studies, it is possible to collect simultaneously emission data from the distribution of the two radionuclides and transmission data from the external source, so that additional imaging time is not required.

Attenuation of 511-keV photons in SPECT imaging is not as significant as for low-energy photon imaging. Nevertheless, Bax et al. (32) studied nine male patients with angiography-documented normal coronary arteries and normal left ventricular function. In these patients, a resting $^{201}$Tl and FDG SPECT was performed. Semiquantitative analysis showed that FDG uptake, similar to $^{201}$Tl uptake, was lower in the inferior and septal area (Fig. 15.1). Thus, the data suggest that attenuation of FDG may also occur in SPECT imaging. However, this is also advantageous for patient studies, as the lower limit of normal of the perfusion ($^{201}$Tl) image may be used to assess the presence of relatively increased FDG upake.

## PATIENT PREPARATION

Because the myocardium uses several substrates (33), including free fatty acids (FFAs), glucose, lactate, ketone bodies, or amino acids, adequate FDG imaging can only be performed if glucose is the main substrate of the heart. In general, there are three approaches to optimize FDG uptake in SPECT imaging: (a) oral glucose loading, (b) glucose-insulin-potassium infusion, and (c) lowering fatty acid levels by nicotinic acid derivatives.

## Oral Glucose Loading

Most cardiac FDG studies have been performed following oral glucose loading (34). Usually 50 to 75 g glucose in an aqueous solution is given. One of the major drawbacks is the occurrence of abnormal glucose tolerance and insulin resistance in a significant proportion of patients with ischemic heart disease (35,36), resulting in inadequate FDG images. Moreover, glucose and insulin levels are not stable during oral glucose loading (37). The presence of impaired glucose tolerance and insulin resistance cannot be determined prospectively at the time of the procedure, but patients with a fasting blood glucose of greater than 100 mg/dL have a high likelihood of having diabetes or impaired glucose tolerance (38). Uptake of FDG can further be enhanced by an additional insulin injection, but the need for frequent blood glucose monitoring and supplemental insulin administration results in significant logistic problems.

## Glucose-Insulin-Potassium Infusion

In nondiabetic patients, a threefold increase in myocardial glucose utilization occurs after a 30-minute infusion of a fixed concentration of glucose-insulin-potassium (GIK) solution (39). Knuuti et al. (40) have demonstrated that superior image quality can be obtained when FDG studies are performed during hyperinsulinemic clamping. A fixed high dose of insulin is administered and glucose is infused to maintain normoglycemia. Potassium is co-infused to prevent hypokalemia. The clamping technique is the standard way to calculate regional myocardial glucose uptake in FDG PET imaging but is a time-consuming and laborious procedure because of the frequent glucose sampling and glucose infusion rate adaptations. An interesting alternative was reported by Martin et al. (41). They performed FDG SPECT imaging after preparation with a fixed concentration GIK infusion administered at a standardized rate of 3 mL/kg/hr, corresponding to an insulin infusion of 1.78 mU/kg/min and a glucose infusion of 10 mg/kg/min. Each patient was primed with an intravenous bolus injection of 5 U regular insulin and 50 mL 20% dextrose immediately before initiation of the GIK infusion. Blood glucose was monitored at 15 and 30 minutes. If blood glucose rose above 200 mg/dL, additional intravenous bolus injections of regular insulin were administered (5 to 10 U). Using this GIK protocol, scan quality was consistently good to excellent, with only 1% of images being uninterpretable (41). This compares favorably to the 2% to 33% incidence of uninterpretable images reported in the literature with oral glucose loading. Standardized infusion of a fixed concentration of GIK may be an effective yet simple method of obtaining consistently good-to-excellent quality FDG cardiac scans.

Uninterpretable FDG scans have been reported in 10% to 28% of diabetic patients (42,43). Consequently, diabetic subjects need to be prepared using a formal or modified euglycemic hyperinsulinemic clamp protocol (40,44–46). Using a modified euglycemic hyperinsulinemic clamp, several investigators have reported excellent image quality in small populations of diabetic patients. This technique is adequate for clinical work but remains labor intensive.

## Nicotinic Acid Derivatives

Knuuti et al. (47) have demonstrated that oral administration of a nicotinic acid derivative (Acipimox) may be an alternative to either oral glucose loading or euglycemic clamping. Acipimox inhibits peripheral lipolysis, thus reducing plasma FFA levels, and has a mechanism of action that is similar to that postulated for nicotinic acids but is 20 times more potent; it also has a longer duration of action as compared to nicotinic acids (48). After oral ingestion, peak plasma levels of the drug are reached within 2 hours (49).

Knuuti et al. (47) have performed a direct comparison between hyperinsulinemic euglycemic clamping and Acipimox. The clamping protocol was performed according to well-described standards (40). For the Acipimox protocol, patients were administered 250 mg Acipimox orally 3 hours before FDG injection, followed by a second dose of 250 mg Acipimox 1.5 hours before FDG injection. As expected, insulin levels were high during clamping and low after Acipimox administration. Plasma levels of FFA were comparably low after Acipimox and during clamping. FDG activity in the myocardium and blood was higher after Acipimox as compared to the clamping protocol. The myocardium-to-blood ratio (frequently used as a measure of image quality) was comparable after both approaches. No side effects of Acipimox (besides flushing) were observed. The myocardial FDG uptake patterns were compared visually and showed no significant differences.

Bax et al. (37) compared all three approaches (Acipimox, clamping, and oral loading) in nondiabetic patients. The oral glucose loading and clamping protocols were performed according to established criteria. The Acipimox protocol was slightly modified from that used by Knuuti et al. (47) in that a single dose of 250 mg Acipimox was administered, and patients received a carbohydrate-and-protein-enriched meal to stimulate endogenous insulin release, thereby further promoting myocardial and peripheral FDG uptake. The myocardium-to-blood activity ratios were comparable after Acipimox and during clamping but significantly lower after oral glucose loading (Table 15.3). The FDG clearance rate from blood was significantly lower after oral loading compared to Acipimox and clamping ($T_{1/2}$ oral load = 16.2 minutes, $T_{1/2}$ Acipimox = 10.7 minutes, and $T_{1/2}$ clamp = 8.1 minutes). Visually, the FDG images were superior after clamping and Acipimox, compared to oral glucose loading. Although Bax et al. (37) included only nondiabetic patients, Knuuti et al. (47) included seven patients with diabetes mellitus type II. In these patients, the image quality was also equivalent after Acipimox administration compared to clamping.

**TABLE 15.3. IMAGE QUALITY IN THREE FDG SPECT PROTOCOLS: HYPERINSULINEMIC CLAMPING, NICOTINIC ACID DERIVATIVES (ACIPIMOX) AND ORAL GLUCOSE LOADING**

|  | M/B ratios | H/L ratios |
| --- | --- | --- |
| Hyperinsulinemic clamping | 2.8 ± 0.8 | 5.8 ± 1.7 |
| Acipimox | 2.9 ± 0.7 | 5.5 ± 1.3 |
| Oral glucose loading | 2.2 ± 0.3* | 4.1 ± 1.3** |

*$p < .05$ versus clamping and acipimox; **$p < .001$ versus clamping and acipimox.
H/L ratio, heart to lung ratio; M/B ratio, myocardium to blood pool ratio.

Limited results with cardiac FDG imaging after Acipimox administration are encouraging, but larger studies are needed in patients with and without diabetes mellitus. Still, the available evidence, although limited, shows that good image quality can be obtained using Acipimox (comparable to clamping and superior to oral glucose loading) and may be sufficient for clinical assessment of viability.

## IMAGING PROTOCOLS

### Sequential Protocols

Identification of hibernating myocardium with FDG can be performed using either sequential or dual-isotope imaging protocols.

### Sequential Acquisition

Both Bax et al. (25) and Burt et al. (26) have demonstrated the ability to identify hibernating myocardium using sequential [201]Tl/FDG SPECT imaging. Data generated by Bax et al. (50) using [201]Tl/FDG imaging to identify hibernating myocardium have been shown to be comparable to results obtained with 13N-NH₃/FDG PET.

### Simultaneous Acquisition

Dual-isotope cardiac studies with FDG/[99m]Tc-MIBI SPECT have been performed to evaluate hibernating myocardium and provide PET-comparable images and results. Delbeke et al. (27) used rest dual-isotope SPECT to detect significant coronary artery disease. FDG/[99m]Tc-MIBI SPECT had a sensitivity of 100% and a positive predictive value of 93%. Similarly, Sandler et al. (28) described the use of rest FDG/stress[99m]Tc-MIBI SPECT to evaluate myocardial ischemia and viability (Fig. 15.2). Dual-isotope SPECT had a sensitivity of 100%, a specificity of 88%, a positive predictive value of 93%, a negative predictive value of 100% and an accuracy of 96% (28). The development of 90-degree dual-head acquisition using high-resolution ultrahigh-energy collimators has

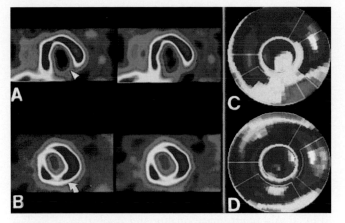

**FIGURE 15.2.** Dual-isotope image of a patient with chronic coronary artery disease and an ejection fraction of 20%. **A:** Two short-axis stress [99m]Tc-MIBI images. **B:** The corresponding rest FDG images. **C:** The perfusion polar map. **D:** The FDG map. After revascularization, the ejection fraction increased to 40%.

permitted cardiac gating with assessment of wall motion and ejection fraction values.

## CLINICAL VALUE OF FDG SPECT

Assessment of myocardial viability with FDG to identify injured but viable myocardium in patients with severe coronary artery disease and ischemic left ventricle (LV) dysfunction, but who are eligible for coronary revascularization, is the most important indication for FDG imaging (51). It has now become clear that impaired LV function is not necessarily an irreversible process, because recovery of LV function after revascularization has been demonstrated, even in severely dyssynergic myocardial regions (52,53). Hibernation and repetitive stunning have been introduced to explain a situation of reversibly impaired LV function (54,55). Hence, in the presence of jeopardized but viable myocardium, improvement of LV function can be expected after revascularization, whereas no improvement will occur when the dysfunction is caused by scar tissue. While patients with a poor LV function are at high risk for perioperative events, any improvement in LV ejection fraction (LVEF) will have a significant impact on their long-term prognosis (56).

It has also become apparent that the assessment of viable myocardium in these patients provides important prognostic information. FDG PET studies have emphasized this issue (57–60). All of these studies were consistent in showing a high cardiac-event rate in patients with ischemic but viable myocardium who did not undergo revascularization. Although FDG PET provides important clinical information in patients with ischemic LV dysfunction, the restricted availability of the technique does not meet the increasing demand (61). The FDG SPECT approach, however, does allow widespread FDG imaging for the assessment of hibernating myocardium.

## FDG PET Versus FDG SPECT

Several studies have consistently shown that there is a good correlation between FDG PET and FDG SPECT in terms of relative uptake of the tracer and the clinical information provided with regard to absence or presence of myocardial viability (23,50,62,63). Figure 15.3 shows the relation between FDG uptake by PET and SPECT. There is a clear linear relation between the two. Figure 15.4 shows an example of a patient undergoing both FDG PET and FDG SPECT. Although image quality and resolution of PET is clearly superior over that of SPECT, the clinical information is the same. Moreover, for prediction of global left ventricular function improvement after revascularization, a large amount of viable tissue needs to be present. Our recent FDG SPECT study has shown that at least 23% of the left ventricle needs to be viable for a significant improvement of the ejection fraction (64). Thus, for cardiac patients, the high resolution of PET may not be a prerequisite.

## Prediction of Functional Recovery by FDG SPECT

In one study, 55 patients with chronic coronary artery disease and LV dysfunction were evaluated with FDG SPECT before revascularization (25). Functional follow-up was obtained 3 months after revascularization. To allow prediction of functional recovery after revascularization on a regional basis, the LV was divided into 13 segments. Resting echocardiography revealed abnormal wall motion before revascularization in 305 segments; 281 of these segments were adequately revascularized. Three months after

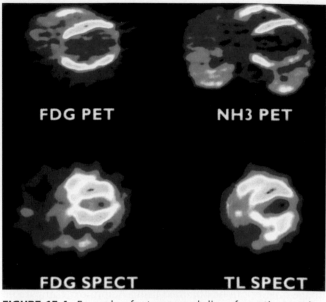

**FIGURE 15.4.** Example of a transversal slice of a patient undergoing $^{201}$Tl/FDG SPECT and NH$_3$/FDG PET. Although the resolution of the SPECT images is clearly inferior to that of the PET images, the presence of viable tissue in the anterolateral region and the presence of nonviable tissue in the apex is clearly shown.

revascularization, 94 segments showed improved function, with 80 segments classified as viable by FDG SPECT. Conversely, 187 segments did not improve in function after the revascularization, with 120 segments classified as nonviable by FDG SPECT. The sensitivity and specificity were thus 85% and 75%, respectively. In a subset of 22 patients with an LVEF <30%, the sensitivity and specificity to predict improvement of regional function were 89% and 72%, respectively. The results are in line with data obtained from a pooled analysis of 332 patients undergoing FDG PET, yielding a sensitivity of 88% and a specificity of 73% (17).

More important than the prediction of regional function improvement is the prediction of global function after revascularization. In the above-mentioned 22 patients with poor left ventricular function, the ejection fraction was also determined before and after revascularization. In 14 patients with three or more viable segments, the ejection fraction improved significantly from 25% ± 6% to 32% ± 6% (*p* <.01). Alternatively, in the patients (*n* = 8) with less than three viable segments, the ejection fraction remained unchanged (24% ± 6% versus 25% ± 6%; nonsignificant). Although the available data were obtained in a small number of patients, FDG SPECT accurately predicts functional recovery after revascularization.

## Comparison of FDG SPECT with Other Imaging Techniques

The most frequently used techniques to assess viable myocardium, besides FDG imaging, are $^{201}$Tl stress-redis-

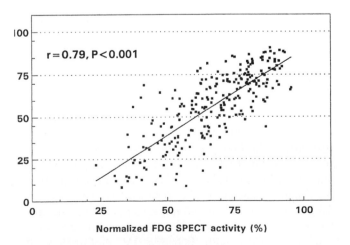

**FIGURE 15.3.** Scatter plot showing the relation between normalized FDG SPECT and FDG PET activity. (From ___, with permission.)

tribution-reinjection scintigraphy, [201]Tl rest-redistribution imaging, rest MIBI imaging, and low-dose dobutamine echocardiography. [201]Tl-stress-redistribution-reinjection imaging (4–7) allows detection of both viability and ischemia, while [201]Tl rest-redistribution (8–11) and rest MIBI (12–16) only permit viability assessment.

Thus far, limited data are available on the comparison between FDG SPECT and the other imaging modalities. One study compared FDG SPECT with [201]Tl reinjection imaging (65). Seventeen patients were studied with both techniques before revascularization. Regional wall motion was assessed by echocardiography before and 3 months after revascularization. The agreement for the detection of viable and nonviable segments between the techniques was modest, being 70%. Both FDG and [201]Tl SPECT reinjection had a high sensitivity in predicting improvement of regional function (89% for FDG and 93% for [201]Tl; Fig. 15.5). The specificity of FDG SPECT, however, was significantly higher than for [201]Tl reinjection (77% versus 43%, *p* <.05). No data are available on the comparison for predicting global function improvement.

Thus far, only preliminary data are available on the comparison between [201]Tl rest-redistribution and FDG SPECT (66). In 24 patients, both techniques were tested against revascularization. Resting echocardiography was used to evaluate regional contractile function before and after revascularization. The sensitivity of FDG SPECT and [201]Tl rest-redistribution were comparable: 89% versus 78%. The specificity of FDG SPECT was higher: 81% versus 59% (Fig. 15.5). Again, no data are available on the comparison for predicting global function improvement after revascularization. Hence, these comparative studies show that FDG SPECT and [201]Tl imaging are equally sensitive in predicting functional recovery after revascularization, but the [201]Tl protocols have a lower specificity and therefore tend to overestimate functional recovery. The low specificity of the [201]Tl protocols are in line with the available literature data. Pooled analysis of published [201]Tl studies in patients undergoing revascularization has detected the same trend (67).

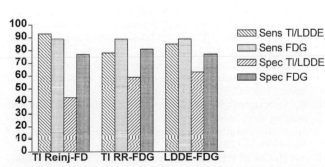

**FIGURE 15.5.** Comparison of the sensitivity and specificity of FDG SPECT with those of [201]Tl stress-reinjection (Tl Reinj), [201]Tl rest-redistribution (Tl RR), and low-dose dobutamine echocardiography (LDDE). Sens, sensitivity; spec, specificity.

Echocardiography during the infusion of low-dose dobutamine is frequently used to identify injured but viable myocardium. Viable myocardium is characterized by the presence of a contractile reserve, i.e., improvement of wall motion in a segment with resting dysfunction (68). Various studies have demonstrated the use of this technique to predict functional recovery after revascularization (67). We studied 17 patients with chronic coronary artery disease and LV dysfunction who underwent coronary revascularization. In these patients, low-dose dobutamine echocardiography was compared with FDG SPECT to detect functional improvement after revascularization. The agreement for the identification of viable and nonviable segments between the techniques was 80%. The sensitivity of dobutamine echocardiography and FDG SPECT to detect improvement of regional function were 85% and 89%, respectively. The specificity of dobutamine echocardiography (to detect absence of recovery of function) was 63%, and for FDG SPECT 77% (Fig. 15.5). No data are available on the comparison between FDG SPECT and MIBI SPECT.

## Improvement of Heart Failure Symptoms After Revascularization

Important from a patient point of view are the findings of Marwick et al. (2) and DiCarli et al. (3) that revascularization of viable tissue, as assessed with FDG PET, was associated with an improvement of exercise capacity and quality of life. Thus, viability assessment has proved to be clinically successful in predicting symptom outcome after revascularization. We have recently performed a study in which 32 revascularization patients with depressed left ventricular function underwent FDG/[201]Tl SPECT and heart failure classification according to the New York Heart Association (NYHA) (64). In 18 patients with three or more viable segments on SPECT, 13 improved their NYHA status by more than 1 grade. In contrast, 11 of the 14 patients with less than three viable segments did not show improvement of heart failure symptoms. Those patients with extensive viable tissue also showed significant improvement of the ejection fraction (28% ± 8% prerevascularization versus 34% ± 9% postrevascularization), in contrast to the patients without extensive viability in whom the ejection fraction remained unaltered at 31% ± 8%. Thus, FDG SPECT is also able to predict improvement of heart failure symptoms.

## Assessment of Prognosis by FDG SPECT

FDG PET studies have shown that FDG imaging may also provide prognostic information on morbidity and mortality. Studies have shown that the presence of a mismatch pattern in patients is associated with a higher morbidity and mortality (57,69,70). Tamaki et al. (69) showed in stable patients with a previous myocardial infarction that the mismatch pattern was the best predictor of future cardiac events, among all clinical, angiographic, and [201]Tl stress-redistribution variables. More importantly, the studies by Eitzman et al. (70) and DiCarli et al. (57) showed that patients with viable tissue who do not undergo revascularization are at risk for the development of cardiac events. In their combined studies, a total of 175 patients with severely depressed ventricular function underwent viability assessment by FDG PET; patients were followed for an average of 13 months. Eighty-three patients were revascularized, and 92 patients were treated medically. The patients were subsequently divided into four groups, depending on the therapy and on the presence or absence of a mismatch pattern. The highest mortality was observed in the group of patients with a mismatch pattern who were treated medically (37% versus 3%, 8%, and 9% in the other groups).

We have recently studied 135 patients with depressed LV function who underwent FDG SPECT imaging. Patients were followed for a mean of 28 months for the hard end points—death and (recurrent) myocardial infarction. Similar to the FDG PET studies, patients were divided into four groups: with and without viability and with and without revascularization. In total, 28 events occurred. Patients with viable tissue who were not revascularized had the highest event rate: 18/30 = 60%. Revascularized patients with viable tissue had a low event rate of 4% (1/26). Similar event rates were observed in patients without viable tissue with and without revascularization, 16% (5/32) and 9% (4/47), respectively.

The results of this study, similar to the FDG PET studies, suggest that viability provides powerful information not only in the prediction of improvement of contractile function, but also in the association with an adverse prognosis. It should be stated, however, that all these studies were based on retrospective analyses of data obtained in patients with poor ventricular function who were often referred for viability imaging.

## CONCLUSION

The introduction of a dual-head scintillation camera equipped with ultrahigh-energy collimators, capable of 511-keV imaging, has permitted FDG SPECT to provide information equivalent to PET for the identification of viable myocardium in patients with chronic ischemic heart disease. The diagnostic value in predicting functional recovery after revascularization and prognosis with FDG SPECT is comparable to the accuracy of FDG PET. The diagnostic accuracy of FDG SPECT is at least equivalent and may be superior to other clinically available viability techniques. Although FDG SPECT has not been studied to the same extent as the other techniques, its potential is such that it may clinically become the modality of choice for evaluating viable myocardium.

## REFERENCES

1. Rahimtoola SH. The hibernating myocardium. *Am Heart J* 1989;117:211–221.
2. Marwick TH, Nemec JJ, Lafont A, et al. Prediction by postexercise fluoro-18 deoxyglucose positron emission tomography of improvement in exercise capacity after revascularization. *Am J Cardiol* 1992;69:854–859.
3. DiCarli MF, Asgarzadie F, Schelbert HR, et al. Quantitative relation between myocardial viability and improvement in heart failure symptoms after revascularization in patients with ischemic cardiomyopathy. *Circulation* 1995;92:3436–3444.
4. Tamaki N, Ohtani H, Yamashita K, et al. Metabolic activity in the areas of new fill-in after thallium-201 reinjection: comparison with positron emission tomography using fluorine-18-deoxyglucose. *J Nucl Med* 1991;32:673–678.
5. Dilsizian V, Rocco TP, Freedman NM, et al. Enhanced detection of ischemic but viable myocardium by the reinjection of thallium after stress-redistribution imaging. *N Engl J Med* 1990;323:141–146.
6. Ohtani H, Tamaki N, Yonekura Y, et al. Value of thallium-201 reinjection after delayed SPECT imaging for predicting reversible ischemia after coronary artery bypass grafting. *Am J Cardiol* 1990;66:394–399.
7. Arnese M, Cornel JH, Salustri A, et al. Prediction of improvement of regional left ventricular function after surgical revascularization. A comparison of low-dose dobutamine echocardiography with [201]Tl single-photon emission computed tomography. *Circulation* 1995;91:2748–2752.
8. Mori T, Minamiji K, Kurogane H, et al. Rest-injected thallium-201 imaging for assessing viability of severe asynergic regions. *J Nucl Med* 1991;32:1718–1724.
9. Ragosta M, Beller GA, Watson DD, et al. Quantitative planar rest-redistribution [201]Tl imaging in detection of myocardial viability and prediction of improvement in left ventricular function after coronary bypass surgery in patients with severely depressed left ventricular function. *Circulation* 1993;87:1630–1641.
10. Alfieri O, La Canna G, Giubbini R, et al. Recovery of myocardial function. The ultimate target of coronary revascularization. *Eur J Cardiothorac Surg* 1993;7:325–330.
11. Charney R, Schwinger ME, Chun J, et al. Dobutamine echocardiography and resting-redistribution thallium-201 scintigraphy predicts recovery of hibernating myocardium after coronary revascularization. *Am Heart J* 1994;128:864–869.
12. Marzullo P, Parodi O, Reisenhofer B, et al. Value of rest thallium-201/technetium-99m sestamibi scans and dobutamine echocardiography for detecting myocardial viability. *Am J Cardiol* 1993;71:166–172.
13. Marzullo P, Sambuceti G, Parodi O. The role of sestamibi scintigraphy in the radioisotopic assessment of myocardial viability. *J Nucl Med* 1992;33:1925–1930.
14. Udelson JE, Coleman PS, Metherall J, et al. Predicting recovery of severe regional ventricular dysfunction. Comparison of resting scintigraphy with [201]Tl and [99m]Tc-sestamibi. *Circulation* 1994;89:2552–2561.
15. Maublant JC, Citron B, Lipiecki J, et al. Rest technetium 99m-sestamibi tomoscintigraphy in hibernating myocardium. *Am Heart J* 1995;129:306–314.
16. Bisi G, Sciagra R, Santoro GM, et al. Technetium-99m-sestamibi imaging with nitrate infusion to detect viable hibernating myocardium and predict postrevascularization recovery. *J Nucl Med* 1995;36:1994–2000.
17. Bax JJ, Cornel JH, Visser FC, et al. Accuracy of currently available techniques to predict functional recovery after revascularization in patients with chronic left ventricular dysfunction: a meta-analysis. *Circulation* 1996;94:I-233(abst).
18. Hoflin F, Ledermann H, Noelpp U, et al. Routine [18]F-2-deoxy-

2-fluoro-D-glucose ([18]F-FDG) myocardial tomography using a normal large field of view gamma-camera. *Angiology* 1989;40:1058–1064.

19. Williams KA, Taillon LA, Stark VJ. Quantitative planar imaging of glucose metabolic activity in myocardial segments with exercise thallium-201 perfusion defects in patients with myocardial infarction: comparison with late (24-hour) redistribution thallium imaging for detection of reversible ischemia. *Am Heart J* 1992;124:294–304.

20. van Lingen A, Huijgens PC, Visser FC, et al. Performance characteristics of a 511-keV collimator for imaging positron emitters with a standard gamma-camera. Eur J Nucl Med 1992;19:315–321.

21. Stoll HP, Hellwig N, Alexander C, et al. Myocardial metabolic imaging by means of fluorine-18 deoxyglucose/technetium-99m sestamibi dual-isotope single-photon emission tomography. Eur J Nucl Med 1994;21:1085–1093.

22. Kalff V, Berlangieri SU, Van EB, et al. Is planar thallium-201/fluorine-18 fluorodeoxyglucose imaging a reasonable clinical alternative to positron emission tomographic myocardial viability scanning? Eur J Nucl Med 1995;22:625–632.

23. Martin WH, Delbeke D, Patton JA, et al. FDG-SPECT: correlation with FDG-PET. *J Nucl Med* 1995;36:988–995.

24. Huitink JM, Visser FC, van Lingen A, et al. Feasibility of planar fluorine-18-FDG imaging after recent myocardial infarction to assess myocardial viability. J Nucl Med 1995;36:975–981.

25. Bax JJ, Cornel JH, Visser FC, et al. Prediction of improvement of contractile function in patients with ischemic ventricular dysfunction after revascularization by fluorine-18 fluorodeoxyglucose single-photon emission computed tomography. *J Am Coll Cardiol* 1997;30:377–383.

26. Burt RW, Perkins OW, Oppenheim BE, et al. Direct comparison of fluorine-18-FDG SPECT, fluorine-18-FDG PET and rest thallium-201 SPECT for detection of myocardial viability. *J Nucl Med* 1995;36:176–179.

27. Delbeke D, Videlefsky S, Patton JA, et al. Rest myocardial perfusion/metabolism imaging using simultaneous dual-isotope acquisition SPECT with technetium-99m-MIBI/fluorine-18-FDG. *J Nucl Med* 1995;36:2110–2119.

28. Sandler MP, Videlefsky S, Delbeke D, et al. Evaluation of myocardial ischemia using a rest metabolism/stress perfusion protocol with fluorine-18 deoxyglucose/technetium-99m MIBI and dual-isotope simultaneous-acquisition single-photon emission computed tomography. *J Am Coll Cardiol* 1995;26:870–878.

29. Patton JA, Sandler MP, Ohana I, et al. High-energy (511-keV) imaging with the scintillation camera. *Radiographics* 1996;16: 1183–1194.

30. Sandler MP, Bax JJ, Patton JA, et al. Fluorine-18-fluorodeoxyglucose cardiac imaging using a modified scintillation camera. *J Nucl Med* 1998;39:2035–2043.

31. Yang DC, Ragasa E, Gould L, et al. Radionuclide simultaneous dual-isotope stress myocardial perfusion study using the "three window technique." *Clin Nucl Med* 1993;18:852–857.

32. Bax JJ, Visser FC, van LA, et al. Relation between myocardial uptake of thallium-201 chloride and fluorine-18 fluorodeoxyglucose imaged with single-photon emission tomography in normal individuals. Eur J Nucl Med 1995;22:56–60.

33. Camici P, Ferrannini E, Opie LH. Myocardial metabolism in ischemic heart disease: basic principles and application to imaging by positron emission tomography. *Prog Cardiovasc Dis* 1989; 32:217–238.

34. Gropler RJ. Methodology governing the assessment of myocardial glucose metabolism by positron emission tomography and fluorine 18-labeled fluorodeoxyglucose. *J Nucl Cardiol* 1994;1:S4–14.

35. Nuutila P, Koivisto VA, Knuuti J, et al. Glucose-free fatty acid cycle operates in human heart and skeletal muscle in vivo. *J Clin Invest* 1992;89:1767–1774.

36. Black HR. The coronary artery disease paradox: the role of hyperinsulinemia and insulin resistance and implications for therapy. *J Cardiovasc Pharmacol* 1990;15(suppl 5):S26–38.

37. Bax JJ, Veening MA, Visser FC, et al. Optimal metabolic conditions during fluorine-18 fluorodeoxyglucose imaging; a comparative study using different protocols. *Eur J Nucl Med* 1997;24:35–41.

38. Bennet PH. Definition, diagnosis and classification of diabetes mellitus and impaired glucose tolerance. In: Kahn CR, Weir GC, eds. *Joslin's diabetes mellitus.* Malvern, PA: Lea and Febiger, 1994: 193–200.

39. Rogers WJ, Russell ROJ, McDaniel HG, et al. Acute effects of glucose-insulin-potassium infusion on myocardial substrates, coronary blood flow and oxygen consumption in man. *Am J Cardiol* 1977;40:421–428.

40. Knuuti MJ, Nuutila P, Ruotsalainen U, et al. Euglycemic hyperinsulinemic clamp and oral glucose load in stimulating myocardial glucose utilization during positron emission tomography. *J Nucl Med* 1992;33:1255–1262.

41. Martin WH, Jones RC, Delbeke D, et al. A simplified intravenous glucose loading protocol for fluorine 18 fluorodeoxyglucose cardiac single-photon emission tomography. Eur J Nucl Med 1997;24:1291–1297.

42. vom Dahl J, Hicks R, Lee FK, et al. Positron emission tomography viability studies in patients with diabetes mellitus. *J Am Coll Cardiol* 1991;121A(abst).

43. Prellwitz J, Vasta M, Sunderland J, et al. Investigation of factors influencing FDG myocardial image quality. J Nucl Med 1991; 32:1039(abst).

44. Bax JJ, Visser FC, van Lingen A. Feasibility of myocardial F-18-fluorodeoxyglucose single photon emission computed tomography in patients with non-insulin dependent diabetes mellitus. *Nucl Med Commun* 1997;18:200–206.

45. Ohtake T, Yokoyama I, Watanabe T, et al. Myocardial glucose metabolism in noninsulin-dependent diabetes mellitus patients evaluated by FDG-PET. *J Nucl Med* 1995;36:456–463.

46. Schelbert HR. Euglycemic hyperinsulinemic clamp and oral glucose load in stimulating myocardial glucose utilization during positron emission tomography. J Nucl Med 1992;33:1263–1266.

47. Knuuti MJ, Yki-Jarvinen H, Voipio-Pulkki LM, et al. Enhancement of myocardial [fluorine-18]fluorodeoxyglucose uptake by a nicotinic acid derivative. *J Nucl Med* 1994;35:989–998.

48. Fuccella LM, Goldaniga G, Lovisolo P, et al. Inhibition of lipolysis by nicotinic acid and by Acipimox. *Clin Pharmacol Ther* 1980;28:790–795.

49. Musatti L, Maggi E, Moro E, et al. Bioavailability and pharmacokinetics in man of Acipimox, a new antilipolytic and hypolipemic agent. *J Int Med Res* 1981;9:381–386.

50. Bax JJ, Visser FC, Blanksma PK, et al. Comparison of myocardial uptake of fluorine-18-fluorodeoxyglucose imaged with PET and SPECT in dyssynergic myocardium. *J Nucl Med* 1996;37: 1631–1636.

51. Ritchie J, Bateman TM, Bonow RO, et al. Guidelines for clinical use of cardiac radionuclide imaging. A report of the American Heart Association/American College of Cardiology Task Force on Assessment of Diagnostic and Therapeutic Cardiovascular Procedures, Committee on Radionuclide Imaging, developed in collaboration with the American Society of Nuclear Cardiology. *Circulation* 1995;91:1278–1303.

52. Haas F, Haehnel CJ, Picker W, et al. Preoperative positron emission tomographic viability assessment and perioperative and postoperative risk in patients with advanced ischemic heart disease. *J Am Coll Cardiol* 1997;30:1693–1700.

53. Elefteriades JA, Tolis GJ, Levi E, et al. Coronary artery bypass grafting in severe left ventricular dysfunction: excellent survival with improved ejection fraction and functional state. *J Am Coll Cardiol* 1993;22:1411–1417.

54. Ross JJ. Myocardial perfusion-contraction matching. Implications for coronary heart disease and hibernation. *Circulation* 1991;83:1076–1083.

55. Vanoverschelde JL, Wijns W, Depre C, et al. Mechanisms of chronic regional postischemic dysfunction in humans. New insights from the study of noninfarcted collateral-dependent myocardium. *Circulation* 1993;87:1513–1523.

56. Mock MB, Ringqvist I, Fisher LD, et al. Survival of medically treated patients in the coronary artery surgery study (CASS) registry. *Circulation* 1982;66:562–568.

57. DiCarli M, Davidson M, Little R, et al. Value of metabolic imaging with positron emission tomography for evaluating prognosis in patients with coronary artery disease and left ventricular dysfunction. *Am J Cardiol* 1994;73:527–533.

58. Yaoita H, Fischman AJ, Strauss HW, et al. Uridine: a marker of myocardial viability after coronary occlusion and reperfusion. *Int J Card Imaging* 1993;9:273–280.

59. Marwick TH, MacIntyre WJ, Lafont A, et al. Metabolic responses of hibernating and infarcted myocardium to revascularization. A follow-up study of regional perfusion, function, and metabolism. *Circulation* 1992;85:1347–1353.

60. vom Dahl J, Altehoefer C, Sheehan FH, et al. Effect of myocardial viability assessed by technetium-99m-sestamibi SPECT and fluorine-18-FDG PET on clinical outcome in coronary artery disease. *J Nucl Med* 1997;38:742–748.

61. Camici PG, Wijns W, Borgers M, et al. Pathophysiological mechanisms of chronic reversible left ventricular dysfunction due to coronary artery disease (hibernating myocardium). *Circulation* 1997;96:3205–3214.

62. Sodi-Pallares D, Disten A, Ponce DL, et al. Polarizing solution in myocardial infarction. *Am J Cardiol* 1968;21:275–276.

63. Srinivasan G, Kitsiou AN, Bacharach SL, et al. [18F]fluorodeoxyglucose single photon emission computed tomography: can it replace PET and thallium SPECT for the assessment of myocardial viability? *Circulation* 1998;97:843–850.

64. Bax JJ, Visser FC, Fioretti PM, et al. Viability on FDG SPECT predicts improvement of LVEF and heart failure symptoms. *Eur Heart J* 1998;19:99(abst).

65. Bax JJ, Cornel JH, Visser FC, et al. Prediction of recovery of myocardial dysfunction after revascularization: comparison of fluorine-18 fluorodeoxyglucose/thallium-201 SPECT, thallium-201 stress-reinjection SPECT and dobutamine echocardiography. *J Am Coll Cardiol* 1996;28:558–565.

66. Bax JJ, Cornel JH, Visser FC, et al. Thallium-201 rest-redistribution SPECT versus FDG SPECT to predict functional outcome after revascularization. *J Nucl Med* 1996;37:59P(abst).

67. Bax JJ, Wijns W, Cornel JH, et al. Accuracy of currently available techniques for prediction of functional recovery after revascularization in patients with left ventricular dysfunction due to chronic coronary artery disease: comparison of pooled data. *J Am Coll Cardiol* 1997;30:1451–1460.

68. Cornel JH, Bax JJ, Fioretti PM. Assessment of myocardial viability by dobutamine stress echocardiography. *Curr Opin Cardiol* 1996;11:621–626.

69. Tamaki N, Kawamoto M, Takahashi N, et al. Prognostic value of an increase in fluorine-18 deoxyglucose uptake in patients with myocardial infarction: comparison with stress thallium imaging. *J Am Coll Cardiol* 1993;22:1621–1627.

70. Eitzman D, al-Aouar Z, Kanter HL, et al. Clinical outcome of patients with advanced coronary artery disease after viability studies with positron emission tomography. *J Am Coll Cardiol* 1992;20:559–565.

# GATED BLOOD-POOL SPECT

**EDWARD P. FICARO**
**JAMES R. CORBETT**

Today gated single photon emission computed tomography (SPECT) has become commonplace, especially in conjunction with imaging of technetium 99m ($^{99m}$Tc)-labeled perfusion tracers. Although generally reliable, abnormal hearts with large regions of severely impaired perfusion may not be reliably assessed using commercially available software. State-of-the-art tomographs are capable of acquiring high-quality gated SPECT studies in as little as 5 to 15 minutes. Unaffected by regional perfusion defects, gated blood-pool (GBP) tomography is ideally suited for the assessment of the abnormal heart. GBP tomography is the logical three-dimensional (3D) extension of planar blood pool imaging. For the first several years after Moore et al.'s (1) initial description of blood pool tomography in 1980, when SPECT imaging systems first became commercially available, there was no software designed specifically for the purpose of acquiring, processing, displaying, or analyzing gated SPECT studies. Reports varied widely in their approach to these tasks (2,3). Not until 1988 was there commercially available software for the acquisition and processing of gated SPECT studies (4,5). Additional options for quantification software are gradually becoming available, and there has been increasing interest in this powerful imaging modality. The theoretical advantages of GBP tomography include the ability to assess wall motion without superimposition of chambers and the potential for assessing chamber volumes without the complicating effects of attenuation (Fig. 16.1) (2,6–8). Like its planar analog, the tomographic technique has been used to assess ventricular ejection fractions and volumes, regurgitant fractions, and regional wall motion including the use of phase analysis for the identification of atrioventricular (AV) nodal bypass tracks (2,8 10). Widespread clinical utilization has been hampered by the limited availability of quantitative software. Affordable workstations can now easily process, quantify, archive, and display these studies in as little as 1 to 2 minutes.

The indiscriminate use of imaging modalities in low-risk asymptomatic populations is not cost-effective or accurate. The preoperative ischemic risk assessment of vascular surgery patients with perfusion imaging and the preoperative cardiomyopathy assessment of liver transplant patients with GBP imaging has clearly demonstrated the futility of the indiscriminate approach (11,12). These same techniques provide invaluable information when applied to properly selected patient populations, i.e., the preoperative assessment myocardial perfusion in high-risk vascular surgery patients and the preoperative and early postopera-

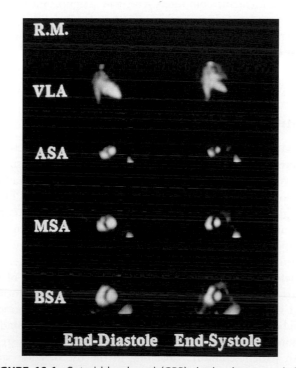

**FIGURE 16.1.** Gated blood-pool (GBP) single photon emission computed tomography (SPECT) tomograms from a normal patient. Shown are vertical long axis (VLA), apical short axis (ASA), midventricular short axis (MSA), and basal short axis (BSA) sections at end-diastole and end-systole. The spleen is seen below and to the right of the left ventricle on the short-axis sections.

E. P. Ficaro and J. R. Corbett: Department of Internal Medicine, Divisions of Nuclear Medicine and Cardiology, University of Michigan Medical Center, Ann Arbor, Michigan 48109.

tive evaluation of biventricular function in cardiac transplant patients (11,13). As Rocco and Pfeffer (14) have pointed out, the current challenge to the nuclear imaging laboratory with respect to the patient with recent myocardial infarction (MI) is the reliable assessment of ventricular function (size, shape, ejection fraction), the presence of residual ischemia, and the presence and extent of viable asynergic myocardium. GBP SPECT has the potential for providing this information, and doing so in a cost- and time-efficient manner.

This chapter reviews (a) practical details regarding the acquisition, processing, display, and analyses of these studies; (b) the validation and early clinical utilization of GBP SPECT; (c) newer methods for the quantitation and display of these studies; and (d) the clinical applications of this imaging modality today.

## METHODS

Early studies with GBP tomography were acquired using single-detector tomographs requiring 30 to 45 minutes for image acquisition alone. Procedures of this duration are a significant impediment to efficient laboratory operations and test the endurance of patients and technical staff. Multidetector SPECT tomographs and high-performance nuclear medicine computers have had a significant impact on image acquisition and processing of gated SPECT in general (15,16). This section discusses methods relating to GBP tomography including patient setup, image acquisition, image processing and reconstruction, and image display and analysis.

## Patient Setup

Minimization of extracardiac motion and artifact-free electrocardiogram (ECG) gating are required for accurate assessments of cardiac function using GBP tomography. Although seemingly the most mundane aspects of SPECT imaging, these are also the most fundamental. Patient comfort and positioning must be assured for successful imaging. Support for head, arms, and low back minimize muscle strain and extend table time. The uncomfortable patient is generally the patient who moves. Patient discomfort often leads to pain and muscle spasm, resulting in patient motion and ECG artifacts. If it is judged that respiratory motion will be a significant problem in a particular patient, a binder around the abdomen should be carefully applied, consistent with patient comfort. Coaching in the use of chest wall breathing rather than diaphragmatic breathing should be provided.

Acquisition times should be minimized by assuring gate integrity and careful attention to acceptance window selection. ECG artifacts are often recognized as premature beats. Some laboratories accept all beats including premature beats

and artifacts and in so doing corrupt the functional information for which the study was intended, generally introducing a bias toward underestimating ventricular function. If bad beats are rejected, one of two consequences occurs: (a) if camera dwell time is not extended for the time of the premature beats or ECG artifacts, count-poor unequally sampled projections are acquired, resulting in image distortion or (b) dwell time and total acquisition time are extended unnecessarily as the acquisition software attempts to acquire each projection for the equal times. Extended dwell time is generally acceptable for a moderate number of premature beats, but is not for ECG artifacts resulting from careless technical effort. The ECG input is critical in gated studies. To ensure an artifact-free signal, the skin should be clean and prepared with alcohol, acetone, or liquid pumice. Electrodes should be positioned on relatively flat surfaces of the body, so that they are unaffected by respiration, head or extremity motion, or camera detector contact. A monophasic R-wave is the input of choice for most gating devices. This can generally be easily approximated with a brief review of the standard 12-lead ECG as a guide for electrode placement from the orientation of the principal QRS vector.

## Acquisition

### Acquisition Protocols

Gated SPECT acquisition software has become readily available (4,16). Essentially, all the features of planar gated acquisition software are now available in tomographic software, including single- or double-buffered bad-beat rejection. It is possible to choose among the storage of only sinus beats, premature beats, postpremature beats, and the separate storage of all three during the same acquisition. Forward and backward gating of the SPECT data necessary for the quantification of diastolic function is now becoming available. With the hardware and software improvements discussed above, the user is faced with a wide and potentially confusing array of variables from which to select. Recommendations for image acquisition protocols are summarized in Table 16.1.

Because of the ever-increasing pressure to maximize efficiency and equipment utilization, most gated SPECT studies today are acquired for only eight frames per cardiac cycle. If qualitative assessments of wall motion are all that is desired or if acquisition time must be kept to a minimum because of patient intolerance, eight frames per cycle will have to suffice. However, at eight frames, ejection fraction measurements will be underestimated by five to ten units (17). Accurate assessments of ventricular function generally requires the acquisition of 16 frames per cardiac cycle (18,19). With modern imaging systems, high-quality 16-frame GBP tomograms can be acquired in 8 to 15 minutes, which is less time than is required for a multiprojection planar study. There are clinical situations where an ejection

## TABLE 16.1. ACQUISITION AND PROCESSING PROTOCOLS

| Protocols | Single or Multidetector |
|---|---|
| **Acquisition protocols** | |
| Dose | 30 mCi $^{99m}$Tc RBCs |
| Energy window | 15% |
| Collimator | LEHRP |
| Acquisition matrix | 64 × 64 |
| Zoom | 1.0–1.45 to 1.0 |
| Pixel dimensions (mm) | ≤6.5 × 6.5 |
| Gating | |
| Frames/cycle | 8–16 |
| Bad-beat rejection | 12–18% window |
| Framing | Forward/backward |
| Orbit | 180° or 360° elliptical/circular |
| Angular step/projection | 3°–6° |
| Time/projection | 30–60 sec |
| **Processing protocols** | |
| Temporal filtering | 1:2:1 |
| Reconstruction filter | Ramp Butterworth |
| Cutoff/order[a] | 0.22 ± 0.05/5.0 ± 1.0[a] |
| Slice thickness | 1 pixel |
| Oblique reorientation | Short and long axis |

[a]If possible, optimize filter function according to power spectrum of images.
LEHRP, low energy, high resolution, parallel hole; RBCs, red blood cells; $^{99m}$Tc, technetium 99m.

fraction underestimated by five to ten units can make a difference in patient management, e.g., serial studies in patients on chemotherapy, or patients with valvular regurgitation or heart failure. This is especially problematic when the magnitude of the artifact cannot be accurately predicted.

The reconstruction of artifact-free gated tomographic data and the accurate quantification of these studies require equal sampling throughout the cardiac cycle at each projection. The use of arrhythmia (bad-beat) rejection is recommended. Although some laboratories choose to accept bad beats in order to minimize acquisition time, in most cases no more than a minute or two is saved. The provision of a stable and artifact-free ECG R-wave input to the gating device is fundamental. If bad-beat rejection is employed, it is important that rejected beats not be counted against acquisition time. This will assure equal sampling (acquisition time) at each projection and the avoidance of artifacts in the reconstructed images. In those systems that do not extend the dwell time at projections where bad beats or ECG artifacts occur, imaged activity is generally normalized for the time acquired. If only a few beats are rejected and the acquisition time is only minimally shortened, this is a reasonable alternative. However, if many beats are rejected and only a few cardiac cycles are actually acquired, the projection data may be so count poor that even when normalized, significant reconstruction artifacts will occur. A 15% to 20% acceptance window will generally provide high-quality studies. Gated tomography is generally not recommended for patients in atrial fibrillation or with other chaotic cardiac rhythm because acquisition times will often be unduly prolonged.

There are many variables from which the user involved in the acquisition and processing of gated SPECT must choose. Ideally, gated studies would be acquired at 3-degree increments over 360 degrees to minimize the occurrence of alias artifacts and geometric distortion. Reasonable compromises that maintain image resolution while minimizing storage requirements and acquisition time include acquisitions with high-resolution parallel hole collimators at 6-degree increments into $64^2$ matrices with hardware zooms providing projection image pixel sizes of 5.0 to 6.0 mm. Greater zooms can result in the truncation of dilated hearts and severe image artifacts. Continuous rotation gated SPECT acquisitions, although still not widely available, should resolve the dead-time problem associated with finer angular sampling.

### Choice of Acquisition Orbits

The majority of SPECT systems sold currently for cardiac imaging are 90-degree dual-detector systems or single-detector systems. Driven by system configuration and the need to keep acquisition times as short as possible while maintaining data adequacy, 180-degree acquisition orbits will generally be the choice today. Acquisition time for 360-degree studies will generally be excessive when single-detector or 90-degree dual-detector systems are employed. Personal preference for the resultant images may affect this choice; i.e., studies acquired over 360 degrees compared to 180-degree studies demonstrate less geometric distortion and fewer reconstruction artifacts (20). The heart appears in a more uniform background. However, even though 360-degree studies are acquired with high-resolution parallel collimators, there is some loss of spatial resolution. When the SPECT system configuration provides the complete 360-degree data set in the same time as required for 180-degree studies (triple-detector or 180-degree dual-detector systems), the choice may be difficult. Elliptical orbits minimize the detector to patient distance, especially over the anterior aspect of the detector path, and provide some gain in reconstructed spatial resolution [1 to 3 mm full width half maximal (FWHM)] (21).

### Acquisition Time

Depending on the injected activity, the number of time frames desired, the choice of 180-degree or 360-degree orbits, and the geometry of the tomographic system used, acquisition times may vary from as brief as 5 minutes to as long as 45 minutes (2,22,23). If multistage imaging during pharmacologic or other interventions is anticipated, such as low-dose dobutamine, then conservative radiopharmaceutical dosing is neither necessary or recommended. The dosimetry of blood pool labeling with $^{99m}$Tc is quite favorable and the dose of 30 mCi or more in large patients is not unwarranted (24,25). Generally, acquisition times of 30 to

45 seconds at each projection will provide high-quality studies, 7 to 12 minutes total for most modern imaging systems. To assure the highest quality labeling, *in vitro* kits are recommended (25).

## Single Detector Versus Multidetector

Multidetector tomographs have had a significant impact on the acquisition of gated SPECT studies. In general, image acquisition can be completed in 7 to 15 minutes. A study acquired for 20 minutes over 180 degrees with a single-detector system, for example, would require only 13.3 minutes for the same data density with a triple-detector system and 10 minutes with a 90-degree opposed dual-detector system. For 20-minute studies acquired over 360 degrees with a single-detector system, 90-degree and 180-degree opposed dual-detector systems will reduce acquisition time to 10 minutes, while triple-detector systems will reduce acquisition time to only 6.67 minutes.

## Processing and Reconstruction

The processing of GBP tomograms is much like that of ungated perfusion tomography with two important exceptions: (a) the potential for temporal filtering and (b) the choice of spatial filters. The acquisition time for all frames (8 to 16) of gated studies is one to two times that generally used for ungated perfusion tomography. Thus, it is not surprising that despite the technetium blood pool label, the individual frames of these studies may be relatively count poor. Because of the temporal relationship of each time frame to the next, there is the potential for temporal filtering. The individual projections are temporally filtered using either simple arithmetic averaging or more complicated Fourier filters (26,27). Either way, image noise is significantly reduced with minimal loss in spatial and temporal resolution. Generally, low-pass Butterworth spatial filters or similar filters work well. Filter frequency cutoffs and orders in about the same range as those employed for high-quality gated technetium perfusion SPECT studies work well. Because of the greater image statistics available with blood pool imaging compared to gated perfusion imaging, GBP SPECT studies acquired using imaging parameters similar to those employed for gated perfusion SPECT can generally be filtered with moderately higher frequency cutoffs (0.02 to 0.05 cycles/pixel higher).

## Display and Analysis

### Display

Gated blood-pool tomograms are often displayed as cine loops of multiple transaxial, long- and/or short-axis sections of the left and right ventricles shown at end-diastole and end-systole, or throughout the entire cardiac cycle. Sectional images can be viewed with or without endocardial surfaces superimposed. Three-dimensional displays have

become available (22,28), and these displays of the cardiac blood pool can be viewed interactively from any perspective, demonstrating motion of the endocardial surface as cine loops, with parametric images color coded for motion or activation, or other variable, or combinations of these display formats (29–31).

Multizone cine displays of long- and short-axis sections chosen to view segments representative of each of the major coronary distributions are effective and quickly generated for both left and right ventricular assessments (Fig. 16.2) (3,32). Typically chosen are midventricular vertical and horizontal long-axis sections, and apical, midventricular, and basal short-axis sections. Care should be taken to avoid the selection of sectional images that are nearly tangential to the myocardial walls from which the chamber of interest completely withdraws during cardiac contraction. This can give a false impression of hyperkinetic regional function. If sectional images are chosen based on the midventricular end-systolic sections, even in small or hyperdynamic hearts, this problems can be easily avoided.

Three-dimensional displays have the advantage of showing the entire ventricle or heart and are unaffected by contractile or translational motion. The two approaches to the identification of endocardial surfaces and the generation of 3D displays are isocount contours and image gradient searches (22,28). Tauxe et al. (33) demonstrated in 1982 that isocount contours can be used to measure chamber vol-

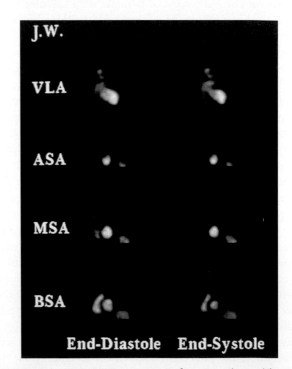

**FIGURE 16.2.** GBP SPECT tomograms from a patient with a massive anterior wall Q-wave myocardial infarction (MI). Note the diastolic deformity and large area of apical anterior dyskinesis especially apparent in the VLA, ASA, and MSA sections. Format same as Fig. 16.1.

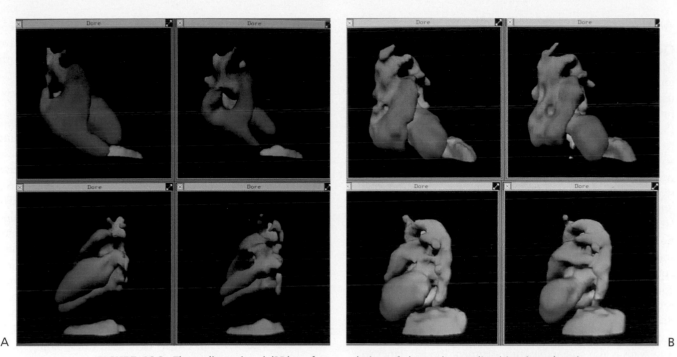

A                                                                                                    B

**FIGURE 16.3.** Three-dimensional (3D) surface rendering of the entire cardiac blood pool and proximal great vessels using the isocount contour approach in studies from a normal patient **(A)** and a patient with a anterior wall Q-wave MI **(B)**. The *upper frames* are seen from the anterior perspective; the *lower frames* are seen from the lateral perspective. Frames on the *left* are at end-diastole; on the *right* at end-systole. Note the symmetric wall motion in the volunteer study and the large anterior aneurysm in the patient study. Patients are same as in Figs. 16.1 and 16.2.

umes with acceptable accuracy. Isocount contours are fast and simple to generate and provide dramatic displays of the entire cardiac blood pool including left and right ventricles and atria (Fig. 16.3). However, the accuracy of quantitative wall motion determinations from isocount contours is questionable (29). If the threshold for the isocontour is set incorrectly, regional wall motion abnormalities near the base of the ventricles may be missed or underestimated. Theoretically more satisfying are endocardial surfaces determined from image gradients. Gradient-determined boundaries should follow the ventricle relatively unaffected by chamber motion and variations in photon flux. Surface determinations based on image gradients are computationally more complex, but accurate (22,32). Gradient-based boundaries are only now being adapted to the right ventricle. Qualitative analysis of wall motion from 3D displays may be approached in much the same way as described below for cine slice displays using similar segmentation and semiquantitative scoring schemes.

The maximal voxel ray trace method described by Miller and Wallis (34,35) is an alternative 3D display method. Unlike the surface rendering approaches discussed above, the maximal voxel ray trace method creates contrast-enhanced planar images from tomographic reconstructions (Fig. 16.4). These displays can provide impressive "three-dimensional" views of the entire cardiac blood pool and the proximal great vessels. Although visually effective, the dis-

plays are not quantifiable. Botvinick et al. (31) have developed an elegant method to encode both amplitude and phase information into volume-rendered displays useful for the study of electrophysiologic activation sequences.

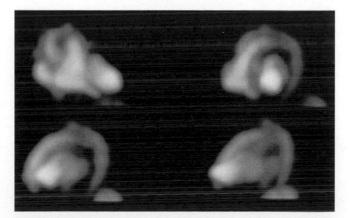

**FIGURE 16.4.** Three-dimensional volume rendering using the maximal voxel ray trace approach. Shown is a GBP SPECT study from a patient with an apical left ventricle (LV) aneurysm. Images are shown in the anterior, best septal left anterior oblique (LAO), steep LAO, and left lateral perspectives at end-diastole. Note the excellent contrast and 3D perspective this display method provides.

*Analysis*

## Qualitative Wall Motion Analysis

Multizone cine displays, quickly and easily formatted for long- and short-axis sections, are often the default technique used to assess wall motion. Semiquantitative scoring systems provide accurate and reproducible evaluations (Fig. 16.5) (5,32). Segmental wall motion is generally scored on a three- to five-point scale. Gill et al. (32) used a five-point system scoring segments from normokinesis (a score of 3) to dyskinesis (a score of −1). The interobserver agreement in this study was good [$r = 0.86$, $y = 0.86x + 0.3$, $p < .0001$, standard error of estimate (s.e.e.) = 0.64]. Other reports using a similar scoring systems have had similar results (2,5). Segmentation of the left ventricle (LV) and assignment of segments to specific coronary vascular distributions is analogous to the approach employed for SPECT perfusion imaging (36). The apex and the distal, midventricular, and proximal segments of each of the four walls of the LV [septal, anterior, lateral, and diaphragmatic (inferior and posterior)] are all scored (13-segment model). Distal and proximal division of each of the four walls is also acceptable (nine-segment model). Finer segmentation (17- to 20-segment models) of the LV blood pool in GBP SPECT studies can be performed but may be unnecessarily tedious. Similar semiquantitative approaches have been applied to surface-rendered blood pool tomograms with favorable results (30,37,38).

## Quantitative Wall Motion Analysis

The methods employed for quantitative wall motion analysis have included endocardial surface tracking from isocount contours or gradient-determined endocardial searches, phase analysis, and regional EF calculations. These quantitative techniques provide objective, reproducible results (Fig. 16.6). Of the methods available for quantitative wall motion analysis, endocardial surface tracking is the method most analogous to those employed for contrast ventriculography (28,29,32,39). However, surface identification and tracking in three dimensions is more complex. Gill et al. (32) defined endocardial boundaries using a second derivative algorithm, and mean percent segmental shortening was determined. Quantitative comparisons between GBP SPECT and contrast ventriculography were highly significant ($y = 0.74x + 8.7$, $r = 0.82$, s.e.e. = 14%). Others have used thresholding techniques in patients with coronary heart disease and left ventricular aneurysms to define surface locations with excellent results (40–42). Because of the relatively poor resolution at the depth of the mitral and aortic valve planes, Faber et al. (29) used higher thresholds for the basal fourth of the ventricle. Tested in a canine model, detected surface points varied by only 1.9 to 3.7 mm compared to the locations of endocardial surface points marked with implanted gadolinium-153 beads. Narita et al. (42) also used variable thresholds with good results in comparison to contrast ventricolography. In their study, thresholds between 45% and 55% were used but were varied based on chamber volume and background activity rather than depth. Faber et al. (22) also employed a 3D gradient search using a spherical cylindrical coordinate system and a 3D extension of the center-line method commonly applied to contrast ventriculography. Compared to gated

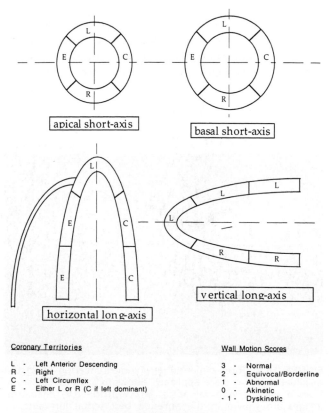

SPECT Segmentation / Territories

apical short-axis

basal short-axis

horizontal long-axis

vertical long-axis

**Coronary Territories**

| | |
|---|---|
| L | - Left Anterior Descending |
| R | - Right |
| C | - Left Circumflex |
| E | - Either L or R (C if left dominant) |

**Wall Motion Scores**

| | |
|---|---|
| 3 | - Normal |
| 2 | - Equivocal/Borderline |
| 1 | - Abnormal |
| 0 | - Akinetic |
| - 1 | - Dyskinetic |

**FIGURE 16.5.** A practical segmentation scheme for the visual semiquantitative analysis of wall motion from GBP SPECT studies labeled according to typical coronary territories.

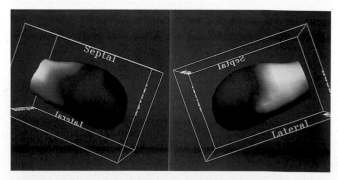

**FIGURE 16.6.** Color-coded endocardial surface maps at end-systole obtained using the gradient search approach and a 3D extension of the center-line method for wall motion quantification. Images viewed from the septal and lateral perspectives from the same patient shown in Figs. 16.2 and 16.3 with a large anterior infarct. Color coding is from white (≥6 mm inward motion) to black (≥2 mm of outward systolic motion).

magnetic resonance studies in humans, the average motion error was only 0.67 mm. Clinical application of this method is promising, but files of normal regional motion will have to be established and tested to ensure clinical accuracy (43).

Phase analysis has been reported with increasing frequency for the analysis of wall motion from GBP SPECT (28,44–48). Most applications of phase analysis to tomographic studies are as simple 3D extensions of the pixel-by-pixel analysis commonly applied to planar GBP studies (49,50). The resultant phase and amplitude data have been displayed as polar maps or color coded on 3D surfaces (44–48). Lee et al. (48) used phase and amplitude polar maps to detect wall motion abnormalities with increased accuracy compared to planar blood pool imaging. Employing an alternate approach, Yamashita et al. (28) calculated the phase of the first harmonic of the length from the endocardial surface to the center of the LV long axis (Fig. 16.7). Although only eight patients were studied, comparisons with contrast ventriculography and planar blood pool imaging were excellent. Abnormal segments generally lagged behind the phase of the global volume curve, while normal segments preceded the global phase. These investigators found this approach to be especially helpful for the septal and diaphragmatic segments.

Although discrepancies have occurred in the analysis of GBP tomographic studies, they have generally been related to the translational and rotational motion of the heart during contraction. Most prone to error have been those methods that rely on voxel-by-voxel analysis of the heart, portions of which may not remain within the field-of-view of many end-diastolic voxels. As has been reported with contrast ventriculography, the quantitative analysis of wall motion is prone to error even when well-defined normal standards are available

for comparison (51,52). Attempts to correct for cardiac translational motion have been frustrated as much by correction technique–introduced error as the error for which the correction was attempted in the first place. The floating axis technique described by Cerqueira et al. (53) in normal volunteers appears promising in the analysis of regional ejection fractions. The application of this technique to patients with abnormal resting wall motion and/or regional diastolic deformities may be a greater challenge.

Regional or sectorial ejection fractions have been employed with good results (44,53–55). This method demonstrated good intra- and interobserver variability; however, comparisons with contrast ventriculography have varied. Barat et al. (54) reported regional ejection fractions that varied from as low as 23.6% to as high as 40.5%. Correlations of regional ejection fractions with contrast ventriculography values provided *r* values from as low as 0.45 at the base to as high as 0.78 in the midanterior wall. More recently, Groch et al. (55) have reported greater success. These investigators compared four different reference models including fixed and floating LV centers and two different segmentation models of the midventricular short-axis sections. They found excellent agreement between GBP SPECT wall motion analysis and coronary angiography (>75% stenosis) (sensitivity 90%, specificity 95%) that was better than either planar blood pool imaging (sensitivity 43%) or contrast ventriculography (sensitivity 57%). In this study, as in Cerqueira et al.'s (53), the floating reference provided the most uniform regional ejection fractions, 78.0 to 79.9. However, the fixed reference at the LV end-diastolic center of mass provided the best sensitivity and specificity.

Increasingly robust methods for the analysis of regional ventricular function are being developed. As these quantita-

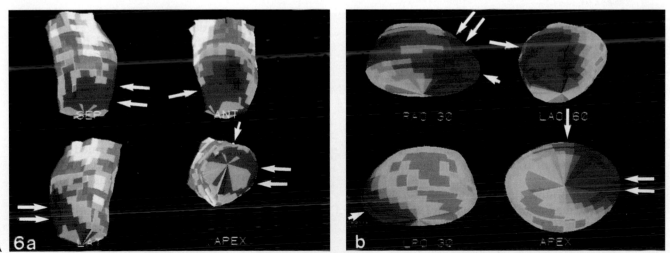

**FIGURE 16.7.** Three-dimensional functional images (3D percent shortening) of a patient with an anterior septal MI. GBP SPECT **(A)** and 3D reconstructed biplane contrast ventriculography **(B)** demonstrate septal *(arrow)*, anterior *(arrows)*, and apical akinesis to dyskinesis and delayed phase. (From Yamashita K, Tanaka M, Asada N, et al. A new method of three dimensional analysis of left ventricular wall motion. *Eur J Nucl Med* 1988;14:113–119, with permission.)

tive methods continue to evolve, aided by ever-increasing computer performance, it is likely that planar blood pool imaging will be largely supplanted in the near future by quicker and more accurate tomographic techniques.

### Left and Right Ventricular Ejection Fraction and Volumes

Quantification of global LV volumes and ejection fractions from GBP tomograms was first described in the early 1980s (33,39,56). The majority of studies performed a surface-rendering operation to define LV volumes of interest. The voxels within the LV volumes of interest are summed at each time frame throughout the cardiac cycle, or at end-diastole and end-systole. When the total number of LV voxels is multiplied by the calibrated volume per voxel, the corresponding LV volume is determined without geometric assumption.

Based on the report in 1982 from Tauxe et al. (33), many studies have employed simple isocount contours at approximately 45% of the peak LV counts to define the LV volumes of interest (2). Others have employed second derivative gradient searches within the individual slices throughout the 3D space occupied by the LV (39,56,57). These methods are more difficult to implement and ensure reasonably smooth and continuous endocardial surfaces. Gradient searches are more readily affected by image noise, and endocardial surfaces based on gradients may include discontinuities that are anatomically impossible (22). Iterative algorithms have proven efficient and more reliable in this regard. The approach described by Faber et al. (57) using a statistical model of the LV to refine progressively gradient-based surfaces provided a significant increment in

automaticity. Further improvements in accuracy, robustness, and automaticity are expected in the near future.

Poor definition of the mitral valve plane due to the inevitable loss of resolution with depth has been one of the major sources of error with all of the methods described above. Some investigators have used time-activity curve analysis of the individual short-axis sections to help define the valve plane (32,53,58,59). These investigators have used the transition point where the slice-by-slice stroke volume switches from positive to negative to define the position of the mitral valve plane at a fixed position in space. Unfortunately, this is inconsistent with the physiology of the heart and the mitral valve plane in particular. Magnetic resonance imaging (MRI) studies have clearly demonstrated the descent of the mitral valve plane by approximately 7 to 15 mm toward the apex during ventricular systole, contributing significantly to the global ejection fraction (60). The availability of higher resolution multidetector tomographs has significantly but incompletely alleviated this problem (Fig. 16.8). Accurate separation of left atrial from left ventricular activity may be a bigger issue with planar imaging than was previously appreciated, leading to an underestimation bias of LV ejection fractions. An intriguing study by Bartlett et al. (61) compared planar with reprojected from SPECT planar blood pool scans. These investigators found that inaccurate definition of the mitral valve plane and separation of left atrium from LV on planar imaging often result in a significant underestimation of LV ejection fractions. Smaller or hyperdynamic hearts, hearts where the left atrium is relatively large in comparison with the LV end-systole volume, or hearts with high ejection fractions, would be expected to be most affected by atrial overlap.

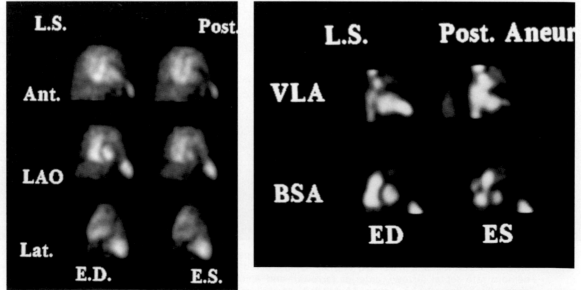

**FIGURE 16.8.** Planar **(A)** and multislice GBP SPECT **(B)** studies from a patient with a posterior infarct. Best seen in the VLA sections is a sharply defined posterior aneurysm.

These considerations call into question the use of planar GBP imaging as a gold standard for GBP SPECT studies.

The right ventricle is generally more superficially located within the thorax than the LV and thus better resolved. A study using a mathematical cardiac torso phantom demonstrated the potential application of GBP SPECT studies to assessments of right ventricle (RV) functions (62). Assessments of RV ejection fractions from GBP SPECT have only recently appeared (63,64). At this time most studies of RV ejection fractions by GBP SPECT have been manual or semi-automatic demonstrations of feasibility. The RV shape is more complex than that of the LV, complicating the design of mathematical models for surface rendering this chamber throughout the cardiac cycle. Significant progress in the study of RV function with GBP SPECT appears close at hand.

## CLINICAL APPLICATIONS

Correlations of GBP SPECT with contrast ventriculography and gated MRI have demonstrated great promise for this imaging technique in the evaluation of global left ventricular function and regional wall motion, including the identification of aneurysms, and quantitative assessments of left ventricular systolic function (2,5,8,32). The application of GBP SPECT studies to the evaluation of patients with AV nodal bypass tracks and patients with valvular regurgitation followed (9,10). The remainder of this chapter reviews the clinical applications of GBP tomography.

### Ejection Fractions and Volumes

The prognostic value of left ventricular ejection fraction and volume measurements in coronary and valvular heart diseases and cardiomyopathies is well established. Measurements of ejection fractions with planar blood pool techniques have been exhaustively validated and are accepted by many as the gold standard for this important variable (18, 65–68). It is well known that variable attenuation significantly complicates the measurement of absolute ventricular volumes using nongeometric count-based methods and planar imaging (69,70). It is less well established but likely correct that the accuracy of global ejection fraction measurements can be seriously compromised by severe regional dysfunction (71). Schneider et al. (71) have convincingly demonstrated that differences in attenuation between the apex and other distal ventricular segments affected by anterior infarcts and the proximal inferoposterior low septal segments affected by inferior-wall infarcts can significantly affect ejection fraction measurements in opposite directions. The deleterious effects of anterior infarcts will be overemphasized while the effects of posterior infarcts will be underemphasized, resulting in under- and overestimation biases, respectively, in LV ejection fraction measurements. GBP SPECT methods sum all the voxels within the ventricle. Because all voxels have the same calibrated volume independent of the degree of attenuation, ventricular volumes determined by this approach are not influenced by the effects of photon attenuation (2,72).

As discussed in the previous section, the accuracy of ventricular ejection fraction and volume measurements with gated SPECT blood pool imaging is well established using either simple isocount contours or other more technically sophisticated endocardial surface rendering methods (Table 16.2). The studies of Bartlett et al. (61) and Schneider et al. (71) discussed above predicted under- or overestimations of LV ejection fractions measured with planar blood-pool

## TABLE 16.2. SUMMARY OF LEFT VENTRICULAR VOLUME AND EJECTION FRACTION RESULTS BY TOMOGRAPHIC GATED BLOOD POOL IMAGING

| Study | End-Diastolic Volume[a] | | End-Systolic Volume[a] | | Ejection | Fraction[a] |
|---|---|---|---|---|---|---|
| | r | SEE (mL) | r | SEE (mL) | r | SEE |
| Gill et al. (32) | 0.94 | 20 | 0.93 | 24 | 0.92 | 0.08 |
| Corbett et al. (2) | 0.90 | 13.4 | 0.93 | 10.1 | 0.92 | 0.07 |
| Stadius et al. (59) | 0.81 | 27 | 0.96 | 12 | 0.92 | 0.04 |
| Caputo et al. (101) | 0.89[b] | 24[b] | — | — | — | — |
| Underwood et al. (8) | 0.91[b] | — | — | — | 0.94 | 0.07 |
| Myers et al. (39) | — | — | — | — | 0.92 | 0.08 |
| Bunker et al. (102) | 0.97 | 23 | — | — | — | — |
| Murano et al. (78) | 0.89 | — | — | — | 0.94 | — |
| Yamazaki et al. (79) | 0.79 | — | 0.95 | — | 0.96 | — |
| Chin et al. (63) | 0.96[b] | 18[b] | — | — | 0.94 | 0.09 |
| Narita et al. (42) | 0.89 | — | 0.94 | — | 0.94 | — |
| Mariano-Goulart et al. (64) | — | — | — | — | 0.93 | 0.06 |

—, not available.
[a]Comparison vs. CVG, planar gated blood pool imaging or gated MRI.
[b]For end-diastolic and end-systolic volumes combined.
CVG, contrast ventriculography; MRI, magnetic resonance imaging; SEE,
Adapted from Fischman AJ, Moore RH, Gill JB, et al. Gated blood pool tomography: a technology whose time has come. *Semin Nucl Med* 1989;19:13 21, with permission.

imaging. A method such as GBP SPECT, unaffected by attenuation or chamber overlap, should be more accurate than planar imaging. Proof of superiority will have to await careful comparisons with other imaging methods such as state-of-the-art gated or fast cine MRI. In addition to its use for the measurement of global variables of ventricular function, GBP SPECT is also highly effective in the assessment of regional function.

## Coronary Heart Disease

### Wall Motion: Chronic Coronary Disease and Myocardial Infarction

Free of chamber overlap, GBP SPECT is well suited for the evaluation of regional ventricular function and wall motion abnormalities. Although planar GBP imaging is an important tool in clinical medicine, it has certain intrinsic limitations. While planar GBP imaging is an excellent method for measuring global ventricular function, it is not as accurate for the identification of regional wall motion abnormalities (2,32,73–75). There is almost always chamber overlap of one or more segments, complicating qualitative and quantitative assessments of regional wall motion. This can be particularly troublesome in the septal and proximal inferior segments. Furthermore, the best septal projection presents the LV foreshortened and viewed variably from above, often with significant left atrial overlap (61). With planar imaging there is limited resolution of ventricular segments and interference from overlapping chambers, particularly in the right anterior oblique (RAO), anterior, lateral, and left posterior oblique (LPO) projections. Wall motion abnormalities can be either missed altogether or assigned to the wrong vascular territory. From its inception, one of the principal clinical applications of GBP SPECT was the evaluation of regional ventricular function (1–3).

Closed loop cinematic displays of the entire cardiac cycle including multiple long- and short-axis sections selected to sample all regions of the LV are now routinely available, generated in seconds automatically or under operator control. Although simple and straightforward, multislice cine displays have proven highly effective and readily demonstrate the diagnostic efficacy of gated SPECT imaging in comparison to contrast ventriculography and planar blood-pool imaging (Fig. 16.9) (2,3,32). Three-dimensional surface rendering approaches provide quantification of endocardial wall motion as well as ventricular volumes and ejection fractions (Fig. 16.10) (22,29,30,37).

The GBP tomographic technique overcomes most of the limitations of planar imaging. These studies permit the assessment of the ventricles without complicating chamber overlap. Further, tomographic data can be easily reorganized for viewing from any perspective, permitting individual ventricular segments to be viewed without interference from adjacent chamber or ventricular segments. Studies comparing

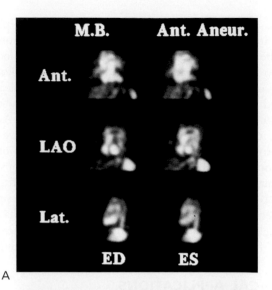

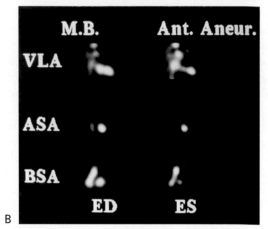

**FIGURE 16.9.** Planar *(A)* and multislice GBP SPECT *(B)* studies from a patient with an apical anterior aneurysm. Format is the same as Fig. 16.8. Note the well-defined apical aneurysm, best seen in the VLA despite well-preserved ventricular function elsewhere.

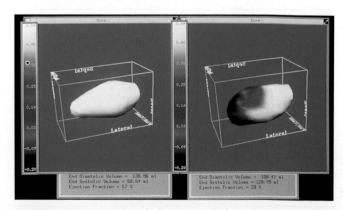

**FIGURE 16.10.** Color-coded endocardial surface maps and global quantitative data from a normal volunteer *(left)* and a patient with a large anterior MI *(right)*. Color-coding is the same as for Fig. 16.6.

GBP SPECT with contrast ventriculography or echocardiography have found almost invariably that the SPECT blood-pool studies identified wall motion abnormalities, including functional aneurysm formation, as well as the compared modalities (2,3,30,32). Two studies comparing gated SPECT, planar GBP studies, and contrast ventriculography with coronary angiography found improved detection of abnormal wall motion (Table 16.3) (2,76). Corbett et al. (2) reported a trend toward improved sensitivity in all three coronary territories. The sensitivity in the left anterior descending distribution and for all coronary distributions combined were significantly enhanced. Metcalfe et al. (76) studied 100 consecutive patients. In patients with prior MI, the detection rates were 95% for contrast ventriculography, 57% for planar, and 90% for GBP SPECT. For patients with coronary disease and no prior MI, the detection rates were 7%, 0%, and 59%, respectively. Overall detection rates were 70% for contrast ventriculography, 40% for planar, and 81% for GBP SPECT. Patients with insignificant coronary disease did not demonstrate abnormalities. Mochizuki et al. (77) studied 50 patients with prior MI using gated thallium 201 ($^{201}$Tl) and GBP SPECT. GBP tomography demonstrated a 94.5% concordance with gated $^{201}$Tl wall motion and a 85% concordance with $^{201}$Tl uptake.

Most of the studies performed in recent years with GBP SPECT have utilized either 3D surface rendering methods or phase analysis to study LV wall motion. Faber et al. (22,38) were among the first to use 3D display and analysis methods with gated tomographic studies, and they demonstrated gains in sensitivity and localization accuracy with this approach. Several studies using 3D surface rendering have utilized simple thresholding at 40% to 50% of the peak activity in the LV blood pool (41,42,78,79). These studies have included patient populations with a high percentage of prior infarcts and have all demonstrated excellent agreement with contrast ventriculography. In these studies,

GBP SPECT always out-performed planar blood-pool imaging for the identification of regional wall motion abnormalities.

Phase analysis has been employed with increasing regularity for the study of wall motion with GBP SPECT in patients with ischemic heart disease and for the localization of AV nodal bypass pathways in patients with Wolff-Parkinson-White (WPW) syndrome (Figs. 16.7 and 16.11) (31,47,48,80–82). As applied to gated tomography studies, phase analysis is a 3D extension of the 2D method commonly used for planar blood-pool imaging. Often the same basic software is simply applied to the gated 2D slices derived from the tomographic study (47,80,81). Cross et al. (81) performed their analyses with phase and amplitude derived from polar maps and comparisons to files from a population of normal controls. Using this approach, they reported increased detection of inferior wall infarcts. Botvinick et al. (31) developed a unique encoded 3D display of volume-rendered blood-pool tomograms with the amplitude data as intensity and the phase data as color. In patients with myocardial infarcts, the 3D images better localized the separation between normal and abnormal wall motion than did the planar-equivalent images.

## Ventricular Aneurysms

The use of GBP SPECT for the assessment of functional aneurysms is a natural extension of the methods for wall motion analysis discussed above (5,32). Assessments of global and regional ventricular function with gated SPECT perfusion imaging may be adversely affected by large severe perfusion defects, with a resulting significant underestimation bias (83). Gated SPECT blood pool imaging is a universally applicable method for the evaluation of global and segmental ventricular function, not compromised by large regions of severely diminished perfusion.

**TABLE 16.3. DETECTION OF WALL MOTION ABNORMALITIES IN PATIENTS WITH CHD: COMPARISON OF PLANAR AND TOMOGRAPHIC METHODS**

|  | No CHD ($n = 10$) | Single Vessel ($n = 55$) | Multivessel ($n = 70$) | All CHD ($n = 125$) |
|---|---|---|---|---|
| Planar (%) | 0 | 40** | 54** | 48** |
| SPECT (%) | 20 | 78 | 90 | 85 |
| CVG (%) | 0 | 62* | 63* | 73* |

*$p < .05$ tomographic method vs. CVG; **$p < .01$ tomographic method vs. planar.
CHD, coronary heart disease; CVG, contrast ventriculography; SPECT, single photon emission computed tomography.
Adapted from Corbett JR, Jansen DE, Lewis SE, et al. Tomographic gated blood pool radionuclide ventriculography: analysis of wall motion and left ventricular volumes in patients with coronary artery disease. *J Am Coll Cardiol* 1985;6:349–358, and Metcalfe MJ, Norton MY, Jennings K, et al. Improved detection of abnormal left ventricular wall motion using tomographic radionuclide ventriculography compared with planar radionuclide and single plane contrast ventriculography. *Br J Radiol* 1993;66:986–993, with permission.

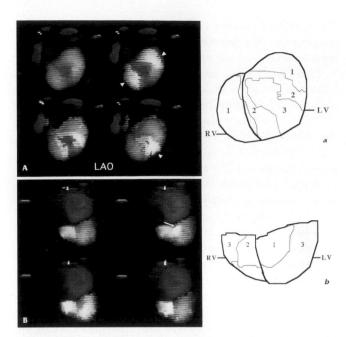

FIGURE 16.11. Patient with a posterior septal accessory pathway. Images are volume-rendered GBP SPECT images viewed from an LAO perspective 18 degrees above transaxial **(A)** and from a posterior perspective 18 degrees below transaxial **(B)**. Images are color coded for phase and intensity coded for amplitude. Phase-angle progression is highlighted in *white*. Activation begins in the posterior septum (*arrow,* **B**), simultaneously reaches the right ventricle (RV) and left ventricle (LV) free walls (*arrowheads,* **A**) and meet in the anteroseptal wall (*arrowhead,* **A**). (From Botvinick EH, O'Connell JW, Kadkade PP, et al. Potential added value of three-dimensional reconstruction and display of single photon emission computed tomographic gated blood pool images. *J Nucl Cardiol* 1998;5:245–255, with permission.

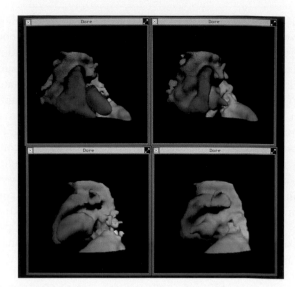

FIGURE 16.12. Three-dimensional surface rendering of the cardiac blood pool using the isocount contour approach from the same patient shown in Fig. 16.8. Format is the same as Fig. 16.3. Particularly well seen on the end-systolic images is a sharply defined posterior aneurysm.

The effect of functional aneurysms on ventricular function, and the negative prognostic implications associated, highlight the need for accurate and reproducible noninvasive methods for their identification and longitudinal assessment (84,85). Several studies with GBP SPECT have reported the identification of ventricular aneurysms (3,6,7). Gill et al. (32) reported that the presence and extent of aneurysms were identified with greater accuracy and confidence than with planar imaging. Meizlish et al. (85), using planar imaging, reported a classification scheme for anterior-wall aneurysms based on the extent of the diastolic deformity and the severity of the associated wall motion abnormality. McGhie et al. (5) adapted that approach to GBP SPECT and the prognostic classification of patients in the first week following MI. Using multislice analysis of GBP SPECT studies, they demonstrated improved detection of aneurysms compared to planar imaging and echocardiography (Figs. 16.8 and 16.9). In addition, they demonstrated significantly lower LV ejection fractions and larger end-systolic volumes in patients imaged early after the acute event. When 3D methods were applied, there was a further improvement in aneurysm detection (Fig. 16.12)

(38). Lu et al. (86) and Yamazaki et al. (79) described excellent visualization of LV aneurysms with increased accuracy compared to planar imaging techniques. Metcalfe et al. (87) studied 30 patients with isolated inferior or anterior MI. Using phase and amplitude analyses and a 3D display technique, these investigators found comparable sensitivities for planar and SPECT imaging in patients with anterior MI (93% and 100%, $p$ = NS) but a significantly increased sensitivity with SPECT in patients with inferior MI (7% and 93%, $p$ <.001). Botvinick et al. (31) used data from phase and amplitude analysis combined with volume-rendered GBP SPECT to image ventricular aneurysms to advantage in comparison with planar-equivalent perspective images alone (anterior, best-septal left anterior oblique, and steep left anterior oblique).

Gaudron et al. (88) and Ertl et al. (89) studied early remodeling and changes in LV volumes following first myocardial infarcts with serial quantitative GBP SPECT. Patients were categorized according to creatine kinase release into small, moderate, and large infarcts. Left ventricular volume index (mL/m²) decreased in patients with small infarcts between 4 days and 4 weeks following the acute event (74.5 ± 4.9 vs. 62.5 ± 3.0, $p$ <.005). Directionally opposite, patient with moderate and large infarcts demonstrated LV dilation at follow-up imaging: moderate (74.6 ± 4.7 vs. 83.6 ± 5.0, $p$ <.0001) and large (71.7 ± 4.8 vs. 90.2 ± 6.5, $p$ <.0001). In both studies, although LV ejection fractions remained depressed on follow-up imaging (4 weeks) in patients with larger infarcts, the stroke volumes normalized as the ventricles dilated without a significant change in filling pressures.

## Pharmacologic Interventions

Matsuo et al. (90) used planar GBP imaging with a combined infusion of low-dose dobutamine and isosorbide dinitrate to identify hibernating myocardium in patients with chronic coronary heart disease and LV dysfunction. In segments with severe asynergy, there was an 85% correspondence with reinjection $^{201}$Tl imaging. With acquisition times of 7 to 15 minutes or less, evaluations of the effects of pharmacologic interventions on global and regional ventricular function are now a clinically realistic possibility using gated SPECT imaging. In patients with coronary heart disease and patients with congestive heart failure, serial measurements of ventricular function may be critical in the selection of mechanical and pharmacologic interventions. Kim and Quaife et al. (43,91) have described the use of quantitative GBP SPECT to assess the effect of long-acting nitrates on ventricular dysfunction prior to and following coronary revascularization. These investigators demonstrated regional improvements or deteriorations in ventricular function pre-revascularization that were predictive of regional functional outcomes. Any pharmacologic intervention that can be sustained for 7 to 15 minutes can be evaluated using these methods. Low-dose dobutamine can be coupled with gated SPECT with impressive results (Fig. 16.13).

### AV Nodal Bypass Tracts

Noninvasive identification of AV nodal bypass tracts and the assessment of ventricular activation sequences have been the aim of several studies employing GBP SPECT (10,31,92–96).

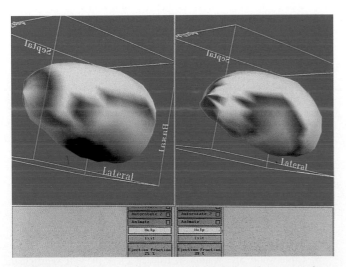

**FIGURE 16.13.** Quantitative 3D endocardial surface maps from a patient with severe multivessel coronary stenoses and a large inferior-lateral MI. Surfaces at end-diastole are color coded for wall motion as seen from perspective below and apical-lateral to the left ventricle (LV). Color coding is from *white* (>6 mm inward motion) to *black* (≥2 mm of outward systolic motion). Images on the *left* were obtained in the basal state. Images on the *right* were obtained during the administration of low-dose dobutamine. Wall motion is seen to improve significantly with a significant quantitative increase in ejection fraction from 25% to 39%.

Assuming acquisition of technically good-quality studies with attention to gating and bad-beat rejection, GBP tomography is well suited to the study of ventricular activation sequences. The entire cardiac blood pool is imaged without chamber overlap. Nakajima et al. (10) were the first to use GBP SPECT for this purpose. They studied 20 patients with WPW syndrome including 14 patients with delta waves. They performed phase and amplitude analyses to identify the site of initial ventricular activation. As confirmed by epicardial mapping at electrophysiologic study and surgery, they correctly identified and localized 12 of 14 (86%) bypass tracts using GBP SPECT imaging. Planar blood-pool studies correctly identified only 8 of 14 (57%) of tracts. Lucas et al. (92) studied seven patients with ambiguous ECG findings for preexcitation. They were able to localize accurately six of seven pathways confirmed at electrophysiologic study.

Botvinick et al. (31), as described above, used phase- and amplitude-encoded volume-rendered studies to localize bypass pathways, particularly advantageous for posteroseptal pathways (Fig. 16.11). Phase angle progression paralleled that of the electrocardiogram. Dormehl et al. (93) and Neumann et al. (94) compressed phase data into 2D parametric images for ease of interpretation. In baboon simulations and patients with WPW syndrome, these methods proved accurate. Although most of these studies were acquired with 16 frames per cardiac cycle, Dormehl et al.'s studies were acquired with only eight frames per cycle. Weismuller et al. (95) used GBP SPECT to study patients with WPW syndrome and patients with ventricular tachycardia. In nine patients with WPW, the site of initial contraction was identical with the site of the accessory pathway found by mapping. In seven patients with ventricular tachycardia, the sites of origin were within 3 cm of the arrhythmic focus by catheter mapping. Clausen et al. (96) applied phase analysis to GBP SPECT to localize arrhythmogenic foci in 85% of 14 patients with WPW and seven patients with ventricular tachycardia. In experimental pig simulations of WPW, these same investigators were able to localize all arrhythmogenic foci within 2 cm of the site of activation. As these methods are further refined, it seems likely that other disorders of cardiac ventricular activation will be approachable.

### Valvular heart disease

In patients with regurgitant valvular lesions limited to one side of the heart, GBP SPECT appears to accurately distinguish patients with regurgitant lesions from those without, and those with mild from those with severe lesions (9). Rigo et al. (97) first reported the use of planar GBP imaging for the quantification of valvular regurgitation. Although highly reproducible, the separation between patients with and without regurgitation when applied to less select patient populations lacked specificity (98). Several variations of this method were reported, including the use of variable rather than fixed regions of interest, the use of stroke-count images generated by the subtraction of end-systolic from end-diastolic images, and the use of the amplitude images from phase analysis (98,99). Overlap of the ventricles with the atria in the best-septal projection used to make these evaluations is a constant source of error. Because of chamber overlap, especially the RV stroke counts are significantly offset by counts filling the right atrium, and the ventricular stroke counts are systematically and quantitatively underestimated. Unfortunately, the magnitude of this underestimation cannot be predicted accurately.

Ohtake et al. (9) reported the use of GBP SPECT as a means of quantifying the LV regurgitant fraction in patients with valvular regurgitation. These investigators studied 14 patients without angiographic regurgitation and 17 patients with left-sided regurgitation. Generating a series of stroke-count images by subtracting end-systolic images from end-diastolic images on a slice-by-slice basis, they measured the left and right ventricular stroke counts without the errors produced by overlapping chambers. The correlation between the gated SPECT and the angiographic regurgitant fractions was very good ($r = 0.821$), and the intercept of the regression equation approached zero ($y = 5.85 + 0.70x$). Unlike previous planar studies, the separation into groups without regurgitation, with mild regurgitation (1–2+), and with severe regurgitation (3–4+), was excellent. In contrast, planar measurements demonstrated substantial overlap between all three groups. The interobserver reproducibility of the SPECT measurements of regurgitant fractions was excellent ($r = 0.964$). Although this approach has not been reported for the assessment of right-sided regurgitant lesions, with the excellent separation of chambers this methodology provides it seem likely that it may be applied successfully.

Delhomme et al. (100) measured left and right ventricular ejection fractions and regional wall motion in 36 patients with mitral valve prolapse (MVP), 15 of whom had complex ventricular arrhythmias. The RV ejection fraction in these patients was decreased compared to controls, especially in patients with mitral regurgitation and complex ventricular arrhythmias (26% ± 7% vs. 40% ± 10%, $p < .001$). Phase analysis demonstrated significantly more heterogeneous RV wall motion as measured by the standard deviation of the phase angles (SDP). In patients with prolapse and complex arrhythmias, phase dispersion was significantly increased, 35 ± 21 degrees (SDP) (MVP and arrhythmias) versus 21 ± 10 degrees (MVP without arrhythmias) ($p < .01$) and 12 ± 5 degrees (controls) ($p < .05$). Left ventricular wall motion also tended to be more heterogeneous in patients with MVP with and without regurgitation, but was not significantly different from controls.

## SUMMARY

The $^{99m}$Tc-labeled blood pool is well suited for gated SPECT acquisitions. Multidetector SPECT systems pro-

vide enhanced system sensitivity and resolution, significantly extending the clinical utility of this underutilized imaging modality. Processing times have been reduced to less than 1 to 2 minutes. Significantly enhanced system sensitivity and resolution, and dramatically reduced processing times have made gated SPECT blood pool imaging a clinically practical imaging modality. The challenge to cardiology to provide accurate, assessable, and cost-effective diagnosis has never been more important (14). GBP SPECT can play an important role in the care of many patient groups, e.g., patients with coronary, valvular, and myopathic heart diseases, and cardiac arrhythmias. The application of this powerful imaging modality appears on the verge of a significant expansion as efficient tools necessary for the rapid, accurate, and reproducible analysis and display of GBP SPECT become available.

## ACKNOWLEDGMENT

The authors would like to acknowledge Mary Dempsey for her assistance in preparing this manuscript.

## REFERENCES

1. Moore ML, Murphy PH, Burdine JA. ECG-gated emission computed tomography of the cardiac blood pool. *Radiology* 1980;134:233–235.
2. Corbett JR, Jansen DE, Lewis SE, et al. Tomographic gated blood pool radionuclide ventriculography: analysis of wall motion and left ventricular volumes in patients with coronary artery disease. *J Am Coll Cardiol* 1985;6:349–358.
3. Underwood SR, Walton S, Ell PJ, et al. Gated blood-pool emission tomography: a new technique for the investigation of cardiac structure and function. *Eur J Nucl Med* 1985;10:332–337.
4. Kahn JK, Henderson EB, Akers MS, et al. Prediction of reversibility of perfusion defects with a single post-exercise technetium-99m RP-30A gated tomographic image: the role of residual systolic thickening. *J Am Coll Cardiol* 1988;11:31A.
5. McGhie AI, Faber TL, Willerson JT, et al. Evaluation of left ventricular aneurysm formation following acute myocardial infarction using tomographic radionuclide ventriculography. *Am J Cardiol* 1995;75:720–724.
6. Maublant J, Bailly P, Mestas D, et al. Feasibility of gated single-photon emission transaxial tomography of the cardiac blood pool. *Radiology* 1983;146:837–839.
7. Tamaki N, Mukai T, Ishii Y, et al. Multiaxial tomography of heart chambers by gated blood-pool emission computed tomography using a rotating gamma camera. *Radiology* 1983;147:547–554.
8. Underwood SR, Walton S, Laming PJ, et al. Left ventricular volume and ejection fraction determined by gated blood pool emission tomography. *Br Heart J* 1985;53:216–222.
9. Ohtake T, Nishikawa J, Machida K, et al. Evaluation of regurgitant fraction of the left ventricle by gated cardiac blood-pool scanning using SPECT. *J Nucl Med* 1987;28:19–24.
10. Nakajima K, Bunko H, Tada A, et al. Nuclear tomographic phase analysis: localization of accessory conduction pathway in patients with Wolff-Parkinson-White syndrome. *Am Heart J* 1985;109:809–815.

11. Eagle K, Coley C, Newell J, et al. Combining clinical and thallium data optimizes preoperative assessment of cardiac risk before major vascular surgery. *Ann Intern Med* 1989;110:859–866.

12. Kryzhanovski VA, Beller GA. Usefulness of preoperative noninvasive radionuclide testing for detecting coronary artery disease in candidates for liver transplantation. *Am J Cardiol* 1997;79: 986–988.

13. Lee KJ, Wallis JW, Miller TR. The clinical role of radionuclide imaging in cardiac transplantation. *J Thorac Imaging* 1990;5: 73–77.

14. Rocco TP, Pfeffer MA. A challenge to the nuclear cardiology laboratory: imaging goals in patients after infarction [editorial]. *J Nucl Cardiol* 1996;3:358–362.

15. Lim DB, Gottschalk S, Walker R, et al. Triangular SPECT system for 3-D total organ volume imaging: design concept and preliminary imaging results. *IEEE Trans Nucl Sci* 1985;NS32:741–747.

16. McGhie AI, Akers MS, Faber TL, et al. Assessment of ventricular topography following acute myocardial infarction with gated tomographic radionuclide ventriculography using a dedicated three-detector tomographic (PRISM 3000). *J Nucl Med* 1989; 30:A770(abst).

17. Germano G, Kiat H, Kavanagh P, et al. Automatic quantification of ejection fraction from gated myocardial perfusion SPECT. *J Nucl Med* 1995;36:2138–2147.

18. Bacharach SL, Green MV, Borer JS. Instrumentation and data processing in cardiovascular nuclear medicine: evaluation of ventricular function. *Semin Nucl Med* 1979;9:257–274.

19. Hamilton GW, Williams DL, Caldwell JH. Frame rate requirements for recording time-activity curves by radionuclide angiocardiography. In: Sorenson JA, ed. *Nuclear cardiology: selected computer aspects.* New York: Society of Nuclear Medicine, 1978:75–83.

20. Knesaurek K, King MA, Glick SJ, et al. Investigation of causes of geometric distortion in 180 degrees and 360 degrees angular sampling in SPECT. *J Nucl Med* 1989;30:1666–1675.

21. Keys JW. SPECT and artifacts: in search of the imaginary lesion. *J Nucl Med* 1991;32:875–877.

22. Faber TL, Akers MS, Peshock RM, et al. Three-dimensional motion and perfusion quantification in gated single-photon emission computed tomograms. *J Nucl Med* 1991;32: 2311–2317.

23. Mazzanti M, Germano G, Kiat H, et al. Fast technetium 99m-labeled sestamibi gated single-photon emission computed tomography for evaluation of myocardial function. *J Nucl Cardiol* 1996;3:S169–171.

24. Du Pont Merck. Package insert: Pyrolite. Billerica, MA: Du Pont Merck, 1991.

25. Mallinckrodt Medical. Package insert: UltraTag RBC. St. Louis: Mallinckrodt Medical, 1992.

26. King MA, Schwinger RB, Doherty PW, et al. Two-dimensional filtering of SPECT images using the Metz and Wiener filters. *J Nucl Med* 1984;25:1234–1240.

27. King MA, Miller TR. Use of a non-stationary temporal Wiener filter in nuclear medicine. *Eur J Nucl Med* 1985;10:458–461.

28. Yamashita K, Tanaka M, Asada N, et al. A new method of three dimensional analysis of left ventricular wall motion. *Eur J Nucl Med* 1988;14:113–119.

29. Faber TL, Stokely EM, Templeton GH, et al. Quantitation of three-dimensional left ventricular segmental wall motion and volumes from gated tomographic radionuclide ventriculograms. *J Nucl Med* 1989;30:639–649.

30. Honda N, Machida K, Takishima T, et al. Cinematic three-dimensional surface display of cardiac blood pool tomography. *Clin Nucl Med* 1991;16:87–91.

31. Botvinick EH, O'Connell JW, Kadkade PP, et al. Potential added value of three-dimensional reconstruction and display of single photon emission computed tomographic gated blood pool images. *J Nucl Cardiol* 1998;5:245–255.

32. Gill JB, Moore RH, Tamaki N, et al. Multigated blood-pool tomography: new method for the assessment of left ventricular function. *J Nucl Med* 1986;27:1916–1924.

33. Tauxe W, Soussaline F, Todd-Pokropek A, et al. Determination of organ volume by single-photon emission tomography. *J Nucl Med* 1982;23:984–987.

34. Miller TR, Wallis JW, Sampathkumaran KS. Three-dimensional display of gated cardiac blood-pool studies. *J Nucl Med* 1989;30:2036–2041.

35. Wallis JW, Miller TR. Volume rendering in three-dimensional display of SPECT images. *J Nucl Med* 1990;31:1421–1430.

36. Maddahi J, Van Train K, Prigent F, et al. Quantitative single photon emission computed thallium-201 tomography for detection and localization of coronary artery disease: optimization and prospective validation of a new technique. *J Am Coll Cardiol* 1989;14:1689–1699.

37. Gibson CJ. Real time 3D display of gated blood pool tomograms. *Phys Med Biol* 1988;33:569–581.

38. Corbett JR, Akers MS, McGhie AI, et al. Wall motion analysis from three-dimensional surface rendered gated radionuclide ventriculograms: comparison with cine slice analysis and coronary angiography. *J Nucl Med* 1990;31:P838.

39. Myers RW, Bails RP, Reed VR, et al. Angiocardiography with the seven-pinhole collimator: evaluation of methodology and accuracy in assessing global and regional left ventricular function. *Clin Nucl Med* 1982;7:151–156.

40. Constantinesco A, Mertz L, Brunot B. Myocardial perfusion and function imaging at rest with simultaneous thallium-201 and technetium-99m blood-pool dual-isotope gated SPECT. *J Nucl Med* 1997;38:432–437.

41. Lu P, Liu X, Shi R, et al. Comparison of tomographic and planar radionuclide ventriculography in the assessment of regional left ventricular function in patients with left ventricular aneurysm before and after surgery [see comments]. *J Nucl Cardiol* 1994;1:537–545.

42. Narita M, Kurihara T, Murano K, et al. Assessment of left ventricular function by gated cardiac blood-pool emission computed tomography using a rotating gamma camera. *Kaku Igaku* 1991;28:51–61.

43. Kim AS, Quaife RA, Meyer DM, et al. Revascularization outcome predicted by regional left ventricular response to nitroglycerin: use of quantitative 3-D wall motion analysis and tomographic ventriculography. *J Am Coll Cardiol* 1992;19 (suppl A):128(abstr).

44. Norton MY, Walton S, Evans NT. Gated cardiac tomography. *Eur J Nucl Med* 1988;14:472–476.

45. Graf G, Mester J, Clausen M, et al. Reconstruction of Fourier coefficients: a fast method to get polar amplitude and phase images of gated SPECT. *J Nucl Med* 1990;31:1856–1861.

46. Mate E, Mester J, Csernay L, et al. Three-dimensional presentation of the Fourier amplitude and phase: a fast display method for gated cardiac blood-pool SPECT. *J Nucl Med* 1992;33: 458–462.

47. Maeda H, Takeda K, Ito T, et al. Improvement in Fourier analysis of gated blood-pool studies using single photon emission computed tomography: methodology and clinical feasibility. *Radiat Med* 1990;8:204–210.

48. Lee HS, Cross S, Norton M, et al. Comparison between planar and tomographic radionuclide ventriculography for detecting inferior wall motion abnormalities. *Clin Radiol* 1998;53: 264–267.

49. Pavel DG, Smyrin S, Lam W, et al. Ventricular phase analysis of radionuclide gated studies. *Am J Cardiol* 1980;45:398(abst).

50. Verba JW, Bornstein I, Alazraki NP, et al. A new computer pro-

gram for the extraction of global and regional behavior of all four cardiac chambers from gated radionuclide data. *J Nucl Med* 1979;20:665(abst).

51. Sheehan FH, Stewart DK, Dodge HT, et al. Variability in the measurement of regional left ventricular wall motion from contrast angiograms. *Circulation* 1983;68:550–559.

52. Sheehan FH, Bolson EL, Dodge HT, et al. Advantages and applications of the centerline method for characterizing regional ventricular function. *Circulation* 1986;74:293–305.

53. Cerqueira MD, Harp GD, Ritchie JL. Quantitative gated blood pool tomographic assessment of regional ejection fraction: definition of normal limits. *J Am Coll Cardiol* 1992;20:934–941.

54. Barat JL, Brendel AJ, Colle JP, et al. Quantitative analysis of left-ventricular function using gated single photon emission tomography. *J Nucl Med* 1984;25:1167–1174.

55. Groch MW, Marshall RC, Erwin WD, et al. Quantitative gated blood pool SPECT for the assessment of coronary artery disease at rest. *J Nucl Cardiol* 1998;5:567–573.

56. Vogel RA, Stern DM, Kirsh DL, et al. Viewer specified projection: a new method of computer display of LAO acquired gated blood pool data in any projection desired. *J Am Coll Cardiol* 1980;45:407(abst).

57. Faber TL, Stokely EM, Peshock RM, et al. A model-based four-dimensional left ventricular surface detector. *IEEE Trans Med Imaging* 1991;10:321–329.

58. Honda N, Machida K, Mamiya T, et al. Two dimensional polar display of cardiac blood pool SPECT. *Eur J Nucl Med* 1989;15:133–136.

59. Stadius ML, Williams DL, Harp G, et al. Left ventricular volume determination using single-photon emission computed tomography. *Am J Cardiol* 1985;55:1185–1191.

60. Young AA, Imai H, Chang CN, et al. Two-dimensional left ventricular deformation during systole using magnetic resonance imaging with spatial modulation of magnetization. *Circulation* 1994;90:740–752.

61. Bartlett ML, Srinivasan G, Barker WC, et al. Left ventricular ejection fraction: comparison of results from planar and SPECT gated blood-pool studies. *J Nucl Med* 1996;37:1795–1799.

62. Pretorius PH, Xia W, King MA, et al. Evaluation of right and left ventricular volume and ejection fraction using a mathematical cardiac torso phantom. *J Nucl Med* 1997;38:1528–1535.

63. Chin BB, Bloomgarden DC, Xia W, et al. Right and left ventricular volume and ejection fraction by tomographic gated blood-pool scintigraphy. *J Nucl Med* 1997;38:942–948.

64. Mariano-Goulart D, Collet H, Kotzki PO, et al. Semi-automatic segmentation of gated blood pool emission tomographic images by watersheds: application to the determination of right and left ejection fractions. *Eur J Nucl Med* 1998;25:1300–1307.

65. Borer JS, Bacharach SL, Green MV, et al. Real-time radionuclide cineangiography in the noninvasive evaluation of global and regional left ventricular function at rest and during exercise in patients with coronary-artery disease. *N Engl J Med* 1977;296:839–844.

66. Dehmer GJ, Lewis SE, Hillis LD, et al. Nongeometric determination of left ventricular volumes from equilibrium blood pool scans. *Am J Cardiol* 1980;45:293–300.

67. Maddahi J, Berman DS, Matsuoka DT, et al. A new technique for assessing right ventricular ejection fraction using rapid multiple-gated equilibrium cardiac blood pool scintigraphy. Description, validation and findings in chronic coronary artery disease. *Circulation* 1979;60:581–589.

68. Dehmer GJ, Firth BG, Hillis LD, et al. Nongeometric determination of right ventricular volumes from equilibrium blood pool scans. *Am J Cardiol* 1982;49:78–84.

69. Links JM, Becker LC, Shindledecker JG, et al. Measurement of absolute left ventricular volume from gated blood pool studies. *Circulation* 1982;65:82–91.

70. Starling MR, Dell'Italia LJ, Walsh RA, et al. Accurate estimates of absolute left ventricular volumes from equilibrium radionuclide angiographic count data using a simple geometric attenuation correction. *J Am Coll Cardiol* 1984;3:789–798.

71. Schneider RM, Jaszczak RJ, Coleman RE, et al. Disproportionate effects of regional hypokinesis on radionuclide ejection fraction: compensation using attenuation-corrected ventricular volumes. *J Nucl Med* 1984;25:747–754.

72. Corbett JR, Rellas JS, Willerson JT, et al. Left ventricular volumes from gated radionuclide ventriculograms: attenuation correction in female and male patients. *J Nucl Med* 1983;24:P27 (abstr).

73. Dewhurst NG, Muir AL. Comparative prognostic value of radionuclide ventriculography at rest and during exercise in 100 patients after first myocardial infarction. *Br Heart J* 1983;49:111–121.

74. Corbett JR, Nicod P, Lewis SE, et al. Prognostic value of submaximal exercise radionuclide ventriculography after myocardial infarction. *Am J Cardiol* 1983;52:82A–91A.

75. Nemerovski M, Shah PK, Pichler M, et al. Radionuclide assessment of sequential changes in left and right ventricular function following first acute transmural myocardial infarction. *Am Heart J* 1982;104:709–717.

76. Metcalfe MJ, Norton MY, Jennings K, et al. Improved detection of abnormal left ventricular wall motion using tomographic radionuclide ventriculography compared with planar radionuclide and single plane contrast ventriculography. *Br J Radiol* 1993;66:986–993.

77. Mochizuki T, Murase K, Fujiwara Y, et al. ECG-gated thallium-201 myocardial SPECT in patients with old myocardial infarction compared with ECG-gated blood pool SPECT. *Ann Nucl Med* 1991;5:47–51.

78. Murano K, Narita M, Kurihara T. [Left ventricular function assessed by multigated blood pool single photon emission computed tomography with 99mTc]. *J Cardiol* 1992;22:245–253.

79. Yamazaki J, Naitou K, Ishida S, et al. Evaluation of left ventricular wall motion and function in patients with previous myocardial infarction by three-dimensional 99mTc-HSAD multigated cardiac pool imaging. *Ann Nucl Med* 1997;11:129–138.

80. Nakata T, Hashimoto A, Kuno A, et al. Sustained right ventricular dyskinesis complicated by right ventricular infarction. *J Nucl Med* 1997;38:1421–1423.

81. Cross SJ, Lee HS, Metcalfe MJ, et al. Assessment of left ventricular regional wall motion with blood pool tomography: comparison of 11CO PET with 99Tcm SPECT. *Nucl Med Commun* 1994;15:283–288.

82. Takahashi M. Assessment of right ventricular function using gated blood pool single photon emission computed tomography in inferior myocardial infarction with or without hemodynamically significant right ventricular infarction. *Kaku Igaku* 1992;29:221–231.

83. Manrique A, Faraggi M, Vere P, et al. T1-201 and Tc-99 MIBI gated SPECT in patients with large perfusion defects and left ventricular dysfunction: comparison with equilibrium radionuclide angiography. *J Nucl Med* 1999;40:905–809.

84. Hutchins GM, Bulkley BH. Infarct expansion versus extension: two different complications of acute myocardial infarction. *Am J Cardiol* 1978;41:1127–1132.

85. Meizlish JL, Berger HJ, Plankey M, et al. Functional left ventricular aneurysm formation after acute anterior transmural myocardial infarction. Incidence, natural history, and prognostic implications. *N Engl J Med* 1984;311:1001–1006.

86. Lu P, Liu X, Shi R, et al. Comparison of tomographic and planar radionuclide ventriculography in assessment of regional left

ventricular function in patients with LV aneurysm before and after surgery. *J Nucl Cardiol* 1994;1.

87. Metcalfe MJ, Cross S, Norton MY, et al. Polar map or novel three-dimensional display technique for the improved detection of inferior wall myocardial infarction using tomographic radionuclide ventriculography. *Nucl Med Commun* 1994;15:330–340.

88. Gaudron P, Eilles C, Ertl G, et al. Early remodelling of the left ventricle in patients with myocardial infarction. *Eur Heart J* 1990;11:139–146.

89. Ertl G, Gaudron P, Eilles C, et al. Serial changes in left ventricular size after acute myocardial infarction. *Am J Cardiol* 1991;68:116D–120D.

90. Matsuo H, Watanabe S, Nishida Y, et al. Identification of asynergic but viable myocardium in patients with chronic coronary artery disease by gated blood pool scintigraphy during isosorbide dinitrate and low-dose dobutamine infusion: comparison with thallium-201 scintigraphy with reinjection. *Ann Nucl Med* 1994;8:283–293.

91. Quaife RA, Kim AS, Meyer DM, et al. Regional left ventricular response to nitroglycerin predicts revascularization outcome: quantitative analysis of gated blood pool tomography. First International Congress of Nuclear Cardiology, Cannes. 1993;abst. 4708.

92. Lucas JR, O'Connell JW, Lee RJ, et al. First harmonic (Fourier) analysis of gated SPECT blood pool scintigrams provides refined assessment of the site of initial activation of accessory pathways in patients with the Wolff-Parkinson-White syndrome. *J Nucl Med* 1993;34:151P(abst).

93. Dormehl IC, van Gelder AL, Hugo N, et al. Gated blood pool SPECT and phase analysis to assess simulated Wolff-Parkinson-White syndrome in the baboon. *Nuklearmedizin* 1993;32: 222–226.

94. Neumann DR, Go RT, Myers BA, et al. Parametric phase display for biventricular function from gated cardiac blood pool single-photon emission tomography. *Eur J Nucl Med* 1993;20: 1108–1111.

95. Weismuller P, Clausen M, Weller R, et al. Non-invasive three-dimensional localisation of arrhythmogenic foci in Wolff-Parkinson-White syndrome and in ventricular tachycardia by radionuclide ventriculography: phase analysis of double-angulated integrated single photon emission computed tomography (SPECT). *Br Heart J* 1993;69:201–210.

96. Clausen M, Weismuller P, Weller R, et al. Abnormal ventricular contraction patterns in patients with arrhythmogenic substrates using three-dimensional phase analysis. *Eur Heart J* 1993;14: 69–72.

97. Rigo P, Alderson PO, Robertson RM, et al. Measurement of aortic and mitral regurgitation by gated cardiac blood pool scans. *Circulation* 1979;60:306–312.

98. Nicod P, Corbett JR, Firth BG, et al. Radionuclide techniques for valvular regurgitant index: comparison in patients with normal and depressed ventricular function. *J Nucl Med* 1982;23: 763–769.

99. Makler PT, McCarthy DM, Velchik MG, et al. Fourier amplitude ratio:A new way to assess valvular regurgitation. *J Nucl Med* 1983;24:204–207.

100. Delhomme C, Casset-Senon D, Babuty D, et al. [A study of 36 cases of mitral valve prolapse by isotopic ventricular tomography]. *Arch Mal Coeur Vaiss* 1996;89:1127–1135.

101. Caputo GR, Graham MM, Brust KD, et al. Measurement of left ventricular volume using single-photon emission computed tomography. *Am J Cardiol* 1985;56:781–786.

102. Bunker SR, Hartshorne MF, Schmidt WP, et al. Left ventricular volume determination from single-photon emission computed tomography. *AJR* 1985;144:295–298.

103. Fischman AJ, Moore RH, Gill JB, et al. Gated blood pool tomography: a technology whose time has come. *Semin Nucl Med* 1989;19:13–21.

# INDEX

# INDEX

Note: Page numbers followed by f and t indicate figures and tables, respectively.